AURAL REHABILITATION

Serving Children and Adults

Fourth Edition

A Singular Audiology Text
Jeffrey L. Danhauer, Ph.D.
Audiology Editor

■ AURAL REHABILITATION ■

Serving Children and Adults

Fourth Edition

Edited by

■ RAYMOND H. HULL, Ph.D. ■

Department of Communicative Sciences and Disorders
Wichita State University
Wichita, Kansas

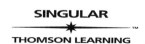

SINGULAR
THOMSON LEARNING

Australia   Canada   Mexico   Singapore   Spain   United Kingdom   United States

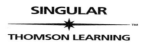

SINGULAR

THOMSON LEARNING

Aural Rehabilitation: Serving Children and Adults, Fourth Edition
By Raymond H. Hull, Ph.D.

Business Unit Director:
William Brotmiller

Acquisitions Editor:
Marie Linvill

Editorial Assistant:
Cara Jenkins

Executive Marketing Manager:
Dawn Gerrain

Channel Manager:
Kathryn Bamberger

Executive Production Editor:
Barb Bullock

Production Editor:
Brad Bielawski

NOTICE TO THE READER

CONTENTS

PREFACE

This is the fourth edition of what has become a popular text in aural rehabilitation. One of the reasons that it has been so popular among professors and students is the logical sequence in which the information is presented, and the ease with which the book can be read by both students and professionals. In other words, even though this book provides comprehensive information on the aural habilitation and rehabilitation of children, and younger and older adults who are hearing impaired, the information is presented in a readable fashion that has immediate theoretical and practical application. The introductory page of each chapter provides a brief outline of the chapter for a quick content overview. Further, the examinations and answer sheets found at the conclusion of each chapter provide a ready-made opportunity for professors to quiz their students on a periodic basis, or to simply allow students to determine on their own whether they understood important points within each chapter.

This book is divided into four parts. The *Introduction* presents information that is fundamental to the provision of services on behalf of all persons who are hearing impaired, including an introduction to aural rehabilitation, an introduction to the handicap of hearing impairment and related terminology, an introduction to hearing aids and their components, a psychosocial, educational, and vocational profile of persons with impaired hearing.

Part II concentrates on children who are hearing impaired. The information centers on the importance of family and their involvement in serving the child who is hearing impaired, considerations regarding amplification for children, the development of auditory skills for children who are hear-ing impaired, language and speech development for children with impaired hearing, and their educational management.

Part III concentrates on adults who are hearing impaired. Chapters in the first section address the impact of hearing impairment on adults, and procedures for counseling; hearing aid orientation; assistive listening devices for adults who are hearing impaired; the history, theory, and application of aural rehabilitation for adults; and strategies for speech conservation on behalf of adults who are hearing impaired. The *second section* of Part III addresses special considerations for older adults who are hearing impaired. The chapters in this section present information on psychosocial factors of aging; the special nature of hearing loss in older adulthood; the impact of hearing loss in older adulthood; counseling the older adult who is hearing impaired; considerations on hearing aid use for older adults; techniques of aural rehabilitation for older adults who are hearing impaired; and programs for the hearing impaired elderly in health care facility environments.

Part IV presents information on the process of evaluating the communicative function of adults who are hearing impaired, their aural rehabilitative needs, and the measurement of their success in aural rehabilitation treatment. Included is an extensive compilation of scales and tests of communicative function for use with adults who are hearing impaired, all of which are found in the appendix.

The Appendix of this book contains the most comprehensive compilation of assessments of communicative function in adults who are hearing impaired found in any text on the topic of aural rehabilitation.

The topics for this fourth edition were by no means arbitrary. Professionals in audiology, speech-language pathology, deaf education, rehabilitation counseling, psychologists and otolaryngologists, along with upper-level undergraduate and graduate students across the United States and Europe were consulted about the topics they felt were important in preparing audiologists and speech-language pathologists to work with children and adults who are hearing impaired. When a general consensus was reached, the fourth edition was designed.

This book covers the topics considered the most important in preparing future professionals to serve children and adults who are hearing impaired. Therefore, a diverse range of vocabulary and sophistication is acknowledged in regard to both the content of the chapters and the book's intended readership. The book has been designed for use by a broad range of readers, primarily upper-level undergraduate students and graduate students in audiology and speech-language pathology, and professional audiologists, speech-language pathologists and deaf educators. Other interested readers include physicians, nurses, gerontologists, vocational rehabilitation counselors, teachers, psychologists, and sociologists.

Preparing this text has, once again, been an enjoyable and rewarding experience. It is hoped that it will continue to be a valuable source of information for serving children and adults who are hearing impaired.

Raymond H. Hull, Ph.D.

CONTRIBUTORS

Dale V. Atkins, Ph.D.
Psychologist in Private Practice
282 North Avenue
Westport, Connecticut 06880

Jill L. Bader, Ph.D.
Executive Director
Hear At Home
2374 South University Blvd.
Denver, Colorado 80210

Frederick S. Berg, Ph.D.
Professor Emeritus
Department of Communicative Disorders
Utah State University
Logan, Utah 84322

Karen A. Dilka, Ph.D.
Associate Professor, Deaf Education
Department of Special Education
Eastern Kentucky University
Richmond, Kentucky 40475

William R. Hodgson, Ph.D.
Professor of Audiology
Department of Speech and Hearing Sciences
The University of Arizona
Tucson, Arizona 85721

Raymond H. Hull, Ph.D.
Professor of Communicative Disorders and
    Sciences, Audiology
Department of Communicative Disorders and
    Sciences
Wichita State University
Wichita, Kansas 67260

Pamela L. Jackson, Ph.D.
Professor of Audiology
Department of Communication Disorders
Northern Illinois University
DeKalb, Illinois 60115

Harriet F. Kaplan, Ph.D.
Professor Emeritus Department of Audiology
    and Speech-Language Pathology
Gallaudet University
Washington, D.C.

Jack Katz, Ph.D.
Professor of Audiology
Department of Communicative Disorders and
    Sciences
State University of New York at Buffalo
Buffalo, New York

Robert K. Lightfoot, M.S.
Audiologist
Birmingham Veterans Administration Medical
    Center
700 South 19th Street
Birmingham, Alabama 35233

Daniel Ling, Ph.D.
Professor Emeritus
Faculty of Applied Health Sciences
The University of Western Ontario
London, Ontario, Canada N6G IHA

Robert McLaughlin[†]

[†]Deceased

James F. Maurer, Ph.D.
Professor Emeritus of Audiology
Department of Speech and Hearing Sciences
Portland State University
Portland, Oregon 97207

Douglas R. Martin, Ph.D.
Associate Professor of Audiology
Director, Program in Speech and Hearing Sciences
Portland State University
Portland, Oregon 97207

Judah L. Ronch, Ph.D.
Executive Director, Brookdale Center on Aging of
    Hunter College
City University of New York
425 E. 25th Street
New York, New York 10010

Joseph J. Smaldino, Ph.D.
Professor of Audiology
Department of Communication Disorders
University of Northern Iowa
Cedar Falls, Iowa 50614

Thomas P. White, M.A.
Assistant Professor of Audiology
Department of Communicative Disorders and
    Sciences
State University of New York at Buffalo
Buffalo, New York

This Book Is Dedicated To
My lovely wife Lucinda,
my daughter Courtney,
my mother, and my dad,
all of whom are at my side through it all.

■ PART I ■

Introduction To Aural Rehabilitation

■   CHAPTER 1   ■

What is Aural Rehabilitation?

■   RAYMOND H. HULL, Ph.D.   ■

Deafness is worse than blindness, so they say—it is the loneliness, the sense of isolation that makes it so, and the lack of understanding in the minds of ordinary people. The problem of the child deaf from birth is quite different from that of the man or woman who has become deafened after school-age or in adult life. . . . But for all of them, the handicap is the same, the handicap of the silent world, the difficulty of communicating with the hearing and speaking world.

Scott Stevenson[1]

The aim of aural habilitative/rehabilitative efforts for the hearing impaired is to overcome the handicap. After discovering a hearing impairment, assessing its type and degree, medical referral by an audiologist is made, expecting that the physician can correct the problem. The referral is made on the premise that the hearing impairment, per se, can be overcome.

If a hearing impairment cannot be medically treated, the audiologist then works with the client to remediate the handicapping effects of the hearing loss and to help the child or adult overcome the communicative, social, and psychological effects of hearing impairment. A team of professionals may also become involved, including vocational rehabilitation counselors, educators, psychologists, sociologists, and speech pathologists, with the audiologist coordinating the team. The client's family will also be involved in the aural rehabilitation treatment process. This task, in its totality, holds tremendous responsibility for all who are involved.

Why, then, is this important area in so many instances presented as a single chapter in books that deal with the subject of hearing impairment? Only recently have entire books been written and published that concentrate on aural rehabilitation. Books that deal with the effects of hearing impairment on children, adults, and aging persons, including approaches to counseling, the psychosocial and vocational impact of hearing impairment,

and approaches for remediation did not exist to any degree until two decades ago.

The three parts of this book provide theoretical and practical information on serving children, adults, and the elderly who have hearing impairment and address the issues and needs unique to each age group.

WHAT IS AURAL REHABILITATION?

What is aural rehabilitation? It has for so many years been discussed from within the framework of speechreading, lipreading, visual communication, auditory training, and other subcategories that we have occasionally strayed from the totality of the habilitative and rehabilitative process.

The first sentence of this chapter stated that, "the aim of aural habilitative/rehabilitative efforts for the hearing impaired is to overcome the handicap." What is the handicap? Elements of hearing impairment may have a great impact on one person, but may not be a handicap to another. One person may remain despondent over his or her partial loss of hearing, but another may rebound and work with vigor to overcome the communication difficulties caused by the hearing impairment. One person may encounter great social handicap from a relatively mild high-frequency hearing impairment, with another who possesses a more severe hearing loss may have only a mild occupational or social handicap. A child with a mild loss of hearing that is not detected until school age may suffer as great a handicap as one who has a greater loss of hearing that was discovered earlier. Two children with equal hearing loss may experience different degrees of impairment, because of the psychosocial and interactive/communicative environment in which they are raised.

[1]From Ballantyne, J. (1977). *Deafness* (p. 215). New York: Churchill Livingstone.

If the catalyst for a psychosocial, educational, and/or occupational handicap resulting from either acquired or congenital hearing impairment could be pinpointed, it would probably revolve around its impact on "communication" and the interference either receptively, expressively, or both caused by a hearing impairment. A child with a severe congenital hearing loss, whether remediation is begun early or late, will have a language deficit to some degree that may impede educational and occupational potential, with language delay the basis for the communication deficit. An adult who acquires a hearing impairment that prevents adequate hearing of the speech of others may become despondent over his or her difficulties in maintaining an occupation or functioning socially. Again, the problem centers on an interference with communication as the result of the auditory deficit.

Aural rehabilitation and the strategies utilized in the process of aural rehabilitation center on the impact of a hearing impairment on communication as experienced by adults and elderly persons who possess it. The majority have probably had normal hearing at some time in their lives and will probably have normal, or near normal, language function. In that regard, the impact of a hearing impairment on communicative function reveals itself from innumerable dimensions and avenues.

Children who have hearing impairments, in the majority of instances, have not experienced normal language and will respond to their hearing loss, their environment, and communication in differing ways. Further, they also have parents, siblings, and other relatives who respond to them and their hearing loss in complex and varying ways.

In relation to acquired hearing loss, each adult and elderly person responds in different ways to the hearing impairment. Each has different demands, either self-imposed or externally imposed. Some will have families who are also affected by the hearing deficit and others will not. For some individuals, their occupations may require precise and in-depth communication with other professionals or clients, with other persons' occupations requiring little communication. Some persons have been greatly involved on a social basis, although others' social lives have revolved around home and family. A Harvard School of Business graduate whose spouse and parents have always had great expectations of him or her for success in the business world may feel a greater impact as the result of acquired severe hearing impairment than one who desires to be a good rancher and who is not required to communicate a great deal on his or her ranch in northern Montana.

Children with hearing impairment are born into families and environments that differ. A child born into a family in which deafness has not occurred before and whose parents become paralyzed and noncommunicating out of self-pity and anger will not fare as well as a child who is born deaf to parents who are also deaf and who accept their child in a nurturing, communicating environment.

SERVING CHILDREN WHO ARE HEARING IMPAIRED

HISTORICAL BACKGROUND

Aural habilitation services on behalf of children have a much longer and more diverse history than services for adults who are hearing impaired. But, much of the history centers on education of people who are deaf and the early oralism versus manualism debates. However, a historical perspective is important in learning about the procedures utilized to serve children who have impairment.

The recorded history of philosophical treatises on hearing impairment, children who are hearing impaired, their apparent ability to learn, and the "methods debate" on how hearing impaired children most efficiently learn language and speech began before the development of Hebrew law—that is, prior to 500 B.C. (Bender, 1981).

One of the first recorded philosophical opinions on the potential of children who are deaf to learn and to speak was rendered by Aristotle (355 B.C.). His theories and philosophies on most topics carried so much weight in his day that others not only hesitated questioning them, but even to venture into the topic areas at all. This situation was particularly disastrous for the hearing impaired, because, interpreted, Aristotle's opinion on the "deaf" was: "Those who are born deaf all become senseless and incapable of reason. Men who are born deaf are in all cases dumb; that is to say, they can make vocal noises, but they cannot speak" (Giangreco, 1976, p.72).

Unfortunately, the words *kophoi,* meaning "deaf", and *eneos* meaning "speechless," had, at the time, taken on the additional meanings of "dumb" and "stupid" in some instances. Therefore, a misinterpretation of Aristotle's statements could have become the interpretation that cast the mold for children and adults who were deaf or hearing impaired for centuries.

By the 16th century, some prominent individuals, primarily priests and physicians, began to challenge the opinions of Aristotle. For example, Giralamo Cardano (1501–1576) of Italy braved the opinion that he could see no reason why people who are deaf could not be taught. In *De inventione dialectica,* Cardano wrote that he had observed a man who was born deaf who had learned to read and write and in that manner could learn and could communicate with others. From that Cordano ventured the opinion that people who are deaf were capable of reason (Farrar, 1923).

During the 17th century, rapid advancements occurred in many areas, particularly in the development of educational philosophy, intellectual growth, political theory, and scientific thought. In relation to people who were deaf, such names as Lock (1632–1704), Francis Bacon (1561–1626), Bonet (1579–1629), Bulwer (1614–1684), and others dominated the scene. The quarrel between John Wallis (1617–1703) and William Holder (1616–1698) concerning the best method for teaching people who were deaf created a beginning of public interest in the area of deafness (Bender, 1981; Giangreco and Giangreco, 1976; and Hodgson, 1953).

During the 18th century, great growth occurred in services on behalf of the individuals who were deaf. Jacob Pereira (1715-1780) was recognized as the first teacher of the deaf in France, with de l'Epee (1712-1789), also of France, being the first person to make deaf education a matter of public concern. He wrote about his work and brought positive attention to the potential of children who are deaf to learn (Bender, 1981; Giangreco, 1976), as did his contemporary Samuel Heinicke (1727–1790) of Germany (Hodgson, 1953). Jean Itard (1774–1838) of France conducted research into the hereditary nature of deafness. He concluded that, indeed, deafness can be inherited, although it can skip generations (Bender, 1981).

In the 19th century, other significant strides were made in the detection and understanding of hearing loss and education of people who are deaf. Some were important to the future of services on behalf of individuals who were deaf in America. The Braidwoods and the Watsons were the operators of nearly all of the schools for the deaf in England, both adhering to an oral method of teaching, emphasizing oral speech (Bender, 1981; Deland, 1931). At the same time, deaf education in France was under the direction of Sicard who emphasized a manual approach to teaching language to children who are deaf (Bender, 1981).

In America, the first school for the deaf, The American Asylum, was begun by Thomas Gallaudet (1781–1851), who is considered to be the father of deaf education in America, a proponent of manualism (Bender, 1981; Giangreco, 1976). So the first school for the deaf in America was manual in orientation. In an effort to begin an oral school in this country, on March 16, 1864, Gardiner Green Hubbard, a concerned and influential citizen, and Samuel Howe, superintendent of the

Massachusetts School for the Blind, petitioned the Massachusetts General Court to incorporate an oral school for the deaf in that state. Governor Bullock of Massachusetts listened to Hubbard. After receiving a letter from philanthropist John Clarke offering $50,000 to establish an oral school for the deaf, Governor Bullock persuaded the state legislature to approve the establishment of a school. It was later named the Clark School for the Deaf and was established in October, 1867 (Bender, 1981).

Alexander Graham Bell strongly influenced the future of services on behalf of children who are hearing impaired in the United States. Bell's mother became deaf because of illness, and Alexander married Mabel Hubbard, who was deaf from scarlet fever in early childhood. When he invented the telephone, Bell also saw its potential for electronically amplifying sound for the hearing impaired. Further, he was moved by the impressive way that his mother and wife were able to communicate without using manual sign. So he openly differed with Gallaudet's manual approach to teaching the deaf. With $200,000 that he received from the Volta Prize for his work with electricity, Bell initiated the Volta Bureau in Washington, DC in 1867. Out of the Volta Bureau arose the Alexander Graham Bell Association for the Deaf.

The debates of Gallaudet and Bell about manualism and oralism remain today. However, those involved in the debates have as their goal the best and most efficient method for language development and communication for children who are deaf.

CURRENT THEORY AND PRACTICE

The 20th century brought more eclectic approaches for the development of language among children who are hearing impaired. Generally, the various approaches had as their goal the utilization of the most efficient sensory avenues available to children with impaired hearing. Although there are sometimes vast differences between the individual philosophies, they are all believed by adherants to be in the best interest of hearing-impaired children. Approaches are generally structured around six primary philosophies, or methodologies (Boothroyd, 1982).

1. **Emphasis on Speech.** This philosophy centers on speech as the avenue for communication to provide a person with the requisite independence that we strive for on behalf of the deaf (Bader, 1997; Calvert & Silverman, 1975; Fry, 1977; Hochberg, Levitt, & Osberger, 1983; Kretschmer & Kretschmer, 1978; Ling, 1978, 1981, 1984a, 1984b; Ling & Milne, 1980; Osberger, Johnstone, Swarts, & Levitt, 1978; Pollack, 1970; Sanders, 1993; Vorce, 1974).

2. **Emphasis On Hearing.** This primarily unisensory approach emphasizes the earliest possible identification of hearing impairment in children and the earliest uses of amplification, so that the child's auditory system can play its natural role in the enhancement of auditory perceptual skills and, thus, the development of speech and language (Boothroyd, 1982). The goal is for hearing to play as great a role as possible in the development of speech and language (Bader, 1997; Boothroyd, 1982; Calvert & Silverman, 1975; Chase, 1968; Hirsh, 1966; Ling, 1980; Ling & Milne, 1980; Markides, 1983; Pollack, 1970, 1985; Simmons-Martin, 1977).

3. **Manual Supplements to Speech.** Cued speech is a manual supplement to lipreading. It is used as a manual supplement to an oral approach to the development of communicative competence (Cornett, 1967; Ling & Ling, 1978).

4. **Emphasis on Language and Communication.** This philosophy emphasizes that the mastery of language, no matter what the mode, is critical for the cognitive, emotional, and social growth of child. It supports total communication and the simultaneous use of hearing, speech, and manual communication. It is believed that the use of manual communication will provide a base for communication and that

speech will emerge out of it, as communicative competencies will be more highly developed (Boothroyd, 1978; Fry, 1977; Groht, 1958; Harris, 1963; Kretschmer & Kretschmer, 1978, 1984; Ling, 1981; Simmons-Martin, 1977).

5. **Cognitive Emphasis.** With this philosophy, a specific modality for language stimulation is deemphasized. The primary concern is placed on providing children who are hearing impaired with optimal opportunities for cognitive skills development. However, proponents generally have their own personal preference about the modality emphasized (e.g., manual, auditory, total) (Blank, Rose, & Berlin, 1978; Boothroyd, 1982; Grammatico and Miller, 1974; Moeller & McConkey, 1984; Stone, 1980; Taba, 1962).

6. **Emphasis on the Child and His or Her Parents.** Successful intervention on behalf of children who are hearing impaired depends, at least to a more than moderate degree, on the emotional well-being of the child, which, in turn, depends on the emotional well-being of the parents (Boothroyd, 1982). No matter how great the expertise of the clinician, parents exert the greatest impact on the social, communicative, and emotional growth of their child (Bader, 1997; Boothroyd, 1982; Lillie, 1969; Luterman, 1987; Mindel & Vernon, 1987; Moses, 1985; Phillips, 1987).

These philosophies are individual approaches that are found to one degree or another throughout the last century. However, it is seldom that one observes a professional who employs a single approach to the exclusion of others. It is, thankfully, most common to observe a wise clinician utilizing the best of several approaches to the benefit of a child and his or her family.

THE POTENTIAL IMPACT OF IMPAIRED LEARNING

In discussing aural habilitation services for children, we are in most instances referring to children who possess hearing losses that are prelingual. According to Boothroyd (1982), these children generally possess a primary impairment of hearing that will, if left untreated, result in other impairments secondary to the hearing loss. For example, if a child possesses a congenital hearing loss that is severe enough to prevent him or her from hearing speech prior to being fitted with a hearing aid, the result may, according to Boothroyd (1982), include any or all of:

1. **A Perceptual Problem.** A child may have difficulty identifying objects and events by their sounds.

2. **A Speech Problem.** A child does not learn the connection between the movements of his or her speech mechanism and the resulting sounds. Consequently, the child has difficulty acquiring control of speech.

3. **A Communication Problem.** A child may not learn his or her native language. The child has difficulty understanding what people say and cannot participate in conversational exchange.

4. **A Cognitive Problem.** Therefore, a child has difficulty acquiring auditory/oral language. Children without language must learn about their world only from concrete aspects, not the elements that normally hearing children use, for example, the abstract elements of language.

5. **A Social Problem.** A child who has hearing impairment as a toddler does not hear the verbal signals signaling that he or she is about to transgress parental limits. At a later age, this child cannot have social rules explained to him or her, unless alternative avenues for communication have been established.

6. **An Emotional Problem.** If a child is unable to satisfy his or her evolving needs through spoken language, unable to make sense of the seemingly precipitous and capricious reactions of parents and peers, and is constantly feeling acted upon rather than feeling in charge, the child may become confused and angry, and may develop a poor self-image.

7. **An Educational Problem.** A child with limited language derives minimal benefit from formal education.

8. **An Intellectual Problem.** A child will be deficient in general knowledge and language competence—both of which are included in a broad definition of intelligence.

9. **A Vocational Problem.** Lacking in verbal skills, general knowledge, academic training, and social skills, the hearing-impaired child will reach adulthood with limited possibilities for gainful employment.

10. **Parental Problems.** The instinctive reactions of parents to a baby's failure to develop language is to withdraw language input and to reduce interaction. When they discover the true nature of the deficit, they may well enter a state of denial and confusion, which reduces their general effectiveness as parents and further undermines the social and emotional development of their child.

11. **A Societal Problem.** The withdrawal of interaction by the parents will be repeated later by society.

THE PROCESS OF AURAL HABILITATION/REHABILITATION

To reduce the potential negative outcomes of a prelingual hearing loss to the extent possible, a comprehensive program of aural habilitation will need to be introduced. In fact, all children with hearing impairment will require habilitative intervention in some form and to some extent. The differences lie in the time of onset of the hearing loss and the impact on language development. The components will include some or all of:

1. **Parental Guidance.** It is critical that the child with hearing impairment have well-adjusted parents, in other words, parents who have overcome the anger, anxiety, and apprehension that they may have felt on diagnosis of their child's hearing loss; who have accepted their child as a child, not as a burden; and who have accepted their role in the development of their child. This requires continuity of support from the day of diagnosis and every step along the way (Sanders, 1993, pp. 228–259).

2. **Audiologic Services.** Early audiological management is extremely important for both the child with hearing impairment and his or her parents. For the child, it is critical that amplification be offered as early as possible. Each day that amplification is not provided is a day lost in auditory development. A hearing aid or hearing aids should be fit. Aid performance must be evaluated by the audiologist who will be involved in services for the child on a long-term basis. The clinician should do all that can be done to make the fitting of the hearing aid(s) a happy occasion. The joy is in observing a child respond and attend to sound, perhaps for the first time, and to celebrate this first day in the hearing life of the child. On the other hand, a solemn and ceremonious atmosphere surely will be reflected in both the child's and the parents' acceptance of the hearing aid(s).

3. **Auditory Development.** This aspect involves providing the child the opportunity to develop an awareness of sounds in his or her environment and to develop the ability to recognize things by the sounds they make; to make judgments about what is heard; to make judgments about where sounds come from; and to use hearing not only for recognizing speech, but for understanding and producing speech.

4. **Cognitive/Language Development.** Even though auditory development cannot be separated from cognitive development, and even though much of what we are doing is involved in the cognitive/linguistic development of the child on an auditory basis, the components involved in language development must be addressed separately. As Boothroyd (1982) observed, we are not only assisting the child to develop a "world model," or a conceptual model of his or her world—the raw materials

from which to construct their internal world models—but also the language required to interact with it and those within it. The child must have access to a rich linguistic environment to not only understand language, but to also express it (See Figure 1-1).

5. **Speech Development.** A child must also have the opportunity for access to speech, no matter what earlier expressive mode for communication was used. Of course, if the child has no access to auditory sensitivity because of the severity of the hearing loss, the child should not be forced to use a form of communication that is doomed to failure. However, if a child appears to have access to the hearing and motor skills that will permit speech development, it should be encouraged in a natural and interactive way. If it is forced and drilled,

speech training may become a dreaded and punishing experience for the child.

AURAL REHABILITATION FOR ADULTS

HISTORICAL BACKGROUND

Following the advent of the field of audiology as an aural rehabilitation service during World War II, it has been interesting to note its progress. Its history is important as we study the process of aural rehabilitation on behalf of adults.

Military aural rehabilitation programs provided the birthplace for the field of audiology. The Veterans Administration expanded the role of the

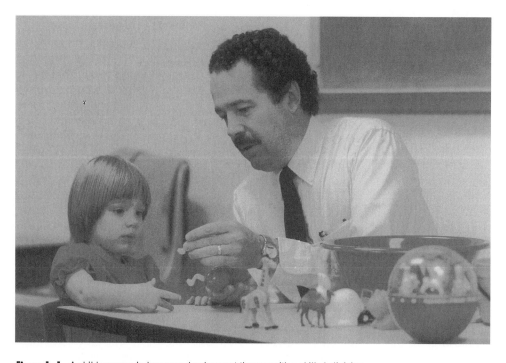

Figure 1–1. A child engages in language development therapy with a skilled clinician.

audiologist and the standards for professionals and equipment. The first training program for audiologists was developed at Northwestern University in the 1940s and programs expanded rapidly through the 1950s and 1960s. As a young profession, growing pains were experienced.

As instrumentation became more elaborate during the 1950s and particularly during the 1960s and the field became more sophisticated through research, there was a shift of emphasis toward pure and applied research and in the medical diagnosis of site of lesion of auditory disorders. It was apparent that the emphasis among the majority of professionals and training programs was turning toward diagnosis, instrumentation, and research and away from aural rehabilitation. Results from an automated piece of equipment or from a research project were more tangible than the emerging signs of improvement in social com-

munication observed in an adult client with hearing impairment.

The course of working with clients with hearing impairment on the improvement of communication skills can be difficult. Interaction with adults or elderly clients with hearing impairment, helping them to deal with the emotional impact of hearing impairment and their frustrations and fears, requires that the audiologist become involved on a close professional basis with clients and their families (Figure 1–2).

Unfortunately in the 1950s and 1960s, research and diagnostics became popular and interest in aural habilitation/rehabilitation of hearing impairment declined. Courses within training programs in the areas of differential diagnosis of auditory problems, speech and hearing sciences, instrumentation, and experimental audiology expanded rapidly and new faculty were hired to

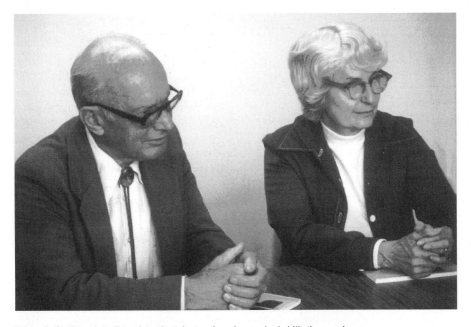

Figure 1–2. Two adults listen intently to instructions for aural rehabilitation services.

teach them. Amid the array of those courses and the blinking lights of the equipment, training programs generally offered a course or two titled Aural Rehabilitation. When it came to finding a faculty member to teach the course, often the lowest ranked faculty member or a doctoral assistant would submit to the task. Students generally reflected the same negativity, not only in regard to the course or courses, but also to aural rehabilitation practicum experiences with children and adults who had hearing impairment.

However in most instances, that attitude does not prevail today. A more humanistic desire to work with people is becoming predominant among practicing professionals and professors of audiology training programs and their students. Prospective students are searching for graduate programs in audiology that permit them to concentrate on learning to provide aural (re)habilitation services, including the fitting and dispensing of hearing aids and other nonhearing assistive listening devices. So our field appears to be achieving a healthy balance.

ACADEMY OF REHABILITATIVE AUDIOLOGY

One of the most positive steps taken during the past three decades toward strengthening the professional stature of aural rehabilitation, the professionals who provide those services, and students in training who desire to provide them after graduation was the origin of the Academy of Rehabilitative Audiology in 1966. The academy has done much to bring about a renewed awareness of the importance of professional training in aural rehabilitation and those services on behalf of children, adults, and elderly clients with hearing impairment.

As procedures for providing aural rehabilitative services for children, adults, and aging persons with hearing impairment become more sophisticated, along with increased emphasis on the need for professional involvement in the fitting and dis-

pensing of hearing aids, the professional prominence of the rehabilitative aspects of audiology continues to expand. But as a primary health care profession, both the diagnostic and habilitative/rehabilitative aspects of audiology must carry an equal share of the responsibility in caring for clients with hearing impairment. This is also true in the conduct of research to discover new and more effective ways of providing those services.

PROCESS OF ADULT AURAL REHABILITATION

DEFINITIONS AND CONSIDERATIONS

What is aural rehabilitation and the provision of aural rehabilitation services on the behalf of adults with hearing impairment? Aural rehabilitation is an attempt to reduce the barriers to communication that result from hearing impairment and facilitate adjustment to the possible psychosocial, educational, and occupational impact of that auditory deficit. In discussing aural rehabilitation, we are generally referring to serving those who had normal to near-normal hearing postlingually, but have sustained hearing loss that will, if left untreated, result in increasing levels of impairment. And, as hearing loss in an equal opportunity impairment, these persons span the age range from younger to older adulthood.

If viewed from the provision of aural rehabilitation services, those services include the facets now detailed.

ASSESSMENT OF HEARING

Assessment of an individual's hearing, per se, and the determination of his or her ability to hear and understand speech are the first important steps in the aural rehabilitation process. In the past, this step may have been the first and last, except for possible referral for a hearing aid if one appeared warranted. Few other avenues for remediation of an auditory deficit were taken. According to Rosen (1967) in an early treatise on aural rehabilitation,

As he [the client] takes leave of the audiologist he knows that he has a hearing problem. . . . It is true that the audiologist may have mentioned lipreading, auditory training, or training in the use of a hearing aid, but probably did not offer those services himself. Furthermore, the advice was likely to be offered half-heartedly, as if the audiologist was really not aware of or convinced of its value. (p. 42)

This attitude is not as widespread as it appeared to be in the early 1960's, but it is still around, to some degree. If the attitude of the audiologist who conducts an audiologic evaluation is such that he or she is not convinced of the value of aural rehabilitative services two things are possible. The individual with the auditory deficit either may not be referred for rehabilitation, or the person may become so discouraged as a result of the audiologist's attitude that, even though a referral is made, the client may not keep the appointment. It is discouraging to find audiologists who apparently entered the field of audiology because it is a helping profession, but who feel uncomfortable when they must relate with people with hearing impairment on a face-to-face basis.

Nevertheless, the accurate assessment of the extent of a hearing deficit, per se, is the first step in the process of aural rehabilitation. With that information, (1) the assessment of the handicapping effects of the hearing loss, (2) the initiation of a hearing aid evaluation, if deemed necessary, and (3) the other steps involved in the aural rehabilitation program can begin.

ASSESSMENT OF THE BENEFITS OF AMPLIFICATION

Assessment of the benefits of amplification for individual clients should be the second step in the aural rehabilitation treatment program, along with, if indicated, the fitting and dispensing of the instruments. Correspondingly, with the hearing aid evaluation, assessment of the handicapping effects of a hearing loss should be made. In that regard, steps 1, 2, and 3 in this sequence must go hand in hand.

An accurate determination of a client's candidacy for a hearing aid can be made by a skilled audiologist who will sift through the audiometric data, including those of speech recognition and the client's dynamic range, and will also assess the emotional and social consequences of each client's hearing loss and his or her communicative needs. The hearing aid evaluation and/or evaluation for other assistive listening devices is only one part of the total aural rehabilitation program, but it is a critical part.

ASSESSMENT OF THE IMPACT OF THE HEARING DEFICIT

Assessment of the impact of the hearing deficit on individual clients, is again, important for formulating a viable aural rehabilitation program based on individual clients' communicative needs. The assessment may include attempts at determining the impact of the hearing loss on an individual emotionally, socially, occupationally, and educationally. In most instances, when dealing with adults and elderly persons with hearing impairment, the potential impact of the hearing deficit on the educational aspects of life may not be the most important. For young school-age adults, it becomes extremely important, as it does for those adults or elderly clients who desire to be involved in continuing education programs for occupational advancement or simply for the enjoyment of learning.

There are, at present, a number of scales and procedures that have been outlined for the assessment of the handicap of hearing impairment on an adult or elderly client. In light of the probability that he or she had normal to near-normal communicative function before onset of the hearing loss, the impact of the hearing loss on the personal lives and occupational or educational goals is, in many ways, a personal thing. Everyone is affected differently.

The results of the audiometric evaluation provide an audiologist with information regarding expected communicative levels resulting from the hearing loss, particularly when observing the shape of the audiogram notations, the degree of hearing loss, and a client's ability to hear and understand speech. A client's response to that hearing loss must be evaluated and taken into consideration as his or her aural rehabilitation treatment program, including the possible fitting and dispensing of hearing aids, is being developed. The perceptive audiologist will be able to observe the more obvious behaviors and respond appropriately to them from the first contact with clients.

Evaluation of the impact of the hearing impairment on adult or elderly clients, then, is an important part of an ongoing aural rehabilitation program. It is, however, a difficult task and one that is probably never finished, since as clients face new situations, their responses to them may differ. As physical, occupational, and personal environments change, so do the responses of persons with hearing impairments. Evaluation, therefore, is ongoing and clients must also be taught to evaluate themselves and their reactions to new communicative environments.

Perhaps the most important component of the evaluation process prior to services and on the decision to terminate them is the client's opinions of his or her ability to function communicatively in his or her own communicating world. Scales and procedures for evaluating communicative functions are discussed in the chapter, "Evaluation in Aural Rehabilitation Treatment for Adults Who Are Hearing Impaired", and are found in the Appendixes of this book.

TREATMENT PROGRAM

A formal aural rehabilitation treatment program is, of course, not separated in any way from the procedures previously discussed, but rather it is an extension of them. It involves ongoing *counseling* to facilitate adjustment to the hearing loss, *facilitating increased efficiency* in communication, including establishment of client priorities in communication, and *developing a treatment program* that targets each individual client's communicative needs. The procedures used may involve efforts toward greater efficiency of the use of a client's residual hearing, greater awareness and use of visual clues in communication, modification of the client's frequented communicative environments, and other specific tasks. The client's family and significant others are important elements in the total process of aural rehabilitation.

The formal treatment program may not be the most important aspect of the aural rehabilitation effort, but for those many clients who can benefit from treatment strategies that may enhance communication in their most difficult environments, it is a critical aspect of the total process. The most successful aural rehabilitation treatment programs are those in which counseling and hearing aid orientation are integral.

INVOLVEMENT OF OTHER PROFESSIONALS

Involvement of other professionals, including the vocational rehabilitation counselor, the social worker, educational personnel, the speech/language specialist, and the psychologist, is important to the ongoing aural rehabilitation program for individual clients who require various services. For elderly clients who reside in a health care facility, involvement of facility personnel is critical. Included may be the activity director, occupational therapist, social worker, nurses,

nurses' aides, and others who are in close contact with the clients.

It is incumbent on the audiologist to call on other professionals to facilitate the rehabilitation process. It is also important to know when the problems an adult or elderly person is facing are beyond the scope of an audiologist's knowledge and skill and to be aware of proper referral sources. As a team leader in the aural rehabilitation process, the audiologist can function as the catalyst in the development of a truly comprehensive rehabilitation program for those clients who require additional services.

INVOLVEMENT OF THE FAMILY

The positive involvement of the family and/or significant others in a client's life can be one of the most strengthening aspects of the aural rehabilitation program, both for the younger and older client. The words "positive involvement" are stressed because involvement by a nonunderstanding family member, or a friend who in the end decides that he or she "does not have the time," or who otherwise does not desire to become involved can be damaging. If a spouse, another family member, or another significant other is to be a part of a client's aural rehabilitation program, it is important that he or she be involved from the time of the initial evaluation, particularly during the period of assessment of the handicapping effects of the hearing loss on the client. As the significant other becomes aware of the impact of the hearing deficit, that person can become an important catalyst in facilitating adjustment and enhancing the communication abilities of the client.

SUMMARY

What is aural rehabilitation? According to Costello et al. (1974), in a classic paper developed by them as members of the Committee on Rehabilitative Audiology of the American Speech-Language-Hearing Association, "Audiologic rehabilitation is designed to assist individuals with auditory disabilities to realize their optimal potential in communication regardless of age, or the age of the person at the onset of the disability" (p. 68).

It is a rewarding process that has as its goal the reduction of the barriers to communication that have resulted from hearing loss. Within the process, a number of professionals may be involved, with the audiologist functioning as the coordinator, or facilitator, of the team. A clients' family will be a critical element in the process.

The process is as complex as the client and the handicapping effects of his or her hearing impairment and, unquestionably, it carries great responsibility. Only those audiologists who are willing to accept that responsibility should provide those services. That means, coming face-to-face with people—children, younger adults, elderly persons, siblings, and the family who require a close professional relationship and a service that will enhance their abilities to function communicatively in a complex and changing world.

REFERENCES

Bader, J. L. (1997). Language development for children who are hearing impaired. In R. H. Hull (Ed.), *Aural rehabilitation* (pp. 121–134). San Diego, CA: Singular Publishing Group.

Ballantyne, J. (1977). *Deafness*. New York: Churchill Livingstone.

Bender, R. E. (1981). *The conquest of deafness*. Danville, IL: Interstate.

Blank, M., Rose, S., & Berlin, L. (1978). *The language of learning: The preschool years*. New York: Grune & Stratton.

Boothroyd, A. (1978). Speech perception and sensorineural hearing loss. In M. Ross & T. Giolas (Eds.), *Auditory management of hearing-impaired children* (pp. 92–101). Baltimore, MD: University Park Press.

Boothroyd, A. (1982). *Hearing impairments in young children.* Englewood Cliffs, NJ: Prentice Hall.

Calvert, D., & Silverman, S. (1975). *Speech and deafness.* Washington, DC: Alexander Graham Bell Association for the Deaf.

Chase, R. A. (1968). Motor organization of speech. In S. J. Freeman (Ed.), *The neuropsychology of spatially oriented behavior.* Homewood, IL: Dorsey Press.

Cornett, R. (1967). Cued speech. *American Annals of the Deaf, 112,* 3–13.

Costello, M. R., Freeland, E. E., Hill, M. J., Jeffers, J., Matkin, N., Stream, R. W., & Tobin, H. (1974). The audiologist: Responsibilities in the habilitation of the auditorily handicapped. *Asha, 16,* 68–70.

Deland, F. (1931). *The story of lipreading.* Washington, DC: The Volta Bureau.

Farrar, A. (1923). *Arnold on the education of the deaf.* London: Francis Carter.

Fry, D. B. (1978). Language development in the deaf child. In F. Bess (Ed.), *Childhood deafness: Causation, assessment and management* (pp. 123–142). New York: Grune & Stratton.

Giangreco, C.J. (1976). *The education of the hearing impaired.* Springfield, IL: Charles C. Thomas.

Grammatico, L., & Miller, S. (1974). Curriculum for the preschool deaf child. *Volta Review, 79,* 19–26.

Groht, M. A. (1958). *National language for deaf children.* Washington, DC: The Alexander Graham Bell Association for the Deaf.

Harris, G. (1963). *Language for the preschool deaf child.* New York: Grune & Stratton.

Hirsh, I. J. (1966). Teaching the deaf child to talk. In F. Smith & G. A. Miller (Eds.), *The genesis of language* (pp. 129–138). Cambridge, MA: MIT Press.

Hochberg, I., Levitt, H., & Osberger, M. J. (Eds.). (1983). *Speech of the hearing impaired.* Baltimore, MD: University Park Press.

Hodgson, K. (1953). *The deaf and their problems.* London: Watts.

Kretschmer, R., & Kretschmer, L. (1978). *Language development and intervention with the hearing impaired.* Baltimore, MD: University Park Press.

Kretschmer, R., & Kretschmer, L. (1984). Habilitation of language of deaf children. In W. H. Perkins (Ed.), *Current therapy of communication disorders: Hearing disorders* (212–235). New York: Thieme-Stratton.

Lillie, S. M. (1969). *Management of deafness in infants and very young children.* Paper presented at the 47th annual international convention, Council for Exceptional Children, Denver, CO.

Ling, D. (1978). Auditory coding and recording: An analysis of auditory training procedures for hearing-impaired children. In M. Ross & T. Giolas (Eds.), *Auditory management of hearing-impaired children: Principles and prerequisites for intervention* (pp. 98–120). Baltimore, MD: University Park Press.

Ling, D. (1980). Early speech development. In G. T. Mencher & S. E. Gerber (Eds.), *Early management of hearing loss* (pp. 128–142). New York: Grune & Stratton.

Ling, D. (1984a). *Early intervention for hearing-impaired children: Oral options.* Boston: College-Hill Press.

Ling, D. (1984b). *Early intervention for hearing-impaired children: Total communication options.* Boston: College-Hill Press.

Ling, D., & Ling, A. (1978). *Aural habilitation: The foundations of verbal learning in hearing-impaired children.* Washington, DC: Alexander Graham Bell Association for the Deaf.

Ling, D., & Milne, M. M. (1980). The development of speech in hearing-impaired children. In F. Bess, B. A. Freeman, & J. S. Sinclair (Eds.), *Amplification in education* (pp. 245–270). Washington, DC: Alexander Graham Bell Association for the Deaf.

Luterman, D. (1987). *Deafness in the family.* Boston: College-Hill Press.

Markides, A. (1983). *The speech of hearing-impaired children.* Manchester, UK: Manchester University Press.

Mindel, E. D., & Vernon, M. (1987). *They grow in silence: The deaf child and his family.* Silver Spring, MD: National Association for the Deaf.

Moeller, M. P., & McConkey, A. J. (1984). Language intervention with preschool deaf children: A cognitive/linguistic approach. In W. H. Perkins (Ed.), *Current therapy of communication disorders: Hearing disorders* (pp. 287–302). New York: Thieme-Stratton.

Moses, K. L. (1985). Infant deafness and parental grief: Psychosocial early intervention. In F. Powell et al. (Eds.), *Education of the hearing-impaired child* (pp. 223–231). San Diego, CA: College-Hill Press.

Osberger, M. J., Johnstone, A., Swarts, E., & Levitt, H. (1978). The evaluation of a model speech training program for deaf children. *Journal of Communication Disorders, 11*, 293–313.

Phillips, A. L. (1987). Working with parents. A story of personal and professional growth. In D. Adkins (Ed.), Families and their hearing-impaired children. *Volta Review, 89*(5), 131–146.

Pollack, D. (1970). *Educational audiology for the limited hearing infant.* Springfield, IL: Charles C. Thomas.

Pollack, D. (1985). *Educational audiology for the limited hearing infant and pre-schooler.* Springfield, IL: Charles C. Thomas.

Rosen, J. (1967). *The role of the audiologist in aural rehabilitation.* Unpublished manuscript, University of Denver.

Sanders, D. A. (1993). *Management of hearing handicap: Infants to elderly.* Englewood Cliffs, NJ: Prentice Hall.

Simmons-Martin, A. (1977). Natural language and auditory input. In F. Bess (Ed.), *Childhood deafness: Causation, assessment and management* (pp. 111–128). New York: Grune & Stratton.

Stone, P. (1980). Developing thinking skills in young hearing-impaired children. *Volta Review, 82*(6), 345–353.

Taba, H. (1962). *Curriculum development: Theory and practice.* New York: Harcourt, Brace and World.

Vorce, E. (1974). *Teaching speech to deaf children.* Washington, DC: Alexander Graham Bell Association for the Deaf.

END OF CHAPTER EXAMINATION QUESTIONS

CHAPTER 1

1. According to the author, the primary objective of aural rehabilitation is to:
   a. assist hearing impaired persons to overcome the handicap of hearing impairment.
   b. diagnose the hearing impairment.
   c. treat the hearing impairment.

2. Which of the following problems might a child who possesses a severe congenital hearing loss experience?
   a. social problems
   b. cognitive problems
   c. emotional problems
   d. all of the above

3. Auditory development is generally defined as:
   a. the physical maturation of the auditory system.
   b. the ability of the client to be aware of and recognize sounds in her or his environment.
   c. structuring an auditory intervention plan for the client.

4. Assessment of an individual's hearing is generally thought of as the first step in the process of aural rehabilitation. According to the author, that assessment should begin with:
   a. the fitting of an amplification device.
   b. determining the extent of a high frequency hearing loss.
   c. determining the ability to hear and understand speech.
   d. determining the impact of one's hearing loss on social issues.

END OF CHAPTER ANSWER SHEET

Name _____ Date _____

CHAPTER 1

1. Which one(s)?   a   b   c

2. Which one(s)?   a   b   c   d

3. Which one(s)?   a   b   c

4. Which one(s)?   a   b   c   d

5. Which one(s)?   a   b   c

6. Which one(s)?   a   b   c   d

7. _____

_____

_____

_____

Circle one

8. True or False?

9. True or False?

10. True or False?

5. The second step in aural rehabilitation should be:
   a. assessment of the type of hearing loss.
   b. assessment of amplification benefits.
   c. assessment of the impact of hearing loss on the individual.

6. Beside the audiologist, another professional (other professionals) who might be involved in the aural rehabilitation process is (are):
   a. the vocational counselor
   b. the social worker
   c. the speech-language pathologist
   d. all of the above

7. In aural rehabilitation programs, the audiologist generally functions as the team leader. What role(s) might he or she play?

8. (True/False) According to the information presented in this chapter, an aural rehabilitation program focuses exclusively on increasing the efficiency of communication.

9. (True/False) All individuals experience an equal degree of handicap from equal degrees of hearing loss.

10. (True/false) Aural rehabilitation programs with all ages of clients are equally enhanced by positive family involvement.

Introduction to the Handicap of Hearing Impairment

Auditory Impairment Versus Hearing Handicap

■   JACK KATZ, Ph.D.   ■
■   THOMAS P. WHITE, M.A.   ■

FUNCTIONAL TERMINOLOGY
   Hearing Level Versus Hearing Loss
   Hearing Impairment Versus Hearing Handicap

RELATIONSHIPS OF TERMINOLOGY

CONGENITAL VERSUS ACQUIRED HEARING LOSS

(continued)

TYPES OF HEARING LOSS
  Conductive Loss
  Cochlear Loss
  Neural Loss
  Central Dysfunction
  Unilateral Versus Bilateral Hearing Loss

WHAT AUDIOMETRIC DATA REVEAL
  Degree of Hearing Loss
  Configuration of Hearing Loss

SPEECH THRESHOLDS AND WORD RECOGNITION

OTHER AUDIOMETRIC TESTS

LIMITATIONS OF AUDIOMETRIC INFORMATION

EDUCATIONAL AND VOCATIONAL CONSIDERATIONS

SUMMARY

To understand the aural rehabilitative needs of a client, a careful interview should be carried out as well as a battery of audiometric procedures. An in-depth interview or questionnaire and specialized diagnostic tests are required to obtain the broadest understanding. In the end, however, there will always be an element of uncertainty. This limitation in precise prediction is due to variations in each client's motivation, alertness, and other factors.

An audiologic assessment permits an audiologist to compare a client's data with that of a control population. Even when accurate audiometric data are obtained, the specialist is left with many questions regarding a person's rehabilitative needs. For example, audiologists do not know with whom the person communicates and if it is within a large lecture hall, over a taxicab CB radio, or if it involves extensive interviews. Tests do not tell clinicians if a child has a well-developed vocabulary and language system or if he or she has optimal classroom conditions. Unless audiologists test further, they will not know how well individuals are able to use visual information to supplement auditory information. Questionnaires can often help the audiologist in gaining a client's perspective and other insights (Kaplan, Bally, & Brandt, 1990; Lamb, Owens, & Schubert 1983).

It is helpful to begin with a discussion of terminology. For example, sometimes cause and effect are confused with measurement and function.

FUNCTIONAL TERMINOLOGY

Some individuals, even professionals, may use the terms *hearing loss, hearing level, hearing impairment,* and *hearing handicap* interchangeably. This is not helpful in understanding the needs of each individual. The following sections delineate these terms.

HEARING LEVEL VERSUS HEARING LOSS

Hearing level (HL) is a measurement made on an audiometer and reported in decibels (S 3.6, ANSI, 1989). Hearing levels obtained in a controlled acoustical environment compare a client's performance to the responses of individuals in a standard population, that is, a population with normal hearing. In essence, it is the dial reading on an audiometer at which an individual responds in a specified manner. *Hearing loss* is be used to indicate the type of problem (e.g., conductive versus sensorineural), or that hearing ability has been lost (Davis & Silverman, 1978). If a person's 40 dB threshold is labeled as a 40 dB HL (*hearing level*), but it was previously known to be −5 dB, then it could also be said that it is a 45 dB *hearing loss.*

HEARING IMPAIRMENT VERSUS HEARING HANDICAP

Hearing impairment is closely associated with *hearing level* and the terms are sometimes used interchangeably. Hearing impairment can also relate to measures that are not in dB, such as word recognition scores. Hearing impairment implies that performance is poorer than normal. It is generally categorized as mild, moderate, or severe. *Hearing handicap* refers to the interference in communication/hearing that results from a *hearing loss.* Thus, the negative influence of a hearing impairment on the person's ability in life situations is the *hearing handicap.* For example, an individual with a hearing level of 30 dB HL may have more difficulty in his or her communicative environment than another individual with a 50 dB HL, because the first person may have greater communicative demands in his or her occupational or personal life.

RELATIONSHIPS OF TERMINOLOGY

The terms just described can best be understood as they relate to individual cases. Two case presentations may clarify their use.

A 42-year-old woman was seen by an audiologist following a sudden onset of tinnitus and hearing loss. The audiometric results revealed a flat sensorineural *hearing loss.* The pure-tone speech-frequency average was 45 dB *hearing level* in each ear. According to a preemployment audiogram, the patient had normal hearing with an average of 8 dB HL in each ear. Thus, there was a 37 dB hearing loss associated with the incident. Her *hearing impairment* is classified as moderate. The actual *hearing handicap* is greater than this because the patient reports considerable difficulty in communicating. The problem is more acute in this case, because the client works as a librarian and people tend to speak softly in libraries.

A 5-year-old child attends a regular kindergarten class. He has normal hearing up to 1000 Hz in each ear, but at this point his thresholds fall off markedly. The *hearing level* at 2000 Hz is 35 dB poorer than his 0 dB HL at 1000 Hz. Although there is a mild *hearing impairment* according to standard classifications, this child has major difficulties in distinguishing high-frequency consonants from one another and in developing age-appropriate verbal concepts. This problem is increased because the child has been placed in a relatively noisy classroom with a teacher who has never had a child who has hearing impairment in her class. In addition, she does not know the special accommodations that should be made for this particular youngster. Thus, the level of difficulty is underestimated when simply looking at the *hearing level*. These concepts are discussed further by Weinstein, Richards, and Montano (1995).

CONGENITAL VERSUS ACQUIRED HEARING LOSS

One factor that influences the effect of a hearing loss is *when* it occurred. Severe congenital or prelingual hearing losses (losses prior to the development of aural speech and language) have a great impact on language, voice, and articulation, because the individual may not develop these skills normally. Such an individual generally does not have constant language stimulation or accurate feedback of his or her own speech production. As an adult, the person may continue to have limitations in language, as well as in voice and articulation. Prelingual hearing disorders also have a more deleterious effect on social, educational, and vocational aspects of a person's life, than if the hearing loss occurred after oral speech and language developed.

The same type of loss at an older age, especially a sudden catastrophic loss of hearing, will be likely to have a profound influence on an individual, but of a much different type. There will be no diminution of the person's language ability and relatively little change in his or her voice quality. However, over a period, articulatory movements will tend to become less precise, typically affecting the high frequency sibilant sounds first. Because the individual is not able to monitor articulation and voice effectively, he or she may compensate for this by increasing their speech volume.

A sudden catastrophic loss is usually more devastating than one of gradual onset in two ways. First, the psychological impact of isolation is much greater because of the suddenness of the onset. Second, the person who has a sudden onset of hearing loss will tend to have difficulty utilizing his or her residual hearing to make fine distinctions among, for example, the sounds of speech. Clients with progressive hearing loss have been able to alter their auditory perceptions in a gradual manner. The person with a sudden loss may not know how to listen for clues to distinguish, for example, the singular form of a word from the plural; whereas the person whose hearing has diminished over time may have developed strategies for doing so.

Obviously, the complex interactions of people, their needs and environments, and the various test indicators provide infinite possibilities about a person who has a hearing loss. Audiometric results give us guidance and general knowledge about a patient, but in the end, they fail to reveal things that the patient or the patient's family can tell an audiologist. The contribution of audiometric test results in predicting hearing handicap is discussed in the following section.

TYPES OF HEARING LOSS

CONDUCTIVE LOSS

Knowing the type of hearing loss can help in predicting the handicap that a client has. For example, *conductive losses*, particularly when the client possesses normal to near normal bone conduction, are associated with good discrimination ability for speech. Clients with conductive hearing loss may achieve very good speech discrimination simply from increased volume. Although the communicative effects of conductive loss in an adult are not as severe as an equivalent sensorineural loss, there is growing evidence that a mild conductive loss early in life may have significant long-term effects (Dalzell & Owrid, 1976; Holm & Kunze, 1969; Secord, Erickson, & Bush, 1988). Furthermore, in some cases, earmold drainage may contraindicate the use of an earmold for the hearing aid, and a conductive overlay on top of a sensorineural problem can complicate the use and types of amplification. (See Figure 2–1 for an example of an audiogram that reveals a conductive hearing loss).

COCHLEAR LOSS

Most cochlear *(sensory)* losses reveal some diminished word recognition ability. There is usually a direct relationship between hearing level and the ability to discriminate speech (Thompson & Hoel, 1962). Therefore, the more depressed the hearing level, the poorer the word recognition score. Disorders of the cochlea produce a variety of audiometric patterns that provide clues to their etiology. Detection of these problems can lead to preventative measures and, thus, minimize any further hearing loss. Most cochlear hearing losses are greater in the high frequencies than in the low frequencies. This is because presbycusis (age-related) and noise-induced hearing loss, the most common

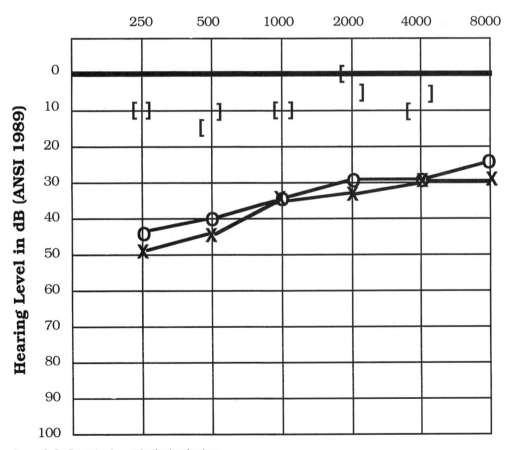

Figure 2–1. Example of a conductive hearing loss.

causes of sensorineural disorder, primarily affect the higher frequency region of the cochlea. On the other hand, cochlear losses associated with Ménière disease, for example, are generally greater in the low frequencies than in the high frequencies. A flat audiometric configuration may be seen in ototoxic-related disorders. These patterns are not mutually exclusive and, thus, may overlap one another.

Another characteristic commonly seen in sensory losses is intolerance for loud sounds (often associated with recruitment). Consequently, this factor must be considered in the use of amplification. In cases with extremely small dynamic ranges, the use of amplification could be contraindicated. That is, some individuals with sensory losses have an intolerance for sounds only slightly above their threshold levels. This might prevent effective use of amplification.

Cochlear losses may also affect the speech and voice of the individual. Because inner ear functioning is decreased, the internal feedback loop is reduced to the extent that the clients are unable to monitor their own speech and voice patterns properly. This can lead to articulation disorder as well as to reduced vocal inflection and quality. This effect is related to the extent and duration of the hearing loss. (See Figure 2–2 for an audiogram that shows a typical sensory [cochlear] hearing loss.)

NEURAL LOSS

The effects of a neural hearing loss, which is caused by a decline in function of the auditory nerve (cranial nerve VIII) and beyond, are generally more a problem of clarity than of sensitivity. Consequently, audiometric findings will usually show more significantly depressed word recognition scores than in cochlear cases with equal pure-tone thresholds. This, in turn, may disrupt not only normal communications, but also the use of a hearing aid that is designed to alleviate the communicative breakdown.

Another characteristic of neural losses is the presence of reflex, or tone, decay or the inability to maintain the audibility of pure tones. For example, Costello and McGee (1967) discussed clients who appeared as either being deaf or aphasic, although their pure-tone thresholds were quite good. These cases were found to have severe discrimination losses and rapid tone decay. It should be noted that many persons with brainstem dysfunction, as well as those with CN VIII losses, have poor discrimination for speech and significant tone decay.

CENTRAL DYSFUNCTION

Peripheral hearing disorders may be due to disease at the conductive, cochlear, or VIIIth nerve levels of the auditory system. Dysfunction in the brain or brainstem results in a central disorder. Although it also might produce a hearing loss, central dysfunction is generally associated with more subtle changes, including figure-ground processing and localization problems. These difficulties may compound the problems associated with a concomitant or coincidental hearing loss; however, central auditory dysfunction, by itself, can produce sufficient difficulty to cause a person to seek evaluation by an audiologist.

Stach (1989) points out that a high percentage of people who fail to benefit from hearing aids, at least among the elderly, have central processing problems. Thus, the audiologist should consider this possibility when an individual does not receive the expected degree of benefit from amplification, or when the amount of auditory disability far outweighs the person's hearing loss as shown on the standard audiometric tests.

UNILATERAL VERSUS BILATERAL HEARING LOSS

The problems produced by hearing loss may be increased or minimized, depending on whether

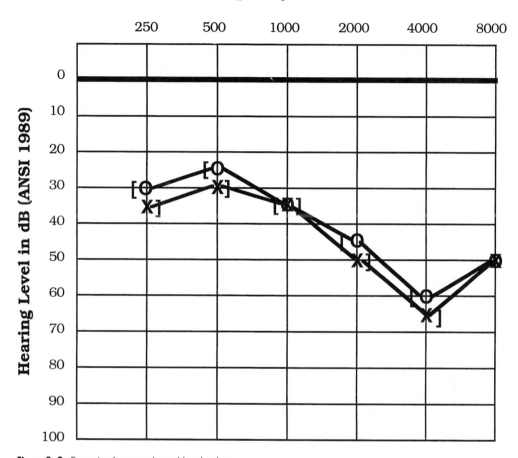

Figure 2–2. Example of a sensorineural hearing loss.

the loss involves one or both ears. The difficulties associated with unilateral hearing impairments generally are not limited to the amount of loss, alone. Although the thresholds in the affected ear are lowered, one would think that if either ear could hear a sound, the individual would benefit fully by its presence. In this way, the better ear would be expected to dominate and greatly reduce the adverse influence of the poorer ear. However, the handicap resulting from a unilateral loss is due

not only to the loss of sensitivity, but even more likely to the imbalance between the ears, which tends to disable important central processes (Jerger, Silman, Lew, & Chmiel, 1993).

Individuals who have unilateral losses often experience some listening problems. One obvious difficulty is the lack of hearing when someone is speaking on the person's impaired side. Two other problems are not as closely linked with the severity of the loss. For one thing, people with unilateral losses can be expected to have trouble in localizing the source of a sound. But, perhaps the most important problem associated with this type of loss is difficulty understanding speech in a background of noise or when the acoustical conditions are poor. Similarly, a person with a unilateral loss who wears a monaural hearing aid tends to lose the benefits he or she might derive from the binaural system. Thus, that person cannot benefit fully from his or her central functions. For example, the person may be unable to separate foreground from background and to locate sounds in space.

Unilateral losses in children, although perhaps not as devastating as hearing lost suddenly in adulthood (Bardon, 1986), have potentially important consequences. A complete journal issue was devoted to the work of Bess and his colleagues, dealing with unilateral hearing loss in children (Bess, 1986). Their work confirms that unilateral losses are associated with poor localization of sound in space, as well as with difficulty on speech-in-noise tasks. The greater the loss in the poorer ear, the greater the difficulty.

WHAT AUDIOMETRIC DATA REVEAL

In their simplest form, hearing disorders can be viewed as changes in sensitivity, frequency range, and fidelity. Sensitivity can be likened to the decibel (intensity) variations produced by an attenuator. A reduced frequency range is similar to the effects of an acoustic filter that selectively impedes the passage of some frequencies and permits others to pass. A lack of fidelity is the distortion caused by the nonlinear transmission of a sound because of the breakdown of either peripheral or central structures.

The influence of sensitivity (degree of loss) and frequency range (configuration) are described first, because they provide the most reliable audiometric information. The disorders of fidelity (clarity),

although vitally important, are not as quantifiable. Fidelity and other factors that are less precise reduce a clinician's ability to predict the handicap from the pure-tone information. The audiologist and the client will be best served when all of the available information is used.

DEGREE OF LOSS

One of several things that audiometric data reveal is the *degree* of loss. This information is important, because it provides a general indication of the handicap a individual may experience. To put hearing threshold levels into perspective, general classifications are shown along with their predicted handicaps in Table 2–1. This permits an audiologist to make general statements about a person's hearing function and probable needs. However, the clinician cannot state with great certainty the specific effects of a loss. Thus, this table should be used only as a guideline, not as an absolute.

Many methods of categorization have been proposed, including those of Davis and Silverman (1978), Green (1978), and Hodgson (1978). The emphasis of each method varies, according to its purpose. These purposes include medical-legal definitions, handicapping effects, rehabilitative needs, and the impact on children versus adults.

The influence of the degree of loss may not be as obvious as it might appear. Generally, the rule of thumb is, the greater the hearing level loss the greater the handicap. However the actual *handicap*, when compared to the *degree* of hearing loss, may vary considerably. Important factors contributing to these differences include personality, intelligence, motivation, occupation, and environmental conditions. Individuals who rely heavily on communicative function for their work, such as salespersons, attorneys, and teachers who possess relatively mild hearing loss may notice significantly greater handicap than those whose jobs are not as verbally demanding (e.g., truck drivers, farmers, industrial workers). Individuals who tend to socialize more (those who go to parties and the theater)

TABLE 2–1. Relationship of Three Frequency Speech Averages to Typical Hearing Difficulties and Amplification Considerations.*

ANSI (1989) Levels In Decibels	Classification	Approximate Discrimination** (%)	Typical Speech Understanding (Unaided)	Typical Adult Amplification Considerations	Typical Child Amplification Considerations
0–24	Essentially normal	92	No significant limitations	Generally none but depends on configuration; high frequency loss may benefit; possible special fittings such as CROS or BICROS	Generally none but preferential seating is recommended; mild gain FM system optional on case by case basis
25–39	Mild	82	Difficulty with faint speech especially from a distance	Recommended based on reported degree of difficulty; mild gain canal and in-the-ear units are appropriate	Preferential seating required; mild gain hearing aid may be considered; in-the-ear or behind-the-ear units recommended based on degree of difficulty; FM systems to be considered
40–54	Moderate	70	Frequent difficulty with normal speech	Frequent to full-time hearing aid use; canal aids useful; in-the-ear and behind-the-ear instruments are more effective; assistive listening devices may be considered	Full-time use of amplification; in-the-ear style is possible but behind-the-ear instrument is preferred; supplemented in school with FM system
55–69	Moderately severe	60	Constant difficulty even with loud speech	Full-time hearing aid use; patient acceptance related to word discrimination ability; behind-the-ear styles most appropriate to yield best performance; direct audio input may be considered	Minimum choice is behind-the-ear units; may require special class and speech therapy; use of FM system is essential
70–89	Severe	36	Severe difficulty; loud or amplified speech might be understood	Full-time binaural hearing aid use; behind-the-ear aid is appropriate style; assistive devices considered, such as closed caption TV decoder	Minimum choice is behind-the-ear instruments; may consider body hearing aid; FM system use is mandatory
90+	Profound	20	Understanding of speech severely limited even with amplification; use of amplification provides mostly environmental and speech clues	Minimum choice is power behind-the-ear instruments; may require body instrument; cochlear implant may be recommended in post-lingually deafened	Powerful behind-the-ear units may be possible; body instrument may prove better consideration; cochlear implant or vibrotactile aids may be considered; often requires special education program

* This information is based in part on that published by Goetzinger (1978). It should be pointed out that this table refers to limitations and needs related to cochlear hearing losses. Conductive, retrocochlear, and central disorders may follow a different pattern of handicap and needs. The three frequency speech average refers to the average dB value for pure tones 500 Hz, 1000 Hz, and 2000 Hz in the better ear. When appropriate, binaural amplification is preferred to monaural.

** W-22 scores at PB-Max for cochlear cases from Thompson and Hoel (1962), and Mongelli (1978).

will notice hearing losses sooner than people who tend to stay home and read, watch television, and relate only to close family members.

The influence of the degree of hearing loss is even more critical in the case of young children in the first few years of life, especially when the problem occurs before the development of language. In cases of profound hearing loss, voice, speech, and language are likely to be substantially influenced. Abnormal breathing patterns and improper use of the vocal folds will influence intonation and stress patterns (Whitehead & Barefoot, 1983). Also, the fundamental frequency of the voice is generally higher than normal (Gilbert & Campbell, 1980). Vocal onset confusions, which result from not knowing how to produce the sounds, affect both a child's understanding and production of voiced and voiceless consonants (Mashie, 1980). Vowels often are substituted for one another and final consonants frequently are omitted (Levitt & Stromberg, 1983).

Less severe hearing losses have correspondingly fewer communicative consequences; however, in any given group there will be notable exceptions. Often, because of unknown reasons, an individual with relatively little hearing will perform especially well. This is most obvious in classrooms for those with hearing impairment in which students with the poorer hearing may perform better in dealing with verbal information than those who possess milder hearing losses. Further, predicting a hearing handicap based on pure-tone thresholds in people who have cochlear implants can be quite perplexing. Even gross generalities do not hold, because of the great dissimilarity between normal or aided hearing versus the electrical stimulation through a cochlear implant.

CONFIGURATION OF LOSS

The shape of an audiogram helps to determine the frequency characteristics of the auditory information an individual receives. When both the audiometric configuration of a client's hearing and the energy distribution of the incoming auditory signals are known, the audiologist can better understand the speech sounds the client is generally able to hear. An audiologist often looks at the client's binaural hearing to determine the sounds that he or she will hear best. This is done by noting the better threshold at each frequency for the two ears. Although this approach is likely a valid one, it is limited in a number of ways. Although it does consider hearing level, it does not consider the locus of lesion, the unilateral/bilateral nature of the loss, and the clarity of the incoming information.

The configuration of hearing loss is considered in the following text as if it were produced by acoustic filtering. Using this approach, the audiologist can obtain important information to better understand a client's communicative abilities and deficits. Other variables that influence performance are discussed later.

Flat Configuration

A flat configuration is seen in a pure-tone audiogram in which there are relatively small differences in thresholds across the audiometric frequencies. However, this does not imply the same exact dB hearing level throughout the audiogram. In fact, slightly sloping and jagged patterns are frequently considered flat because they are not extreme enough to be classified as high- or low-frequency curves. (See Figure 2–3 for an example of an audiogram with a "flat" configuration.)

The audiologist can assume that a flat loss will limit the input evenly across the frequencies. The major energy component of speech is in the low frequencies (250 to 500 Hz). Despite the power of those frequencies, they contain relatively little information for identifying words. There is little speech energy in the high frequencies. In the normal listener, essentially complete and accurate intelligibility comes from the frequencies 300 to 3000 Hz. The frequencies of speech that contribute most to intelligibility are between 1000 and 3000 Hz (Hodgson, 1978). This information can help

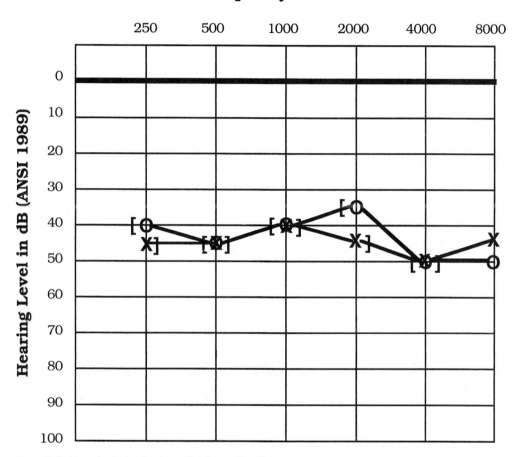

Figure 2–3. Example of a hearing loss with a flat configuration.

clinicians to understand hearing loss as a "filter effect." Because speech contains little high-frequency energy, a flat loss is likely to affect the high-frequency information most severely and the low-frequency information least of all.

High-Frequency Configuration

Although a flat configuration tends to impact heavily on the high-frequency portion of speech signals, a high-frequency loss has an even greater effect. This type of loss is analogous to a filter with a sharply sloping reduction for the high frequencies. In other words, the low frequencies are passed on to the listener, with the high frequencies impeded and not heard or heard less well. (See Figure 2–4 for an example of an audiogram that depicts a high-frequency hearing loss.)

A person with a predominantly high-frequency hearing loss is keenly aware of speech and environ-

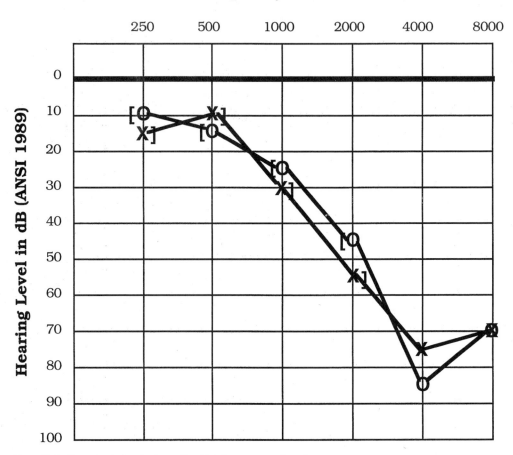

Figure 2–4. Example of a hearing loss with a high-frequency configuration.

mental sounds that contain a preponderance of low-frequency energy. Thus, he or she is able to hear such life-saving sounds as a car horn or a verbal warning, but misses nuances, confuses words, and may not understand the punch lines of jokes. These individuals also have difficulty in locating the source of a sound, understanding speech from another room, and blocking out background sounds.

When there is a major difference between a person's hearing in the low and middle frequencies versus those in the upper frequency range, this difference may create a problem for the audiologist in planning appropriate amplification. The specific frequency at which a loss drops off is most important, especially if it is within the speech frequencies.

Individuals with high-frequency losses are often accused of hearing just what they want to hear or simply of not paying attention. For example, they may easily recognize their names and familiar phrases from low-frequency components, but fail to understand when the language or concepts become complex or abstract. Furthermore, their level of understanding can be expected to fall sharply when the listening environment is noisy or otherwise distracting.

Low-Frequency Configuration

Low frequency audiometric configurations are the least common and have the fewest disadvantages. Low frequency information is the most powerful and the most expendable portion of the speech signal. Thus, from a simple filter effect, the patient retains the most important part of the frequency range and should have good discrimination for speech. The one exception to this rule is when the low-frequency loss is associated with brainstem pathology, which may result in reduced speech discrimination. Even in those instances, the client's voice is generally unaffected and articulation usually remains normal. (See Figure 2–5 for an example of an audiogram that shows a low frequency hearing loss).

Saucer-Shaped Configuration

Occasionally, a saucer-shaped audiometric curve is observed. This pattern is characterized by better thresholds for the high and low frequencies than for those in the midrange. Thus, the sounds that are most important for speech recognition are diminished the most. Although this configuration of loss would appear to be extremely handicapping, we often find good speech thresholds and very good speech recognition scores. This may be because saucer-shaped losses are frequently congenital in nature. Therefore it is likely that, over the years, affected individuals refine their ability to derive phonemic cues from the higher and lower frequency information. (See Figure 2–6 for an example of an audiogram that depicts a saucer-shaped hearing loss.)

SPEECH THRESHOLDS AND WORD RECOGNITION SCORES

Standard speech threshold and discrimination (recognition) tests are administered to understand a person's hearing ability under optimum conditions (such as those found in a sound-treated environment and spoken by an excellent speaker). The expected relationship between pure-tone thresholds and word recognition scores can be estimated by way of the percentage scores obtained to help identify those who have excessive difficulty with speech clarity (Dubno, Lee, Klein, Matthews, & Lam, 1995). Suprathreshold measures such as most comfortable loudness (MCL) and uncomfortable loudness (UCL) tests can be administered to help predict how comfortably an individual will handle amplified speech (e.g., a hearing aid).

Good speech recognition, along with a moderate speech threshold and a wide dynamic range of comfortable listening, encourages audiologists to think that an individual will be relatively easy to fit with a hearing aid. However, poor word discrimination with very poor pure-tone thresholds may complicate achieving excellent aided results. The hypersensitivity to moderate levels of speech may call for complex solutions to enable the individual to fully benefit from amplification.

Because standard speech threshold and discrimination measures generally employ single word tasks, they are not representative of normal conversation and do not include background noise, or use a professional speaker. The measures do not take into account the context of conversations, inflections, and visual cues. Thus, a variety of speech measures is needed to accurately represent a person's performance under normal listening conditions. The Central Institute for the Deaf's Everyday Speech Sentence lists (Davis & Silverman, 1978) and the Harvard Psycho-Acoustic Laboratory (PAL) question-and-answer type materials are often used for testing longer speech strings (Hudgins, Hawkins, Karlin, & Stevens, 1947).

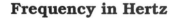

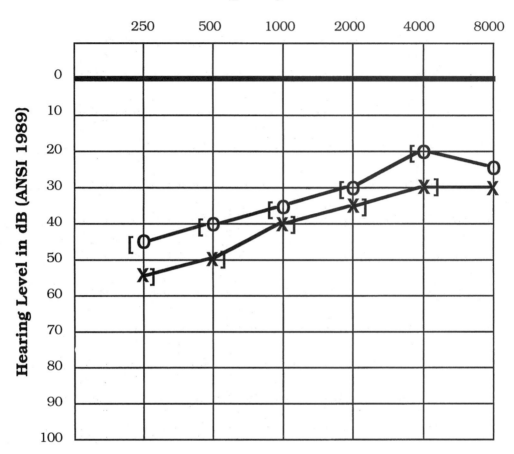

Figure 2–5. Example of a hearing loss with a low-frequency configuration.

Early tests of speech recognition failed to address the difficulties experienced by people with losses that primarily involved the high frequencies. This problem has been resolved somewhat by the use of tests such as the California Consonant Test (Owens & Schubert, 1977), a multiple-choice procedure that requires careful attention to high frequency consonant sounds.

The evaluation of young children poses additional challenges to an audiologist. Speech threshold and recognition measures generally require modification, if they can be used at all. If time tested materials such as the Haskins Phonetically Balanced Kindergarten Word Lists (PBKs) (Haskins, 1949) or the Word Intelligibility by Picture Identification test (WIPI) (Ross & Lerman, 1970) are not successful, informal procedures can be employed.

OTHER AUDIOMETRIC TESTS

A group of other audiometric tests, many of more recent origin, is available to the audiologist to pro-

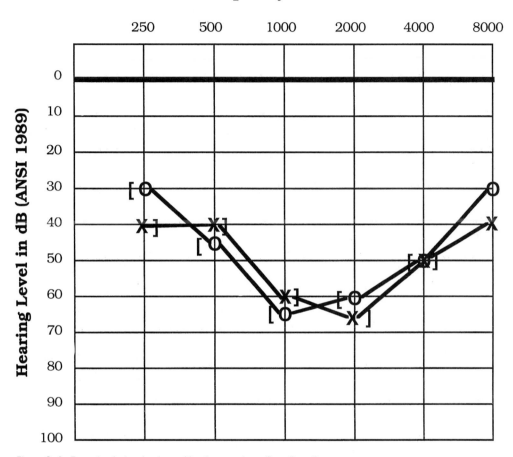

Figure 2–6. Example of a hearing loss with a "saucer shaped" configuration.

vide a better understanding of the client. Acoustic immittance measurements are of great value in determining the need and type of rehabilitative services for an individual. Tympanometry, which measures the mobility of the tympanic membrane, permits determination of the status of the middle ear. If a middle ear problem, such as otitis media, exists, then medical referral is warranted. Acoustic reflex thresholds may delineate the maximum possible output level of a hearing aid for an individual who cannot communicate his or her intolerance for loud sounds (Keith, 1979).

Another important procedure that is useful for young children and the difficult-to-test is the auditory brainstem response (ABR). Although hearing aid evaluations with those who can communicate effectively do not need such elaborate procedures to verify the benefit of a hearing aid, this might be necessary for young children and others who may not provide reliable responses to other test stimuli. ABR audiometry utilizes minute electrical potentials that can be measured on the scalp to monitor the activity of the acoustic nerve and central auditory system when auditory signals are presented to the ears. The audiologist can assess the levels at which the auditory system produces acceptable electrical responses from the CN VIII and brainstem. This will help an audiologist to ascertain if there is a functional auditory system when the child is too young to respond accurately, if an aid might be of benefit, and at what level the aid should be set.

A number of behavioral tests also can be of importance when assessing a patient for rehabilitation. Tests of central function may explain why a particular individual does not fully benefit from amplification (Stach, 1989). When central tests show that one ear is especially deficient (regardless of the peripheral test performance), then the other ear might be considered more strongly for amplification.

Tests that provide speech signals embedded in competing noises may be used as a more realistic measure of performance in real life situations. The Synthetic Sentence Identification (SSI) (Speaks & Jerger, 1965) and the Speech Perception in Noise (SPIN) (Kalikow, Stevens, & Elliot, 1977) tests are particularly applicable for this purpose.

LIMITATIONS OF AUDIOMETRIC INFORMATION

Audiometric data can accurately describe a person's hearing status, but cannot reveal with any precision how well an individual gets along in his or her personal and professional communication environments. The specifics and complexities of real-life situations are too idiosyncratic for audiologists to make accurate predictions about how each complex individual will perform or react (Hargus & Gordon-Salant, 1995). Thus, audiologists can make assumptions and generalizations, but they must validate them through interviews and informal testing. Certain information may never be known. The following examples illustrate these uncertainties.

CASE 1

A college student inadvertently pushed a cotton swab through his tympanic membrane. He was tested audiometrically over time until his hearing levels improved to a level of about 10 dB poorer than his normal ear. At this point, both ears were within normal audiometric limits. After 5 years, the client continues to feel that the hearing deviation has affected him greatly. He is annoyed because the two ears hear differently and he is highly distracted by background noise.

CASE 2

At the other end of the continuum is a child who has severe-to-profound hearing impairment but who performs better than other individuals with normal hearing could be expected to perform. He excels in foreign languages, plays a musical instrument, and communicates without obvious handicap when facing the speaker at a distance of not greater than 15 feet. We believe that this is due, in large measure, to early binaural amplification and a mother who had been determined that her child would develop normal speech and language.

EDUCATIONAL AND VOCATIONAL CONSIDERATIONS

EDUCATIONAL

The child or young adult who has hearing impairment will be faced with limitations in a mainstreamed classroom perhaps more than any other setting. Despite the numerous potential advantages of integrating a child with a hearing impairment into a typical class, the challenge may be considerable. By definition, school is a setting in which new information and unfamiliar concepts are presented. Unlike the rest of the class, the child or adult who has auditory impairment must attempt to determine what was said and then deal with it at the cognitive level that the teacher intended.

In recent years, many forms of assistive listening devices have become available to help people who are limited in their auditory function to pursue their education along with normally hearing individuals. These devices and approaches are discussed in greater length elsewhere in this textbook.

VOCATIONAL

As in the classroom, the workplace provides many challenges to a person who has hearing impairment. People choose careers that are suited to their abilities but which may be affected by their limitations. Hearing-impaired individuals generally avoid jobs that require intensive communication. However, in recent years we have seen a growing number of students who are disabled enter fields that were in earlier years considered out of their reach. For example, individuals who are partially sighted or have hearing impairment now become physicians and lawyers. New vocational opportunities make the need for efficient and innovative management strategies even greater than in the earlier times when a person's options were more severely limited by his or her hearing impairment.

SUMMARY

In this chapter we have discussed the implications of audiometric findings on the needs of individuals who have hearing impairment. Much information can be obtained from basic audiometric procedures that shed light on the auditory status and auditory capabilities of these people. This, in turn, helps in developing a rehabilitative plan that can address their communicative needs.

Although audiometric data provide crucial information in understanding a client's problems, the audiologist must also be aware of the test limitations. It is often difficult to generalize from formal tests to a person's day-to-day life. To fill those gaps, audiologists must seek information from interviews, questionnaires, and other sources.

REFERENCES

American National Standards Institute (1989). *American National Standard Specifications for Audiometers.* (53.6), New York; Author.

Bardon, J. I. (1986). Unilateral sensorineural hearing loss: From the inside out, a patient's perspective. *The Hearing Journal, 39,* 13–17.

Bess, F. (Ed.). (1986). The unilaterally hearing-impaired child. [Special issue]. *Ear and Hearing, 7*(1), 1–54.

Costello, M. R., & McGee, T. M. (1967). Language impairment associated with bilateral abnormal auditory information. In A.B. Graham (Ed.), *Sensory processes and disorders* (pp. 86–97). Boston: Little Brown.

Dalzell, J., & Orwid, H.L. (1976). Children with conductive deafness: A follow-up study. *British Journal of Audiology, 10,* 87–90.

Davis, H., & Silverman, S. R. (1978). *Hearing and deafness.* New York: Holt, Rinehart & Winston.

Dubno J., Lee, F., Klein, A., Matthews, L., & Lam, C. (1995). Confidence limits for maximum word-recognition scores. *Journal of Speech and Hearing Research, 38,* 490–502.

Gilbert, H. R., & Campbell, M. I. (1980). Speaking fundamental frequency in three groups of hearing-impaired individuals. *Journal of Communicative Disorders, 13,* 195–205.

Goetzinger, C.P. (1978). Word discrimination testing. In J. Katz (Ed.), *Handbook of clinical audiology* (pp.149-158). Baltimore, MD: Williams & Wilkins.

Green, D. (1978). Pure tone testing. In J. Katz (Ed.), *Handbook of clinical audiology* (pp. 98–109). Baltimore: Williams & Wilkins.

Hargus, S., & Gordon-Salants, S. (1995). Accuracy of speech intelligibility index predictions for noise masked young listeners with normal hearing and for elderly listeners with hearing impairment. *Journal of Speech and Hearing Research, 38,* 234–243.

Haskins, H. (1949). *A phonetically balanced test of speech discrimination for children.* Unpublished master's thesis, Northwestern University, Evanston, IL.

Hodgson, W. R. (1978). Disorders of hearing. In P. Skinner & R. Shelton (Eds.), *Speech, language and hearing* (pp. 457–470). Reading, MA: Addison-Wesley.

Holm, V.A., & Kunze, L.H. (1969). Effect of chronic otitis media on language and development. *Pediatrics, 43*, 833–839.

Hudgins, C. V., Hawkins, J. E., Karlin, J. E., & Stevens, S. S. (1947). The development of recorded auditory tests for measuring hearing loss for speech. *Laryngoscope, 47*, 57–89.

Jerger, J., Silman, S., Lew, H., & Chmiel, R. (1993) Case studies in binaural interference: Converging evidence from behavioral and electrophysiologic measures. *Journal of American Academy of Audiology, 4*, 122–131.

Kalikow, D. N., Stevens, K. N., & Elliott, L. L. (1977). Development of a test of speech intelligibility in noise using sentence materials with controlled word predictability. *Journal of Acoustical Society of America, 61*, 1337–1351.

Kaplan, H., Bally, S. J., & Brandt, F. (1990). Communication Self-Assessment Scale Inventory for Deaf Adults. *Journal of the American Academy of Audiology, 2*, 164–182.

Keith, R. (1979). An acoustic reflex technique of establishing hearing aid settings. *Journal of the American Auditory Society, 5*, 71–75.

Lamb, S., Owens, E., & Schubert, E. (1983). The revised form of the Hearing Performance Inventory. *Ear and Hearing, 4*, 152–157.

Levitt, H., & Stromberg, H. (1983). Segmental characteristics of speech of hearing-impaired children—Factors affecting intelligibility. In I. Hochberg, H. Levitt, & M.J. Osberger (Eds.), *Speech of the hearing-impaired: Research, training, and personnel preparation* (pp.32–41). Baltimore, MD: University Park Press.

Mashie, J. J. (1980). *Laryngeal behavior of hearing-impaired speakers.* Unpublished doctoral dissertation, Syracuse University, Syracuse, NY.

Mongelli, C. (1978). *Central auditory involvement in two geriatric populations measured with the staggered spondaic word test.* Unpublished manuscript, University of California, Santa Barbara.

Owens, E., & Schubert, E. (1977). Development of California Consonant Test. *Journal of Speech and Hearing Research, 20*, 463–474.

Ross, M., & Lerman, J. (1970). A picture identification test for hearing impaired children. *Journal of Speech and Hearing Research, 13*, 44–53.

Secord, G. J., Erickson, M. T., & Bush, J. P. (1988). Neuropsychological sequelae of otitis media in children and adolescents with learning disabilities. *Journal of Pediatric Psychology, 13*, 531–542.

Speaks, C., & Jerger, J. (1965). Method of measurement of speech identification. *Journal of Speech and Hearing Research, 8*, 185–194.

Stach, B. (1989). Hearing aid amplification and central processing disorders. In R. E. Sandlin (Ed.), *Handbook of hearing aid amplification. Vol. II, Clinical considerations* (pp. 87–111). Boston: College-Hill Press.

Thompson, G., & Hoel, R. (1962). Flat sensorineural hearing loss and PB scores. *Journal of Speech and Hearing Disorders, 27*, 284–287.

Weinstein, B., Richards, A., & Montano, J. (1995). Handicap versus impairment: An important distinction. *Journal of the American Academy of Audiology, 6*, 250–255.

Whitehead, R. L., & Barefoot, S. (1983). *Air flow characteristics of fricative constants produced by normally hearing and hearing impaired speakers.* Unpublished manuscript, National Technical Institute for the Deaf, Rochester, NY.

END OF CHAPTER EXAMINATION QUESTIONS

CHAPTER 2

1. Audiologists make use of standard speech threshold and speech recognition tests to _____.

2. A person who possesses a conductive hearing loss may achieve very good speech recognition simply by_____.

3. As with other diagnostic information, audiometric data have inherent informational limitations. Describe three.

4. Severe congenital or prelingual hearing losses have a great impact on _____, _____, and _____ because an individual does not develop these skills without usable hearing.

5. Describe and explain the difference between (a) hearing loss and (b) hearing handicap.

6. Describe and explain the difference between (a) hearing level and (b) hearing loss.

7. Describe and explain the difference between (a) hearing impairment and (b) hearing handicap.

8. According to the authors, although a *flat* frequency configuration hearing loss tends to impact heavily on the high-frequency portion of speech, a high frequency hearing loss has an even greater adverse effect. Why?

9. The handicap resulting from a unilateral hearing loss is due not only to the loss of sensitivity, but also to the _____.

10. Both the classroom and the workplace provide many challenges to persons who have hearing impairment. From the information obtained in this chapter, describe four of those challenges.

END OF CHAPTER ANSWER SHEET

Name   Date

CHAPTER 2

1. _____

_____.

2. _____

_____.

3. a.

   b.

   c.

4. _____ , _____

_____ , and

_____

5. a.

   b.

6. a.

   b.

7. a.

   b.

8. _____

_____

_____

_____.

9. _____

_____

10. a.

b.

c.

d.

A Psychosocial, Educational, and Economic Profile and Vocational Rehabilitation Counseling for the Hearing Impaired and Deaf

■ PAMELA L. JACKSON, Ph.D. ■
■ KAREN A. DILKA, Ph.D. ■

*THE VOCATIONAL IMPACT OF HEARING IMPAIRMENT
AND VOCATIONAL REHABILITATION COUNSELING*
The Vocational Rehabilitation Process
Case Studies
Discussion of Case Studies
Combining Vocational Rehabilitation and Audiology

SUMMARY

Loss of hearing is the most common of all physical impairments. Yet until recently it has received little attention in terms of the possible psychosocial and economic handicaps that it can impose on the life of an individual. In 1974, Schein and Delk published a classic treatise reflecting the results of the National Census of the Deaf Population in a comprehensive book, *The Deaf Population of the United States.* This work presented much data that describe the extent and the characteristics of the hearing-impaired population. However, that information is well beyond 25 years old. More recent information can be obtained from publications by the National Center for Health Statistics.

PREVALENCE OF HEARING LOSS

Figure 3–1 summarizes prevalence and prevalence rates for hearing losses occurring at various ages, noting changes that have occurred between 1971 and 1991 and emphasizing the extent of the overall problem. An increase in incidence figures is apparent if the data are compared to past figures. For example, in the early 1930s, the prevalence rate for severe hearing loss was reported as approximate-

ly 1 per 1,000. The 1971 rate, however, reported by Schein and Delk (1974) indicated a rate for prevocational (prior to 19 years of age) deafness of 2 per 1,000 or, more exactly, 203 individuals who are deaf per 100,000.

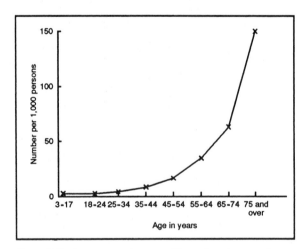

Figure 3–1. Average annual age-specific number of persons 3 years of age and over who cannot hear and understand normal speech per 1,000 persons: United States, 1990–91 (National Center for Health Statistics, March, 1994).

This doubling of the rate in 40 years is attributed to three factors: (1) possible inaccuracies in past counts, (2) differences in definitions that alter the population sampled, or (3) an actual increase in the occurrence of deafness. Although all of these do play a part, it is important to add that survival rates of high-risk infants have also increased in recent years and will contribute to an overall increase in the number of adults with impaired hearing who in the past might not have survived beyond early childhood.

According to a report by the National Center for Health Statistics (1994b), the rate per 1,000 persons in the U.S. who cannot hear and understand normal speech was 2.7 per 1,000 for youth ages 3–17 years, rising sharply at about 55 years of age until it reached 150.1 per 1,000 for persons age 75 years and older. Those figures are seen in Figure 3–1.

The incidence figures presented in Table 3–1 present clear differences among age groups as compared to the earlier Schein and Delk (1974) data. For example, figures from the National Center for Health Statistics (1994a) indicate that only 5% of children and young adults between age 3 and 17 years had some degree of hearing impairment. However, that accounts for more than 4 million children and young adults. The same data suggest that between age 18 and 44 years, 23% possess hearing impairment, which accounts for another 7 million. Between age 45 and 64 years, the estimated incidence rises to 29%, which accounts for another 8 million persons with impaired hearing. At age 65 years and beyond, the incidence is estimated at 43%, or approximately 15 million persons. According to the National Center for Health Statistics (1994b), among the latter 43%, approximately one-half were among the 65–74 year age group, and one-half were among those who are age 75 years and beyond.

It is interesting to note that comparing the information from the 1971 Health Interview Survey (National Center for Health Statistics, 1975) with the statistics from the 1994 National Center for Health Statistics report, the number of persons with hearing impairment was estimated to be 53.40% greater than the 13.2 million persons reported to have hearing loss in 1971. According to the National Health Interview Survey (NHIS) report (1994a), a significant proportion of this increase was probably due to the increase in the aging population during the 23 year period.

According to the National Center for Health Statistics (1994), in 1971 there were 69 persons per 1,000 population with hearing impairment, and in 1991, the incidence was 86.1 per 1,000. And the NHIS (1994) report stressed the relationship between aging and hearing loss (National Center for Health Statistics, 1994a), indicating that as the population ages, the incidence of hearing loss within the total population will likewise increase since hearing loss generally accompanies the process of aging. Table 3-1 presents comparative data on the number of persons of various ages with impaired hearing between 1971 and 1991.

INFLUENCES OF HEARING LOSS

FAMILY INCOME

According to the report by the National Center for Health Statistics (1994), persons with severe hearing loss were more frequently found in families with an annual income of less than $10,000, and less frequently found in families with incomes of $50,000 and more. According to that survey, 24.9% of persons with no hearing impairment were found in families earning $50,000 or more, and only 16% of those with hearing impairment were in that income group.

EMPLOYMENT STATUS AND TYPE OF OCCUPATION

More persons with impaired hearing are unemployed than those with average hearing (National Center for Health Statistics, 1994a; Reis, 1993),

TABLE 3–1. Population, prevalence, crude and age-adjusted prevalence rates, and change since 1971 for persons 3 years and over with reported hearing loss: United States 1971, 1977, and 1990–1991 average annual.

Item	1971	1977	1990–1991
All persons 3 years of age and over (in thousands)	191,602	202,936	235,688
Prevalence of hearing trouble (in thousands)	13,228	14,240	20,295
Percent increase in prevalence since 1971	—	7.7	53.4
Number with hearing trouble per 1,000 persons	69.0	70.2	86.1
Percent increase in prevalence rate since 1971	—	1.7	24.8
Age-adjusted number with hearing trouble per 1,000 persons[1]	75.5	73.6	86.1
Percent change in age-adjusted prevalence rate since 1971	—	−2.5	14.0

[1]The 1971 and 1977 prevalence rates are age-adjusted to the average 1990–1991 population.

Reprinted with permission from the *National Center For Health Statistics. U.S. Department of Health and Human Service*, March,1994.

ranging from 77.6% of persons with a severe hearing impairment, to 29% among those without hearing impairment. Utilizing the Bureau of Census categories of occupations, persons with moderate-to-severe hearing loss are significantly underrepresented in occupations related to sales, service, and administrative support. Only around 37% of persons with hearing impairment were found in those types of occupations.

The economic problems of adults who have severe hearing impairment appear to involve both unemployment and underemployment. A large part of the problem may be attributed to the myths concerning deafness and hearing impairment and ignorance by many employers about the capabilities of those with hearing impairment. In a survey of Baltimore manufacturing firms, 32% of the employers indicated that deafness was the disability that would most likely prevent them from hiring an applicant. Total deafness ranked fourth after total blindness, mental retardation, and epilepsy (Fellendorf, Atelsek, & Macklin, 1991) in relation to their perception of degree of handicap. (See Figure

3–2 for information on the comparative employment status of those with impaired hearing.)

Studies cited by Meadow-Orlans (1985) present some interesting information on employment and employability of deaf workers in Europe, the Netherlands, and Scandinavia. Beuzart (1982) found that in one inquiry in France, 50% of workers lost their jobs upon onset of deafness. Others remained, but earned lower salaries. A survey by Thomas and Herbst (1980) found 236 respondents were significantly "less happy at work" than matched hearing controls. Breed, van den Horst, and Mous (1981) found members of a Dutch hard-of-hearing organization were most likely to do "lonely" work, away from their hearing conterparts.

Meadow-Orlans (1985) cites two studies in detail that elaborate on the impact of hearing loss on a person's economic future. Those include a study by Kyle and Wood (1983) that consisted of an interview with 105 persons ages 25 through 55 years with onset of hearing loss in the previous 10 years. According to Meadow-Orlans (1985), 91% of those persons could, with their hearing aid(s), "hear

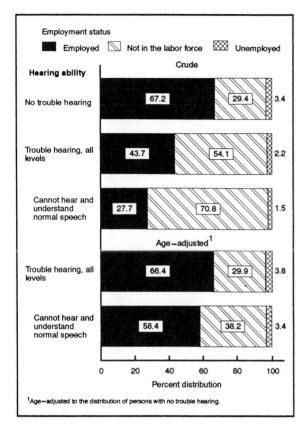

Figure 3–2. Average annual crude and age-adjusted percentage distribution of persons 18 years of age and older by employment status, according to hearing ability: United States, 1990–1991 (National Center for Health Statistics, March, 1994).

normal speech across a room." Despite their usable hearing, 35% "felt that promotion at work was relatively impossible." Sixty-three percent of persons who were prelingually deafened felt the same, compared with only 16% of those who possessed normal hearing. Kyle and Wood (1983) state that acquired hearing loss affects the quality of working life more than the level of earnings. In this study, it was found that when the workers discovered their hearing losses, only 39% informed their employers.

Another study described in detail by Meadow-Orlans (1985) involved adults in greater London who had hearing impairment. The study was conducted by Thomas, Lamont, and Harris (1982). All subjects were of employment age and had hearing loss greater than 60 dB. The study involved interviews with the workers and surveys. Representative responses by the workers as it relates to the impact of their hearing loss on their ability to work included (1) difficulty coping with the public, (2) difficulty with the telephone, (3) difficulty doing their job, (4) difficulty with colleagues, (5) being given less responsibility, and (6) altered job assignments.

The impact of hearing loss on vocational success and job satisfaction varies with the person involved, interacting with the degree of loss. Needless to say, however, hearing loss can have a negative impact on a person's job and on vocational satisfaction.

EDUCATION

For persons 18 years and older, the number of persons with less than 12 years of education increases proportionately with the degree of hearing loss (National Center for Health Statistics, 1994). The discrepancy between those who attend college and those who do not widens proportionately with degree of hearing loss. That is, as hearing loss increases, the number of persons attending college proportionately decreases (Adams & Benson, 1994). (See Figure 3–3 for information on the comparative educational status of those who possess impaired hearing).

MARITAL STATUS AND LIVING ARRANGEMENTS

Among persons with severe hearing loss, comparatively few have never been married as compared to persons with normal hearing, that is, only 8.2% (Adams & Benson, 1994). However, when comparing persons more than age 18 years who have

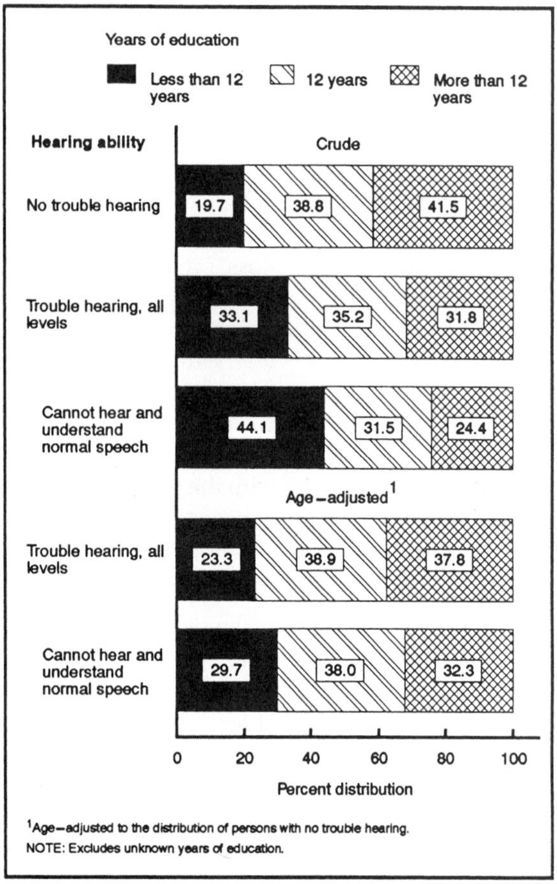

Figure 3–3. Average annual crude and age-adjusted percentage distribution of persons 18 years of age and older by years of education, according to hearing ability: United States, 1990–1991 (National Center for Health Statistics, March, 1994).

severe hearing loss with those who have normal hearing, more in the hearing loss category are found to have been divorced, widowed, separated, or married but not living with a spouse (National Center for Health Statistics, 1994a), that is, 27.8% as compared to 20.3% among persons with normal hearing. Further, more persons with hearing loss that interferes with hearing and understanding speech in the age 18 years and above range live alone (23.4%) as compared to those with normal hearing (12.4%) (Adams & Benson, 1994). Figure

3–4 presents comparative information on marital status for those with impaired hearing.

BIRTHS

Fewer children are born to women who are deaf than to normal hearing women. The reason for this is not clear, but it may perhaps be related to the marital status that the survey by the National Center for Health Statistics (1994b) listed as most prevalent among those with severe hearing loss. Those with severe loss tended to be divorced, widowed, separated, or never married. Among those who become parents, children born into families in which at least one parent is prevocationally deaf have normal hearing 88% of the time (Reis, 1993).

SUMMARY OF THIS SECTION

The information presented in this section offers an emerging profile of the psychosocial, educational, and economic characteristics of the population of persons who have hearing impairment or deafness. It must be stressed that this is a changing profile. In light of new educational opportunities, improved training programs for professionals who work on behalf of persons who are deaf or have hearing impairment, and the emergence of advocates for the rights of the handicapped, the profile will be altered. Hopefully, in time, the differences created by a loss of hearing will be minimized.

THE VOCATIONAL IMPACT OF HEARING IMPAIRMENT AND DEAFNESS, AND VOCATIONAL REHABILITATION COUNSELING

The purpose of rehabilitation is to provide comprehensive services to individuals with mental, physical, sensory, or emotional handicaps with the intent that they will "attain usefulness and satisfaction in

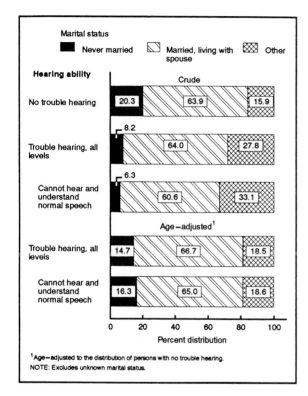

Figure 3–4. Average annual crude and age-adjusted percent distribution of persons 18 years of age and over by marital status, according to hearing ability: United States, 1990-1991 (National Center for Health Statistics, March 1994).

life" (Wright, 1980, p. 3). This broad definition asserts that determination of a recipient's goals and objectives will vary along a continuum from those who have achieved independent living skills to those who have achieved gainful employment. The rehabilitation process encompasses a series of prioritized steps tailored to the unique needs and circumstances of each individual client. Therefore, the associated time limit for successful completion of the rehabilitation process will depend on the extent and diversity of designated services. The expectation for accomplishment of a client's initial goal(s) is correlated with his or her stamina, capabilities, motivation, and support base, which includes his or her family and significant others.

Unfortunately, the deaf/hard-of-hearing population does not have equivalent sociological, educational, and linguistic advantages that are inherent in the hearing society. Undoubtedly, this is because a hearing loss, regardless of the type of remedial treatment proposed, significantly restricts the acquisition and comprehension of information that is readily accessible to the hearing majority. Divisional gaps deepen with demographic data indicating inferior educational and socioeconomic status of persons with hearing loss compared to their hearing counterparts (Phillipe & Auvenshine, 1985; Schein & Delk, 1974; Wooton & Mowry, 1986). To complicate the situation further, members of this minority group do not necessarily have homogeneous characteristics. For example, school environments, parental acceptance and leadership, exposure to cultural experiences, onset and degree of loss, and most importantly self-esteem are all variables that affect individual growth and development. Hence, the accumulation of the listed factors compounds any career dynamics associated with occupational choice, mobility, adjustment, and work-related functions.

The literature regarding technological advancements in business and industry is replete with references that detail the rapid changes and breakthroughs in industrial mechanization. The forecast of career profiles reflects this shift, with a move from manual labor toward administrative and executive positions. Concurrently, a concentrated effort must be made by all professionals serving individuals who are deaf or hard-of-hearing to empower and prepare them to take advantage of these trends.

VOCATIONAL REHABILITATION PROCESS

The structural framework of vocational rehabilitation is mandated by public law (PL 93-112, Rehabilitation Act of 1973, & PL 93-516, Vocational Rehabilitation Act of 1973) and consists of specific phases of implementation.

PRELIMINARY PHASE

The preliminary phase combines (1) client referral, (2) an intake interview, and (3) evaluations to determine the client's eligibility or potential for employment. Two critical components are (1) the interview in which valuable personal, educational, vocational, and financial information is collected; and (2) an aggregate of evaluations (medical, audiological, visual, vocational, and psychological) to assess a client's physical, mental, and work-related abilities and limitations. Consideration of appropriate testing instruments and administration procedures with persons who are deaf/hard-of-hearing predominates in this phase of the rehabilitation process. A wide range of communication possibilities and cultural experiences collectively influences the sequential movement of preparation toward vocational achievement. Emphasis is placed on individual assets and liabilities. However, regardless of a client's circumstances, the listed requirements must be met to receive further specialized assistance through the government program.

1. The individual is mentally, physically, or sensory impaired or disabled.
2. The disability creates a barrier or handicap to attainable employment.
3. The individual will obtain and sustain employment on completion of services provided by vocational rehabilitation.

DEVELOPMENT OF INDIVIDUALIZED REHABILITATION PLAN

The next phase entails the development of an individualized written rehabilitation plan (IWRP) to focus on pertinent occupational goals and establish a course of action. Vocational guidance, under the direction of a vocational rehabilitation (VR) counselor, is imperative at this stage to develop a realistic perspective regarding preparation, duration of the task, extent of provisions, and financing.

At this juncture, the client and counselor jointly decide on career aspirations, orientation, timeliness, and procedures.

The data gathered on job placement for persons with hearing loss consistently indicate that they tend to be underemployed rather than unemployed (Schroedel, 1987; Steffanic, 1982; Williams & Sussman, 1976). Job stereotyping and employer discrimination have contributed to this situation (Phillips, 1975). Individuals who are deaf/hard of hearing are predominantly hired in the operative and clerical areas (El-Khiami, 1986). Therefore, there is a severe underrepresentation of persons who are deaf/hard-of-hearing in what are considered to be high-status professions (Schroedel, 1987).

RESTORATION PHASE

Although all phases of the vocational rehabilitation program compose essential elements, the categories of restoration and training are exclusively oriented to the needs of the client and, therefore, considered the core of the process. Auditory devices such as hearing aids, telephone accessories, and other assistive equipment/appliances for communication or personal management are necessary. Additionally, medical, surgical, or prosthetic intervention may be necessary, as well as the correction of visual problems to enhance clients' communicative effectiveness via sign language and/or lipreading. Another option might be classes to improve the communication techniques of auditory training and speechreading, manual communication systems, and/or American Sign Language (ASL) when they will assist the client.

TRAINING PHASE

As the client progresses, formal training begins. Training activities will vary for the person who is deaf/hard-of-hearing, depending on the results of previous evaluations and his or her occupational interests. Support services are interwoven throughout the rehabilitation process. However, access to information provided during training is crucial to the application of new skills. Individuals who are deaf/hard-of-hearing may derive benefit from the availability of interpreters, oral or manual. Other auxiliary resources may be requested for full participation in community or educational settings. Notetakers and tutors also facilitate instruction and learning for a person with hearing loss.

EMPLOYMENT PHASE

For a client who has more severe hearing impairment or deafness, the final phase of vocational rehabilitation solidifies the original plan by the formulation of a tangible conclusion—employment or independence. Job opportunities will have, at this point, been solicited and placement of the client proceeds. Continual observation provides the counselor with insight into the success or failure of the arrangement. Clients' freedom to express themselves and be understood by management contributes to their performance level. Both client and employer satisfaction determine which procedures a counselor will select for follow-up sessions. If the situation is unfavorable, then an attempt to gain employment elsewhere is investigated. It must be noted that provisions need to be made in each phase to disqualify a client from services and from receiving further assistance through vocational rehabilitation, if extenuating circumstances arise.

ROLE OF THE REHABILITATION COUNSELOR

The vocational rehabilitation process is designed to offer counseling and personal or career consultation at all phases of a client's program. At times, the counselor's role involves intensive therapeutic interaction with the client to resolve personal issues that interfere with the ultimate goal of employ-

ment. Therefore, demonstrated proficiency in the preferred language of the individual who is deaf/hard-of-hearing, irrespective of the mode or method, creates an atmosphere of trust and respect vital for a positive client-counselor rapport. Rehabilitation counselors provide direction, supervision, and advocacy for a client while arranging, organizing, and monitoring the delivery of an array of services. These responsibilities cover a gamut of vocational, educational, and professional transactions (operations).

CASE STUDIES

The following vignettes are presented to illustrate the diversity of service alternatives within the realm of vocational rehabilitation and the individualization embedded in the system. The three clients described represent a spectrum of the deaf/hard of hearing population whose needs are interwoven into the IWRP. The ability of the rehabilitation counselor to tailor the IWRP is one of the unique strengths of the rehabilitation process.

ACQUIRED HEARING LOSS

REHABILITATION

Wendy was a skilled home economics teacher. She had enjoyed teaching high school students for 12 years. Her goal was to continue teaching for 13 more years and then retire with her husband. As Wendy was driving to work one morning she had a serious car accident and was hospitalized for several weeks. Although she recovered from her physical injuries, Wendy was left with a severe bilateral sensorineural hearing loss. This traumatic experience left Wendy angry and frustrated. Her acquired hearing loss created obstacles that were extremely difficult with which to cope both emotionally and physically. Wendy tried to return to work only to discover she no longer had control of her classes and could not communicate with her students or colleagues. Subsequently, Wendy chose to give up her teaching position.

Wendy's home life was also affected by her postlingual loss of hearing; family relationships were strained because of the lack of spontaneous communication or compensatory techniques. Misunderstandings frequently arose and she began to remove herself from social gatherings with family and friends. Feeling isolated and seeking alternatives, Wendy decided to contact a local organization for those with hearing impairment. She was eventually referred to a vocational rehabilitation counselor, from whom she gained information about her hearing loss and opportunities for revised career development.

After the initial interview and application procedure, Wendy was sent to an otologist for a thorough examination of the hearing mechanism and to her family physician for a medical update. The next step entailed an audiological evaluation to assess the extent of the hearing loss sustained in the accident and an ophthalmological evaluation to ascertain the integrity of her visual system. With relevant information obtained from the audiologist, Wendy became aware of a wide range of assistive devices, hearing aids, and communication strategies to enhance adjustment to her hearing loss.

Wendy met all the necessary requirements for eligibility for vocational rehabilitation and proceeded to develop, in conjunction with the counselor, an individualized written rehabilitation plan. Wendy identified an aspect of home economics she wanted to pursue (fashion editor) and the IWRP document detailed her new career direction, including training, resources, essential materials, a proposed schedule of activities, and anticipated outcomes. It was recommended that Wendy return to the audiologist to purchase bilateral hearing aids. She also inquired about the purchase of a telephone device for the deaf (TDD) and a lighting system for her house, so she would know when the doorbell or telephone rang. Vocational Rehabilitation approved and paid for these items on

Wendy's behalf. Concurrently, arrangements were made for Wendy to enroll in an auditory training and lipreading class sponsored by a local speech and hearing clinic. Wendy's preference was to continue to use an oral method of communication, and the instruction was designed to maintain speech production and diminish the frustration of adjustment to auditory stimuli. Vocational Rehabilitation contributed financial support to Wendy's endeavors; however, the amount was based on her income and economic status reports.

The relationship between Wendy and her counselor developed into a warm, respectful exchange of thoughts, ideas, and information. Communication became less of a challenging task and more of a relaxed acquisition of messages. Personal and career counseling were an integral part of Wendy's IWRP.

The onset of a sudden hearing loss can evoke emotional turmoil which an individual is not psychologically prepared to manage without the help of a professional trained in the area of hearing loss. Gradually, Wendy began to acknowledge and ultimately accept her disability. She gained confidence in her communication abilities, focusing on the positive aspects of change. This significant progress was due, in part, to the effective guidance and monitoring techniques employed by her vocational rehabilitation counselor.

Through specialized courses, Wendy studied interior design. She assumed responsibility for payment of all supplies and materials for the courses; however, she was reimbursed for tuition by her local office of Vocational Rehabilitation. Wendy finished the program within 1 year and later found employment at a woman's publishing company. The VR counselor proceeded to conduct an in-service for the manager of the publishing company on practical communication strategies and disseminated similar information to departmental employees. Wendy's goals were consequently achieved in a 2-year time frame, resulting in an occupational shift and successful rehabilitation closure.

CONGENITAL HEARING LOSS

HABILITATION

Dustin was born with a profound bilateral sensorineural hearing loss. The cause of his prelingual hearing impairment was traced to maternal rubella. As a senior in high school, Dustin attended the state school for the deaf and his preferred mode of communication was American Sign Language (ASL). Dustin's strong academic performance, talent as an artist, and interest in drafting led him to explore the field of architecture. With encouragement from his high school principal, Dustin arranged an appointment to discuss future educational/career goals with the vocational rehabilitation counselor.

Dustin applied to several universities and was accepted by two. His final decision was to attend an institute recognized for its highly acclaimed architectural school. The VR counselor explained the procedure to request a sign language interpreter for classes. The week of his arrival, Dustin contacted Disabled Student Services on campus and submitted his semester itinerary. He noticed a circular tacked on the bulletin board announcing a tutorial program on English proficiency for second-language learners. English was always a laborious subject for Dustin, yet he clearly understood the importance of English competency. Therefore, with an avid endorsement from the VR counselor, Dustin applied for the private instructional sessions.

Vocational Rehabilitation subsidized Dustin's educational expenses, including interpreting services for extracurricular activities. Costs for interpreting and notetaking in the classroom setting were absorbed by the university. Incidentals were furnished by Dustin's parents and he commuted to and from school, which decreased the overall financial obligation incurred by both the agency and his family. The only stipulations for receiving aid were the maintenance of a cumulative grade-point average consistent with program standards and enrollment in the minimum semester credit hours equivalent to full-time status. Dustin was responsible for contacting the counselor regarding any changes to this agreement.

During the summer months, Dustin worked for a small architectural company. Because his co-workers did not have an understanding of the cultural or linguistic aspects of sign language, the VR counselor authorized an interpreter for several weeks to facilitate communication. This gave Dustin an opportunity to become familiar with his surroundings and foster an atmosphere of fluent, spontaneous interaction.

When Dustin graduated, he continued to receive vocational rehabilitation services, including interpreter assistance for interviews and tools to construct a portfolio. After Dustin secured a position with a large architectural firm, an interpreter was requested to orient Dustin to his duties and establish a positive rapport with other employees. The VR counselor conducted in-service presentations and dispensed information regarding methods of communication with adults who have hearing impairment. Dustin's work-related progress was confirmed by his supervisor, and within several months he was successfully released from the vocational rehabilitation process.

GENETIC CONDUCTIVE HEARING LOSS—APERT SYNDROME

INDEPENDENT LIVING

Stanley was born with an autosomal dominant disease diagnosed as Apert syndrome. He had multiple handicapping conditions, including a moderate hearing loss (SRT of 50 dB HL), skull and facial malformations, decreased cognitive capacity, fusion of the hand and toe digits (syndactyly), and spina bifida. Stanley's extremely high forehead and facial anomalies were primary indicators of the genetic syndrome at birth. Therefore, Stanley received early medical, otological, and audiological intervention.

Throughout the developmental years, Stanley underwent numerous surgeries to correct the cranial and facial anomalies. The multidisciplinary management team also performed several operations on Stanley's hands and feet to separate the digits. However, only the thumb and smallest finger could be detached from the solid mass. This allowed Stanley to manipulate objects, even though he did not have optimal functioning of his hands. Otological intervention was necessary to improve his hearing acuity for the acquisition of speech and language. The stapes footplate was removed and a prosthesis put in place; however, further reconstructive surgery to remediate his hearing loss was not possible. After treatment, Stanley had an audiological evaluation that signified an increase in his hearing ability to within the mild range. Simultaneously, Stanley was fitted with a bone conduction hearing aid.

Education for Stanley was difficult. His mobility was restricted because of his spina bifida and, therefore, he used a wheelchair. During his school years, he was assigned to a self-contained classroom for the trainable mentally handicapped and later transferred to the district's vocational setting. Stanley enjoyed the hands-on work that was expected of him in this new environment. The precision with which he assembled products was recognized by his teachers. The quality of his workmanship was consistently above average. Prior to graduation, Stanley's instructor contacted the VR counselor, starting the vocational rehabilitation process. Stanley was 21 years old.

Diagnostic data were collected regarding Stanley's medical, audiological, educational, and vocational history. Fortunately, current information was available in all these specialty areas, expediting the determination of eligibility. The years of training and work experience gained at the vocational school were noted for consideration when Stanley's future placement was discussed. Together with scores from a battery of work sample evaluations to measure Stanley's occupational aptitudes and input from the immediate family, an IWRP was developed. This document focused on independent living skills and extended employment at a sheltered workshop.

It was decided that a combination of community resources would benefit Stanley in his pursuit of independence. An occupational therapist taught Stanley functional self-care tasks. This helped him attain a higher level of autonomy within the family unit. The services of a physical therapist were contracted to administer a therapeutic exercise program aimed at strengthening body parts, enhancing circulation, and reducing the possibility of muscular atrophy. Of course, it was apparent to Stanley's family that he would always need additional support, as he had multiple disabilities affecting his mental, physical, and emotional health. Restorative devices allowing freedom of movement were purchased, including an automatic wheelchair and a contemporary bone conduction hearing aid. These items were deemed essential for Stanley to cope constructively with the barriers in the environment. This significant expenditure of money was shared by Vocational Rehabilitation and Stanley's parents.

Job placement at a local sheltered workshop for rehabilitation clients complied with Stanley's IWRP objectives. He was tentatively accepted at the facility and a conference was scheduled for the VR counselor and appointed supervisor to exchange relevant competency-based information. A brief transitional period from school to work was allotted before actual training sessions were set up. Stanley's performance was assessed for several weeks. It was eventually established that he met the criteria for extended employment. The counselor remained in contact with the center until closing Stanley's file. Follow-up conferences were positive and his supervisor reported he was an asset to the facility.

DISCUSSION OF THE CASE STUDIES

As indicated in the case studies, a distinction is evident between the terms, rehabilitation and habilitation. The first implies that an individual becomes disabled because of a medical condition or an injury, after possessing work-related skills. In contrast, the latter term signifies that the individual has a congenital disability and must be introduced to the complexities of employment. Although these terms are used synonymously throughout the literature, the difference is considerable when selecting appropriate facilitative methodology.

Wendy, Dusty, and Stanley obviously have very different needs, idiosyncratic qualities, and lifestyles. Optimally, a vocational rehabilitation counselor will develop a plan for the delivery of services that accentuates each recipient's aptitudes and talents. Often this will require unlimited resources and a longer period of training than is usually allocated for completion of the VR process. Consequently, the enormous challenge facing both client and counselor necessitates a creative and flexible program to derive maximum benefits that will lead to a profitable future.

COMBINING VOCATIONAL REHABILITATION AND AUDIOLOGY

Networking between professionals, their sponsoring agencies, and organizations affiliated with hearing loss is a powerful tool for the collection and dissemination of information. Most VR counselors recognize networking as the key to a smooth vocational transition for the client who is deaf or hard-of-hearing. It expands client opportunities and negates bias factors that have, in the past, prohibited the participation of those with hearing loss. Networking breaks down the barriers involved in professional "turf guarding" and allows for positive interaction and valuable input into the rehabilitation process (Woodrick, 1984). Without this cooperative working relationship among service providers, the client will have delayed progress due, in part, to external matters beyond his or her control. Additionally, the lack of com-

munication and/or miscommunication between professionals interrupts the continuity and flow of services. In return, this affects a client's personal motivation and has a profound impact on the client's perspective toward specialized personnel. Confidence in the system and associated professionals begins to deteriorate. Therefore, prompt and accurate information, exchanged in an efficient and timely manner, eliminates conflict and unnecessary obstacles. Through the avenue of networking, many of these intrusive problems can be avoided or resolved.

Given the continuum of audiological needs exhibited by persons with hearing loss, the role of the audiologist is significant in all phases of the vocational rehabilitation process. Considering the proliferation of new developments in technology, the audiologist's knowledge and expertise is vital to programming success. Contemporary hearing aids and devices are capable of refining a client's auditory skills and enabling each individual to develop strategies for the enhancement of overall communication.

A VR counselor cannot possibly keep abreast of the latest improvements in hearing aids and devices and, for this reason, must regularly consult with the audiologist. This is especially true for adult clients who have recently acquired a hearing loss. Most often the VR counselor is the client's first contact, so most likely the counsellor has not been introduced to these sophisticated instruments. The client, therefore, may require in-depth counseling by the audiologist. It becomes apparent in these particular situations that the charge for both professionals is interrelated, with counseling and supervision as shared responsibilities. However, the VR counselor and audiologist's complementary roles come from distinctive knowledge bases from which each can solicit useful information. The VR counselor is accountable for the client's vocational habilitation/rehabilitation program, whereas the audiologist's focus is primarily on the auditory/communicative aspects of rehabilitation.

SUMMARY

The placement and retention of individuals who are deaf/hard-of-hearing in quality work environments is the ultimate goal of vocational rehabilitation. Counselors are trained in the area of deafness to diligently seek out new frontiers for employment, to liase with other professionals, and to provide assistance to clients in their efforts to obtain personal and occupational independence. The underlying commonality that VR counselors share is the advancement of people who have hearing impairment into the labor market.

REFERENCES

Adams, P. F., & Benson, V. (1994). Current estimates from the National Health Interview Survey, 1993. *National Center for Health Statistics, 13,* 181.

Beuzart, J. G. (1982, November). *Deafened workers in France: Characteristics and conditions.* Paper presented at the International Congress of Audiophonology, Besançon, France.

Breed, P. C., van den Horst, A. P., & Mous, T. J. M. (1981). Psychosocial problems in suddenly deafened adolescents and adults. In Hartmann (Ed.), *Congress report.* Hamburg, Germany: First International Congress of the Hard of Hearing.

El-Khiami, A. (1986). Selected characteristics of hearing-impaired rehabilitants of general VR agencies: A socio-demographic profile. In D. Watson, G. Anderson, & M. Taff-Watson (Eds.), *Integrating human resources, technology and systems in deafness: Proceedings of the Tenth Biennial Conference of the American Deafness and Rehabilitation Association* (pp. 136–144). Silver Spring, MD: American Deafness and Rehabilitation Association.

Fellendorf, G., Atelsek, F., & Macklin, E. (1971). *Diversifying job opportunities for the adult deaf.* Washington, DC: Alexander Graham Bell Association for the Deaf.

Kyle, J. G., & Wood, P. L. (1983). *Social and vocational aspects of acquired hearing loss.* Final Report to the Ministry of Social Concern. Bristol, England: School of Educational Research Unit, University of Bristol.

Meadow-Orlans, K. P. (1985). Social and psychological effects of hearing loss in adulthood: A literature review. In H. Orlans (Ed.), *Adjustment to adult hearing loss* (pp. 35–58). San Diego, CA: Singular Publishing Group.

National Center For Health Statistics (1975). Persons with impaired hearing: United States. *Vital and Health Statistics, 10,* 101.

National Center For Health Statistics (1994a). Current estimates from the National Health Interview Survey, 1990. *Vital and Health Statistics, 10,* 1991, 181.

National Center For Health Statistics (1994b). Prevalence and characteristics of persons with hearing trouble. Series 10. No. 188. Data From *The National Health Survey.* DHHS, PHS, 5–10.

National Health Interview Survey (1994). Prevalence and characteristics of persons with hearing trouble: United States, 1990-1991. *Vital and Health Statistics, 10,* 188, 1–8.

Phillipe, T., & Auvenshine, D. (1985). Career development among deaf persons. *Journal of Rehabilitation of the Deaf, 19,* 9–17.

Phillips, G. B. (1975). Specific jobs for deaf workers. *Journal of Rehabilitation of the Deaf, 9,* 10–23.

Reis, P. (1993). Hearing ability of persons by sociodemographic and health characteristics: United States, 1993. *National Center for Health Statistics. 10,* 140.

Schein, J. D., & Delk, M. T., Jr. (1974). *The deaf population of the United States.* Silver Springs, MD: National Association of the Deaf.

Schroedel, J. G. (1987). The educational and occupational aspirations and attainments of deaf students and alumni of postsecondary programs. In G. B. Anderson & D. Watson (Eds.), *Innovations in the habilitation and rehabilitation of deaf adolescents: Selected proceedings of the Second National Conference on Habilitation and Rehabilitation of Deaf Adolescents* (pp. 117–139). Afton, OK: American Deaf Adolescent Conference.

Steffanic, D. J. (1982). *Reasonable accommodation for deaf employees in white collar jobs* (Monograph 10). Washington, DC: United States Office of Personnel Management Office of Research and Development.

Thomas, A., & Herbst, K. (1980). Social and psychological implications of acquired deafness for adults of employment age. *British Journal of Audiology, 14,* 76–85.

Thomas, A., Lamont, M., & Harris, M. (1982). Problems encountered at work by people with severe acquired hearing loss. *British Journal of Audiology, 16,* 39–43.

Williams, W., & Sussman, A. E. (1976). Social and psychological problems of deaf people. In A. E. Sussman & L. G. Stewart (Eds.), *Counseling with deaf people* (pp. 13–29). New York Deafness Research and Training Center.

Woodrick, W. E. (1984). Utilization of existing potential programs and facilities for serving multihandicapped deaf persons in region IV. *Journal of Rehabilitation of the Deaf, 18*, 17–20.

Wooton, S. C., & Mowry, R. L. (1986). A follow-up study of hearing-impaired vocational rehabilitation clients closed successfully by a state VR agency. In D. Watson, G. Anderson, & M. Taff-Watson (Eds.), *Integrating human resources, technology and systems in deafness: Proceedings of the Tenth Biennial Conference of the American Deafness and Rehabilitation Association* (pp. 410–419). Silver Spring, MD: American Deafness and Rehabilitation Association.

Wright, G. N. (1980). *Total rehabilitation.* Boston: Little Brown.

END OF CHAPTER EXAMINATION QUESTIONS

CHAPTER 3

1. In 1994, the National Center for Health Statistics reported that the prevalence rate of severe hearing loss was _____ for youth ages 3–17 years.
   a. 9.1 per 2,500
   b. 9.3 per 15,000
   c. 2.7 per 1,000
   d. 1.5 per 2,000

2. People with a hearing loss may miss out on which of the following?
   a. group interaction
   b. social knowledge
   c. career development
   d. all of the above

3. The amount of people with hearing loss has nearly _____ in the past 40 years.
   a. doubled
   b. tripled
   c. quadrupled
   d. decreased

4. (True or False) A hearing impairment affects all aspects of the individual's life.

5. (True or False) Loss of hearing is the most common physical impairment experienced by people in the U.S.

END OF CHAPTER ANSWER SHEET

Name   Date

CHAPTER 3

1. Which one(s)?   a   b   c   d

2. Which one(s)?   a   b   c   d

3. Which one(s)?   a   b   c   d

4. Circle one: True   False

5. Circle one: True   False

6. a.

   b.

   c.

   d.

7. _____

   _____

   _____

   _____

8. a. _____

   _____

   _____

   b. _____

   _____

   _____

c. _____

_____

_____

9. _____

_____

_____

_____

6. Describe four areas in your own life which would be changed if you had hearing loss.

a.

b.

c.

d.

7. After reading the reasons given for the increase in the incidence of hearing loss given in this chapter, give another reason why you believe there has been such a large increase.

8. List three job situations where it would be impossible to work if you had a severe hearing loss, and tell why.

a. _____

b. _____

c. _____

9. Choose an area of life in which a person might have difficulty (school, work, home, shopping, etc.) and describe what changes could be made to accommodate his or her hearing impairment.

■ CHAPTER 4 ■

Introduction to Hearing Aids and Amplification Systems

■ JOSEPH J. SMALDINO, PH.D. ■

In-the-canal
Completely-in-the canal
Implantable Hearing Aids
Cochlear Implants
Middle Ear Implants
Bone-anchored Hearing Aids

EARMOLD ACOUSTICS

PROGRAMMABILITY AND DIGITAL SIGNAL
PROCESSING

SUMMARY

Hearing aid selection and assessment are important components of the process of hearing habilitation/rehabilitation. An impaired auditory system typically involves reduced function in the perception of intensity, differentiation of frequency, and/or analysis of the temporal components of incoming sound. When that incoming sound is speech, the impaired system can affect the development of normal speech and language or significantly reduce ability to accurately perceive speech (Sanders, 1993; Smaldino, 1995). Primarily, these impairments are produced by loss of receptor cells in the cochlea and/or reduction in the number of neurons in the auditory nerve and are permanent. The function that remains is residual hearing and it is the goal of hearing aid selection procedures to enable the hearing-impaired individual to use all of the residual hearing potential that remains.

This discussion of hearing aids includes (1) basic components, (2) electroacoustic properties, (3) types of aids, (4) earmold acoustics, (5) implantable aids, and (6) programmability/digital signal processing. Consideration of hearing aid selection, assessment philosophies, and procedures

in regard to children is in Chapter 6. Hearing aid orientation guidelines for adults is discussed in Chapter 13 and other hearing aid considerations in older adults are found in Chapter 20. A thorough discussion of other assistive listening devices can be found in Chapter 14.

HEARING AID COMPONENTS

Modern hearing aids are very complex signal processing devices. However, there are basic components that compose all hearing aids. A basic hearing aid circuit block diagram is pictured in Figure 4–1. The actual components of a hearing aid are shown in Figure 4–2. Each component modifies the incoming signal in prescribed ways. All of the components working together result in the frequency and intensity response characteristics of a given hearing aid.

All hearing aids amplify sound for the listener. Acoustic waves entering at the hearing aid microphone are converted into electrical signals that mimic the pressure variations of the sound waves.

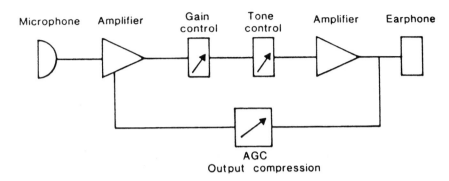

Figure 4–1. Diagram of a basic hearing aid circuit.

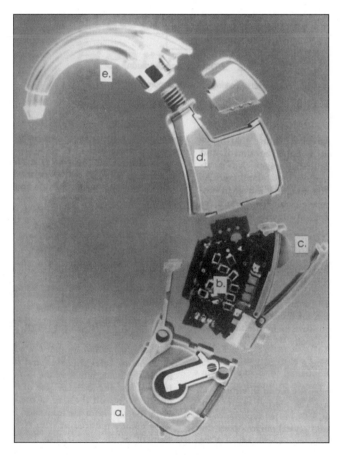

Figure 4–2. Actual hearing aid components. a) Microphone. b) Amplifier components. c) Battery compartment. d) Receiver. e) Earhook. (Courtesy of Telex Communications, Inc.)

The electrical signal from the microphone is amplified by the amplifier section of the hearing aid and delivered to the receiver of the aid, which converts the electrical signal back into its acoustic form to be heard by the listener. Along the way, the user can adjust various aspects of the amplification process, the person fitting the aid sets some aspects, and some are automatically adjusted by the hearing aid circuitry. The overall goal of a hearing aid fitting is to make sound audible and clear, without exceeding a person's level of comfortable listening

THE MICROPHONE

Sound energy is transduced (changed) to electrical energy by the microphone. Although different kinds of microphones, such as magnetic and ceramic, have been used in hearing aids over the years, the electret microphone is the most versatile and is used in virtually all modern hearing aids. According to Killion and Carlson (1974), the electret microphone offers (1) an excellent response to a wide range of frequencies, even at low intensities, (2) low sensitivity to mechanical vibration, and (3) low noise. Figure 4–3 is a diagram of an electret microphone.

An electret microphone is made from a permanent electrically charged element (the electret). A very thin metallically coated diaphragm is suspended just above the electret material. As sound waves strike the diaphragm, the vibration causes a fluctuating charge to be generated, which is amplified by a transistor in the microphone housing and is delivered to the next hearing aid component.

Microphones are classified as *omnidirectional* and *directional*. Directional microphones are more responsive to sound from the front and are useful in helping the hearing aid user hear better in noise by allowing the user to point the microphone toward the wanted signal and away from the unwanted noise.

Some hearing aids are equipped with a telecoil (T-coil) for telephone use. The telecoil bypasses the microphone by picking up electromagnetic energy produced by a telephone or induction loop and directing it to the hearing aid amplifier.

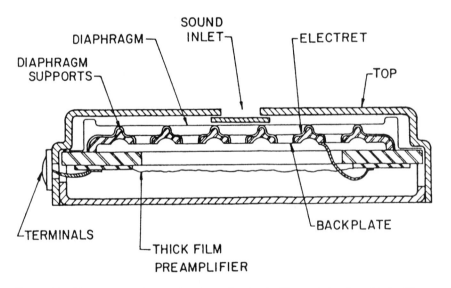

Figure 4–3. Diagram of an electret microphone. (Reprinted with permission from M. S. Killion, Etymotic Research, 61 Martin Lane, Elk Grove Village, IL 60007.)

THE AMPLIFIER

The electrical signal from the microphone is small and must be strengthened to be useful to a hearing aid user. Before development of the integrated circuit (IC), the amplifier was the largest hearing aid component. The integrated circuit amplifier increases the signal intensity by combining transistors and other components on a very small silicon chip.

The components are interconnected, which permits a wide variety of eletroacoustic characteristics to be specified for a particular hearing-impaired user. For instance, differing amounts of amplification (gain) can be prescribed, or certain frequencies can be amplified, which specifies the frequency response of the amplifier, or the maximum amplification permitted by the amplifier can be set to accommodate various degrees of loudness discomfort.

In modern hearing aids, several IC amplifiers can be combined on a silicon chip to provide even greater ability to modify the electroacoustic characteristics. Some of these circuits permit programming of characteristics to suit the needs of a user in a variety of listening situations. Also, automatic features are included that permit the hearing aid response to vary depending on the acoustic environment without manual user controls. The most sophisticated amplifiers incorporate digital signal processing, which allows a broader range of signal modification to better match a client's needs. Figure 4–4 is an example of a hearing aid amplifier.

Basic amplifier electroacoustic performance can be adjusted using specific controls. Typically, there is a control to regulate the volume and others to change the frequency response and maximum output of an aid. Advanced amplifier circuits have additional controls and some aids have circuits specifically designed to prevent squealing (feedback).

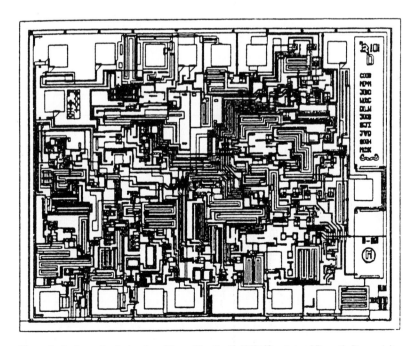

Figure 4–4. Example of a hearing aid amplifier, the K-AMP. (Courtesy of Etymotic Research.)

THE RECEIVER

The receiver works like a microphone in reverse and converts an electrical signal to an acoustic signal to be received by the ear. Most modern hearing aids incorporate an internal air conduction receiver that is connected by tubing to the outside of the hearing aid case or to the earmold. External air conduction receivers are also found in body-worn instruments and are coupled directly to the earmold. Air conduction receivers are generally of the balanced-armature magnetic type, because these can faithfully reproduce an amplified wide band signal and can be constructed in an extremely small package (Staab & Lybarger, 1994). Figure 4–5 is a diagram of a receiver.

The alternating electrical signal from the amplifier causes the electromagnetic field around the armature to change strength and be more or less attracted to the permanent magnets. As the armature is attracted to the diaphragm, the movement of the armature causes the diaphragm to vibrate and produce sound. Bone conduction receivers are used when factors contraindicate the use of air conduction receivers. These receivers are designed to directly vibrate the skull and may have less desirable electroacoustic performance than air conduction receivers.

BATTERIES

The power source for the increased signal strength and output produced by the amplifier is the battery. Modern hearing aids are typically powered by zinc-air or mercury batteries. Long shelf life and less environmental impact make the zinc-air batteries more desirable. Its batteries are basically containers of stored power, the rate at which the hearing aid drains the stored power will determine how long a battery lasts. The storage capacity of a battery is rated as mAh (milliampere-hours), and each hearing aid circuit consumes at a certain mAh rate. Usually the greater the gain and output demands placed on the hearing aid circuit, the greater its current consumption and the shorter the battery life. To extend battery life in this type of aid, a larger battery is needed for increased storage capacity. Hearing aids with lower current drain requirements can use smaller batteries with

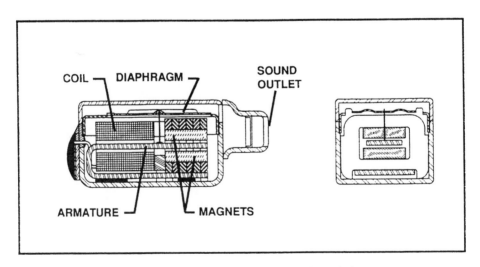

Figure 4–5. Diagram of a hearing aid receiver. (Courtesy of Knowles Laboratories.)

less storage capacity. Table 4-1 shows the relative storage capacity of batteries from the smallest #10A to the largest #401. Most recent hearing aids use the newest and smallest #5A battery.

ELECTROACOUSTIC PROPERTIES OF HEARING AIDS

To select a set of hearing aid components that will meet the needs of a specific hearing-impaired person, knowledge of how the hearing aid compo-

TABLE 4–1. Relative Voltages and Life of Common Hearing Aid Batteries.

Battery Type	Nominal Voltage Volts	Capacity mAh
Zinc-air 5A	1.4	30
Zinc-air 10A	1.3	50–60
Zinc-air 230	1.3	50–60
Zinc-air 536	1.3	50
Silver 312	1.5	37–40
Mercury 312	1.3	45–60
Zinc-air 312	1.3	100–120
Silver 13	1.5	75–80
Mercury 13	1.3	85–100
Zinc-air 13	1.3	170–230
Silver 76/675G	1.5	180–190
Mercury 675	1.3	180–270
Zinc-air 675	1.3	400–550
Mercury 401	1.3	800–1300

To estimate battery life:

$$\text{Hours} = \frac{\text{Milliampere hours (mAh)}}{\text{Current drain (mA)}}$$

Example: the 312 Zinc-air type battery has a capacity of 110 mAh. A hearing aid with current drain (mA) at 0.5 mA will give approximately 220 hours usage.

Source: Reprinted with permission from Staab, W., & Lybarger, S. (1994). Characteristics and use of hearing aids. In J. Katz (Ed.), *Handbook of clinical audiology* (p. 669). Baltimore, MD: Williams & Wilkins.

nents will affect a signal is crucial. As the hearing aid selection process often involves a comparison of hearing aid performance, a standard method of comparing key amplification properties allows comparison across circuits and manufacturers. Currently the American National Standards Institute (ANSI S3.22, 1987), *Specification of Hearing Aid Characteristics*, provides the standard measuring techniques for linear hearing aids, with ANSI S3.42, 1992, *Testing Hearing Aids With a Broad Band Noise Signal*, specifying the techniques for nonlinear aids. The standards are revised periodically as hearing aid technology changes. Additional tests are also performed in the actual client's ear (real-ear measurements) using actual use settings to verify the adequacy of the fitting. Although these measurement standards are reviewed in detail here, important electroacoustic properties of hearing aids are briefly discussed.

SATURATION SOUND PRESSURE LEVEL (SSPL)

Saturation sound pressure level (SSPL) is the maximum sound pressure level that can be produced by a hearing aid when the input signal to the hearing aid is at a high level. The SSPL is usually set below the point at which a user considers the sound to be uncomfortably loud. ANSI S3.22, 1987 specifies that the SSPL-90 measurement should be made with the volume control of the hearing aid at maximum and a 90 dB SPL input signal. The high frequency average SSPL-90 (HFA SSPL-90) is the SSPL-90 averaged for the frequencies 1000, 1600, and 2500 Hz.

ACOUSTIC GAIN

The *gain* of a hearing aid is determined by measuring its output across the frequency spectrum when compared to the level of the sound input to the hearing aid. Gain is a measure of how much the sound is amplified by a hearing aid. *Hearing aid gain* is determined by the capabilities of the amplifier and the degree to which the user adjusts the volume control, among other things. For example, persons with severe-to-profound hearing losses will require more acoustic gain than persons with a mild hearing loss. ANSI S3.22, 1987 specifies that the gain is measured with the volume control turned full on and the input set to 50 or 60 dB SPL. The high frequency average acoustic gain (HFA full-on gain) is the gain averaged for the frequencies 1000, 1600, and 2500 Hz.

FREQUENCY RESPONSE

Under normal listening conditions, hearing aid users will not turn their volume control to its full-on position, as is required to measure the acoustic gain according to ANSI S3.22. As a result, the actual shape of the gain across frequency curve, or *frequency response* of the hearing aid, may depart from the shape obtained during the acoustic gain measurements and not provide an accurate description of how a hearing aid will perform in actual use. ANSI S3.22, 1987 describes a reference test gain position to be used with a 60 dB SPL input to the hearing aid across frequency to arrive at a realistic frequency response for the hearing aid. The frequency response curve can be repeated to visualize the effect of changing hearing aid characteristics or making control adjustments. Figure 4–6 depicts the frequency/intensity response curves of a typical hearing aid using the methods specified in ANSI S3.22.

DISTORTION

If the signal delivered by the hearing aid to the ear of the user contains sounds that were not present at the hearing aid microphone, the hearing aid system is said to have added *distortion* to the input signal. It is generally agreed that distortion reduces the clarity and perhaps the intelligibility of speech and should be minimized in an amplifica-

Standard Frequency Response 007 HX-RPC-1

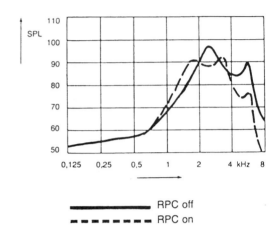

Figure 4–6. Plot of ANSI frequency response and output characteristics of a hearing aid. (Courtesy of Siemens Hearing Instruments.)

tion system. One characteristic of hearing aid component malfunction is high levels of distortion. ANSI S3.22, 1987 specifies ways to measure a type of distortion referred to as harmonic distortion. Other types of distortion, including intermodulation and temporal, may prove to be important in the future.

TYPES OF HEARING AIDS

Early electrical hearing aids were bulky and required large batteries to furnish the power needed to run them. By 1955, the invention of the transistor allowed engineers to design aids that were dramatically smaller. Subsequent miniaturization in the size of microphones, receivers, and batteries plus the development of integrated circuits has permitted the development of ever-smaller hearing aids. This trend toward miniaturization has been driven by the public's desire for the "invisible hearing aid." Unfortunately, as hearing aids have shrunk in size, they have become less flexible, although future designs may remediate this shortcoming.

Modern hearing aids come in a wide range of types. The suitability of a particular type depends on the shape of the user's outer ear, circuitry requirements, and age, among others. Hearing aids can be classified as body-worn, eyeglass, behind-the-ear (BTE), in-the-ear (ITE), in-the-canal (ITC), completely-in-the-canal (CIC), and implantable. Figure 4–7 shows examples of hearing aid types.

BODY-WORN

Body-worn and eyeglass hearing aids make up less than 2% of hearing aid sales (Hearing Industries Association [HIA], 1992). Body-worn aids

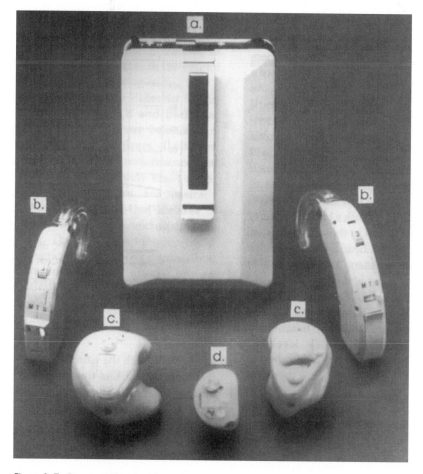

Figure 4–7. Representative examples of hearing aid types: (a) body aid; (b) eyeglass hearing aid; (c) behind-the-ear (BTE) hearing aid; (d) in-the-ear (ITE) hearing aid; (e) in-the-canal (ITC) hearing aid. (Courtesy of Telex Communications, Inc.)

have a receiver that is separated from the rest of the hearing aid by a lengthy cord. The separation enables the aid to provide sufficient gain without feedback to persons with extreme hearing loss. Because of the size of body-worn aids, circuitry compromises are usually not necessary; therefore the aids typically allow for many features and adjustments. Batteries can be larger to accommodate the larger current drain required of a high-gain hearing aid.

EYEGLASS

According to Berger (1984), eyeglass hearing aids accounted for 50% of hearing aid sales in 1959. Typically the microphone, amplifier, and receiver were built into the eyeglass temple or sidepieces. A major drawback of the type was that the wearer was forced to wear his or her glasses when the hearing aid was to be used.

BEHIND-THE-EAR

Behind-the-Ear (BTE) hearing aids are designed to fit behind the pinna. The size requires little circuit compromise, and the aids frequently come equipped with several electroacoustic adjustment controls. They are available in many styles, sizes, and configurations for hearing loss from the mild to profound categories. They can easily be adapted for use with classroom amplification and so are frequently used for children.

IN-THE-EAR

In-the-Ear (ITE) hearing aids are self-contained packages that fit within the concha and ear canal, with all of the components located in the concha section of the pinna. This positioning of the hearing aid is not only more invisible, but takes advantage of the natural sound enhancements produced by the pinna and possibly the ear canal

(Staab & Lybarger, 1994). The ITE hearing aid was made possible by the development of smaller electret microphones, smaller receivers, and smaller yet longer-lasting batteries. The cosmetic appeal of the all-in-the-ear concept has led to wide acceptance of this design over the bigger and more conspicuous BTE. Although the ITE is compact, it is large enough to include such options as the telecoil, frequency and output controls, and feedback controls, although size limits the flexibility that can be built into the aid. This style currently makes up about 60% of hearing aid sales (HAI, 1992).

IN-THE-CANAL

In-the-Canal (ITC) hearing aids were conceived with further miniaturization of the microphone, receiver, and battery. They are self-contained and fit into a small section of the concha and the ear canal. Most of the hearing aid components fit into the concha section, but some reside in the ear canal section. This position in the ear takes advantage of natural high frequency resonance of the pinna, unblocked concha, and deep ear canal insertion. The smaller receivers used in the ITC provide more high frequency response than the larger receivers found in the ITE (Staab & Lybarger, 1994). Although less visible than the ITE, their smaller size further limits the circuits and controls that can be built into the aid. The small size also makes them inappropriate for older clients and persons with disabilities who have dexterity or visual problems, which would make handling of the small aids and batteries difficult. This style currently makes up about 20% of hearing aid sales (HAI, 1992).

COMPLETELY-IN-THE-CANAL

Completely-in-the-canal (CIC) hearing aids are the newest innovation in the hearing aid marketplace. They are self-contained and fit completely within the external auditory canal. Because they are inserted deeply in the ear canal they terminate very close to the tympanic membrane. An example of an a CIC hearing aid is shown in Figure 4–8.

This deep CIC insertion provides a number of acoustic benefits to the user. The aids are more cosmetically pleasing, because they are nearly invisible; termination close to the eardrum permits less gain and output to be needed for a given loss, and gain availability is enhanced; and the deep insertion reduces the "head in a barrel" effect (occlusion), provides a secure fit, allows normal use of the telephone, reduces wind noise, makes feedback less likely, and reduces the amount of cerumen that can clog hearing aid receivers (Staab, 1992).

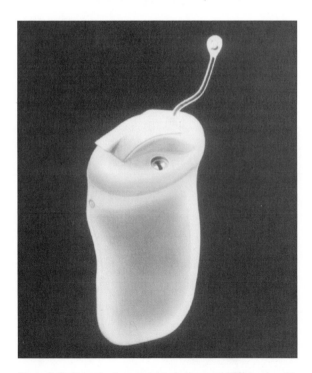

Figure 4–8. Example of a completely-in-the-canal (ITC) hearing aid. (Courtesy of Unitron Industries.)

The small size of the CIC hearing aid does severely constrain the circuits and controls that can be built into the aid. Until recently, for example, volume controls were difficult to incorporate into a CIC design. Most recently a programmable CIC has been introduced into the marketplace and it is likely that flexibility will improve as component miniaturization continues. Because the aid fits completely in the ear canal, some persons with small canals are not able to use these small devices.

IMPLANTABLE HEARING AIDS

As the name implies, this category of hearing aid requires a surgical implantation of part of the aid into the auditory pathway. Typically, the electronics, battery, and microphone are not implanted and require a connection to the implanted transducer in the auditory pathway.

Cochlear Implants

This type of aid converts sound to electrical impulses that are delivered through an electrode that has been surgically placed within the cochlea. The electronics process the acoustic signal and encode it into electrical patterns that can used to directly stimulate the auditory nerve. The implanted individual must undergo a learning process to efficiently interpret patterns of sound.

Historically, cochlear implants were reserved for post-lingually deafened individuals who could not benefit from traditional amplification. However, implants are also being used successfully with children with profound congenital hearing impairment, or who have been deafened adventitiously. Additional information on the use of cochlear implants can be found in Chapters 6 and 7 in this text.

According to Larky (2000), candidacy criteria for referral of **adults** for a cochlear implant typically requires (1) a 70 dB or greater hearing loss for frequencies 500, 1000, and 2000 Hz; (2) aided or unaided word recognition scores of poorer that 30%; and (3) unsuccessful trials of hearing aids for more than 2 months. For **children** to be candidates for cochlear implantation, the child must (1) possess a hearing loss of 90 dB or greater at frequencies 500, 1000, and 2000 Hz in both ears; (2) have had an unsuccessful trial of appropriately fitted hearing aids; (3) demonstrate failure to progress in speech-language-listening development based on therapist, teacher, parent report; (4) not respond to his or her name while wearing hearing aids in a quiet environment; and meet other requirements. Figure 4–9 is an illustration of a typical cochlear implant.

Middle Ear Implants

These aids use a magnet, piezoelectric crystal, or other driving device to physically vibrate the tympanic membrane or one of the middle ear ossicles. According to *The Hearing Review* (Tech reports, 1999), middle ear implants are designed for per-

sons with a moderate-to-severe hearing loss and who for whatever reason, do not or cannot benefit from air conduction hearing aids.

Bone-Anchored

These aids use a vibrator that is surgically affixed into the skull. Sound causes the skull to vibrate and the individual hears by bone conduction. The bond-anchored hearing aid was developed by Nobel Biocare Medical Systems. The BAHA uses a sound processor attached to a small titanium implant that is placed in the temporal bone. The temporal bone, then, provides a pathway for sound to the cochlea without involving the ear canal (Tech reports, 1999).

EARMOLD ACOUSTICS

Careful ear impressions are necessary to accurately reproduce the geometry of the ear canal, prevent acoustic feedback, and ensure user comfort.

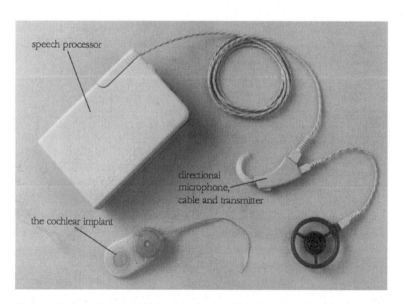

Figure 4–9. Illustration of a typical cochlear implant. (Courtesy of Cochlear Corporation.)

Earmolds can be fabricated from ear impressions into many different types and can be made of hard to very soft plastic. Figure 4–10 shows examples of earmold types.

Earmold acoustics are important to understand, because they can be used to modify the response of the aid to better fit the needs of a user. However, the marketplace shift to ITE, ITC, and CIC hearing aid styles limits the acoustic modifications that were once possible. Nonetheless, BTE hearing aids still require an explicit earmold and tubing coupling to the ear, which can be modified to change the sound delivered through the aid to the ear canal. Some of the modifications can also be applied to hearing aid styles for aids that reside in the concha or ear canal.

As can be seen in Figure 4–11, the frequency response of a hearing aid can be dramatically modified using different earmold acoustic modification techniques (Killion, 1980).

These changes in hearing aid response are often necessary to fine tune a hearing aid response to a user's residual hearing. The techniques in common use can be categorized as: (1) **Venting** (pri-

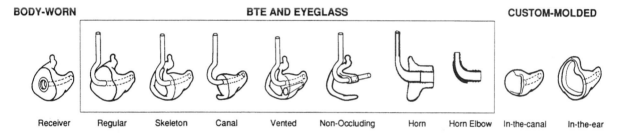

Figure 4–10. Examples of different types of earmolds. (Reprinted with permission from Staab, W. & Lybarger, S. (1994). Characteristics and use of hearing aids. In J. Katz (Ed.), *Handbook of clinical audiology* (p. 691). Baltimore, MD: Williams & Wilkins.)

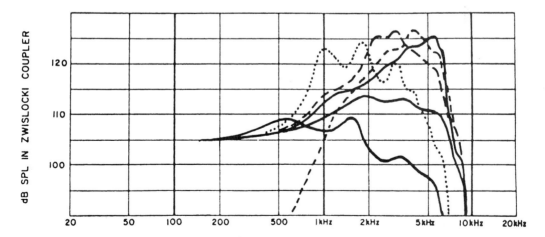

Figure 4–11. Example of the range of frequency response changes which can be produced by a single hearing aid with six different earmolds. Reprinted with permission from Killion, M. C. (1980). Problems in the application of broadband hearing earphones. In G. Studebaker & I. Hochberg (Eds). *Acoustical factors affecting hearing aid performance* (p. 259). Baltimore, MD: University Park Press.

marily affecting the low frequencies) is the making of an opening through the hearing aid from the outside to the ear canal, usually parallel with the receiver tubing of the hearing aid. The diameter of the hole may range from 0.065 mm to simply release pressure against the eardrum when inserting the earmold, up to a 3mm diameter, where maximum acoustic effects are expected. (2) **Damping** (influencing mostly the midfrequencies) works by inserting occluding devices that restrict the flow of acoustic energy at specific frequencies depending on the resistance and the location of the damping device in the tubing or earmold. They are frequently used to reduce the gain when peaks occur in the frequency response. (3) **Horn Effects** (affecting primarily the high frequencies) is an increase in the volume of the ear canal end of an earmold. This increase in volume acts much like a "horned" musical instrument to emphasize certain frequencies depending on the size and shape of the "horn" (Killion, 1976; Libby, 1981).

The diameter and length of the tubing used in the earmold type can also produce major changes in the frequency response. Although the acoustic effects of earmold modifications are somewhat predictable, obtaining a desired result is often done by trial-and-error and can be a lengthy process.

PROGRAMMABILITY AND DIGITAL SIGNAL PROCESSING

Until recently, all hearing aids came with relatively fixed electroacoustic characteristics selected to generally meet the residual hearing needs of the user. Fine tuning of these devices was sometimes difficult and so an approximate fitting to the user's needs was often considered acceptable. Some modern hearing aids are designed to have a wide variety of electroacoustic characteristics built into them, along with a *programming function*, which allows the aid to be finely tuned to the needs of a user. Electronic control of the electroa-

coustic modifications is more predictable than purely acoustic modification through earmold changes. Until recently, most programmable hearing aids were programmed using a computer (programming was digital), but the actual functioning of the aid did not convert the acoustic signal into digital form (so the amplification remained analog). The newest programmable aids employ both digital programming digital signal processing during amplification. These offer an increasing selection of processing options to more precisely meet the amplification needs of each client.

A diagram of a programmable hearing aid is shown in Figure 4–12. Typically the user's audiometric data is input into a computer program that makes calculations for desirable electroacoustic characteristics based on established predictive equations. The hearing aid dispenser selects additional features that are required by the dynamics of the hearing loss and user needs. Given the different combinations of gain, output, frequency response, output limiting, and number of channel combinations possible, the dispenser has literally thousands of aids to choose from to meet user needs. In the most sophisticated aids, multiple programmable memories are built in, which allows the user to switch from one set of electroacoustic characteristics to another to maximize the characteristics for particular listening situations. Of course, if the user's hearing and listening needs change, the programmable aid can be reprogrammed without the purchase of an entirely new aid.

SUMMARY

Designing and fitting hearing aids to enable the hearing-impaired individual to use all of the residual hearing potential that remains has been and continues to be a challenge. Advances in hearing aid technology have allowed us to come closer

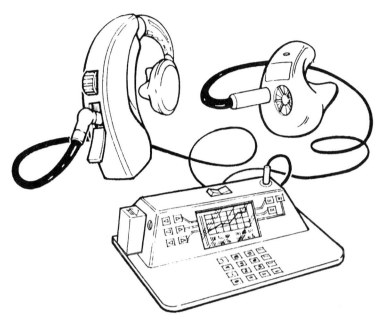

Figure 4–12. Diagram of a programmable hearing aid. (Courtesy of Danavox.)

than ever to meet the challenge, but our understanding of how to repair a broken auditory system is still incomplete. As more is learned about the function and dysfunction of human hearing, it is a certainty that hearing aids will be designed to utilize that knowledge.

REFERENCES

American National Standards Institute (ANSI). (1987). *Specification of hearing aid characteristics*. ANSI S3.22-1987. New York: Author.

American National Standards Institute (ANSI). (1992). *Testing hearing aids with a broad-band noise signal*. ANSI S3.42-1992. New York: Author.

Berger, K. (1984). *The hearing aid: Its operation and development*. Livonia, MI: The National Hearing Aid Society.

Hearing Industries Association (HIA). (1992). *Statistical report for the quarter ending December. New units sold by type and origin*. Washington, DC: Author.

Killion, M. (1976). Experimental wide bandwidth hearing aids. *Journal of the Acoustical Society of America, 59,* S62 (A).

Killion, M. (1980) Problems in the amplification of broadband hearing aid earphones. In G. Studebaker & I. Hochberg (Eds.), *Acoustical factors affecting hearing aid performance* (pp. 121–132). Baltimore, MD, University Park Press.

Killion, M., & Carlson, E. (1974). A sub-miniature electret microphone of new design. *Journal of the Auditory Engineering Society, 22,* 237–243.

Larky, J. (2000). Who is a cochlear implant candidate? Criteria for referring patients. *The Hearing Journal, 53,* 6, 38–42.

Libby, E. (1981). Achieving a transparent, smooth, wideband hearing aid response. *Hearing Instruments, 32,* 9–12.

Sanders, D. (1993). *Management of hearing handicap.* Englewood Cliffs, NJ: Prentice Hall.

Smaldino, J. (1995). Speech perception processes in children. In C. Crandell, J. Smaldino, & C. Flexer (Eds.), *Sound-field FM amplification: Theory and practical applications* (pp. 220–232). San Diego, CA: Singular Publishing Group.

Staab, W. (1992). The peritympanic instrument: Fitting, rationale and test results. *The Hearing Journal, 45,* 21–26.

Staab, W., & Lybarger, S. (1994). Characteristics and use of hearing aids. In Katz (Ed.), *Handbook of clinical audiology* (pp. 657–722). Baltimore, MD: Williams & Wilkins.

Tech reports. Update on implant technology Part 2: Implantable hearing aids. (1999). Hearing Review, 6, 12, 13, 33, 34.

END OF CHAPTER EXAMINATION QUESTIONS

CHAPTER 4

1. What is the overall goal of a hearing aid fitting? Briefly describe that goal.

2. Most hearing aids utilize an earmold. In general acoustical terms, what does an earmold do?

3. The author describe five (5) different types of hearing aids in this chapter. What are they? What are their benefits and limitations?

4. Define the following terms, and describe how they contribute to the overall function of a hearing aid.

   a. Saturation sound pressure level

   b. Acoustic gain

   c. Frequency response

   d. Distortion

5. In regard to types of hearing aids, which one currently is the most popular in relation to the numbers fit and sold in the U.S.? _____.

6. Define the following terms as they relate to earmold acoustics:

   a. Venting

   b. Damping

   c. Horn effects

END OF CHAPTER ANSWER SHEET

Name _____ Date _____

CHAPTER 4

1. _____

   _____

   _____

   _____

2. _____

   _____

   _____

   _____

3. _____

   _____

   _____

   _____

   _____

4. a.

   b.

   c.

   d.

5. _____

_____

_____

_____

_

6. a.

 b.

 c.

PART II

Aural Habilitation: Children Who Are Hearing Impaired

Family Involvement and Counseling in Serving Children Who Are Hearing Impaired

■ DALE V. ATKINS, Ph. D. ■

Acknowledging that one's child has hearing impairment is a long and difficult process that no one, aside from another parent of a child who is hearing impaired, can fully understand. It is the first and most important fact that each professional needs to accept before, during, and after provision of service to any family. This chapter presents information on the families of children who have hearing impairment, the family role in the support of the children, and the involved role of the professional with families behalf of the children who have hearing impairment.

PRELIMINARIES FOR THE PROFESSIONAL

There is much that professionals can do to help in the navigation of an unfamiliar and confusing road. Whether trained as teachers, doctors, speech and language pathologists, audiologists, or counselors, professionals must always be mindful of who they are and what their role is in the process of working with parents and children. Professionals may wish to make their client's pain go away, they may wish to fix everything, see themselves as saviors, miracle workers, persons on whom parents rely to cope better with their situation. They may, intentionally or not, raise parents' expectations based on their own desire to have everyone feel better.

Certainly, it is well within a professional's realm to be encouraging, hopeful, and positive in spirit. *It is not within a professional's realm to promise what cannot be delivered.* Early in this author's career of working with families of children who have hearing impairments, a mother of a happy, popular, highly communicative 12-year old girl who used total communication (i.e., a combination of sign language, voice, and audition) kept insisting that her daughter mostly use her voice instead of signing when talking with me. Afterward, in my private conversation with the mother, she said she felt like a failure whenever her daughter chose not to speak. When asked why, she replied, "I'll never forget the first professional I met in the field of deafness. She was a therapist who told me that if I worked hard enough, my daughter would speak as well as any normal child. You know, I devoted my entire life to trying to teach her to speak well. Since she doesn't, I feel as if I didn't do enough."

Another family has been waiting for life to return to the way it was before their son lost his hearing at age 26 months. The father, on reflection of the doctor's words, recalled him saying, "Things will be as good as new; even better because you all have survived such a terrible trauma." Contrary to what the doctor predicted, things were far from better. The household was in chaos and the older, 6-year old brother felt confused, abandoned, and neglected because of his parents' involvement with the younger boy. They were waiting for things to go back to "the way it was." It was already more than 4 years and the family was still trying to sort out their lives. Things were hardly "as good as new."

Professionals must be mindful that each person's experience is unique and that discovering that one's child has hearing impairment changes each person in some way. In all families, parental actions are heavily influenced by various factors, among which are the child's responses. Also vital are the parents' family backgrounds and interpersonal stories, how they were raised, marital harmony or discord, finances, chronic or acute stresses and means of dealing with them, strengths and support of friendships, expectations for themselves and their children, knowledge about and attitude toward hearing impairment, maturity, and attitude toward life's challenges. There are cultural differences in how persons with disabilities and their families are perceived (Yacobacci-Tam, 1987).

How professionals see themselves and interpret their roles will greatly affect the course of treatment for a family as a whole and a child, individually. Helping people to approach their lives from a perspective of strength and expediting their discovery and utilization of their own inner resources, while sorting out the maze in which they find themselves is within the professional's domain. The rate at which a family's progress occurs is outside the professional's domain and is determined by the persons, themselves, and their response and interaction with the long process of healing, coping, and living. Specialists need to be unintimidating, cooperative teammates who have chosen a field of study and have developed considerable experience and training in specific areas, but who are open to learning from the people who have come for help. They must present themselves as human beings who have selected a particular profession and, as a result, have accumulated some knowledge. He or she cannot be all-knowing, superior, or condescending. Rather, professionals must embark eager to learn in a partnership with people whom they view positively and respectfully.

PRELIMINARIES FOR THE FAMILY

The family is a primary, powerful emotional system that shapes and influences the lives of its members. In systems theory, the family is conceptualized as a dynamic unit. The theory posits that family relationships are interdependent and mutually interactive; change in one part of the system stimulates compensatory change in other parts. Erikson (1964) found that the stability of a family hinges on the complicated and sensitive pattern of emotional balance and interchange. The behavior of each member affects and is affected by the behavior of other members. Families are the greatest potential resource for personal well-being, as well as for psychological distress.

Luterman (1979) states that in families with children who are disabled, the family as a whole may initially attempt to adjust to the disability without changing the existing family structure. However, members may eventually reach a point where they cannot continue to meet previous social, economic, and personal roles and expectations, and where they may become dissatisfied with their relationships with each other. A role organization crisis may occur that is associated with elevated tension, in which delicately balanced family priorities may shift. Siblings may be expected to take over adult responsibilities and the quality and frequency of recreational activities may change; Grandparents may shy away from sharing child care responsibilities or may offer help and be rejected. Previously earmarked finances may need to be budgeted for the funding of hearing aids, tactile stimulators, private therapy, or attendance at conferences. Long-standing friendships may be critically scrutinized and personal time and energy all but disappear. When family disequilibrium persists and parents feel particularly stressed, there is a risk of severe personal or relational problems developing.

All too often, the actual issues that are troubling a family are not addressed and symptoms rather than causes are confronted. In a rather typical example, a father in one family became increasingly more involved in his work after the diagnosis of his son's hearing impairment. He attended evening work meetings, traveled more, and accepted business-related phone calls at home. Whenever he would attend a clinic appointment, invariably, someone from his office would call. This put a severe strain on his relationship with his wife. She felt she was alone and they argued frequently. The symptoms appeared to indicate marital distress, but, in truth, the man needed to become totally absorbed in his work to get his mind away from the pain he was experiencing about his child who was hearing impaired and to reassure himself of his importance. The father needed to believe that he could still control much of his world even though he felt helpless over not being able to change his son's hearing impairment.

THE ROLE OF THE PROFESSIONAL

INTERACTIONS WITH THE FAMILY

In the beginning of a professional association, the professional does not know the people seeking help (parents or children), and they (the parents and children) do not know the professional. Professionals are viewed as "the experts." The danger of this for professionals is that they may maintain the parents' expectation of them and forget that they, too, are involved in a learning process. This "halo effect" is a dangerous illusion for a professional who does not understand the lengthy process in which the parents are immersed. Parents desperately need to know they are not lost, that their family, particularly their child, will be okay. They desire reassurance about the decisions confronting them. Parents are thrown into a new world and are required to make serious decisions for and about their child, based on recommendations of many professionals.

Even before a child's hearing aids arrive, the parents need to select one of many early intervention programs representing different philosophies. "What should we do?" What would you do if you were in my shoes?" asks the overwhelmed parent. The professional is often, during these moments, viewed as much more than human and asked to make decisions for the parents about their family's future. The professional's job is to not make decisions for the family, but rather to help the parents become sufficiently comfortable and informed so that they can make their own decisions. It is a difficult position to be in because of the nature of the counseling required.

COUNSELING

As speech and language pathologists, teachers and audiologists are not trained to be professional counselors, social workers, or psychologists, thus they sometimes feel inadequate to deal with the range of emotional responses they encounter while performing the service for which they *were* trained. Many of these professionals feel competent working with children, but find themselves interacting at arm's length with the child's parents, as well as siblings, grandparents, and caregivers. Frequently, an entire family (extended and nuclear) will show up for an appointment and the professional feels unprepared to handle the different people and the various emotions expressed.

It is essential that a clinician understand that his or her role is not to become a counselor. However, to be more proficient, the professional does need to be sensitive to and unafraid of the multifaceted nature of their work, which is simultaneously content- and emotion-based. Both aspects are equally important to the success of the interaction. At times, content may be more to the fore, but that does not mean that emotional underpinnings are absent.

THE PROFESSIONAL AS COUNSELOR

To enable professionals to feel prepared for these encounters, it is useful for them to learn basic counseling theories, with the understanding that they will, for the most part, be dealing with a well-patient model.

Unlike in psychotherapy, where the main goal is to help reorganize and reinterpret a client's intrapersonal conflicts which may be characterized by anxieties, depression, guilt, confusions, or ambivalence, counseling in this context is done with psychologically normal individuals who are presently trying to confront and cope with a major, or series of major disruptions in their lives. (Clark, 1990, p. 5)

Counseling is supportive and builds on renewed insights into the person, his or her family, goals, and specific aspects of their lives. For a more intense examination of the various models and their use with a population that has hearing impairment, the reader is referred to the works of Harvey (1989), Luterman (1979), and Rollin (1987). One can attempt to be familiar with a variety of theories and then blend them, depending on the need of a client and the situation.

Whatever a professional's orientation, no response will compensate for the loss that the family is going through. The gaping hole cannot be filled by words. The hurt may be soothed, over time—

usually years. Professionals must be active and involved listeners, committed to the process; active in that they encourage parents to express their emotions and the circumstances underlying those emotional states; involved in that they recognize when questions need a direct, informal response. It is essential to be straightforward yet compassionate and empathetic, confident yet neither pompous nor omniscient, respectful of the family and sensitive to their plight and concerns, so that the family will be able to perceive and accept the professional as a viable and trustworthy partner.

Trust has more chance of developing if a professional learns the parents' personal hopes and their goals for themselves and their children. These people have a lot to teach. Refraining from making assumptions is vital for a professional. The extent to which the news of a hearing impairment affects a family can only be discovered by listening to and observing *each* particular family. Yet, the professional can view them against a backdrop of knowledge that has been garnered from other families.

EMOTIONAL RESPONSES OF FAMILIES

Among research and observation of families of children who have hearing impairment, professionals find that, in the area of emotional response, these families experience reactions similar to those of children who have other disabilities. The response cycle is not unlike that experienced by any person involved in grieving a major loss. For years, this process was likened to that described by Elisabeth Kübler-Ross (1969) in *On Death and Dying*. Predictable stages were described as shock, recognition, denial, acknowledgment, and constructive action. Because parents lost the child they had envisioned, their task at hand is to adapt to the thought and reality of life with this different child. What was previously normal suddenly undergoes reassessment. Somehow, a new normalcy needs to be established. There is an ending to the relationship with the child who was believed to have normal hearing and a beginning of a new relationship with the child who has hearing impairment. With neither warning nor preparation, the parents are thrust into an unfamiliar world filled with information and people they would have gone a lifetime without confronting. To add to the predicament, there really is no choice. They enter this world reluctantly and apprehensively. The professional's function at this point is to serve as a supportive guide through the maze.

This process of parental grieving is different from that of losing a child completely. It is also unlike the discovery that one's child has a more visible disability that may have been obvious at birth. Deafness is referred to as "the invisible handicap" and, thus, the extent of the disability is not known to most people. Additionally, as deafness is rarely discovered at birth, parents initially bond with the child whom they believe is 100% all right. They sing, talk, and, in general, relate to the baby as if there were normal function. When the suspicion that the child may have a hearing problem is confirmed, there is, understandably, much sadness, guilt, anger, and remorse on the part of the parents and other family members. These feelings frequently appear and reappear over the years, although the families rebuild their lives and deal with their loss constructively. It is essential that parents go through, rather than avoid, the mourning process. "It enhances their parental capacity for satisfaction in childrearing" (Leigh, 1987). Dr. Nancy Miller, in her book, *Nobody's Perfect* (1994), describes four stages of adaptation experienced by parents of children who have disabilities. These stages are familiar to parents of children with hearing impairments. They are dynamic, nonlinear, and often overlap. They are: surviving, searching, settling in, and separating. Each stage has its own set of experiences and reactions that go along with them for each person.

HEARING THE NEWS

Often, on hearing the news, parents question their ability to parent a child, feel unprepared, and don't know what to do. They question everything they do know about their child and wonder if they will ever relate to this different child from whom they feel estranged and with whom they imagine they will be unable to communicate. Previously held feelings of competency about their own parenting skills are called into question as they begin to worry about what will happen to their children, their relationship, and their family. One mother mused: "I knew that music was my whole life and I had spent so much time thinking about how great it would be to have a child to sing with. I played soothing classical music during my pregnancy, sang all the time while he was an infant, and brought him every musical toy that I could find. I truly do not know what I'm supposed to do. I'm just so utterly sad." On the recent discovery of his fourth child's hearing impairment, one father lamented, "I don't think I can rely on anything I did with my other kids to be right. I don't know how to deal with Mickey since he cannot hear me. How will I discipline him? How will I find out what he wants? I'm questioning everything I ever knew about children, because I see how much I don't know." The overwhelming sense that they will not know what to do or that there is too much to learn and they are not equipped to handle all that will be required can cause some parents to question everything they know about children.

To help parents realize their full potential, their initial perceptions of weakness and helplessness must be gradually and consistently replaced by confidence and competence. The clinician's role is to enable parents to work effectively with a child, while providing objective, individualized support, guidance, and critique. The professional's role changes over time. At first, their words are the only words of guidance and instruction that are available to the family. Later, they serve as a sounding board.

It is at this point that the message "child first and foremost" needs to be conveyed to parents gently and consistently. Usually, parents focus on the aspect of their child that is impaired rather than focusing on the whole child. This is a natural response. It is up to the professional to relate to the child as a child first, considering the hearing impairment second. Even though the family sees the professional for issues regarding the hearing impairment, the nature of the professional's interaction, questions, and manner should be that of a person interested in the functioning of a whole child within a whole family. A mother of a newly diagnosed 20-month-old daughter insisted that whenever her husband interacted with their daughter, that he wear the microphone for her FM unit. At times he resisted, especially when he wanted to "rough house" with his daughter. This incited tension between the couple. She felt she was the only one working with Angela, while he was just there for the fun. The mother felt they did not have time to "fool around." Without realizing it, the mother sent disapproving messages to her husband, so that he felt his way of relating to his daughter was not valuable. Much of his time was not engaged in "teaching language", therefore, it was deemed unimportant. She felt he was not giving his daughter anything that she needed. He claimed, "I don't do as well as my wife does in the structured setting. At least I can still develop a relationship with my daughter. Isn't that worth something?" Intuitively he knew that he was right, but the pressure of needing every waking hour to be involved in a structured language experience had taken over and dictated their lives. The valuable, delicate balance had not yet been struck.

FEELINGS, DOUBTS, AND QUESTIONS

Feelings are complex and confusing. Doubts abound. Questions are asked. Some are unanswerable, thus adding to the frustration and the sense of feeling unfamiliar and incompetent. Parents of newly diagnosed children frequently report feeling numb. They are overwhelmed with a horrible sense of disbelief and shock and unable to process information they are given about hearing loss, audiograms, hearing aids, educational options, and state support services, while attempting to look attentive with tears welling up or running down, fighting enormous lumps in throats, resisting nausea and a generalized feeling of being in another place or time zone, with people who are unfamiliar (Buscalia, 1975; Featherstone, 1980; Moses, 1985).

Maria Forecki (1985) recounted her experiences with her son, Charlie, who has hearing impairment, in *Speak to Me*. She recalled her initial experience this way:

Mourning manifested itself in not wanting to speak to Charlie, or anyone else. I unplugged my radio and refused to watch television. I surrounded myself with the absence of sound so as to make sound not exist. It was impossible to live with the fact that Charlie could not experience sound. (p. 29)

One father described hearing the news this way:

It was as if I was knifed in my stomach; my insides were threatened to come out and the more I tried to hold them in, the more I lost control. The audiologist just kept staring at me with a shocked expression on his face. I must have looked like something had snapped inside of me . . . in fact, it did.

Delivering bad news is something most of us are not comfortable with. At various stages in the families' journey they will meet many professionals who will be in the position of delivering, if not bad, then difficult news. The first person to confirm the parents' suspicion of hearing impairment is usually a pediatrician, otologist, or audiologist. Although the news may be delivered gently and tactfully, it may not be received in that way.

Many professionals perceive their role to be one of delivering news and then asking the parents for questions. When the parents do not ask any, the professional assumes all is understood as it was presented and continues to talk. It is useless to deliver news and information, if you do not validate that it is received and understood. Yet when the news is difficult, professionals often avoid the very probing that is necessary, not wanting to "upset" the parents more. The professional must make a serious and consistent effort to listen to what is and what is not being said. Whenever professionals are in the position of delivering news, they must be conscious of several factors, among which are environment, participants, timing and sequencing, language or symbols, strength ability, and resources (Kroth, 1987). Because the sorrow of having a child who has hearing impairment is often chronic, professionals need to be supportive and mindful of these factors throughout the years of their interactions with parents. One mother thought aloud:

Sometimes, today, 15 years later, I still feel like I did at that first meeting with the audiologist. When I hear important information about Jackie, my emotions get in the way of my being able to listen attentively, and I have a hard time hearing what is being said. I guess because we have been through so much, people expect me to have an unfeeling filter through which I hear all of the facts. It just isn't so.

If a professional is furnishing information, it is imperative that attempts be made to assist the parents in feeling less overwhelmed by making enough time to give information and to answer questions. Language needs to be carefully chosen and words that may be unfamiliar should be explained. Few situations are more intimidating to parents than listening to professionals talk about their child, using words that are unfamiliar. In the area of hearing impairment, where there are unfamiliar terms and symbols (e.g., interpreting an audiogram), handouts should be provided with terminology, phrases, and definitions, with resource sheets and pamphlets readily available. Parents need time to ingest what is discussed.

They need to be assured that a follow-up meeting or phone call is scheduled to ensure clarification of points made.

ENHANCING COMMUNICATION BETWEEN PROFESSIONALS AND PARENTS

Because much of the information that is presented may or may not be heard or processed, it is essential to frequently review what has been previously discussed. One mother tape recorded every session she had with the otologist and audiologist so that she could review the tape with her husband who was unable to attend many of the appointments with her. As her child grew up, tape recording became a useful habit. She taped teachers' meetings and individualized educational plan (IEP) sessions. Some professionals she encountered were uneasy, but she countered by saying that she wanted to concentrate on what was being said, wanted to feel free to ask questions, and wanted to have time to review all of the answers when she was in the privacy of her own home. Professionals who feel comfortable with this idea can expand it by providing prerecorded tapes of the information to be covered or by taping their sessions and giving the parents the audiotape. Additionally it is helpful to furnish families with a packet of information sheets, booklets, lists of national and local organizations and resources, and books for home study and sharing with family members. The information packet should be available in as many languages as the community served. This practice is especially helpful when parents travel a great distance and the likelihood of frequent follow-up meetings or immediate contact with other parents is slim.

Realizing that only a portion of a message is going to be received is an important lesson for all professionals. Messages, particularly those that are not entirely welcome, are frequently distorted as they are filtered through our thoughts and feelings. Whenever professionals are in the position of giving news to parents, they must be aware that parents also need to hear what the possibilities are for their children and for their families. One father remembers:

The therapist seemed so upbeat, hopeful, and positive. It helped us because, like us, our friends and family were all so down and grief-stricken. Every conversation we had was about Joey and his hearing. Heaven knows what was happening in other aspects of our lives since it seems now that we didn't deal with anything else. We were sad, but we also wanted to do something constructive.

Referring to his own participation he said:

I realized that I began to enjoy the sessions because I was learning while I was getting to know Joey in a different way. Instead of focusing on the fact that he could not hear, I began to think of ways I could broaden his ability to hear. It became exciting. That is when I began to feel hopeful.

Families seem to do better when they are confident that a professional is familiar and current with different educational programs. Visiting area schools and keeping up professional associations with those in the same and related fields is helpful for the clinician's personal and professional growth. It is invaluable when sharing knowledge with families. Professionals who attend conferences and participate in workshops designed for parents can develop a sensitivity to the situation faced by those parents. Teachers who visit local hearing aid dispensers and hearing and speech centers at local hospitals and clinics where families receive services have a better chance of connecting with families and understanding the complex network with which the families interact. Too often, parents are the link in a large network of services. When they discover that professionals are unacquainted or unfamiliar with one another, their confidence in the professionals and the system can wane. If they perceive that there is a larg-

er, interconnected structure of which they are a part, they feel less isolated.

EXCHANGING ROLES

A strategy at seminars and workshops is to encourage parents and professionals to assume the role of the other when involved in a particular problem-solving exercise or sensitivity-training role play. By reversing roles, empathy is likely to develop, and the process of working together can be accomplished more smoothly. In one such exercise, a speech-language pathologist expressed anger over a parent's tardiness for her son's sessions. The clinician interpreted this chronic lateness as the mother's resistance to having her son in therapy. When the speech-language pathologist took the role of the mother, she discovered that the mother needed to travel two hours on public transportation to attend therapy. After discovering this, the pathologist became more alert to such situations in her clients' lives. In this case, there was an effort to address the problem directly, enlisting a community ride service, which helped to ease the transportation problem.

It is essential for professionals to develop sensitive communication skills that consider a family's needs and comfort. Professionals who work with children who have hearing impairment and their families are involved with them in searching for solutions to their problems. The overriding message the professional can convey is that the family *will* be able to cope, and the professionals the parents encounter will make their task easier. Parents' existing coping skills may enable them to deal with their situation better than professionals expect. Conversely, developing coping skills may be what is needed to facilitate better adjustment and, therefore, the professional's role may be enlarged to include helping parents discover how to efficiently negotiate the maze of people, places, and things related to and about hearing impairment. Additionally professionals can help them incorporate family and friends into their lives in ways that can be beneficial to them and their families. Finally, professionals can help provide a safe place where families can see and explore their fears and develop the courage to deal with them.

PARENT SUPPORT GROUPS

Most professionals know the value of connecting families with other families who are in similar situations. At times, there may be initial reluctance by clients to meet other parents. Perhaps talking to one professional is all a family can handle at the moment. Perhaps meeting with other parents is too threatening, too definite an acknowledgment that they have a child who has hearing impairment. But the eventual sharing that occurs among families is potentially the most therapeutic and healing remedy that any family can undertake. Bonds of friendship, understanding, empathy, and humor form among families who, under "normal" circumstances would not have met. They give one another strength as well as hope. Helen Keller wrote:

We bereaved are not alone. We belong to the largest company in all the world—the company of those who have known suffering. When it seems that our sorrow is too great to be borne, let us think of the great family of the heavy-hearted into which our grief has given us entrance, and, inevitably, we feel about us their arms, their sympathy, their understanding. (Keller, 1954, p. 56).

It is the parents who grow together, leaving behind feelings of helplessness and despair, as they try jointly to make sense out of the new world into which they have reluctantly been thrust.

Professionals must encourage attendance at parent support groups and if none exist, commit to starting such a program with one or two interested families. These discussion groups augment parent-to-parent phone connections; membership in organizations; attendance at panel discussions featuring parents of teenagers and young adults who are hearing impaired, older children who are hearing impaired, grandparents, and siblings; and interaction with adults and professionals who have hearing impairment. All are of inestimable value in the adaptation of families with children who have hearing impairment.

It is other parents who can offer solace when a grandparent appears to favor one child over another and the parents do not know how to address this with their own parents. It is other parents who understand what it is like when a child who has hearing impairment is not asked for "playdates" by the neighborhood kids. It is other parents who can talk openly about their feelings of neglecting their other children in favor of the child who is hearing impaired, because the "need" is greater. Other parents can truly understand the difficulty of not having the time or energy for their spouses or their children. They can notice other parents placing expectations on the hearing siblings in the family to behave maturely, accepting responsibilities beyond their ages.

Parents in a parent group can organize a "Sibling Day," arrange to have all of the families meet at a picnic site, emphasize the "normalcy" of their families so that the siblings can see other families with children who wear hearing aids (Atkins, 1987). These events help families and siblings, in particular, feel less isolated. It is in a parent group that parents can let their hair down and not have to be "supermom" or "superdad." It is in a parent group that parents can discuss what it is like to have one's personal and familial identity quickly transformed into the "father of" or "family with the deaf kid," recognizing that wherever they go people look at them and make assumptions, sometimes asking questions, sometimes not, sometimes offering suggestions, sometimes not. One mother received nods of recognition from group members when she said, "Running to the market used to be so easy. Now when I take Alex, everyone in the check-out line stares at his hearing aids. One woman asked if he was listening to a Walkman. I'm embarrassed to tell you that I said "Yes!"

Only other parents can identify with the sinking feeling when every eye in the store is on you when your child has a tantrum. Upon reflections of his daughter's tantrum in a toy store, one father admitted:

It is worse when your kid is deaf, because when she closes her eyes and pulls her hearing aids out of her ears there really is no way to reach her. While I am waiting for her to calm down, it seems like everyone in the store has passed me and I'm convinced they think I am the most incompetent father in the world.

It is also parents who are going through a similar process who can encourage other parents to be patient while witnessing the progress of their friends' children and not seeing any discernible change in their own children:

Sometimes when we see my sister's kids, I can't help feeling envious of her. She has it all so easy! We were pregnant at the same time, planned it so that the cousins would be close and play together, and now I wonder how they will ever get along. I don't want my nephew to feel that Billy is a drag to be around.

Another mother commented:

Years ago when I saw other mothers playing with their children in the park I would feel intensely jealous. Now I know that many of my friends envy my relationship with my daughter because we really are close. Maybe that has to do with how hard we have worked at communicating. I needed a lot of patience.

OTHER FAMILY MEMBERS

In addition to parent support groups as a means of assisting parents to adapt to life with a child with hearing impairment, parents also benefit from acknowledgment by professionals that there are other important influences in their lives. Attending to the needs of their child who is hearing-impaired is often dominant, but it is not the only important aspect in their lives. Relationships with other children in the family, spouses or significant others, grandparents, friends, and the relationship with one's self need to be addressed.

PARENTS AND SIBLINGS

Other children in the family fare better when their needs are also recognized, when they are included in family decisions, and when they are spoken to openly and honestly about what has transpired and what is happening in their family. Explanations take time and need to be repeated and broadened as children grow and develop. Books written for and about sibling issues are available, and most professionals welcome brothers and sisters attending an occasional session so that they can become informed, participate if they care to, and "listen" through hearing aids. Siblings can help in very specific ways, thus alleviating some of the pressure felt by the parents. It is imperative to remember at all times, however, that the responsibility for the child who has hearing impairment, whether about lessons or care, does not lie with a sibling. In addition to making brothers and sisters feel welcome and important, professionals can offer correct, easy explanations embellished by pictures, filmstrips, and the actual apparatus that is used for testing, while providing answers to questions that help siblings respond when their friends ask them questions about hearing loss.

Professionals and parents can organize the "Sibling Days" devoted to the education and involvement of brothers and sisters. Age-appropriate information can be shared about facts and myths about hearing impairment, family adjustment issues, and coping techniques for specific situations. Children of all ages need to know that they are not responsible for their brother or sister's hearing impairment. They need to be reassured that their school performance, for example, is unrelated to their brother's or sister's. A 44-year-old teacher of children who have hearing impairment remembered her own household:

Everyone made such a fuss when Kristen did well in school. If she got a "B" it was cause for celebration. I was happy for her too, but sometimes I would have liked some recognition for my hard work. Granted, things came easier for me because I had my hearing, but school was still hard. I had a straight "A" report card throughout high school and it was as if it was expected. I was the model kid. I know my folks had enough on their minds. I didn't want to add to their heartache, so I never brought them my problems.

To help siblings face their own feelings, parents need to be encouraged to provide full, age-appropriate explanations, with emphasis on the feelings the family and siblings are experiencing. This is particularly beneficial when helping siblings deal with feelings of sadness, guilt, disappointment, confusion, anger, jealousy, overprotection, fear, embarrassment, responsibility, pride, love, comfort, interest, concern, tolerance, patience, and sympathy. Encouraging siblings to express their feelings is difficult for some parents, if they, themselves, have been avoiding their emotions. Allowing children to express their feelings is a gift.

It is also worthwhile to know the parents' perception of their normally hearing child's role in relation to the sibling who has hearing impairment. Is the parental perception communicated to the sibling? If so, by what means? If not, is this a problem for the sibling? Most children need to know that the feelings they are having are okay. Parents do not need to do anything except listen nonjudgementally and lovingly.

When parents attempt to deal openly with their own feelings related to having a child with a hearing loss, they are more likely to be able to address the issue with their other children. Some are unable to do this. One mother who was deep in grief interpreted her normal hearing daughter's "needy requests at bedtime" for "another glass of water and just one more story and please straighten out the dolls" as the daughter's willful attempt to be uncooperative and a pest. The daughter, however,

realized that this was the only time during the entire day that her mother spent any time alone with her. She was determined to extend those moments as long as she could, even if her mother became impatient with her. It was better than nothing.

One father observed that his only chance to be with his children occurred when he returned from work in the evening and on weekends. He tried to divide his time so that he could have separate time with each of the children while still maintaining family time:

I try to make everyone feel important, emphasizing not only what they do for themselves, but what they do for each other. I try to have them develop pride in how they help one another. Everyone gives to everyone else in this household. Dana teaches us things and we teach her things. That's just the way it is. I expect the same behavior out of all the kids. It is just harder to get Dana to understand what I expect. What's funny is that frequently, the older kids understand Dana better than I do, and they are the ones who help me understand what she is trying to say. I have to be careful though, that they are not always used as her interpreter. I don't want her to become too dependent on them. They really do look out for her though.

This father noticed many aspects of sibling interaction within his own family. Siblings in all families serve many roles—friends, playmates, caregivers, teachers, models, interpreters, socializers, and confidants. The challenge in families with children who have hearing impairment is to try to accentuate the positive aspects of sibling relationships, promote healthy bonding, while encouraging each child to develop his or her individuality and to feel good about themselves as valuable, contributing members of the family. Their role in the family is as important as any other child in the family. Their needs are as significant. When parents are unable to be totally available to all of their children, they can enlist the help of friends or family members who may be eager to help, but may not otherwise know what they can do.

GRANDPARENTS

Grandparents are often a source of support for families of children who have hearing impairment. Sometimes the diagnosis facilitates the healing of old family wounds because of the need. Like parents, grandparents also have expectations for their grandchildren. They, too, have dreams about their relationship and how it will develop. One woman said:

When my daughter was pregnant I fantasized about how I would tell my grandchild stories about our life before we came to America. My English isn't very good, so I thought I would teach her Spanish and she would become bilingual and travel with me to Mexico and meet her relatives. Now I worry that she will not understand me. How will I talk to her?

This grandmother needed reassurance that she was not inadequate. The love and caring that she wanted to give her granddaughter could still be transmitted effectively. She continued to talk to her granddaughter. Instead of withdrawing, she helped to encourage attendance at meetings of Spanish-speaking grandparents. Her involvement with her granddaughter was invaluable and a close relationship developed.

If grandparents live nearby, they can play a more consistent role in the lives of their grandchildren, especially in the case of single-parent households. Their support of their children and their "extra pair of hands" can, in some families, enable parents to cope successfully with their situation. It behooves the professional to understand the role that grandparents have undertaken and interact with them respectfully and in accordance with their position. When a grandparent cares for a child all day while the parent is at work, it is advisable that both the parent and the grandparent be involved in lessons and any informational sessions that may be scheduled. This important relationship between parents of the child who has hearing impairment and their own parents is one that is a potential source of support or one that is a potential source of stress. Without a doubt, it comes under scrutiny when a child is diagnosed as hearing impaired.

PARENT SELF-CARE

Encouraging parents of children who have hearing impairment, particularly mothers, to take care of themselves, physically, mentally, emotionally, and spiritually is of utmost importance. For women who work outside of their homes, the conflicts surrounding caring for their children and caring for themselves is profound. Arranging time off from work to attend professional meetings and appointments is frequently difficult and can cause distress, even with the most understanding employers and co-workers. One mother stated, "My performance on the job diminishes, and taking care of my own needs doesn't even make the list of 'things to do'." Another mother reflected:

My boss was wonderful to me when I discovered Hillary's hearing loss, but now I feel I have to make up the time. People assume that once you get hearing aids, and your child is enrolled in a program, your involvement is virtually over, and you can return to your 9 to 5 job. I feel apologetic when I ask for time off to visit school programs, audiologists, and to attend a mothers' group. The mothers' group is really for me and me alone, but I can't attend regularly because it meets in the daytime. Almost all of the things that I have to do for Jenny take place during working hours. Believe me, as much as I love my job, if I did not *have* to work I would not.

Single mothers are not the only ones who have difficulty with inflexible work schedules that clearly add to the stress in their lives. Every parent who works outside of the home needs to take into account the time it takes to travel between appointments. Professionals need to be as flexible as possible when scheduling sessions, if the goal is to have parents participate.

THE LONG PROCESS

PROFESSIONAL VERSUS PARENTAL EXPECTATIONS

Professionals are sometimes unaware of the time it takes for parents to see results and believe that a particular method will work for their child. Because auditory technology has come so far in the last several years, professionals in the field of hearing impairment have tremendous confidence in the value of hearing aids and auditory stimulation. This confidence is frequently conveyed to parents, but the context of an appropriate time frame is not. It is helpful to communicate a variety of examples illustrating the kinds of responses that have been observed with other children, so that the family has a framework within which to work. Many parents have no way of knowing that learning to attend auditorily is a process that takes years. As assurances cannot be given, parents are asked to proceed on faith. Professionals implore them to be patient.

However, it is not only parents who become impatient for their children to begin showing progress. Professionals, at times, have a specific time frame in which a parent's acceptance of the hearing loss is supposed to fit. At a meeting of several professionals who had contact with one family, one commented: "This mother has been denying her son's deafness long enough." Another added, in a particularly frustrated way, "I can't handle this father's anger any longer. He really should be moving on; he's known about his son's hearing loss for two years already!" Their frustration demonstrates that sometimes professionals have their own internal requirements for the "rate of recovery." But what about a mother who was doing fine with her daughter's deafness, in fact was the mother most often found comforting and helping other parents in a parent group? She was thrown into a tailspin when her mother died and she began mourning the loss of her daughter's hearing all over again. The knowledge that she was now on her own, without her own mother to take care of her (even though the mother had lived 2,000 miles away) was enough to stimulate her bereavement again. Subsequent losses are felt more severely; previous losses may be reexperienced more intensely.

COMING TO TERMS

It is imperative that both professionals and parents are mindful of the emotional seesaw of frustration, fear, anger, denial, recognition, and adaptation. Families who overidentify with their children may attribute to them aspects of life that may be inappropriate. "Deaf people are so isolated, Annie will never be able to make friends." This mother's comment reflects her own pain and does not take into consideration Annie's personality, ability to socialize, communicate, or interact. Coming to terms with one's own feelings as separate from those of one's child and the child's situation takes time and experience. Accepting one's feelings, no matter what they are, is imperative to establishing a healthy relationship with one's self and one's loved ones, especially one's children. Acceptance of one's feelings is a positive precursor to acceptance of one's situation. Adapting to life with a child who has hearing impairment means accepting change. By nature, some of us do this better than others, but all of us have the ability to learn.

SUMMARY

There are numerous and varied aspects to the adjustment to life with a child who has hearing impairment. Parents and professionals need to work together to help families find a balance that suits them. Whole families can learn much about themselves as individuals and as a family unit. Among the many challenges they face is that of discovering and tapping their inner resources. This is a long process requiring courage, strength, and patience.

REFERENCES

Atkins, D. (1987). Siblings of the hearing-impaired: Perspectives for parents. In D. Atkins (Ed.) *Families and their hearing impaired children* (pp. 32–45). Washington, DC: Volta Bureau.

Bevan, R. (1988). *Hearing-impaired children: A guide for concerned parents and professionals* (pp. 3–13). Springfield, IL: Charles C. Thomas.

Buscalia, L. (1975). *The disabled and their parents: A counseling challenge.* Thorofare, NJ: C. B. Slack.

Clark, J. (1990, Spring/Summer). Counseling in communicative disorders: A responsibility to be met. *Hearsay, 12,* 4–7.

Clark, J., & Martin, F. (1994) *Effective counseling in audiology: Perspectives and practice.* Englewood Cliffs, NJ: Prentice Hall.

Erikson, E. (1964). *Childhood and society.* New York: W.W. Norton.

Estabrooks, W. (Ed.) (1994). *Auditory/verbal therapy for parents and professionals.* Washington, DC: Alexander Graham Bell Association for the Deaf.

Featherstone, H. (1980). *A difference in the family: Life with a disabled child.* New York: Basic Books.

Forecki, M. (1985). *Speak to me.* Washington, DC: Gallaudet College Press.

Harvey, M. (1989). *Psychotherapy with deaf and hard-of-hearing persons.* Hillsdale, NJ: Lawrence Erlbaum.

Keller, H. (1954). *The story of my life.* Garden City, NY: Doubleday. [Originally published 1903].

Kroth, R. (1987). Mixed or missed messages between parents and professionals. In D. Atkins (Ed.) *Families and their hearing impaired children* (pp. 1–10). Washington, DC: Volta Bureau.

Kübler-Ross, E. (1969). *On death and dying.* New York: Macmillan.

Leigh, I. (1987). Parenting and the hearing impaired: Attachment and coping. In D. Atkins (Ed.) *Families and their hearing impaired children* (pp. 11–21). Washing-ton, DC: Volta Bureau.

Luterman, D. (1979). *Counseling parents of hearing-impaired children.* Boston: Little Brown.

Miller, N. (1994). *Nobody's perfect.* Baltimore: Paul H. Brookes Publishing Co.

Moses, K. (1985). Infant deafness and parental grief: Psychosocial early intervention. In F. Powell, T. Finitzo-Hieber, S. Friel-Patti, & D. Henderson (Eds.), *Education of the hearing-impaired child* (pp. 115–127). San Diego, CA: College-Hill Press.

Rollin, W. (1987). *The psychology of communication disorders in individuals and their families.* Englewood Cliffs, NJ: Prentice-Hall.

Yacobacci-Tam, P. (1987). Interacting with the culturally different child. In D. Atkins (Ed.) *Families and their hearing impaired children* (pp. 46–58). Washington, DC: Volta Bureau.

END OF CHAPTER EXAMINATION QUESTIONS

CHAPTER 5

1. From the information in this chapter, describe what *is* and *is not* the role of the professional when navigating parents of a disabled child.

2. A professional should not _____.

   a. encourage

   b. be hopeful

   c. be positive in spirit

   d. promise outcomes of services

3. Briefly describe "systems theory" in counseling.

4. A "role organization crisis"

   a. causes family members to become dissatisfied with family relationships

   b. causes elevated tension

   c. causes siblings to take on additional responsibilities

   d. causes family members to adjust to a disability

5. What is the goal of the audiologist in counseling the family of a hearing impaired individual?

6. Name the four stages of adaptation experienced by parents of children with disabilities.

   a. _____

   b. _____

   c. _____

   d. _____

END OF CHAPTER ANSWER SHEET

Name _____ Date _____

CHAPTER 5

1. _____

   _____

   _____

2. Which one?   a   b   c   d

3. _____

   _____

   _____

4. Which one?   a   b   c   d

5. _____

   _____

   _____

6. Which one?   a   b   c   d

7. Which one?   a   b   c   d

8. _____

   _____

   _____

9. _____

10. Which one?   a   b   c   d

7. A message the audiologist should stress to the parent of a hearing impaired child is:

   a. child first and foremost

   b. focus mainly on the child's impairment

   c. a structured language setting is not necessary for language development

   d. both a and b

8. Briefly describe why parent support groups and family involvement are important when coping and dealing with a disabled child.

9. Professionals must be _____ when scheduling sessions if the goal is to have parent participation.

10. A way for parents to "come to terms" with their child's disability is to:

    a. identify with their child's disability

    b. accept their feelings as their own

    c. show patience only as needed

    d. not separate parent/child feelings

Considerations and Strategies for Amplification for Children Who Are Hearing Impaired

■   WILLIAM R. HODGSON, Ph.D.   ■

Children who wear hearing aids are not a homogeneous group. There is a world of difference between the needs of a child with profound congenital hearing loss, an older child with acquired sensorineural loss, and a child with a small, fluctuating conductive loss. A child with profound congenital loss faces an almost insurmountable obstacle of learning to use minimal residual hearing and of acquiring speech and language through the use of partial auditory clues to supplement those available through vision. An older child with sensorineural loss, although having the advantage of normal language and speech, faces social stigma associated with hearing loss and hearing aid use, and the task of learning in a noisy classroom with an impaired sensory system. The child with small hearing loss, perhaps a fluctuating conductive disorder, may have the handicap unrecognized, misunderstood, or underestimated and there may be difficulty developing the discipline required for effective hearing aid use.

Because children with congenital losses are the most visible and perhaps the most common of this disparate group, the majority of this chapter is devoted to them. However, attention is also given to the very different but also severe problems of children in the other two groups.

During the last 20 years, significant changes have occurred in the etiologies of hearing losses in children. Hearing losses from maternal rubella and problems associated with RH-factor incompatibility have been substantially reduced. The prevalence of hearing losses from unknown causes remains at 40% of identified cases (Upfold, 1988). Increased availability of genetic counseling may have had some impact on the prevalence of hereditary disorders. These factors have led to a reduction in the number of severe and profound hearing losses and the proportional increase in the number of mild and moderate losses. The latter are not being identified and aided at an early enough age (Matkin, 1984).

Significant improvements have been made in miniaturization and flexibility of hearing aids. Digital and programmable hearing aids have improved accuracy and flexibility of fitting, but still amplify unwanted noise along with the desired speech signal. Better identification procedures for children with smaller hearing losses, better techniques for preventing hearing losses, and smarter hearing aids are goals to work for in the immediate future.

EARLY IDENTIFICATION AND ADEQUATE EVALUATION

Amplification is the foundation on which the structure of aural habilitation for hearing-impaired children is built. If the structure is to be sound, the hearing loss must be detected early in life, so children can learn the meaning and utility of sound, can develop language and speech, and can acquire an education—although all auditory stimuli are filtered through an impaired sensory system. Therefore, the impact of an impairment must be minimized as early as possible through amplification, stimulation, and training in use of residual hearing.

Additionally, early identification is vital to provide time for parents to progress through a sequence of events commonly reported to occur in the parents of hearing-impaired children. Those include disbelief, grief, anger, and acceptance. Because of the crucial role parents must play in habilitation of a hearing-impaired child, they must also have time to acquire the knowledge that will make them an effective part of the aural habilitation team.

As cochlear implants continue to improve, parents are faced with an early decision to consider an implant versus conventional amplification. Issues include the greater cost of the implant, the long-term intensive training vital to an implant program, and the difficulty of preoperatively predicting the degree of success. On the positive side is the possibility of achieving better understanding of speech than would be likely with conventional hearing aids. It is important that a team of professionals evaluate each child and educate parents in the process of deciding which habilitation route to take.

IMPORTANCE OF EARLY AMPLIFICATION

The negative effects of sensory deprivation in children born with profound hearing loss may be both physiologic and behavioral. Evans, Webster, and Cullen (1983) reported incomplete maturation in the central auditory nervous system associated with auditory deprivation in animals. An "unaided ear effect" has been established in children with bilateral hearing losses who are fitted monaurally versus binaurally. Hurley (1999) reported significant reduction in word recognition ability in subjects' unaided ears relative to scores in the aided ears. The delay in language, speech, and educational development in children with congenital hearing losses is well documented (Northern & Downs, 1991).

Children who acquire hearing loss may also experience delay in language, speech, and educational development dating from the onset of the loss. The time between onset of loss and the fitting of amplification may increase resistance to acceptance of amplification. Because of all these factors, fitting and use of amplification must begin as soon as possible. A prerequisite for use of amplification is detection and evaluation of the hearing loss.

STRATEGIES FOR IDENTIFICATION AND EVALUATION

Physiologic measures, such as auditory brainstem response (ABR) testing and otoacoustic emissions (OAE) testing provide the most accurate results in infants under 6 months of age (ASHA, 1997). These measures add materially to the quantification of hearing loss in young children (Harrison & Norton, 1999; Jacobson, 1985). Beyond 6 months of age, behavioral methods for the identification and

evaluation of hearing loss in infants and young children become increasingly useful and include conditioned orientation reflex audiometry (Suzuki & Ogiba, 1961), visual reinforcement audiometry (Liden & Kankkunen, 1969), and conditioned play audiometry. These techniques have the advantages of eliciting frequency-specific information and of being applicable to either unaided or aided testing. Therefore, in addition to quantification of the hearing loss, the amount of functional gain delivered by a hearing aid can be evaluated. Using behavioral assessment methods, Wilson and Thompson (1984) established that reliable estimations of hearing status can be established for children under 1 year of age.

Although skilled clinicians experienced in the evaluation of young children can obtain useful estimates of hearing sensitivity, evaluation is an ongoing process involving continued refinement of original estimates (Figure 6–1). Final determination of the exact extent and fine details of an auditory impairment for each ear is usually not completed until a child is 2 or 3 years of age. This consideration calls for fitting of hearing aids that are flexible enough to be modified appropriately as more is learned about a child's hearing loss.

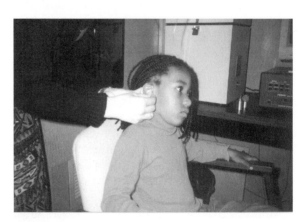

Figure 6–1. Great skill is required to correctly fit a child with a hearing aid.

Fortunately, hearing aids that can be substantially modified in gain, maximum output, and frequency response are available and should be used when fitting young children.

Immittance measures also help to identify the presence of conductive components, as well as giving information about the sensorineural system (Guidelines for screening, 1989). In addition to usefulness in the initial diagnostic process, immittance measures should always be part of ongoing audiologic monitoring to detect development of conductive disorders that may require treatment and that can render an otherwise appropriate hearing aid fitting inadequate. When a hearing-impaired child is identified, language development should be evaluated. This information may be useful in estimating the degree of handicap associated with the hearing loss and in mild hearing loss may help to suggest whether or not a hearing aid is needed. Information regarding language development can be solicited from parents or teachers and receptive language level can be assessed by a scale such as the revised Peabody Picture Vocabulary Test (Dunn & Dunn, 1981).

The clinician should also be alert for the possibility of impairments in addition to hearing loss that may complicate the aural habilitation plan. Wolff and Harkins (1986) reported additional problems such as visual impairment, mental retardation, and learning disabilities in 30% of hearing-impaired children. A parent questionnaire, such as the Min-nesota Child Development Inventory Profile (Ireton & Thwing, 1974), provides information about gross development, motor development, self-help ability, and personal-social development, in addition to receptive and expressive language development. Low profiles in areas outside language development indicate the need for additional evaluation to explore for the possibility of multiple handicaps.

Children with significant hearing losses must learn to use vision for clues that a defective auditory system cannot provide. For this reason, screening of a child's visual acuity is important and good visual health care must be maintained. This consideration is particularly important, as some causes of hearing loss are also associated with visual abnormalities.

It is important that preschoolers and children in regular classes from kindergarten onward enjoy a good hearing conservation program designed to prevent the development of hearing loss (through awareness of the hazard of noise exposure, for example). Screening audiometry is part of a good school hearing conservation program for identifying hearing losses that develop during the school years (Guidelines for identification audiometry, 1985). School hearing conservation programs are also still needed for another purpose: to detect unilateral as well as small, long-standing hearing losses that may be undetected until a child starts school.

PARENT COUNSELING AND EDUCATION

Without the understanding, acceptance, and commitment of parents or other primary caregivers, aural habilitation of a hearing-impaired child cannot be successful. First, parents must understand the nature and implications of hearing loss. Hearing is generally taken for granted and the general public knows substantially nothing about how ears function. Parents must learn how the ear works and what can go wrong to understand their child's hearing problem. Carney and Moeller (1998) reviewed studies that found that family counseling enhanced realization of treatment goals for children with hearing impairment.

Early reactions of parents to the statement that their child has hearing impairment are likely to be emotionally driven and result in rejection of the statement, as well as feelings of doubt, anxiety, and guilt. A starting point for reducing these negative emotions is an explanation of auditory function, along with discussion of the potential of residual hearing to be realized through successful aural habilitation. The advantages and limitations of amplification must be thoroughly discussed, for parents will know nothing more of hearing aids than they know of the basic auditory processes.

Many questions must be answered regarding groundless fears that parents may have. Parents should be assured that there is no causal relationship between deafness and intelligence. Research indicates a similar distribution of performance IQ scores in the hearing-impaired and hearing populations (Vernon, 1968). Audiologists should keep in mind, however, that hearing loss associated with some etiologies may be accompanied by brain damage or other organic disorders. For example, these problems have been substantiated in meningitis and the postmaternal viral syndromes (Mindel & Vernon, 1987).

In addition, parents should be made aware of the genetic origin of some hearing disorders. Hopefully, those who carry these traits will learn about the probabilities of having hearing-impaired children. In this way, they can make an informed decision.

Positive professional support and encouragement must accompany instruction as parents learn to accept a hearing problem and commit themselves to a long-term program of aural habilitation. Development of a goal-oriented program that includes the acquisition and successful use of hearing aids can reduce the anxiety, guilt, and feeling of helplessness as parents learn about hearing loss and what can be done.

HEARING AID EVALUATION AND FITTING

After hearing evaluation has established hearing levels, the next step before hearing aid fitting is medical clearance. Hearing aids are currently classified as medical devices and federal regulations require medical clearance prior to fitting hearing aids on children (Food & Drug Administration, 1977). This regulation should be conscientiously followed to facilitate the general otologic health of each child, to look for correctable disorders, and to establish that there are no medical contraindications for hearing aid use. Following the initial medical examination and fitting of hearing aids, regular otologic examinations should be part of the aural habilitation plan. This practice will help to ensure good otologic health and reduce the probability of encroaching conductive disorders: for example, ear wax or middle ear problems, which can cause further damage to a child's hearing or render the selected amplification units inadequate.

SELECTING ELECTROACOUSTIC CHARACTERISTICS FOR CHILDREN

Several prescriptive procedures designed to specify overall gain, gain-versus-frequency, and maximum output have been developed for use in fitting linear hearing aids. Most incorporate modification of the half-gain rule suggested by Lybarger (1963), who observed that adults with sensorineural loss preferred hearing aid gain that amounted to about one-half of their hearing loss. Subsequently, other individuals (Berger, Hagberg, & Rane, 1977; Byrne & Tonisson, 1976; McCandless & Lyregaard, 1983) modified the half-gain rule to reduce overamplification of low frequencies and to make other adjustments to maximize audibility of speech.

With the increase of hearing aids that use various kinds of compression amplification, newer procedures have been developed. For example, Cornelisse, Seewald, and Jamieson (1995) and Dillon (1999) reported strategies for fitting nonlinear hearing aids. Additionally, various computer software programs are available to facilitate hearing aid fitting. In general terms, all of the procedures aim to make as much as possible of the aided speech spectrum comfortably audible. This goal is clearly important for children learning new vocabulary on a daily basis.

MODIFICATIONS OF PRESCRIPTIVE PROCEDURES FOR CHILDREN

Each prescriptive procedure can be adapted for use in hearing aid evaluation and selection for children, although some call for loudness judgments that very young children cannot make. The following paragraphs suggest ways in which prescriptive procedures designed for adults can be modified to be appropriate for evaluation for children.

Probe-Tube Microphone Measurements

Of particular interest in evaluating the function of hearing aids on children is the use of probe-tube microphone measurements. Once a hearing loss is established and a hearing aid is selected, the probe-tube system can be used as an objective measurement to quickly and definitively determine the real-ear performance of the hearing aid. Desired changes in response can then be made and again measured, with the process continuing until the ideal response is realized (Figure 6–2). These measures are much faster than behavioral testing, during which a child may become restless, and inattentive before the evaluation is completed. Hawkins, Morrison, Halligan, and Cooper (1989) have presented a plan to use probe-tube microphone measurements to evaluate hearing aids in children. They reported success in their goal of amplifying and packaging the long-term speech spectrum into a child's residual hearing.

Electroacoustic Performance

The relationship between hearing aid electroacoustic performance as measured in the 2 cm³ coupler and the human ear is not very good when adult ears are considered, because of coupler-real ear differences. This disparity may be increased in a child's ear (Seewald & Scollie, 1999). Because of the smaller size of a child's ear canal relative to the adult, greater sound pressure levels (SPLs) will be generated in a child's aided canal. Jirsa and Norris (1978) reported SPLs about 5 dB greater in the canals of preschool children relative to that of adults. Although these values may be accurate on average, they cannot account for the considerable variability in the volume of ear canals of different children. A decided advantage of probe-tube measures in hearing aid evaluations is the measure of the SPLs actually generated in ear canals under aided conditions. Actual real-ear measurements may be difficult to obtain in infants and very young children because of movement and vocalization. Moodie, Seewald, and Sinclair (1994) described an alternative method for predicting real ear hearing aid performance in young children, employing real ear-to-coupler transformation values.

Amplification-Induced Threshold Shift

There appears to be a remote possibility of further change in the hearing of children who wear hearing aids because of exposure to high sound levels. Sporadic accounts of individual cases appear in the literature. Rintelmann and Bess (1977) surveyed the literature on this topic and conducted their

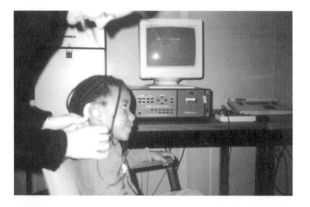

Figure 6–2. A child having real-ear measurements conducted on her hearing aid.

own investigation. They concluded that sufficient evidence existed regarding isolated instances of amplification-induced threshold shift to justify careful limitation of maximum outputs according to the degree of loss and to emphasize the importance of careful audiologic monitoring. Subsequently, a federal regulation was enacted requiring a warning to accompany hearing aids whose maximum output exceeds 132 dB SPL, that the hearing aid may be hazardous to residual hearing (Food & Drug Administration, 1977).

Concerned about the possibility of damage to a hearing-impaired child's remaining hearing through amplification-induced threshold shift, Matkin (1986) recommended the following SPL limits for maximum output of hearing aids: (1) with profound loss, 125 dB; (2) moderate loss, 120 dB; and (3) mild loss, 110 dB. He further recommended that 5 dB be subtracted from these values when fitting preschool children. More specifically, Skinner (1988) recommended that 6 dB be subtracted from the otherwise appropriate maximum output for infants to 2 years of age and that 3 dB be subtracted for children between the ages of 2

and 5. It should be noted that Kawell, Kopun, and Stelmachowicz (1988), in a study of LDLs in children, did not find systematic differences between children older than 7 years and adults, and concluded that there may be no reason to reduce maximum output of the hearing aid for older children beyond the levels necessary for adults.

Maximum Discomfort Levels

Maximum output values are usually selected when fitting hearing aids for adults by determining loudness discomfort levels (LDLs) and selecting output levels below a patient's LDL. Young children cannot report LDLs reliably and it may be necessary to select output values based on those found to be uncomfortable on subjects with loss of hearing sensitivity comparable to that of the child in question. Estimated levels may be obtained by reference to the average LDLs obtained from subjects as a function of the magnitude of sensorineural loss. LDLs from one study (Kamm, Dirks, & Mickey, 1978) are shown in Table 6–1. It should be remembered that these are values from adult sub-

TABLE 6–1. SPLs at 25, 50, and 75 Percentile for LDLs in 178 Subjects with Sensorineural Hearing Loss (Adapted from Kamm et al., 1978)

Stimulus	Hearing Threshold in dB HL re: 1969 ANSI Norms				
	10 dB or better	11–30 dB	31–50 dB	51–70 dB	Greater than 70 dB
500 Hz					
75%	115.5	113.4	117.0	>124	>124
50%	106.5	109.1	106.0	120.0	>124
25%	97.5	102.5	100.5	115.5	>124
2000 Hz					
75%	108.0	115.0	108.6	>124	>124
50%	102.0	104.3	102.4	112.3	121.5
25%	97.5	98.4	98.0	108.0	114.0

Source: Adapted from Effect of Sensori-neural Hearing Loss on Loudness Discomfort Level by C. Kamm, D. Dirks, and R. Mickey, 1978. *Journal of Speech and Hearing Research, 21,* 668–681.

jects and appropriate corrections should be made, as previously discussed. In addition, the investigators reported considerable variability in LDL for subjects in each hearing loss group, necessitating caution when using the averages to limit hearing aid output.

Finally, it should be noted that appropriate procedures may permit assessment of LDL in older children. Kawell et al. (1988) reported reasonably reliable LDL measures on children as young as seven years. They used five loudness categories from "too soft" to "hurts." Although listening to signals at various levels, children judged loudness by pointing to pictures of human faces whose expressions represented typical reactions to each of the five loudness levels.

BINAURAL AMPLIFICATION

It is generally recognized that most adults with bilateral hearing loss and aidable hearing in each ear perform better with two aids than with one. Advantages include improved localization ability, reduction of the head shadow effect one obtains with one hearing aid, improved audibility of speech in noise (the squelch effect), more natural "three-dimensional" sound quality, and the ability to set the volume controls at a lower level because of binaural summation (about 5 dB, according to Byrne, 1981). However, some hearing-impaired individuals appear to function better with one hearing aid than with two, possibly because of defects in the central auditory system that prevent the interaction of signals coming from each ear as they ascend in the central pathways.

Adults may be able to judge whether they function better with two aids, but small children cannot. Skinner (1988) suggests careful observation while a child is aided with one versus two aids to evaluate the ability to localize and to respond to speech with each aid alone, plus language and speech development during trial periods of monaural and binaural amplification.

As mentioned earlier, evidence is accruing that a hearing impaired ear, left unaided, may be subject to deterioration in word recognition ability as a result of auditory deprivation. Silverman and Silman (1990) reported that in two adult cases there was a reduction over time in word recognition scores in the unaided ears relative to the performance of the aided ears. Moreover, on eventual binaural fitting, there was significant improvement in the performance of the previously unaided ears. Additionally, Gelfand and Silman (1993) reported a reduction in word recognition scores in the unaided ears of a group of monaurally fitted subjects, whereas they observed no such reduction in the ears of a similar group of binaurally fitted subjects.

TYPE OF HEARING AID

Conventional Hearing Aids

As is the case with adults, when fitting children, decisions must be made about the type or style of hearing aids. Concern about cosmetics plays a large role when adults are fitted. The same will be true for older children and for the parents of younger children. This concern must be considered, for aids considered stigmatic may not be worn. However, every attempt should be made to reduce these concerns on the part of a child and parents, so that appropriate amplification is the primary basis on which the decision of hearing aid type is made.

Beauchaine, Barlow, and Stelmachowicz (1990) point out that behind-the-ear hearing aids are ideal to meet many of the special amplification needs of children, in that they permit frequent earmold remakes, simplify provision of loaner instruments, provide strong telecoils and connections for direct audio input, and are available with directional microphones. Today, behind-the-ear aids are available with sufficient power and flexibility to fit most hearing losses. They offer the advantage of ear-level hearing, which may be important in binaural functions and reduction of clothing noises and cord problems previously associated with body-type aids. However for the very young child, it is easier for parents to see and manipulate controls of body aids. Body-type amplification is more feasible for an infant before the child sits and walks. For the child who requires extremely high gain, serious feedback problems may limit effective am-plification if behind-the-ear aids are used. For example, Matkin (1984) reported that 8 of 11 preschoolers surveyed were receiving inadequate gain from ear-level aids, because the volume controls were turned down to avoid feedback problems.

To receive maximum gain without feedback, earmolds must be well designed and frequently replaced. Full-shell earmolds should be used and earmolds made of soft material are reported to reduce feedback problems (Seewald & Ross, 1988). Additionally, soft earmolds reduce the risk of injury, if a child falls or is struck on the head. Especially with ear-level aids, frequent replacement of earmolds is necessary to maintain adequate gain without feedback. Constant monitoring of gain and earmold adequacy is necessary. Matkin (1984) suggests that children younger than 3 may need new earmolds at 3-month intervals to maintain an adequate seal.

As children grow older, particularly as they approach adolescence and changes in size and shape of the external ear are reduced, cosmetic concerns may lead them to ask for in-the-ear aids. Such a change is justifiable, if the hearing loss is appropriate for this type of aid, remembering that in-the-ear aids generally do not provide as much overall gain or high-frequency amplification without feedback and that the cost of recasing in-the-ear aids as a youngster's ear changes shape and size is greater than that of replacing earmolds.

Non-Hearing Aid Assistive Listening Devices For Children

Hearing-impaired children, especially those with more serious losses, should not be confined to con-ventional, wearable amplification. Systems used in the classroom and others designed for personal use and generally classified as "assistive listening devices" are designed to improve signal-to-noise ratio and reduce effects of reverberation by moving a system's microphone closer to the person who is speaking.

Examples include the **FM radio transmitting-receiving unit** designed for either classroom or personal use. Behind-the-ear hearing aids are now available with built-in FM receivers so that the aid can be used as a conventional amplifier, as an FM receiver only, or with both input modes activated. In the latter case, a child can hear his or her own amplified voice while still maintaining a favorable signal-to-noise ratio for the primary signal. Another common unit is the **induction loop** system, which sends an electromagnetic signal from a person speaking to a child's hearing aid. It is necessary that the selected hearing aids be compatible with the classroom or personal units that are used. That is, if an induction loop system is to be used in the class or in the home, the child's hearing aids must have induction coils ("telephone switches, or T-coils") that pick up the electromagnetic signals. These coils should be evaluated to ensure appropriate function, as hearing aids may operate quite differently with induction coil function than when the microphone is the input transducer.

The child's hearing aids should have input jacks to hardwired external microphones that can be located close to the mouth of the person speaking. An example of such an aid, with direct audio input via an external microphone, is shown in Figure 6–3. The result will be vastly improved signal-to-noise ratio, when the hardwired arrangement is feasible. Moreover, when FM transmitting-receiving units are used, the hearing aid can be wired directly to the FM receiver output. Alternatively, a neck-worn loop can deliver the signal to a hearing aids' induction coils via electromagnetic energy, but the hardwired arrangement is preferable, as each additional transduction of the signal increases the chances for reduced quality or increased noise.

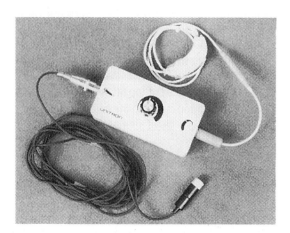

Figure 6–3. Hearing aid with "hardwired" external microphone. (Courtesy of Unitron Industries.)

Consistent with a child's age and auditory needs, other assistive devices, such as **telephone and television aids,** should be introduced. The former may consist of telephone amplifiers or visible print-outs of telephone messages (TTDs). In the latter case, various systems improve pickup of TV audio. The signal may be sent directly to a child's amplification system via hardwire, FM, or induction loop. These arrangements avoid amplification of room noise. For more severely impaired children a **close-captioned decoder** will reveal on the TV tube the printed subtitles that are available on many TV programs as appropriate. A complete amplification program should consider these, and many other alerting, warning, and auditory devices which are available.

LEARNING EFFECTIVE HEARING AID USE

Three principles ensure effective hearing aid use by a child: (1) the parents must learn how to operate and care for hearing aids; (2) the child must learn and assume responsibility for hearing aid use and care, learning as soon as possible optimum setting of controls and reporting of hearing aid problems; and (3) an effective monitoring system must be in place involving the audiologist, the parents, the child, and others, such as teachers, who are a part of the aural habilitation team.

DUTIES OF PARENTS AND CHILDREN

Parents, and children as they are able, must become aware of the physical components and functioning of a hearing aid. They must learn to operate the switches, rotate the volume control, and replace the battery. Prior to first hearing aid use, all concerned should be warned of the toxic nature of batteries and the danger of accidental ingestion. Parents should be instructed to call their doctor if a battery is accidentally swallowed and should be given the National Battery Hotline number, (202) 625-3333, which they can call for help.

Parents must learn how to place the earmold in the ear and remove it. They should be assisted in teaching their child to assume this responsibility as early as possible.

Care and maintenance of the aid and troubleshooting of simple problems must be learned by the parents and assumed by the child in a graduated fashion, beginning with the concept of responsibility for the hearing aids.

Beyond learning the physical aspects of hearing aid manipulation and care, parents and the child must learn good hearing aid use through effective listening strategies. They must learn to survey the environment and assess factors that contribute to or detract from successful communication. They must learn to help the hearing aid by moving closer to desired speech signals and further away from interfering noises. They must learn to reduce background noise levels when possible, and to adjust hearing aids' volume controls for maximum intelligibility in various noise levels. They must even learn the degree of assertiveness necessary to inform those who talk to them of the presence of the hearing loss and how to improve communication by getting the hearing impaired child's attention before speaking, limiting conversation to line-of-sight situations when possible, speaking more slowly, and interpreting signs that indicate if these strategies to improve communication are being successful or if additional effort is needed.

Of vital importance, a program of hearing aid monitoring must be developed involving the audiologist, the parents, the child, and others who are in frequent contact. With remarkable consistency, surveys taken over the years to determine how well hearing aids worn by children are functioning have shown that at any given time about half of them were defective or set inappropriately (Blair, Wright, & Pollard, 1981; Gaeth & Lounsbury, 1966; Porter, 1973).

These surveys also suggest little knowledge on the part of parents about hearing aid function. For example, in the early Gaeth and Lounsbury study, when asked how long the batteries in the child's aid lasted, 9% of the parents answered longer than a year. 11% were more honest and admitted that they didn't know. Although it is of great importance that parents learn to monitor the hearing aids and help to keep them operating well, it is most critical that a child learn to assume this responsibility, as the wearer is the only person who can monitor hearing aids full-time.

The guide provided in Table 6–2 may be helpful to assist parents in a daily check of the child's hearing aids, and, in addition, whenever problems are suspected. Initially, the audiologist should instruct parents and provide supervised practice in this hearing aid check, and parents should instruct

TABLE 6–2. The Hearing Aid Check.

1. *Visual inspection of aid, tubing, and earmold.* Each should be clean and free of wax. All can be wiped clean with a dry tissue. The earmold and tubing can be removed from the earhook of the aid, washed in warm soapy water, rinsed, and dried completely. Afterwards, the earhook, not the hearing aid, should be held firmly while the tubing is replaced. If the tubing is discolored, cracked, dry and brittle, or loose where it fits into the earmold or onto the earhook, a trip to the dispenser is needed to replace the tubing.

2. *Battery check.* The battery should deliver its specified voltage, which can be learned from the dispenser, and discarded if this is not the case. It should be free of corrosion, as should be the battery case.

3. *Listening check on the parental ear.* Using the hearing aid stethoscope or a custom earmold, the parent should ascertain that speech is understandable through the aid, that speech quality has not deteriorated from its usual level, that there are no unexpected noises generated by the aid, and that the expected loudness is delivered when the volume control is rotated. While turning the volume control, the parent should ascertain that there are no scratchy noises or dead spots. Speech should smoothly grow louder as the volume control is rotated. The parent should tap the case of the aid and listen for intermittency, suggesting loose battery contacts. Additionally, with body aids, the cord where it inserts into the aid and into the earphone should be twisted gently, for the same purpose. Problems in any of these areas necessitates a visit to the dispenser.

4. *Listening check on the child's ear.* Separately, each aid should be inserted and the volume control rotated to the level recommended by the audiologist. Feedback (squealing) should not occur. Parents should learn that feedback results when too much sound leaks out of the aided ear canal and re-enters the hearing aid microphone. Causes of feedback at recommended volume control setting are: (1) wax in the ear canal that reflects too much sound back to the hearing aid; (2) an incompletely inserted earmold; (3) loose connections along the sound delivery route between hearing aid, earhook, tubing, and earmold; (4) an earmold that no longer fits well enough to create an adequate seal; and (5) internal, which occurs when the acoustic isolation between the hearing aid microphone and earphone is destroyed. Additionally, feedback can occur momentarily when a hand is cupped over the hearing aid or the child stands close to a wall or other reflecting surface. The listening check on the child's ear should be completed by making sure the child can hear and understand speech in the usual fashion, consistent with the amount of hearing loss which is present.

the child to assume this responsibility if normal hearing is not a requisite.

Some equipment is needed for this hearing aid check. For listening to the hearing aid, the parent will need a hearing aid stethoscope or a custom earmold that fits the parental ear. These are shown in Figure 6–4. A voltmeter for testing the battery is useful. Batteries have been improved until they deliver almost their full voltage until near the end of their life and then die suddenly. Therefore a battery that delivers anything less than its specified voltage should be discarded and spare batteries should always be carried, in case a battery dies between hearing aid checks. Figure 6–5 illustrates an inexpensive battery tester. As shown in Figure 6–6, a small brush and a wire loop may be helpful to remove accumulated wax from the sound channel of the earmold. Also illustrated is a hand syringe, which is useful to dry out tubing after the earmold has been removed and washed. Fluids other than water should not be used on the earmold and, of course, the hearing aid, itself, should never be exposed to fluids of any kind.

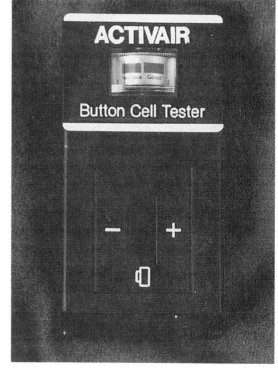

Figure 6–5. Battery tester. (Courtesy of Activar.)

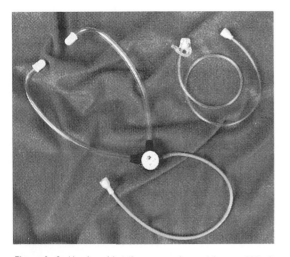

Figure 6–4. Hearing aid stethoscope and parental ear mold for hearing aid listening check. (Courtesy of Hal-Hen.)

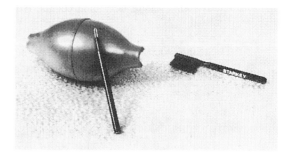

Figure 6–6. Brush and wire loop for removing wax from ear mold and hand syringe for cleaning water and debris from ear mold tubing. (Courtesy of Starkey Electronics.)

Parents must learn, and assist their child in learning, simple hearing aid troubleshooting procedures that may correct some problems and prevent a visit to the dispenser when problems arise. Some of these are presented in Table 6–3. Parents should not try to go beyond these simple procedures and should never attempt to open the case to repair the aid.

Finally, as hearing aids are expensive and repairs or replacement are costly, parents and the child must learn certain fundamentals of care and maintenance. Some of these are detailed in Table 6–4.

SUMMARY

For children born with hearing loss, early identification and amplification are crucial, since amplification is the foundation on which aural habilitation is built. Today, behavioral and electrophysiological test batteries can reliably establish the existence of hearing loss even in infants, and estimate magni-

TABLE 6–3. Hearing Aid Troubleshooting.

Symptom	Possible Causes
No sound	Off-on switch may be set to off or to the T-coil (telephone) position. Battery may be wrong kind, dead, or inserted backwards. Corrosion on the battery contacts may be responsible and may be cleaned gently. There may be a mechanical blockage of the sound route, such as perspiration in the tubing, which may be dried with a hand syringe after the tubing is removed from the earmold. Aids fitted with acoustic filters are particularly prone to this problem, as the filter consists of a very small opening that is easily blocked. If the problem persists, a drying kit can be purchased, into which the aid can be placed each night. The earmold sound channel may be blocked by wax, which can be removed with the wire loop described earlier. It is possible, with the aid on the ear, that a kink or twist may close the tubing and block sound, necessitating correct placement or a new tube.
Weak sound	Weak battery, sound channel partially blocked by moisture or wax, or the tubing may be bent partially closed. These problems can usually be corrected by the parents. If these causes are not evident, there may be an internal problem requiring repair by the dispenser.
Intermittent sound	Loose battery caused by bent contacts. With body aids, broken cords or loose connections may be the problem. Solutions are best left to the dispenser.
Loudness does not change appropriately as volume control is rotated. Volume control rotation may be accompanied by noise, no change in loudness, or a sudden loudness at a given rotation.	Dirty or broken volume control, requiring repair by the dispenser.
Unnatural sound quality or noise	Remembering that all hearing aids sound different than unamplified speech and that some audible noise is present in normal function, the parent must learn to discern abnormalities that develop. Dirty controls can produce noise and turning them back and forth may dislodge the dirt responsible for the problem. Unnatural sound quality may result from a nearly dead battery or from an inappropriately set tone control. Other noise and quality problems require attention by the dispenser.
Feedback (squealing)	Earmold incompletely inserted, volume control set above recommended level, loose connections between earhook, tubing, and earmold. These problems may be solvable by the parents. Other causes of feedback, for which parents must seek help, are wax in the ear canal and poorly fitting earmolds. Internal feedback can be diagnosed by removing the earhook and holding a finger over the sound outlet while rotating the volume control on. If the feedback is internal, the squealing will persist.

TABLE 6–4. Hearing Aid Care and Maintenance.

1. Do not drop the aid. Today's hearing aids are more resistant to shock than earlier models, but a long fall onto a hard surface may damage the case or contents. It is a good practice to sit on the bed or other soft surface when inserting or removing the aid.

2. Moisture, heat, and dirt damage hearing aids. Therefore, the aid should be removed before taking showers or applying hair spray. If the child forgets and takes a dip in the pool while wearing the aid, a trip to the dispenser is necessary. As mentioned elsewhere, a kit that contains a drying agent is available from the dispenser, if moisture from perspiration is a problem. Opening the battery cases after removal of the aids each evening may permit some drying out and will ensure that the aids are turned off. Batteries should be removed if the aids are to be unused for a period of time. The aid should never be left in a really hot place such as a window sill or the dashboard of a car.

3. Ear molds and their tubing can be removed from the earhook of the aid and washed. A hand syringe is useful to blow water out of the tubing before replacing it. Brushes and wax picks should be used to keep the ear mold sound channel and vents free of wax. Small "pressure equalizing" vents are especially liable to become occluded by wax, and a broomstraw may be helpful to clean them. A wire should not be used, especially with soft ear molds, because vents are not always straight and the material is easily damaged.

4. A safe place should be reserved to keep the aids when they are not in use. Longtime audiologists have witnessed the problem of temporarily or permanently lost hearing aid, or aids damaged or completely ingested by the family dog. As an additional safeguard, parents may want to consider purchasing insurance for the hearing aids.

5. Parents should institute a regular schedule of visits to the audiologist where, in addition to evaluation of the child's hearing, the performance of the aids and integrity of the ear molds can be evaluated. Retubing of the earmolds and minor repairs to the aids may prevent development of more serious problems.

tude and configuration. After fitting with hearing aids, a period of continuing evaluation and modification of amplification characteristics will follow. For this reason, it is important to prescribe flexible hearing aids with provision for considerable modification in electroacoustic characteristics. At the same time, parents must learn about hearing and hearing loss, the advantages and limitations of amplification, and become dedicated to the long-term habilitation process.

Parents must learn efficient use of amplification, including the physical manipulation of hearing aids and environmental strategies for effective listening. They must learn about the care and maintenance of hearing aids, how to assess functioning of aids, and how to detect problems and correct them, when possible. The child who uses the aids must assume all of these responsibilities as soon as possible. There must also be in place an effective program for monitoring the hearing aids' function and regular audiologic and otologic attention to the aids and the child's hearing.

REFERENCES

Beauchaine, K., Barlow, N., & Stelmachowicz, P. (1990). Special considerations in amplification for young children, *Asha, 32,* 44–46, 51.

Berger, K., Hagberg, E., & Rane, R. (1977). *Prescription of hearing aids: rationale, procedures, and results* (4th ed.). Kent, OH: Herald Publishing House.

Blair, J., Wright, K., & Pollard, G. (1981). Parental knowledge and understanding of hearing loss and hearing aids. *The Volta Review, 83,* 375–382.

Byrne, D. (1981). Clinical issues and options in binaural hearing aid fitting. *Ear and Hearing, 2,* 187–193.

Byrne, D., & Tonisson, W. (1976). Selecting the gain of hearing aids for persons with sensorineural hearing impairments. *Scandinavian Audiology, 5,* 51–59.

Carney, A., & Moeller, M., (1998). Treatment efficacy: Hearing loss in children. *Journal of Speech, Language, and Hearing Research, 41,* 61–84.

Cornelisse, L., Seewald, R., & Jamieson, D. (1995). The input/output (I/O) formula: A theoretical approach to the fitting of personal amplification devices. *Journal of the Acoustical Society of America, 97,* 1854–1864.

Cox, R. (1985). Hearing aids and aural rehabilitation: A structured approach to hearing aid selection (1985). *Ear and Hearing, 6,* 226–239.

Dillon, H. (1999). NAL-NL1: A new procedure for fitting non-linear hearing aids. *Hearing Journal, 52*(4), 10–16.

Dunn, L., & Dunn, L. (1981), *Peabody Picture Vocabulary Test—Revised.* Circle Pines, MN: American Guidance Service.

Evans, W., Webster, D., & Cullen, J. (1983). Auditory brainstem responses in neonatally sound deprived CBA/J mice. *Hearing Research, 10,* 269–277.

Food and Drug Administration (1977). Hearing aid devices—Professional and patient labeling and conditions for sale. *Federal Register, 42,* 9286–9296.

Gaeth, J., & Lounsbury, E. (1966). Hearing aids and children in elementary schools. *Journal of Speech and Hearing Disorders, 31,* 283–289.

Gelfand, S. & Silman, S., (1993). Apparent auditory deprivation in children. *Journal of the American Academy of Audiology, 4,* 313–318.

Guidelines for identification audiometry (1985). *Asha, 28,* 49–52.

Guidelines for screening for hearing impairment and middle ear disorders (1989). *Asha, 31,* 71–77

Harrison, W., & Norton, S. (1999). Characteristics of transient evoked otoacoustic emissions in normal-hearing and hearing-impaired children. *Ear and Hearing, 20,* 75–86.

Hawkins, D., Morrison, T., Halligan, P., & Cooper, W. (1989). Use of probe tube microphone measurements in hearing aid selection for children: Some initial clinical experiences. *Ear and Hearing, 10,* 281–287.

Hurley, R. (1999). Onset of auditory deprivation. *Journal of the American Academy of Audiology. 10,* 529–534.

Ireton, H., & Thwing, E. (1974). *Minnesota Child Development Inventory.* Behavior Science Systems.

Jacobson, J. (Ed.). (1985). *The auditory brainstem response.* San Diego: College-Hill Press.

Jirsa, R., & Norris, T. (1978) Relationship of acoustic gain to aided threshold improvement in children (1978). *Journal of Speech and Hearing Disorders, 43,* 348–352.

Kawell, M., Kopun, J., & Stelmachowicz, P., (1988) Loudness discomfort levels in children (1988). *Ear and Hearing, 9,* 133–136.

Kamm, C., Dirks, D., & Mickey, M. (1978). Effect of sensorineural hearing loss on loudness discomfort level. *Journal of Speech and Hearing Research, 21,* 668–681.

Liden, G., & Kankkunen, A. (1969). Visual reinforcement audiometry in the management of young deaf children. *International Audiology, 8,* 99–106.

Lybarger, S. (1963) *Simplified system for fitting hearing aids.* Canonsberg, PA: Radioear Corp.

Matkin, N. (1984). Wearable amplification: A litany of persisting problems. In J. Jerger (Ed.), *Pediatric audiology* (pp 125–145). San Diego: College-Hill Press.

Matkin, N. (1986). Hearing aids for children. In W. Hodgson, (Ed.), *Hearing aid assessment and use in audiologic habilitation* (3rd ed., pp 170–190). Baltimore: Williams and Wilkins.

McCandless, G., & Lyregaard, P. (1983). Prescription of gain/output (POGO) for hearing aids. *Hearing Instruments 34* (1), 16–17, 19–21.

Mindel, E., & Vernon, M. (Eds.) (1987). *They grow in silence: Understanding deaf children and adults* (2nd Ed.). Boston: College-Hill Press.

Moodie, K., Seewald, R., & Sinclair, S. (1994). Procedure for predicting real-ear hearing aid performance in young children. *American Journal of Audiology 3,* 23–31.

Northern, J., & Downs, M. (1991). *Hearing in children* (4th ed). Baltimore: Wiliams and Wilkins.

Porter, T. (1973). Hearing aids in a residential school. *American Annals of the Deaf, 118,* 31–33.

Rintelmann, W., & Bess, F. (1977). High-level amplification and potential hearing loss in children. In Bess, F., *Childhood deafness: Causation, assessment and management* (pp. 267–293). New York: Grune and Stratton.

Seewald, R., & Ross, M. (1988) Amplification for young hearing impaired children. In Pollack, M., *Amplification for the hearing-impaired* (3rd ed., pp. 213–271). Orlando, FL: Grune and Stratton.

Seewald, R., & Scollie, S. (1999), Infants are not average adults: Implications for audiometric testing. *Hearing Journal, 52*(10), 64–72.

Silverman, C., & Silman, S. (1990). Apparent auditory deprivation from monaural amplification and recovery with binaural amplification: Two case studies. *Journal of the American Academy of Audiology, 1,* 175–180.

Skinner, M. (1988). *Hearing aid evaluation.* Engelwood Cliffs, NJ: Prentice Hall.

Suzuki, T., & Ogiba, Y., (1961) Conditioned reflex audiometry. *Archives of Otolaryngology, 74,* 192–198.

Upfold, L. (1988). Children with hearing aids in the 1980s: Etiologies and severity of impairment. *Ear and Hearing, 9,* 75–80.

Vernon, M. (1968). Fifty years of research on the intelligence of the deaf and hard-of-hearing. A survey of literature and discussion of the implications. *Journal of Rehabilitation of the Deaf, 1,* 1–11.

Wilson, W., & Thompson, G. (1984). Behavioral audiometry. In J. Jerger (Ed.), *Pediatric audiology* (pp. 1–44). San Diego, CA: College-Hill Press

Wolff, A., and Harkins, J. (1986). Multihandicapped students. In Schildroth & M. Karchmer (Eds.), *Deaf children in America* (pp. 55–82). San Diego, CA: College-Hill Press.

END OF CHAPTER EXAMINATION QUESTIONS

CHAPTER 6

1. What three principles ensure effective hearing aid use for a child?

   a. _____

   b. _____

   c. _____

2. According to the chapter author, what is the foundation upon which the structure of aural habilitation is built?

3. (True/False) There is no causal relationship between deafness and intelligence.

4. What are the five advantages of two hearing aids with a bilateral hearing loss?

   a. _____

   b. _____

   c. _____

   d. _____

   e. _____

5. (True/False) Parents should turn the majority of their child's aural habilitation program over to the audiologist.

6. Children with profound congenital hearing loss can acquire speech through:

   a. visual cues

   b. using their residual hearing

   c. manual communication

   d. both a and b

END OF CHAPTER ANSWER SHEET

Name _____ Date _____

CHAPTER 6

1. a. _____

   b. _____

   c. _____

2. _____

   _____

   _____

3. Circle one: True   False

4. a. _____

   b. _____

   c. _____

   d. _____

   e. _____

5. Circle one: True   False

6. Which one?   a   b   c   d

7. _____

8. Circle one: True   False

7. _____ percent of hearing losses are from unknown causes.

8. (True/False) Cosmetics should not play a role in fitting children with hearing aids.

Development of Auditory Skills in Children Who are Hearing Impaired

■ JILL L. BADER, M.A. ■

APPROPRIATE AMPLIFICATION
　　Hearing Aids
　　Cochlear Implants

ELEMENTS OF AUDITORY DEVELOPMENT
　　Detection
　　Discrimination
　　Identification
　　Comprehension
　　Creating a Listening Environment
　　Parent-Child Interaction
　　A Full Range of Listening Experiences

(continued)

AURAL INFANT INTERVENTION MODEL
  The Process of Therapy
  Other Components of Therapy

SUMMARY

Auditory development is the process by which children learn to recognize and understand auditory signals available to them. Aural (re)habilitation programs for young children with limited hearing must promote the optimal use of residual hearing by development of the auditory modality for acquisition and maintenance of spoken language. Children's optimal use of residual hearing requires: (1) early identification of hearing loss, (2) consistent use of appropriate amplification, (3) parents committed to the belief that their child's auditory capacity can be developed, and (4) an educational program with skilled professionals equally committed to the same belief.

A holistic approach to children's auditory-speech-language development ensures parallel development of children's cognitive, socio-emotional, motor, and self-help abilities (Cole & Mischook, 1986). This approach enhances the integration of auditory listening skills with cognitive experiences and social interactions throughout a child's day. It is a child's use of, not amount of, residual hearing that is valuable for functional communication. In the preschool years, it is the parent who becomes the primary habilitative agent for maintaining a child's hearing aids and structuring an auditory learning environment rich with listening experiences and expectations.

This chapter outlines the stages and levels of auditory development. Appropriate amplification is briefly discussed, with the critical role played by parents and professionals in the aural (re)habilitative process of children under 3 years dealt with at length.

APPROPRIATE AMPLIFICATION

The first step toward optimal development is early identification, as a child's capacity for language learning is at its peak in the first 3 years. Significant difficulty in acquiring spoken communication skills can be encountered, especially by a child with a severe-to-profound hearing loss that goes undetected through the early first few months of life (Cole & Mischook, 1986). Building on the dramatic deprivation studies of the early 1960s, more recent evidence further supports the probability of functional or even physiological atrophy from a lack of early auditory stimulation. Although early auditory deprivation is not impossible to overcome, early identification greatly facilitates the integration of auditory information with the other sensory information a young infant receives. Early identification usually results in early amplification, but does not always ensure optimal selection or consistent use. The consistent use of functional, appropriately selected hearing aids or a cochlear implant (discussed later in this chapter) is the second necessary step to optimal auditory development.

HEARING AIDS

Hearing aid selection is far from an exact science and requires the collaborative expertise of audiologist, parent, and educator. The audiologist offers the knowledge of a variety of hearing aids' capabilities and the skill to conduct a full audiologic assessment. The parents provide the intimate knowledge of their child's response patterns and will be responsible for the maintenance and their child's consistent use of the hearing aids. The educator ideally possesses a combined understanding of speech acoustics, child development, and family dynamics (including the diagnosis reaction discussed in Chapter 5). This professional combination of skills affords parents the appropriate guidance and encouragement necessary for their family's health and their child's optimal development.

Once hearing aids are recommended and purchased, regular evaluation of hearing aids must be ongoing. Availability of a number of earmold modifications also can assist some hearing-impaired children in a variety of ways. As young children's auditory responses expand and become more consistent, acoustic horns and filters or different shapes and materials used in earmolds may be beneficial.

Properly fitting earmolds are of the utmost importance to ensure maximum gain from powerful aids. A poor acoustic seal can produce feedback and lead parents to decrease the volume to solve the annoying problem. This solution allows parents to avoid the headache or embarrassment in public places, but the child loses the auditory information that links the child to him or her world. An even more common solution by parents of newly diagnosed infants is to remove the hearing aids altogether. Infants and toddlers are active, wiggly little creatures who dislodge the best fitting earmolds many times a day. Parents, still adjusting to their new role as parents of a hearing-impaired child, may be clumsy with earmold insertion or simply glad for a temporary reprieve. In the immediate postdiagnostic state, parents and children require the encouragement of a supportive educational (re)habilitative program.

Hearing aids should be purchased with the necessary adaptation for FM use, which can be an important contributor to promoting auditory development. FM systems allow a consistent optimal auditory input of the parent's voice free of masking by background noise. The use of FM systems during early learning years can accelerate children's use of their residual hearing and often generates a greater recordable frequency range later in life (Ling, 1984). As children enter the toddler and preschool years, the FM system can be used for a good portion of each day. FM systems can also be adapted for use with cochlear implants.

COCHLEAR IMPLANTS

Children who demonstrate no auditory progress after an extended period of consistent hearing aid use and appropriate aural (re)habilitation, may be candidates for a cochlear implant. These children's aided and unaided responses remain the same or nonexistent over time and with training. A lengthy discussion of cochlear implants is not possible here, but many articles describing implant devices, surgical and programming procedures, and noted auditory benefits to young children can be found in current publications. A cochlear implant represents the most advanced form of audiologic technology available and allows sound reception for this small subgroup of profoundly deaf children. Intensive aural (re)habilitation for implant children who are congenitally deaf is absolutely critical, because of years of preoperative auditory deprivation.

It cannot be overemphasized that hearing aids and/or cochlear implants must be worn and in good working order for a young child to learn how to use them. However, simply providing a child with hearing aids does not ensure that he or she will learn to listen, anymore than buying a child a bike guarantees learning to ride. Learning to listen requires time, attention, and practice, and adults who create an environment conducive to a child's development of audition.

ELEMENTS OF AUDITORY DEVELOPMENT

Normal development of audition proceeds through the same stages for hearing and hearing-impaired children alike, albeit at a slower pace for the latter. The hearing-impaired infant must wait for identification and consistent, optimal amplification of the hearing loss before he or she can embark on what Pollack (1985) describes as the first "Listening Year."

During the first year of life, infants develop an affective bond with parents, who reinforce the infants' social, motor, and vocal responses to auditory events. As parents attach communicative intent to these responses, an infant begins to associate sounds with their source and meaning. For at least a full year, toddlers then attempt verbal reproductions of the sounds they have heard. Those sounds include their own babble, which Fry (1978) describes as functionally important to integrating the auditory and kinesthetic feedback functions in the brain. The development of that auditory feedback mechanism is the means by which children learn to approximate adult forms of spoken language. Naturally, more speech dimensions are available to children with more hearing and to those children who are appropriately amplified.

The key elements to auditory development include (1) detection, (2) discrimination, (3) identification, and (4) comprehension.

DETECTION

Detection involves children becoming aware of sound and learning to attend to sounds. At the detection level, the child simply responds to the presence or absence of sound. For most hearing-impaired children, this only happens with amplification and through parents who have learned to draw their child's attention to the linguistic and nonlinguistic sounds in his or her environment. In this way, parents represent their child's first feedback mechanism. *The most important job of a parent is to assist their hearing-impaired child to attend and respond to speech* (Simmons-Martin 1981).

DISCRIMINATION

Discrimination develops as children learn to perceive the differences in sounds. Suprasegmental discriminations of intensity, duration, pitch, and timing appear first. Children can discriminate, for example, that their parent's conversation conveys excitement before they can understand the cause or content of their parent's excitement. Children at the discrimination level also discover that different objects, people, and situations have different sounds associated with them. Discrimination allows children to tell whether auditory patterns are the same or different from others. How sounds differ and what the sounds mean comes later in the developmental schema.

IDENTIFICATION

Identification is the stage at which children can repeat or point to a representation of a specific set of sounds. Identification does require memory, but not understanding of the sounds. For example, children can identify a toy cow in response to "moo-o-o" and a toy pig to "oink," simply because one is a long set of sounds and the other is short. However, with only this long versus short identification ability, a child may also identify another toy animal (i.e., a sheep) that also represents a long set of sounds (i.e., "baa-a"), but which is not semantically correct to the auditory signal presented (i.e., "moo-o"). This occurs because the child has not yet gained comprehension of a sound's specific meaning or identification of the specific sounds.

COMPREHENSION

Comprehension of acoustic signals sent to a child by the linguistic and nonlinguistic sounds in his or her environment is the final and most complicated stage of auditory development. At this stage, children must be able not just to repeat an auditory set, but to also demonstrate that they understand the meaning of sounds received. Erber (1982) stated that a child's demonstrations of comprehension are "usually referenced to his or her knowledge of language."

Very young children will initially use nonverbal behaviors to indicate their understanding. Specifically, when a parent hurriedly says "Let's go bye-bye," a child may wave or go get his or her coat. This child, on a detection level, is aware that sound exists. On a discrimination level, the child knows that the parent is in a hurry and the tot's identification skills allow the child to look to the parent as the source of sound, even before linguistic skills allow him or her to repeat a verbal approximation to "bye-bye." Finally, the comprehension and understanding that the child gives, completes the cycle of connecting sound to meaning. The auditory stimulus (i.e., "Let's go bye-bye") has integrated with cognitive functioning (i.e., the memory of the experience of going bye-bye) and elicited an appropriate motor response (i.e., waving).

This lengthy process of auditory development begins with attention and ends in comprehension. The very best hearing aid selection will not totally compensate for the hearing loss or guarantee the child's acquisition of spoken communication through audition. Audition must be viewed as the desirable primary modality for (re)habilitation, but not the only modality available. *Hearing aids can enhance the child's hearing, but the act of listening is a behavior that must be learned.*

CREATING A LISTENING ENVIRONMENT

The world of a child in utero is far from silent. The auditory system (cochlea) becomes functional for hearing at around 7 months prenatally (Furuhjelm, Ingelman-Sundberg, & Wirsen, 1986) and the amniotic fluid provides a better source of sound conduction than air does after birth. One might say that neonates emerge with almost a fourth of a year of listening in their experience! No research is yet available with which one can draw conclusions about the influence of prenatal auditory experiences, so our discussion is confined to the postnatal period.

The Listening Environment

Parents and, later, educators are primarily responsible for a listening environment that neither limits the quality nor quantity of a child's auditory experiences. Prior to receiving hearing aids, the sensorimotor child has experienced how things look, feel, taste, and smell without integrating how things and people sound, as well. After receiving hearing aids, a child must attach new auditory information to past perceptions and to his or her future learning experiences through an imperfect input system. Vygotskii (1962) explained that parents direct their child's attention to certain aspects of experiences and thereby determine the way a child perceives and responds to their world.

Nonlinguistic Listening Environment

Parents of a hearing-impaired infant must direct their child's attention to the auditory aspects of ongoing daily experiences as soon after hearing aid fitting as possible (Figure 7–1). For the young infant, directing attention to sound is a difficult, but necessary task. Parents can enhance their infant's ability to make auditory responses by controlling the sound distractions in their home. For example, the running of a nearby dishwasher or television

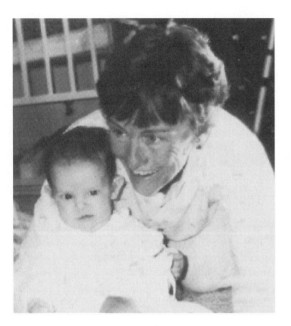

Figure 7–1. The development of listening skills must involve both child and caregiver.

during mealtime should be delayed. The use of the radio or stereo should be confined to nonconversational periods of the day. The acoustic quality of language input, impoverished by the hearing loss, is thereby increased for an infant's reception, when parents provide a noise-controlled environment.

The parents' heightened awareness of sound also allows them to draw their child's attention to the numerous common everyday environmental sounds (i.e., toaster, running water, toilet, garage door, etc.) that parents take for granted in their home. For the very young inattentive toddler in the first listening year, association of those sounds with their source and meaning requires focused attention and repeated exposure.

Dunst (1981), Simmons-Martin (1981), and van Uden (1979), have all described an effective strategy whereby parents and teachers "stage" or "structure" situations to ensure that auditory learning events occur and reoccur daily. For exam-

ple, parents may instruct frequent visitors to ring the doorbell two or three times before expecting an answer, thus allowing ample opportunity for parents to direct their child's attention to the sound until the day the child responds spontaneously. Parents can stage bathtime so that a child's hearing aids are not removed until after the child has had a chance to listen to the language of undressing, the bath water running, and the toys splashing into the tub. Parents can learn to apply this staging strategy to virtually every moment of their child's day, given the professionally guided practice necessary to the creation of an optimal listening environment.

Linguistic Listening Environment

Although attention to nonlinguistic auditory events is certainly a worthy component to a child's aural (re)habilitation, the primary focus must be on linguistic events, as the ultimate goal for a child is spoken language competence. An optimal listening environment is linguistically rich when parents provide a running verbal commentary on the people, objects, and activities in their child's life. These verbal descriptions are simple, meaningful, interesting, and repetitive phrases and sentences. They match the child's thoughts, feelings, and interests. Such acoustic input affords children phonemes and words in a prosodic envelope steeped with the suprasegmental features available auditorily to nearly all hearing-impaired children. It is those features that will first be imitated by young children and will maintain a child's natural-sounding voice quality and that contribute to intelligibility into adulthood.

PARENT–CHILD INTERACTION

Because early optimal auditory learning requires an exchange between a child and an adult, learning will be broadened and accelerated by a positive parent/child relationship. The young hearing-impaired infant must be viewed as an active participant in audition capable of increasing his or her contributions to the communicative exchanges that develop between parent and child. Many investigators cite turntaking exchanges, wherein parents and child alternate the role of "speaker" and listener, as precursors to language and social development. Balanced turntaking is achieved by parents who follow their child's lead, interact on the child's level, and match their child's pace of interaction (Mahoney & Powell, 1986). The resultant reciprocity and synchronization in the parent/child dyad increases mutual enjoyment (Brazelton, 1986) and provides a solid foundation for auditory learning.

A FULL RANGE OF LISTENING EXPERIENCES

The final component to creating a listening environment for young children is to provide a full range of listening-learning experiences. This cannot be achieved in the preschool years without the help of parents. A wide variety of experiences, shared by a monitoring parent, will greatly expand a child's learning horizons. Fortunate is the hearing-impaired child who has been given the opportunity to learn to listen to the sounds of the circus, the carwash, a whisper, a parade, and the singing of Christmas carols.

As the critical period for learning is in the first three years of life, the provision of an optimal listening environment must not be left to chance. Caring, skilled professionals must help parents establish positive interaction patterns with their toddler that promote the quality and quantity of learning situations necessary to optimal auditory development.

A Listening Attitude

Perhaps the single most critical criterion to a child's auditory success, once consistent appropri-

ate amplification is in place, is the ongoing interaction with at least one significant adult who believes in that child's ability to hear. This attitude will dictate adult expectations of the child and subsequently how the child grows to view him or herself. To the general public, the word "deaf" is viewed as synonymous with "cannot hear." Most hearing parents emerged from that group on the day of diagnosis when someone told them that their child was deaf. Therefore, professionals should model for parents an attitude that gently expects children to listen, hear, and speak. Within the first few months of intervention, parents need to make a conversion from the general public's attitude of "cannot hear" to "can hear with training and proper amplification." Whether or not a parent comes to believe that their child can hear and, therefore, can learn to listen and speak, will contribute greatly to the choice of methodology and of professionals employed for their child's (re)habilitation (Figure 7–2).

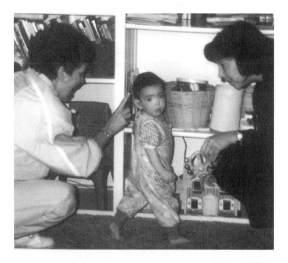

Figure 7–2. Aural habilitation can be an enjoyable and challenging experience for both the child and the clinician.

AURAL INFANT INTERVENTION MODEL

Auditory responses, especially from infants and toddlers unsophisticated to the world of behavioral audiometry, cannot always be obtained in the audiologists' clinical setting. Young children exhibit auditory responses first in familiar settings with familiar adults. Because infant and parent are bound in an inseparable dyad, aural (re)habilitation is most effective when it goes through the parent to the child. Infant (re)habilitation programs, therefore, must simulate the most conducive environment possible for both optimal parent and child responses. That first learning environment is the home.

The preferred infant intervention model is a home demonstration center. This model operates aural (re)habilitation programs in a center-based house with a modestly furnished kitchen, living room, baby's bedroom, and bathroom. A center-based advantage of professional control over the physical environment and availability of training materials is not sacrificed to provide the comfortable "home" environment advantage of home-based programs. The Home Demonstration Center offers a warm, safe, stimulating learning environment for both parent support group sessions and individual parent-child therapy.

Auditory learning is most effective during a child's ongoing daily activities (Erber, 1982, Simmons-Martin, 1981). Moreover, a child's integration of audition into their everyday life is the ultimate goal. At a Home Demonstration Center, children are immediately at ease to interact naturally and learn to listen while watering flowers, unloading the dishwasher, fixing lunch, getting dressed, or mopping up spills. Participation in these simulated daily household chores, with the guidance of a trained professional, allows sensorimotor children to learn by doing (Northcott, 1972, Piaget, 1952), and parents to modify their behaviors more effectively by being placed in a doer rather than an observer role (Brazelton, 1986).

Strategies learned and practiced by parents at a Home Demonstration Center can then easily be transferred into their own daily activities at home. It is in the pleasures of being dressed, fed, and played with that infants establish socially communicative skills that help in the acquisition of language and stimulate the elements of auditory development.

Parents gain confidence in their own competence to influence their child's optimal development when they receive reinforcement for effective parenting skills from a trained professional during parent-focused (re)habilitation. A professional's expertise in a child-centered program may benefit the child for an hour or two a week, *but optimal progress occurs when children have parents who have been helped to develop their own expertise with their child all day long, everyday—not by becoming teachers, but by becoming confident, competent parents!*

THE PROCESS OF THERAPY

Detection

Since detection is the first auditory skill children must acquire, initial therapies focus on parents gaining detection-stimulating strategies. Parents are asked to keep their child's hearing aids on through all waking hours, use clear, well-articulated speech, reduce the background noise (Estabrooks, 1994), and stay within a 3-foot distance from their child's hearing aid and to be on hearing aid level. The latter has been named by the author as "The Yardstick Strategy" and is one of a long list of strategies taught to parents. This list includes: (1) attention-getting strategies (primarily, drawing attention to sound) and imitation of sounds ("vroom, vroom"); (2) naming of sounds ("That's a motorcycle."); and (3) alerting to sound (using a bright expression and halting activity to say "Daddy heard that!")

During a therapy session in the Home Demonstration Model described earlier, parent and child might be fixing lunch at the kitchen table. The on-looking (but not directly involved with the child) therapist prompts the parent to listen for sound that may occur. Then the therapist turns on an electric mixer, microwave, or kitchen-counter TV. When a sound occurs, the therapist coaches the parent to cue the child to attend ("Listen" while pointing to their ear), adopt an alerting expression as they name the sound ("Mommy hears the microwave"), and to imitate the sound ("Ding"). Parents are guided to take their child to the sound, point to the source of the sound as they name it ("That's the microwave."), and then repeat the sound.

At the end of therapy, parents sit with their child and record sounds with a picture and written representation in a little notebook. The child carries the book between home and therapy each week, so parents can add to it daily at home.

In the detection stage, conditioned play responses are classically taught by a therapist at a table with blocks or pegs. The preferred method, however, is to coach the parent through some everyday activities internal to which they can condition the child to give a response to an auditory stimulus. For example, parents might tote pajamas, diapers, and so on to an evening therapy at a Home Demonstration Center and give their child a bath. They can practice the alerting response scenario (described earlier) to the water getting turned on and off. They can line bath toys on the edge of the tub and help condition their child to push a toy in only when they hear mommy or daddy say something ("Push it in." or "Make it splash.").

Helping parents become confident in their own competence can make a 1-hour weekly therapy session explode into 7 days a week, 12 hours a day of auditory stimulation for the child! In addition, the bonding between parent and child increases. The child begins to respond better to parents and to sounds in his or her world, which encourages the parent to accelerate their stimulation, which helps the child develop quicker. The attitude conversion begins.

OTHER COMPONENTS OF THERAPY

This therapy model for a child's first 2 years of life trains parents to proceed through (1) discrimination, (2) identification, and (3) comprehension listening skills within an everyday context. Children learning the suprasegmentals, for example, need parents who use interesting auditory patterns. "Ah-o" could be used whenever things fall, break, or spill. "Oooo, that hurts. Ow!" for bangs and bruises. "Whee," "Up up up we go," and "Danger!" become a way of life for parents of children with hearing impairments. Working on long versus short (duration) can be as simple as "Up, up, up, up, up" versus "down." Imagine the fortunate child who hears those phrases each time he or she gets picked up or put down or goes up and down a flight of stairs!

By the time children reach stage (4), the segmental stage of auditory identification of mono- versus duosyllabic words, they will have parents who engage them in helping unload the groceries (grapes, pear, milk, bread versus apple, butter, ketchup, french fries). At the Christmas holiday, decorating the tree with star, lights, and wreath versus snowman, tinsel and reindeer versus candy cane, Santa Claus, and nutcracker can be more highly motivating than the best of a "sit-down-therapy" session.

Cochlear Implantation

Since this author provides auditory development services on behalf of a large number of successfully implanted young children, information is included on this important topic. Cochlear implantation requirements are broader than before and, in many parts of the world, cochlear implants may be placed in children during the first few months of life. It is becoming more commonplace to observe very young children with cochlear implants, even binaural implantation.

Cochlear implants offer children full access to sound within normal hearing ranges. In that regard, then, quality auditory-intensive training in the infant and preschool years should afford the vast majority of limited-hearing children to be educated alongside their hearing peers. However, they need support and guidance from professionals with holistic approaches to auditory and other learning domains.

SUMMARY

It is critical that professionals involved in the auditory (re)habilitation of very young children have a broad base of knowledge about child development, speech acoustics, and family dynamics. This can be meshed with the specificity of strategies parents must learn to enhance a child's listening and language development. *Listening is not an isolated skill and a child's auditory development must not be approached in a segmented way.*

Each child's unique family system and the dyadic interaction patterns therein must be assessed by the infant habilitator. Internal to that knowledge, the professional can guide parents to establish appropriate expectations, to capitalize on auditory learning opportunities that arise naturally during a child's daily routines, and to stage situations that accelerate their child's progress through the levels of auditory development.

During those first three critical years, aural (re)habilitation programs must regard the family as an entity, not just the child. Parents make a huge commitment of time and energy to aural (re)habilitation that helps their child integrate listening into daily life as they become active members of the hearing world. Parents need the support and guidance from professionals whose holistic approach balances auditory learning with the parallel development of the child's other learning domains.

REFERENCES

Brazelton, T. B. (1986). *Infants and mothers*. New York: Dell Publishing Co., Inc.

Cole, E., & Mischook, M. (1986) . Auditory learning and teaching of hearing impaired infants, *Volta Review, 88*, 67–81.

Dunst, C. J. (1981). *Infant learning*. Hingham, MA: Teaching Resources.

Erber, N. P. (1982). *Auditory training*. Washington, DC: Alexander Graham Bell Association for the Deaf.

Estabrooks, W. (1994). Auditory/verbal therapy. Washington, DC: Alexander Graham Bell Association for the Deaf.

Fry, D. B. (1978). The role and primacy of the auditory channel in speech and language development. In M. Ross & T. Giolas (Eds.), *Auditory management of hearing impaired children* (pp. 55–71). Baltimore, MD: University Park Press.

Furuhjelm, M., Ingelman-Sundberg, A., Wirsen, C. (1986). *A child is born* (pp. 116–117). New York: Dell Publishing.

Ling, D. (1984). (Ed.). *Early intervention for hearing impaired children: Oral options*. Boston: College Hill Press.

Mahoney, G., & Powell, A. (1986). *A teacher's guide* (Transactional Intervention Program Monograph No. 1).

Northcott, W.H. (1972). (Ed.). *Curriculum guide: Hearing-impaired children birth to three years—and their parents*. Washington, DC: Alexander Graham Bell Association for the Deaf.

Piaget, J. (1952). *The origins of intelligence in children* (M. Cook, Trans.). New York: International Universities Press.

Pollack, D. (1985). *Educational audiology for the limited hearing infant and preschooler*. Springfield, IL: Charles C. Thomas Publisher.

Simmons-Martin, A. (1981). Acquisition of language by under-five including the parental role. In A. M. Mulholland (Ed.), *Oral education today and tomorrow* (pp. 253–273). Washington, DC: A. G. Bell Association for the Deaf.

van Uden, A. M. J. (1979). Hometraining service for deaf children in the Netherlands. In A. Simmons-Martin & D.R. Calvert (Eds.), *Parent-infant intervention* (pp. 165–177). New York: Grune & Stratton.

Vygotskii, L. (1962). *Thought and language* (E. Hanfmann & G. VaKaf Trans.). Cambridge, MA: MIT Press.

SUGGESTED READINGS

Cole, E. B. (1992). *Listening and talking*. Washington, DC: Alexander Graham Bell Association for the Deaf.

Cole, E., & Gregory, H. (Eds.). (1986). Auditory learning. *Volta Review, 88,* pp. 26–31.

Erber, N. P., & Hirsh, I. J. (1978). Auditory training. In H. Davis & S. R. Silverman, *Hearing and deafness* (4th ed.) . New York: Holt, Rinehart, and Winston.

Fisher, E., & Schneider, K. (1986). Integrating auditory learning at the pre-school level, *Volta Review, 88,* 83–92.

French-St. George, M. (1986) . What does speech sound like to the hearing impaired? *Volta Review, 88,* 109–120.

Ling, D. (1976). *Speech and the hearing-impaired child: Theory and practice*. Washington, DC: Alexander Graham Bell Association for the Deaf.

Ling, D. (1986). Devices and procedures for auditory learning. *Volta Review, 88,* 19–28.

Northern, J. L., & Downs, M. P. (1978). *Hearing in children* (2nd ed.). Baltimore, MD: Williams & Wilkins.

Stone, P. (1983). Auditory learning in a school setting: Procedures and results. *Volta Review, 85,* pp. 47–52

Stone, P., & Adams, A. (1986). Is your child wearing the right hearing aid? Principles for selecting and maintaining amplification. *Volta Review, 88,* 45–55.

Vaughan, P. (Ed.). (1981). *Learning to Listen*. New York: Beaufort Books.

END OF CHAPTER EXAMINATION QUESTIONS

CHAPTER 7

1. List the key elements of auditory development that are presented in this chapter.

2. Explain the importance of a "listening attitude" in auditory development.

3. Discuss five ways in which parents can facilitate the development of auditory skills in their child who has hearing impairment.

   a.

   b.

   c.

   d.

   e.

4. Explain the function of the aural infant intervention model.

5. What is meant by a "holistic" approach to children's auditory-speech-language development, and how would you integrate this approach in therapy (aural habilitation)?

6. A child who points to a cow when a parent says "moo-oo-oo" is demonstrating

   a. detection

   b. discrimination

   c. comprehension

   d. identification

7. A child who turns her or his head toward a door that has been slammed is demonstrating

   a. detection

   b. discrimination

END OF CHAPTER ANSWER SHEET

Name   Date

CHAPTER 7

1. _____

2. _____

3. a. _____

   b. _____

   c. _____

   d. _____

   e. _____

4. _____

5. _____

6. a. _____

   b. _____

   c. _____

   d. _____

7. a. _____

   b. _____

   c. _____

   d. _____

8. a. _____

   b. _____

   c. _____

   d. _____

9. a. _____

   b. _____

   c. _____

   d. _____

10. a. _____

    b. _____

    c. _____

    d. _____

c. comprehension

d. identification

8. For the child who has hearing impairment, the act of listening.

   a. is not possible

   b. evolves naturally once hearing aids are in place

   c. depends on lipreading

   d. must be learned

9. The primary focus in aural rehabilitation for young children is on

   a. exposing the child to everyday environmental sounds

   b. maximizing linguistic output

   c. teaching the child to use a hearing aid

   d. the adult modeling and the child repeating words

10. The cochlea becomes functional for listening

    a. during the first trimester

    b. during the second trimester

    c. during the third trimester

    d. when it is stimulated at birth

■ CHAPTER 8 ■

Language Development for Children Who Are Hearing Impaired

■ JILL L. BADER, M.A. ■

DEFINITIONS AND TERMS
  Communication/Language

THREE COMPONENTS OF LANGUAGE
  Semantic Content
  Syntactic Form
  Pragmatic Use

HIERARCHICAL DEVELOPMENT OF LANGUAGE
  Receptive Language
  Expressive Language

GENESIS OF LANGUAGE
  Birth to 6 Months
  6 to 12 Months
  12 to 18 Months

(continued)

18 to 24 Months

24 to 48 Months

4 to 5 Years

TRANSACTIONAL BREEDING GROUND

IMPACT OF HEARING LOSS

A SAMPLE THERAPY SESSION

PARENTS AND CHILDREN NEED THE ACTIVE ROLE

IMPACT OF GRIEVING ON PARENT/CHILD INTERACTION

SUMMARY

Language development, like auditory development discussed in Chapter 7, must be viewed within the context of a child's overall developmental profile, including the learning environment provided in early childhood. The current focus, for those of us involved in facilitating the receptive and expressive language development of young hearing-impaired children, must be directed toward a global view. This vantage point allows a treatment focus on auditory and language learning in relation to a child's other developmental areas, physical health status, and the family system within which a child will learn. Acquisition of language is enhanced by integration of the emerging auditory, social, motor, self-help, and cognitive functionings and stimulated by the transactional relationship parents form with their infants. As audition is the most efficient sensory modality for initial development of functional verbal communication skills during the first 3 years of life (Ling, 1976; Pollack, 1985) those hearing impaired children, regardless of degree of hearing loss, who can use hearing as their main avenue of learning must be given the (re)habilitative opportunity to do so. Erber (1972) states that audition has also proven to be a complementary skill to lipreading (and vice versa), which is a valuable avenue of effective communication for some children.

As the (re)habilitative process begins, *parents* are the primary focus of the professional's attention. It is the parents who have gone into crisis. It is parents who make some of their most important decisions when they are least equipped with information and emotional stability. As the (re)habilitative process unfolds, parents need a great deal of professional guidance to establish effective and mutually satisfying interactions with their child. The rich linguistic climate required for a preschool hearing-impaired child to acquire language depends first on the child's parents.

This chapter describes the components of language, outlines the stages of language development, and presents a sample therapy activity in the aural rehabilitative process. Because the grieving process concerns all professionals involved with the family, a brief comment on this is included. It is hoped that the reader will see the integration of the relationship of a child's learning domains, the level of parent competence, and the efficacy of professional guidance, all of which shape the process of language acquisition for preprimary hearing-impaired children.

DEFINITIONS AND TERMS

COMMUNICATION/LANGUAGE

Communication is defined here as the exchange of ideas, information, and feelings between two or more individuals. Spoken language is *the orderly arrangement of verbal symbols to convey meaning*. Each part of the definition reflects what decades of psycholinguistic research and (re)habilitative discussion have established as the three basic components of language: (1) *Meaningful symbols* refers to the **semantic content** (Bloom & Lahey, 1978) of language, (2) *orderly arrangement* is the **syntactic form** of language, and (3) *conveyance* is the **pragmatic use** that must be functional (Simmons-Martin, 1981) with relation to the context in which it is spoken. Therefore, this chapter refers to the three basic components of language as: (1) semantic content, (2) syntactic form, and (3) pragmatic use. *Spoken language* falls within either a receptive or expressive realm. Simply defined, *receptive language* is the information that a person receives with comprehension. *Expressive language* is the information sent to a listener.

THREE COMPONENTS OF LANGUAGE

Language is truly three-dimensional and multifaceted. For young children learning language, these components must mesh in an integrated fashion (Bloom & Lahey, 1978) to achieve conversational competency (Stone, 1988). The components of language are separated here for brief examination, but are learned by people interdependently (Bruner, 1983).

SEMANTIC CONTENT

Semantic content is the element of language that concerns meaning. As cognition's linguistic component, semantics involves much more than sheer acquisition of word meanings. It involves meaning of words related to other words in sentences that represent relationships between people/actions/objects.

During the first 2 years of a child's life, parents follow a conversational model, which begins at birth with short, simple, interesting, redundant, comprehensible sentences (Snow, 1977b). The semantic simplicity of parents' verbal interactions with their infants clearly indicates their intent to match the infant's ability to receive meaning. Infants must extract meaning from their actions before attempts at expressive language can begin. Nonverbal counterparts (i.e., positioning, pointing, proximity, visual gaze, etc.) therefore become the first semantic carriers and continue into adulthood to exert a communicative influence. It is from those nonverbal frames, established between parent and infant, that mastery of even the simplest form of verbal self-expression emerges (Bruner, 1975).

Riding in the rumble seat of nonverbal language behaviors are suprasegmental features that are semantically laden. These phonological aspects include **intensity, pitch, timing, intonation,** and **duration**. Suprasegmentals are understood and imitated by infants before they demonstrate comprehension of words. With the possible exception of pitch, these suprasegmental features are available to profoundly hearing-impaired children and carry the emotion of communication on an acoustic waveform. Simmons-Martin

(1981) described intonation as "the vehicle one rides to syntax."

SYNTACTIC FORM

The form component of spoken language includes **syntactic, phonologic,** and **morphologic features** that parents choose to enhance meaning. Syntax composes the grammatical rules one applies to alter words and arrange them into orderly, meaningful sentences in an orderly fashion (Pollack, 1985). Every language has its syntactic rules governing the order of adjectives, nouns, and verbs; but, describing form requires phonologic and morphologic descriptions, too.

Morphological inflections (e.g., *ed, ing, ly*) or single sounds (phonemes) carry their own unique set of rules and acoustic elements that vary in the combinations chosen for use. The act of choosing the form of sentences directed to a young child is dictated to some degree by the parents' perception of their child's cognitive and linguistic abilities (Bruner, 1975). This leads us to the third component of language, pragmatic use.

PRAGMATIC USE

Pragmatics, the least tangible component of language, has a socially related ingredient that involves the contextual appropriateness, functionality, and intent of language. Parents' simplification of their language from typically adult complex words and forms for use with infants is pragmatically controlled by their perception of their young listener's level of understanding (Van Uden, 1981).

Pragmatic use is also controlled by parental intent. For example, a speaker uses *"an* authority" when intending a nonspecific, one-of-many authorities and if he desires to direct one's attention to a specific authority, he or she chooses *"the* authority." If a vocal stress is added to the article, **"the,"** it is communicated that the speaker believes that authority to be the best among many. Furthermore, if that someone is **the** authority him or herself, then humor or sarcasm may be intended as well. The correct use of articles is listed among the most common errors of verbalizations of hearing-impaired children (Erber, 1982). That articles gain their semantic value from their syntactic use, which is pragmatically controlled, may serve to explain this phenomenon more than the low acoustic feature aspect.

HIERARCHICAL DEVELOPMENT OF LANGUAGE

RECEPTIVE LANGUAGE

Receptive language develops from an ever-increasing awareness of and attention to the verbal signals to which a child is exposed. Those features of language to which a child attends are likewise imitated. Although this stage of receptive language development is not yet connected to meaning, a child is absorbing information. The comprehension stage is reached when children can behaviorally demonstrate understanding. These ongoing cyclic stages are the means by which children and adults process the components of language.

EXPRESSIVE LANGUAGE

A child's expressive language passes through orderly predictable stages of development, each of which appears for a fairly short period and then becomes an integral part of the next stage. During the first year of life, infants' vocalizations begin with reflexive crying and cooing and proceed to babbling consonant/vowel chains, then combinations. This verbal exercise cultivates the ability to imitate increasingly complex prosodic patterns used by parents. When these imitative vocalizations carry meaning and intent, they begin to approximate single words. Single words lead, in turn, to inflected jargon, wherein children combine the babble and suprasegmental imitations into long vocalizations that over time are interspersed with single words. As single words increase, children combine 2 words, then 3, together into telegraphed phrases that eventually become part of complete sentences.

GENESIS OF LANGUAGE

Children are introduced to language at the moment of birth, even before caregivers direct conversation to them. A neonate embarks on a quest for neurological organization that requires sensorimotor refinement before the child can process or produce spoken language.

During the first 2-year sensorimotor period, language emerges from the thoughts a child has about the objects and people in his or her immediate experience (Figure 8–1). The infant picks up toy keys to feel, taste, hear, and see. Through the

infant's senses, he or she has inferred meaning related to an object. Parents accompany their child's sensory experiences with linguistic symbols. Over time and with repeated exposures, a child attaches the verbal symbol ("keys") to an object. The child's thought now has receptive language. Expressive production by the child of that linguistic symbol will soon follow.

So, young children's language stems from thought and that thought has its roots in the child's experiences. Because a sensorimotor child's thought is extremely concrete and self-referenced, so is the first language understood and later expressed by the child.

BIRTH TO 6 MONTHS

During the first 6 months of life there is no symbolic representation. An infant's expressive verbal language proceeds from reflexive random vocalizations toward more purposeful sounds cooed with socioemotional intent. He or she socially engages caregivers by initiating vocalizations direct-

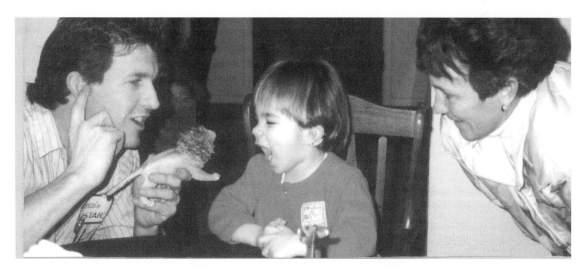

Figure 8–1. Language development occurs through interactive communication with parents and siblings.

ly at others to express displeasure. These vocalizations contain patterns other than crying and are primarily vowels, although consonant/vowel babble chains do emerge. An infant's nonverbal language is far more advanced than verbal communication and includes reaching, directed visual gaze, and body positioning.

6 TO 12 MONTHS

Receptive language development proceeds from a reflexive point, as well. The startle responses of infants in the first month of life become quite deliberate and are directed toward the source of sound. By the 6th month, they are followed by a social smile. A child not yet identified as having a significant hearing loss may not have heard auditory signals well enough to search for the location of a sound and, instead, may exhibit the social smile as a response only to the visual presence of an object or caretaker. Measurement tools of receptive language development evidence a prominence of social as well as auditory response behaviors. The 6-month-old demonstrates a general contextual understanding (angry versus friendly versus danger) that is conveyed through the suprasegmental features of language. A child has also attached meaning to words with situational clues like "bye-bye" as evidenced by his or her emerging nonverbal response of a social waving behavior. The hearing-impaired child fortunate enough to have full-time hearing aid use during this time benefits from the accompanying auditory and language labels for the sensorimotor experiences.

12 TO 18 MONTHS

By the end of the first year of life, a toddler's behaviors have become coordinated, goal-directed, and imitative. A full year of object orientation and attention toward the effect of actions on a child's environment will have contributed to the development of symbolic representation of objects independent of self. With the development of internal language, the toddler can carry the memory of familiar objects and people when they are not present and demonstrate receptive comprehension of concrete verbal labels for them. The toddler begins to coordinate nonverbal behaviors of pointing, reaching, and looking from an object to a parent and back to the object again to communicate his or her social intent. These nonverbal manifestations of cognitive growth and increased social awareness dictate parents' continued use of naming ("That's a bunny.") and descriptive language ("It's so soft.") strategies in verbal interactions with the child. As a toddler's imitative powers mature, his or her verbal contributions of intonational parameters of conversations increase. Motoric imitations of the physical actions of speech gesture games (patty cake and peek-a-boo) soon are accompanied by the highly audible prosodic features of parents' verbal expressions. The 1-year-old may delight his or her parents by speaking first words and taking first steps all at once. A motor preoccupation with newly gained walking and climbing skills can decrease the toddler's quantity of vocalizations for a few weeks. It is important that parents of hearing-impaired children be forewarned of this natural phenomenon, lest they assume the possibility of a progressive loss of hearing or decreased efficacy of intervention.

18 TO 24 MONTHS

As the sensorimotor toddler actively explores his or her way to 18 months of age, a new separation of people-oriented acts and object-oriented acts is gained. The toddler begins to use communicative behaviors (e.g., pointing, nodding, vocalizing, eye contact) more frequently with people, and motoric behaviors (e.g., grasping, tasting, manipulating) more often with objects. As a toddler, the earlier repetition of object manipulatory acts now yields to social pleasure gained from imitation of people's acts. These imitations are often repeated to re-engage an adult in joint play. Object permanence allows the 18-month-old child to carry out verbal requests for an object not in direct view.

Receptively, the 18-month-old who is gaining on symbolic representation can match objects to pictures and identify pictures when they are named. The child appears to understand more and more words each week. By 18 months, the toddler has an expressive vocabulary of approximately 20 words and babbles intricate inflections, which evidence increased consonant use. Pointing and gesturing now have a vocal counterpart. Babbling and nonverbal imitations abound, with verbal imitations being less frequent and not yet semantically connected. As the toddler moves into the second half of his or her second year of life, these parroted vocal imitations provide a household echo.

Imitations and gestural representations (e.g., holding telephone to ear, hugging baby doll, putting shoe to foot) explode in the last few months of the second year period, allowing the world of make-believe to emerge. There is an increased interest in books and pictures, which now carry meaning for the child and can be connected to objects and word labels. The prosodic rhythms of nursery rhymes and fingerplays lure the 2-year-old to an accelerated level of repetition.

The 1-year-old's babble that bred a handful of single words is temporarily superceded by the 20-month-old's practice of suprasegmental jargon. This jargon often accompanies a 2-year-old's fantasy play. It is characterized by inflectional similarities to adult conversations, but with a noted lack of intelligible words.

At 18 months, the normal hearing toddler can imitate two-word phrases and many environmental sounds. By 22 months, four-word phrases are often imitated, but not spoken spontaneously. Nouns, verbs, and modifiers all appear in a child's expressive vocabulary, but are still used as noun labels (e.g., food may be called "banana" or "eat").

Receptively, this toddler can give appropriate responses to a series of two to three simple, but related commands. The child appears to listen to the meaning and reason of language utterances, not just to words or sounds, as receptive word vocabulary grows steadily.

The semantic focus of parents' and toddlers' verbal interactions during the first 2 years of a child's life results in the use of spontaneous two-word "telegraphs" about the objects, actions, and events with which he or she is actually involved. These concrete utterances reflect the cognitive level of concrete thought. Telegraphic utterances require verbal expansion by the parent that adds syntactic fill-ins. The use of correct word order gives form to the semantic intentions (Bloom & Lahey, 1978) that the child formerly could only express suprasegmentally through pitch, inflection, and intensity.

24 TO 48 MONTHS

During the third year of life, the child embarks on development of "Wh" question forms (Brown, 1973). The child's expressive language gives clear evidence of morphological additions of pronouns, prepositions, articles, plurals, and word endings. The 2-year-old's verbal use of pronouns and plurals demonstrates his or her social possessiveness. The child is no longer content with one block, but desires all the "blocks" that are "mine!" Prepositions come to life as the motorically coordinated and socially independent toddler goes in, under, around, and behind things in his or her world. Phonemic features gain clarity of articulation and most basic syntactic forms are used, although errors are frequent and telegraphic phrases are still present.

Receptively, the child demonstrates word associations and categories. Conceptually and linguistically, the child understands size, shape, color, and location. A preoperational child whose thinking is becoming representational demonstrates comprehension of early number concepts and is able to talk about things not physically present. The child's learning remains experience-based and the range of opportunities afforded the child serves as a learning catalyst.

4 TO 5 YEARS

During the fourth and fifth year of life, the three interwoven components of language (semantic content, form, pragmatic use) are expanded and refined. This transformational period of language development coordinates with a child's increased comprehension of attribution, quantity, causality, and time concepts. The child engages his or her semantic knowledge of word meanings and calls an umbrella an "underbrella." McNeill's LAD (language acquisition device) (McNeill, 1966) illustrates how semantically and syntactically sensible words can work pragmatically in context, but nevertheless be incorrect.

A child of this age has gleaned the generalities of form rules and may simply apply them universally. For example, as time concepts emerge, children learn that the morpheme "ed" is added to action words which describe events that have already happened (e.g. "I throwed it in the sink.") The well-intentioned parent who attempts to correct form errors, may say (e.g., "No, you threw it. Threw.") only to have their transformational LAD simply apply the same rule again (e.g., "I threw it in the sunk!"). How complex this task of language learning! For the hearing impaired child who may have no auditory information available from these visually and acoustically low morphological endings, the progress toward linguistic competence becomes even more challenging.

TRANSACTIONAL BREEDING GROUND

The first three years of life represent the critical period to acquire language and the interactional

patterns that provide the foundation stones of conversational competence. As active, information-seeking infants become neurologically organized and integrated, their learning is molded by the experiences afforded them through their senses in interactions with adults. Infant research in the 1980s confirmed these interactions between parent and infant to be transactional in nature, because both participants alternate the roles of initiator and responder.

The infant exhibits a behavior (e.g., cries without stopping), which elicits a response from the parent ("Oooh, Mommy's coming," followed by going to and picking up the infant). The quality of that response and the speed with which it occurs, over time, shapes an infant's subsequent response (cries, but then pauses to listen for mom's voice/footsteps or feel her uplifting arms).

Conversely, parents initiate a behavior (e.g., Mommy calls child's name and says "There's my happy boy!"), which elicits a response (e.g., smiling) from the infant, which, in turn, triggers the parents' subsequent response (Mommy repeats the compliment and expands it to "There's my happy boy! See that big smile?").

A child with an impaired auditory sense is receiving impoverished data about his or her world through the prediagnostic period of no amplification, or the postdiagnostic period of inconsistent or inappropriate amplification (Friedlander, 1979). The hearing-impaired infant and toddler, therefore, proceeds to experience his or her world with auditorily diminished semantic connectors to the transactional patterns and learning concepts being formed.

IMPACT OF HEARING LOSS

Professional peer pressure for audiological advancement toward earlier identification and ever-improving amplification is a natural result of knowledge about aural input and language development. Despite audiologic advancements, an appalling number of children are still not identified in the first year of life, when critical milestones of emotional bonding should occur.

Consider how a hearing loss can impact the parent/child transaction in the example just given, and an infant does not hear mother call or walk toward the crib. The baby continues to cry and, as nothing short of mother appearing visually or picking him or her up physically halts the crying, mother ceases in a few days to call her child at all. Furthermore, because mother does not yet know her infant cannot hear her, she may begin to perceive her child as her "fussy baby," instead of her "happy baby."

The auditory signals that contribute to the bonding of parent and child (Bowlby, 1982) that typically progressively increase between parent and child, diminish and, in some cases, actually disappear altogether with parents of a hearing-impaired child who fail to make those parent-reinforcing responses. When this occurs, one critical ingredient of auditory stimulation for the child's optimal listening environment is omitted. Restoration of those stimulating behaviors from parents must be an early goal in the habilitative process.

Even with the benefit of appropriate amplification, auditory signals initiated or sent in response by a parent out of a child's hearing range will go unnoticed by the hearing-impaired infant/toddler. This lack of response may be misinterpreted by a parent as emotional apathy or mental inability. Moreover, when the auditory signals of endearment that bond human beings together go undetected by a hearing-impaired infant, the outcome will neither promote the child's self-worth nor reap the parents' desired cuddly response from their infant. Undetected signals of danger could have even more disastrous consequences.

Infant (re)habilitation programs, therefore, must strive to help parents understand this transactional phenomenon and modify, not cease, their stimulating behaviors. Speech and hearing professionals classically only address auditory implications of behavior. For example, they might help

parents resume calling to their child at a 3', then 6', then 9' distance as they approach a fussing infant. This author is suggesting that professionals have more global insight and address psychosocial implications during intervention. Parents need professional help to understand that their child may be a "happy baby" when they call to the infant inside 6' where the baby can hear and that "fussy baby" behaviors beyond 6' are a function of the child's audiogram and *not* personality.

Transactional intervention, thereby, prevents the erosion of mutually satisfying interactions that bond parents to children, that teach children appropriate behaviors to communicate effectively later in life, and that help parents form realistic expectations and perceptions of their child.

A SAMPLE THERAPY SESSION

Armed with the knowledge of the components and stages of the language that children with hearing impairment need to acquire, professionals must immerse themselves in the transactional nature of infant aural (re)habilitation. Therapy sessions must be planned around the daily sensorimotor activities that, as Ling says in Chapter 9 are "part and parcel of everyday communication" for a child and his or her parent. Those activities include fixing meals, dressing, undressing, putting away groceries or laundry, decorating for holidays or birthdays, yardwork, playing, and planting. Because of the nature of such activities, a Home Demonstration Center is the model preferred over a clinic, hospital or school.

A therapy activity can be any daily household routine that is done during a family's everyday life. For the sake of this discussion, putting away groceries is used. The therapist prepares a bag or two of grocery items (preferably real ones in dealing with very young children) before the parent and child's arrival. After a brief welcome and reminder to the parent of the goals targeted for the session, the parent and child engage in the task of putting away the items in the bag.

At an early stage, one language goal for the child might be to vocalize on demand. The therapist might suggest that the parent use the attention-getting strategy of controlling objects by bringing forth one item at a time and a language strategy of giving it to the child to put away only after he or she vocalizes. A simultaneous goal for the parent might be to name objects and use descriptive language strategies. The therapist would encourage the parent to name and describe each item as it is taken from the bag. For example: "That's soup. Ugh, the soup is heavy!"

If necessary or desired by the parent, the therapist can model the technique with the child one or two times before the parent takes over. As the parent proceeds through the activity, the therapist is reinforcing the parent by saying things like, "I like how you're remembering to name each item. In fact, sometimes you repeat the name 2 or 3 times. That really helps [child] learn the names of things." When the child slams the cabinet closed after putting away the soup and the parent points to her ear and says to the child, "Mommy heard that! Bang! That was loud!" the therapist has opportunity to applaud the parent again for drawing her child's attention to a sound, naming the sound, and describing the sound.

Even though language goals change and become more complex over time, activities such as unloading groceries can continue to be employed. When language goals include learning categories, the parent can instruct the child to put away a fruit or a vegetable. Children learning to count can count the apples before they put them in the refrigerator crisper. Children learning prepositions can put the bread *in* the drawer, the ketchup *on* the shelf, and the soup *behind* the jelly. Auditorily discriminating "in the drawer versus on the door" is a worthy goal for any hearing impaired child.

The key here is *not* the activity, but the strategies taught a parent to orchestrate the activity—any activity. Once a parent learns to draw his or her child's attention to sound, name, and describe ob-

jects and events or control background noise, for example, they can help their child learn language while doing almost anything. Take caution that parents are **not** being trained to be a therapist, but rather as highly effective, competent parents who assist their child in learning to listen and speak 7 days a week 14 hours a day while having fun in the context of everyday life!

PARENTS AND CHILDREN NEED THE ACTIVE ROLE

Preschool children learn by doing (Northcott, 1977) and it is the parents who control whether their child will be an active participant or passive observer in learning experiences. Many parents need help to let their child be actively involved in even very simple daily tasks, such as cooking, cleaning, turning things on and off, stirring, opening, and unloading.

Prior to a child's third birthday, parent-focused intervention dictates that a parent also be in the active interactive role with his or her child, while the professional, at a close distance, "coaches" parents through the activity. Although the professional may step in periodically to model a particular strategy of behavior management or speech/language/auditory stimulation, the ultimate goal is for parents to gain confidence in their own competence. Parents, like their young conversational partner, learn by doing, not by watching others. Therapists, on the other hand, gain valuable insight watching parents interact with their children.

Communicative behaviors acquired transactionally in the first few months of life are predominantly nonverbal, but nevertheless critical precursors to spoken language. Parents can learn to match their infant's attention, imitate their behaviors, and "read" their child's thoughts. A synchrony of pace and emotion occurs as parents become increasingly tuned in to their infant. Parents soon can match their child's thoughts, actions, and perceptions with spoken language descriptors appropriate to their child's focus of attention. Non-verbal imitative games lead to verbal turntaking games. Children's language thus emerges from warm, mutually pleasurable, social transactions with their parents (Figure 8–2).

IMPACT OF GRIEVING ON PARENT/CHILD INTERACTION

Grieving parents can unwittingly undermine their own relationship with their child and with subsequent intervention. Parents in denial about their child's disability may delay the early consistent use of hearing aids and the beginning of active auditory-verbal stimulation. Depressed parents may seriously limit their communication with their spouse or their child's exposure to

those natural prosodic intonation patterns so critical to an infant's early understanding of language. Luterman's (1987) contention that "parents of hearing impaired children are the first clients" is valuable from both a linguistic and family health perspective.

Support groups and, in some cases, individual counseling are key components to the rehabilitative process. Certainly, teachers and therapists should not attempt to become counsellors, but neither should they abdicate their role in facilitating grieving. Because grieving is appropriate and necessary for parents receiving "bad" news, it must be viewed as a positive phenomenon by the professionals who work most frequently with the parents.

The grieving states of **anger, depression, denial, guilt,** and **anxiety** all are experienced by the

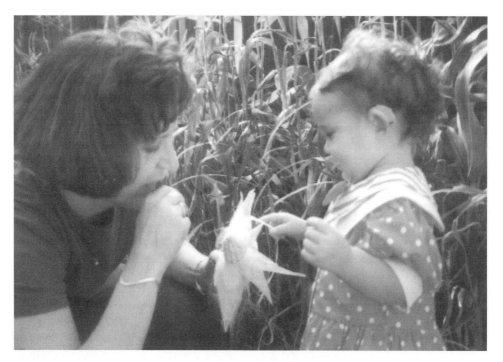

Figure 8–2. Parents are primary partners in language development for their hearing impaired children.

parents who arrive each week for therapy. These feeling states are commonly viewed as undesirable conditions. In actuality, they are the very conditions which (if professionally guided) will ultimately afford families the desired healthy adjustment to their child's diagnosis.

Consider denial, which buys people the time needed to find the internal strengths and external supports to meet the challenges ahead. When parents are in denial, therapists have a golden opportunity to verbally acknowledge a parents' internal strengths as they are discovered each week in therapy (e.g., "Good job, Mom! You seem to be able to read your child's thoughts and that will really help you match the language you use with what your child is thinking. I won't even have to teach you that!")

As therapists become acquainted with parents, they also can identify external supports, such as a supportive extended family, a caring next door neighbor, a deep religious faith, or a trusted pediatrician. Helping parents focus on and add to those external supports (e.g., introducing them to a parent of another child) is part of a therapist's role. When parents feel confident that they have the strength and supports necessary, they give up their denial.

Therapists need to exercise the same patience with parents that they have with children! All too often, as Dale Atkins explains in Chapter 5 of this text, professionals can impose their own "rate of recovery" on parents by their attitude. Each of the grieving states serves a positive purpose in parents becoming confident in their own competency. So, therapists need to welcome the grieving states!

For example, anxiety mobilizes energy. Energy is a very positive, desirable commodity, especially for the parent of a child with a profound hearing impairment. A therapist who has adopted the recommended positive attitude toward grieving, specifically the anxious parent, will help that parent identify and focus energy on his or her feeling. For example, the teacher says, "Wow, you sound really worried. What are you worried about?" The parent responds, "I am afraid there won't be the special teachers to help my child when they get to school." The teacher acknowledges the parents' individual strength by saying, "Aren't you clever to be thinking about the future for your child?" and steers that parent to use their energy to visit a program for older children and suggests they might want to talk about that at support group this week. *Parents, then, can use their grieving to grow.*

SUMMARY

Professionals involved in the audiologic (re)habilitation of young hearing-impaired children require a broad base of knowledge about child development, speech acoustics, and family dynamics into which can be meshed the specificity of strategies to enhance a child's listening and language development and to facilitate the parents' grieving process.

Early intervention is best served by addressing a family's emotional agendas with the same aggressiveness employed in fitting amplification, because parents are responsible for the wealth or poverty of their child's experiential base. Optimal language development in young children is accelerated by warm, nurturing transactional relationships with parents and, later, by teachers who can follow a child's lead in experiential exploration of his or her world.

The length of auditory deprivation can be as devastating to a child's language development as the diagnosis of deafness is to the emotional health of the child's primary language input source—the child's parents. Consistent, appropriate amplification for the child, individualized grief counselling for parents and early transactional parent-focused intervention, are parallel first steps in the audiological (re)habilitation of young hearing-impaired children.

Parents need many hours of guided interaction with their child to learn to take advantage of everyday activities. Devoted effective parents and professionals working together, help children gain the communicative competence needed for full participation in an integrated society in later years.

REFERENCES

Bloom, L. & Lahey, M. (1978). *Language development and language disorders.* New York: John Wiley and Sons.

Bowlby, J. (1982). *Attachment and loss* (2nd ed.). New York: Basic Books.

Brazelton, T. B., Koslowsk, B., & Main, M. (1974). The origins of reciprocity: The early mother-infant interaction. In M. Lewis & L. A. Rosenblum (Eds.), *The effect of the infant on its caregiver* (pp. 138–152). New York: Wiley.

Brown, R. (1973). *A first language: The early stages.* Cambridge, MA: Harvard University Press.

Bruner, J. (1975). The ontogenesis of speech acts. *Journal of Child Language, 2,* 1–21.

Bruner, J. (1983). *Child's talk: Learning to use language.* New York: W. W. Norton.

Erber, N. P. (1972). Speech envelope cues as an acoustic aid to lipreading for profoundly deaf children. *Journal of the Acoustical Society of America, 51,* 1224–1227.

Erber, N. (1982). *Auditory training.* Washington, DC: Alexander Graham Bell Association for the Deaf.

Friedlander, B. (1979). Finding facts of value and value in facts. In A. Simmons-Martin & D. Calvert (Eds.), *Parent-infant intervention: Communication disorders* (pp. 114–132). New York: Grune & Stratton.

Ling, D. (1976). *Speech and the hearing-impaired child: Theory and practice.* Washington, DC: Alexander Graham Bell Association for the Deaf.

Ling, A. H. (1976). The training of auditory memory in hearing-impaired children: Some problems of generalization. *Journal of the American Audiological Society, 1,* 150–157.

Luterman, D. (1987). *Deafness in the family.* Boston: College-Hill Press.

McNeill, D. (1966). Developmental psycholinguistics. In F. Smith & G. A. Miller (Eds.), *The genesis of language* (pp. 15–85). Cambridge, MA: MIT Press.

Northcott, W. (1977). *Curriculum guide: Hearing impaired children birth to three years, and their parents.* Washington, DC: Alexander Graham Bell Association for the Deaf.

Pollack, D. (1985). *Educational audiology for the limited-hearing infant and preschooler.* Springfield, IL: Charles C. Thomas.

Simmons-Martin, A. (1981). Acquisition of language by under-fives including the parental role. In A. M. Mulholland (Ed.), *Oral education today and tomorrow* (pp. 253–273). Washington, DC: Alexander Graham Bell Association for the Deaf.

Snow, C. (1977a). The development of conversation between mothers and babies. In *Talking to children: Language and acquisition.* New York: Cambridge University Press.

Snow, C. (1977b). Mother's speech research: From input to interaction. In C. Snow & C. Ferguson (Eds.), *Talking to children: Language input and acquisition.* New York: Cambridge University Press.

Stone, P. (1988). *Blueprint for developing conversational competence: A planning/instruction model with detailed scenarios.* Washington, DC: Alexander Graham Bell Association for the Deaf.

van Uden, A. M. J. (1981). Hometraining service for deaf children in the Netherlands. In A. Simmons-Martin & D. R. Calvert (Eds.), *Parent-infant intervention* (pp. 165–177). New York: Grune & Stratton.

SUGGESTED READINGS

Anisfeld, M. (1984). *Language development from birth to three.* Hillsdale, NJ: Lawrence Erlbaum Associates.

Bloom, L., & Lahey, M. (1978). *Language development and language disorders.* New York: John Wiley & Sons, Inc.

Brown, R., & Bellugi, U. (1964). Three processes in the child's acquisition of syntax. *Harvard Educational Review, 34,* 133–151.

Bruner, J. (1978). The role of dialogue in language acquisition. In A. Sinclair, R. Jarvella, & W. Levelt (Eds.), *The child's conception of language* (pp. 212–222). New York: Springer-Verlag.

Dunst, C. J. (1981). *Infant learning.* Hingham, MA: Teaching Resources.

Grant, J. (1987). *The hearing impaired: Birth to Six.* Boston: Little, Brown.

McArthur, S. H. (1982). *Raising your hearing-impaired child: a guideline for parents.* Washington, DC: Alexander Graham Bell Association for the Deaf.

Piaget, J. (1952). *The origins of intelligence in children* (M. Cook, Trans.). New York: International Universities Press.

Vygotskii, L. (1962). *Thought and language* (E. Hanfman & G. Vakar, Trans.). Cambridge, MA.: MIT Press.

White, B. L. (1975). *A guide to the physical, emotional, and intellectual growth of your baby.* Englewood Cliffs, NJ: Prentice-Hall.

White, B. L. (1985). *The first three years of life.* New York: Prentice Hall Press.

END OF CHAPTER EXAMINATION QUESTIONS

CHAPTER 8

1. Discuss the parents' role in the three basic components of language: (a) semantic content, (b) syntactic form, and (c) pragmatic use.

2. Briefly describe the difference between receptive and expressive language. Give an example of each.

3. Give three examples of how parents might suspect that their child possesses a hearing loss.
   a.
   b.
   c.

4. Preschool children learn best by
   a. observing
   b. hearing
   c. doing
   d. none of the above
   e. all of the above

5. The most efficient sense that is utilized in the initial development of functional verbal communication skills during the first 3 years of life is
   a. hearing
   b. sight
   c. touch
   d. all of the above

6. _____refers to the orderly arrangement of verbal symbols to convey meaning.
   a. communication
   b. spoken language
   c. receptive language
   d. none of the above

END OF CHAPTER ANSWER SHEET

Name   Date

CHAPTER 8

1. a. _____

   b. _____

   c. _____

2. _____

   _____

   _____

   _____ .

3. a. _____

   b. _____

   c. _____

4. Which one(s)?   a   b   c   d   e

5. Which one(s)?   a   b   c   d

6. Which one(s)?   a   b   c   d

7. Circle one: True   False

8. Circle one: True   False

9. Circle one: True   False

10. Circle one: True   False

7. (True/False) Between the ages of 6-12 months, an infant's expressive verbal language is geared towards more purposeful sounds that possess socio-emotional intent.

8. (True/False) Receptively, the 12 month old who is gaining on symbolic representation can match objects to pictures and identify those pictures when they're named.

9. (True/False) During the 24-36 month stage, children embark on the "wh" question forms.

10. (True/False) According to the author, during a therapy session, one should avoid activities that are similar to the sensorimotor activities that are part of everyday communication.

■ CHAPTER 9 ■

Speech Development for Children Who are Hearing Impaired

■ DANIEL LING, Ph.D. ■

SPEECH AS A SENSORY-MOTOR PROCESS

THE RATIONALE FOR PROMOTING SPOKEN
LANGUAGE

THE SPEECH ACHIEVEMENTS OF CHILDREN WITH
HEARING IMPAIRMENT
    Speech in the Context of Spoken Language
    Factors Affecting Speech Development

CRUCIAL BASES FOR OPTIMAL SPEECH
DEVELOPMENT
    Early Detection of Hearing Impairment
    Provision of Appropriate Sensory Aids: Devices and
       Speech

(continued)

For several centuries, children with various degrees of hearing impairment, including many who were totally deaf, have been taught to communicate through the use of spoken language. Nowadays, speech development is included on the curricula of most special schools and classes for hearing-impaired children. The extent to which such teaching succeeds depends not only on the characteristics of the children enrolled, but also on the importance assigned to speech in any given educational program and on the relative competence of the professionals undertaking the work (Markides, 1983).

Until the years immediately preceding World War II, speech development among children with hearing impairment was promoted mainly by teachers of the deaf in the course of their classroom work. Among the most famous of such teachers was Alexander Graham Bell (1907), who contributed many specific speech teaching techniques to the field. In more recent years, speech-language pathologists and, to a lesser extent, audiologists have become increasingly involved in developing spoken language skills, often working in clinical settings with very young children and their parents.

SPEECH AS A SENSORY-MOTOR PROCESS

Speech acquisition is a perceptual as well as an oral process. Perception pervades speech communication. For people to understand the speech addressed to them, they must, through the ears, the eyes, and/or the skin, be able to detect, discriminate, and identify sufficient information in the spoken message to permit them to comprehend it. For acquiring accuracy of expression, a talker also requires some form of sensory feedback involving conscious or unconscious awareness of the sensations generated in the act of talking. The sensory modalities that are most appropriate for the development of speech vary from one child to another, mainly according to the degree of hearing impairment and the type of educational or habilitation program that has been or is being, followed (Boothroyd, 1982; Ling, 1988; Reed, 1984).

The work of teachers of speech for those with hearing impairment up to about 50 years ago was based almost exclusively on speechreading, the use of tactile cues, and awareness of internal feedback cued by kinesthesia (Silverman, 1983). Now, as a result of research and the technology developed during the past few decades, much more is known about spoken language and its acquisition. Hearing impairment can be identified at birth or even before birth and speech communication skills can be enhanced by working with parents and their hearing-impaired children during the earliest stages of infancy. Modern speech development procedures are supported by ever-more sophisticated devices and strategies to measure hearing and to provide amplification. One can now, through the use of cochlear implants, stimulate the neural receptors in the inner ear of children who would formerly have had to function as totally deaf individuals, thus permitting many of them to perceive a great deal of spoken language and other acoustic stimuli in their environments. During recent years it has also become possible to

transmit speech to the skin through wearable vibrotactile and electrotactile devices (Blamey & Clark, 1985; McGarr, 1989; Proctor, 1984; Sherrick, 1984). As a result, we are now in a much better position than at any other time in history to promote the development of speech communication skills among hearing-impaired children (Lauter, 1985).

THE RATIONALE FOR PROMOTING SPOKEN LANGUAGE

Speech skills are strongly associated with superior educational achievements (Jensema & Trybus, 1978); and educational achievements, in turn, are strongly influenced by how effectively children can read and use English (Hanson, Liberman, & Schankweiler, 1984). In reviewing the evidence relating to speech and memory, Quigley and Paul (1984, p. 50) concluded that "speech recoding is important to reading development" and that "faithful representation of English structure seems to be particularly sensitive to speech recoding."(p. 50) At a more general level, it is clear that individuals with hearing impairment who can communicate through the use of spoken language, whether or not they also use sign, have many advantages. They can interact more freely with other members of society, most of whom talk. They can, therefore, function more independently in most of the everyday situations that they are likely to meet in employment, leisure, and family life (Subtelny, 1980).

Legislation and social awareness have improved the lot of most hearing-impaired people in western societies, but, even so, the advantages lie with those who can talk. With spoken language, opportunities for higher education are less restricted, a more extensive range of careers is open, and there is greater security of employment. Those who can talk also face fewer limitations in the personal and social aspects of their lives (Silverman, 1983). To talk poorly rather than well can, however, be disadvantageous to individuals with hearing impairment in their employment. Doggett (1989), for example, found that there was a high correlation between employers' ratings of the comprehensibility of speech and their ratings of a person's independence, likeability, and competence. Her hearing-impaired subjects received poorer ratings than those who were native or foreign speakers, and the poorest ratings were given to the poorest speakers.

THE SPEECH ACHIEVEMENTS OF CHILDREN WITH HEARING IMPAIRMENT

The speech of children with moderate (50–70 dB HL) or severe (70–90 db HL) hearing impairment usually reflects the quality of their auditory management. Such children, when appropriately aided and stimulated, are able to acquire much of their spoken language spontaneously through the use of their residual hearing (Ling, 1988). The speech of profoundly (>90dB HL) hearing-impaired children tends to reflect not only the type of information provided by the device(s) a child is using (hearing aid, cochlear implant, and/or tactile aid), but also the amount and quality of systematic teaching received (see Figure 9-1). The more profoundly hearing impaired the child, the more difficult it is to acquire speech spontaneously. In general, the more profound the degree of hearing impairment, the greater the amount of formal speech teaching a child will require to acquire spoken language (Markides, 1983).

Various levels of speech and spoken language achievement by children with impaired hearing have been reported in the literature. On the one hand, the many advantages of early perceptual-oral treatment have led some profoundly hearing-impaired children to acquire normal or near-normal speech (Ling & Ling, 1978; Ling & Milne,

1981). On the other hand, several large-scale demographic studies have shown that, overall, there has been scant improvement in the average standards of speech production by hearing-impaired school children during recent years despite technical and educational advances in speech science and allied fields (Wolk & Schildroth, 1986). There is clearly a great deal of unrealized potential for better speech and language among children who are hearing-impaired.

SPEECH IN THE CONTEXT OF SPOKEN LANGUAGE

The traditional method of teaching speech to children with hearing impairment has been to develop the production of sound patterns largely in isolation and then to combine them to form syllables, words, and sentences. But, during the last few decades, authors such as Calvert and Silverman (1975, 1983); Ewing and Ewing (1964), and Vorce (1974), among others, have recognized that some speech skills can, under conditions that favor speech reception and language learning, usually be acquired spontaneously by many such children. Accordingly, authors such as Clark (1989), Cole (1990), and the writer (Ling, 1988) have advocated a greater focus on promoting the acquisition of speech in the context of spoken language as it is used in natural communication. Their views are strongly supported by numerous other writers in the Volta Bureau's 1992 monograph on speech production in hearing-impaired children and youth edited by Stoker and Ling (1992).

Individual differences among children with hearing impairment are often greater than those among children who hear normally because degree and age at onset of hearing impairment are additional and important variables affecting development. Consequently, no one type of speech development program can possibly suit the needs

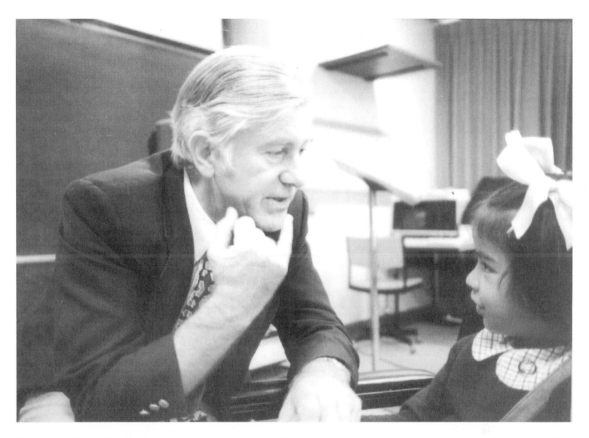

Figure 9–1. The quality of speech of a hearing impaired child reflects not only the device worn, but also the systematic level of teaching received.

of all such children. Some, with appropriate parental participation and professional support, can learn to hear (and even overhear) people talking to them and around them and, by this means, acquire most of their speech and spoken language skills much as normally hearing children do (see Bader, Chapters 7 and 8). Others require highly organized training to develop effective speech communication (see Ling, 1976, 1988; Stone, 1988). Most require at least some remedial help to gain mastery over the production of certain sound patterns, for abnormalities commonly develop in the

speech of children whose hearing impairment is severe (about 70–90 dB HL) or profound (>90 dB). Remedial help is usually focused on particular speech patterns and on strategies for their carryover into everyday communication practices.

Carryover from lessons to life is least difficult to orchestrate when speech lessons and speech-language therapy closely relate to real life conditions. It is most difficult to manage effectively when lessons or therapy are organized around the use of devices and procedures that are not part and parcel of everyday communication (Ling, 1988, pp.

250–255). Generalization problems facing children who are hearing-impaired can, therefore, if inappropriate devices are used extensively and exclusively in formal teaching or therapy, become even more serious than those facing normally hearing children who have language deficits. A far-reaching analysis of issues affecting generalization from lessons to life has been undertaken by various writers in a clinical forum section of *Language, Speech and Hearing Services in Schools* (Fey, 1988).

FACTORS AFFECTING
SPEECH DEVELOPMENT

Both intrinsic and extrinsic factors influence the acquisition of speech skills among children who have hearing impairment. Factors that are intrinsic to each child cannot, in general, be changed or greatly improved through direct intervention. These include unaided sensorineural hearing levels, age at onset of hearing impairment, visual acuity, integrity of or damage to the central nervous system, integrity of or damage to the peripheral speech mechanisms, and so on.

Extrinsic factors may be defined as devices, procedures, people, and life experiences that, either by design or chance, affect the development of children's communication skills. They include hearing aids, cochlear implants, tactile aids, glasses, socioeducational practices and experiences, environmental communication modes, parents' management skills, teacher/clinician competence, availability of support personnel, and the extent and type of children's contacts with peers (Ling, 1989). Orchestration of such extrinsic factors so that they operate most effectively to enhance the development of spoken language skills should be regarded as an extremely important part of any speech development program. To be optimally effective, developmental and remedial speech training programs for children who have hearing impairment cannot be confined within the walls of a clinic or classroom or to professionals' involvement within their normal working hours.

CRUCIAL BASES FOR OPTIMAL
SPEECH DEVELOPMENT

EARLY DETECTION OF
HEARING IMPAIRMENT

During the past few decades, the use of computers has become widespread in the fields of speech, language, and hearing (Curtis, 1987). They have allowed development of the various forms of electrophysiological hearing tests that are now in widespread clinical use, not only as diagnostic tools, but also for screening the hearing of children at birth (Jerger, 1984). Further relatively recent and highly significant contributions to tests of hearing in early infancy have been the development of the immittance battery (Popelka, 1981), and visual response audiometry (Wilson & Thompson, 1984). Such tests, together with the use of probe-tube microphone systems in hearing aid selection, permit the effective use of hearing aids or other sensory aids with more and more children from a few months of age (Jerger, 1984; Stelmachowicz & Seewald, 1990).

When spoken language development begins in the first year of life rather than later, children cannot only be provided with more natural exposure to their mothers' spoken commentaries on objects and events that interest them, but can monitor and preserve the quality of much of the reflexive vocalization and repetitive babble they produce during the first year of life (Oller, Eilers, Bull, & Carney (1985). Such auditory or alternative sensory access to their own early utterances promotes the children's production of an extended range of vocalization (Mischook & Cole, 1986). It also provides them with the essential foundations for feedback on the quality of their voices and the accuracy of the spoken language that they will later acquire (Ling & Ling, 1978). The ultimate development of children's spoken language has long been known to be most effectively triggered by appropriate stimulation during the first few years of life (Friedlander, 1970; Fry, 1966; Lenneberg, l967; Studdert-Kennedy, 1984). Music and song, well within the perceptual capacity of most children who have hearing impairment, is a recommended part of such stimulation (Estabrooks & Birkenshaw-Fleming, 1994)

The acoustic environment of most homes approaches the ideal for speech acquisition by children under a year of age. With carpets on the floors, relatively little noise is created by movement. With drapes at the windows and soft furnishings around the house, reflection and reverberation of sounds are at minimal levels in most rooms. Most important, however, is that mothers are usually quite close to their infants when they are talking to them. Conditions that predominate in most homes thus make for clear speech signals at babies' ears—signals that are not degraded by background noise. Speaking while a child is within earshot is clearly an essential for auditory learning (Ling, 1981).

After their first year, children's acoustic environments are less stable. As they become able to move over considerable distances without help from or contact with their mothers, they tend to have less speech addressed to them at close quarters. Nevertheless, young children are more frequently at home in good acoustic conditions than out and in noise. The emphasis in early speech habilitation over the past few decades has, therefore, shifted to the guidance of parents rather than direct intervention with infants. Descriptions of exemplary programs having such emphasis have been provided by the several contributors to a book edited by the writer (Ling, 1984a). Many ways in which parents can be involved in the aural habilitative process are discussed by Atkins in this volume (see Chapter 5).

PROVISION OF APPROPRIATE SENSORY AIDS: DEVICES AND SPEECH

The three senses through which we can gather information about speech are audition, vision, and touch. When aided hearing does not provide adequate sensory information about speech, vision and touch can be used as supplementary or alternative sensory channels. Cochlear implants and tactile aids, both of which became generally available as recently as the 1980s, are now quite frequently prescribed as alternatives to hearing aids for children who have little or no residual hearing over all or part of the frequency range of speech. Either type of instrument can be of single or multichannel design and both vibro- and electrotactile devices are available. No currently available cochlear implant or tactile device can compensate fully for severe, profound, or total deafness so, like hearing aids, they are most effective when used to supplement speechreading (DeFilippo, 1984; Pickett & McFarland, 1985).

Some children use both a hearing aid and a cochlear implant, and many children who hear nothing beyond 1000 Hz find that a multichannel tactile device or frequency transposition (see Figure 9-2) will supplement aided audition in speech perception. These devices and what they can contribute to children's speech and spoken language acquisition have been presented in detail in a book by the writer (Ling, 1988), and are also discussed by others in this volume. The selection of appropriate sensory aids (hearing aids, cochlear implants, and tactile devices) will depend on the needs of individual children. To use any one of them to the utmost effect in developing speech skills, the teacher/clinician must be thoroughly familiar with the acoustic properties of speech, know exactly what speech patterns a given sensory aid can be expected to provide for each particular child, ensure that the sensory aids for each child have been appropriately selected and adjusted, and see that the devices are consistently used under good acoustic conditions.

VISION AND SPEECH

Speechreading is the art of understanding the visual cues that occur as talkers move their tongues,

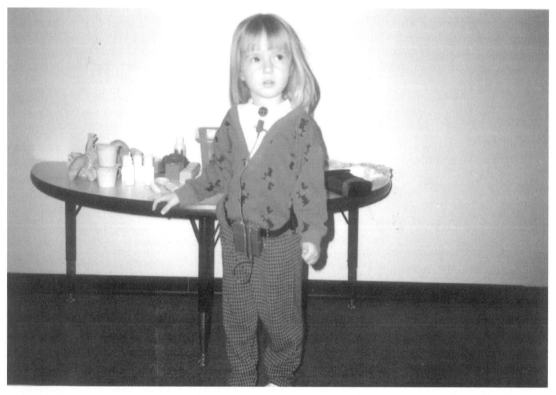

Figure 9–2. Frequency transposition provides increased accessibility to sounds that otherwise may not be heard by a child with a hearing impairment.

lips, and jaws and produce related facial expressions and body postures in the act of speaking (Ijsseldijk, 1988). Unfortunately, only comparatively degraded information on speech production is available through speechreading. This is because there are no visible correlates of some speech patterns. For example, vocalization (the use of voice), prosody, and nasality cannot be perceived through speechreading alone, because adjustments and positions of the larynx, tongue, and velum are partially or completely obscured by the lips and the teeth. Thus, there are severe limitations to learning speech through visual imitation. Also, several other sounds share visual patterns

and, on this account, are frequently confused (see DeFilippo & Sims, 1988; Dodd & Campbell, 1987).

Although speechreading by itself provides a very impoverished signal it is, nevertheless, a natural and often effective supplement to hearing in the development of spoken language. This is because the cues that speechreading provides, such as those relating to place of consonant production, can usefully augment a message that is heard only in part (see Erber, 1972). Many of the sensory aids such as tactile devices and cochlear implants produced in recent years serve or have been designed to supplement speechreading. If vision is to be used in helping children who have hearing impairment to talk, the teacher or clinician must know exactly what components, if any, of a given speech pattern can be clearly seen and how such components complement the information provided by the sensory aid or aids used by each individual.

Numerous visual aids, some involving sophisticated technology, have been produced to enhance children's speech production in the course of clinical training. However, there are at least three major problems inherent in their use. *First*, visual displays that represent the complete speech signal are hard to perceive, whereas simpler displays poorly represent the dynamic nature of communicative speech. *Second*, because they provide information that is quite unlike that required for communication in everyday life, it becomes essential for the teacher or clinician to design and supervise an extensive range of generalization procedures to ensure that speech skills acquired through the use of such devices are carried over into children's meaningful use of spoken language. *Third*, teaching through reference to a visual representation of only part of the normally complex speech signal has to be done under the close supervision of a professional, if one skill is not to be learned to the detriment of another. Although one can easily show that children can learn particular skills through the use of visual speech training aids (and it is on this account that they are recommended), there have been no convincing studies demonstrating that the use of such devices leads to improved speech communication abilities in the everyday lives of children. It is difficult to promote the carryover of speech skills into everyday life when they are learned through strategies that are not primarily based on interpersonal communication (Perigoe & Ling, 1986).

EARLY INTERVENTION

To be optimally effective in developing perceptual-oral communication, professionals and parents must adopt developmental strategies for speech perception and speech production that differ according to each child's unique sensory capacities and needs. Special attention to such needs should, ideally, be initiated from the first few months of life. Such early intervention in which parents become the primary agents in the process of fostering their children's development is discussed in Chapters 5, 6, 7, and 8 in this volume.

Topics such as audition, speechreading, hearing aids, speech development, language development, technology, education, parent guidance, and early intervention inevitably tend to be discussed in separate chapters. Unfortunately, this gives many readers the false impression that activities related to such topics may also be treated as distinct when helping children develop speaking skills. Nothing could be further from the truth. Programs that do not integrate all aspects of habilitation can impede rather than encourage progress in the acquisition of perceptual-oral communication.

Children can acquire optimal speech communication skills only when they use personal hearing aids and/or other selected sensory aids during all waking hours. A further requirement is that the speech addressed to children relates closely to their cognitive levels, motor development, self-help skills, and personal and social experiences. Such experiences normally abound in the meaningful situations that pervade the activities of everyday living (Grant, 1987; Ling & Ling, 1978). Early speech development should not be based initially on the formal teaching of particular speech patterns, but on children's desire to communicate through speech and on their approximations to adult sentence patterns in the various areas of discourse—conversation, narration, questions, explanation, and description (Ling, 1988).

The first step in the process of learning speech informally will usually result in vocalizations in which desirable intonation contours rather than consonants or vowels are imitated. Appropriate perception and production of segmental features are likely to follow naturally under such circumstances, if, according to their individual needs, children are using acoustic hearing aids, more than one sort of sensory information, or another sort of sensory aid. Even with children who start their program somewhat later—for example at age 3 or 4—developing speech through the meaningful use of spoken language in interactive situations is likely to result in later speech skills that are superior to those developed through more formal teaching (Ling, 1988).

SYSTEMATIC PROGRAMMING

Many different levels of skill have to be acquired before intelligible words can appear (Murry & Murry, 1980). Just as a variety of vocalizations and canonical (repetitive) babbling patterns precede speech in normally hearing babies so do such prespeech patterns help to lay the foundations for the speech of children who have hearing impairment. Just as control of a wide range of vowels and diphthongs precedes mastery of most consonants and blends in the speech of normally hearing children, so do they create a similar groundwork for consonant production in those with hearing impairment. The order of speech pattern development presented in the model described and discussed by Ling (1988) appears to be optimal for both informal and (the later) formal development and remediation of speech among children with hearing impairment. The model suggests that speech development should be promoted in seven somewhat overlapping sequential stages, progressing from control of vocalization, to production of prosodic patterns, vowels and diphthongs, consonants differing in manner, consonants differing in place, consonants differing in voicing, to consonant blends (clusters).

Such organization can save substantial amounts of time and increase efficiency, because systematic programming ensures that behaviors that are prerequisites for the production of any given pattern are already present and that new skills can be developed that relate to skills that have been previously acquired. For example, children who, on account of their hearing impairment, have failed to develop a /g/ spontaneously, can, as explained by Ling (1988), more easily learn to produce the sound through reference to the production of /b/ and /d/ than through description, direct imitation, or any other strategy (see following discussion).

EVALUATION

Children's potential for learning to talk should, particularly during the early stages of habilitation, be assessed mainly through ongoing evaluation in the course of treatment in a program that features wholehearted commitment to the development of spoken language. Many factors contribute to young children's speech acquisition and, apart from a relatively few essentials such as hearing levels and basic oral-peripheral function, the aspects cannot be assessed simply through formal clinical evaluation. For example, it is only following parental counselling, education, and support services that one can determine the extent to which they are able to help their children. Also, it is only when children have sufficient experience of speech reception through an appropriate sensory aid that their capacities for speech recognition can be assessed. In short, diagnostic training under optimal conditions is a prerequisite for a valid prognosis and the planning of therapy or teaching (Cole & Gregory, 1986).

Evaluation of both speech reception and speech production are essential aspects of any program directed toward children's speech development. Tests of either aspect can be norm-referenced (designed and standardized to permit comparisons) or criterion-referenced (designed to determine what skills a particular child has acquired). The latter tests provide the most appropriate guides for therapy or teaching. To evaluate speech reception abilities, one must have tests that determine if children can detect, discriminate, and identify the elements of speech (prosodic features, vowels and consonants) as well as tests that determine how well running speech is perceived. Audiological tests of these types have been discussed by Beasley (1984) and by Bess (1988). Such tests, as currently performed, however, can provide but part of the necessary information, as speech reception measures must also encompass appraisal of children's performance not only with hearing aids, but with cochlear implants, tactile aids, speechreading, or a combination of these (see Geers & Moog, 1989).

Various tests of speech production are available, and procedures that measure speech intelligibility through listener judgments and rating scales are commonly used in research studies (Subtelny, 1980; Wolk & Schildroth (1986). For therapy and teaching purposes, however, one needs to use tests that permit the assessment of each child's ability to produce both the elements of speech (vocalization, suprasegmental features, vowels, and consonants) and to use speech meaningfully in everyday discourse. Only if one can identify the precise deficits in place, can one select the most appropriate remedial measures to overcome them. The Ling (1976) Phonetic Level and Phonologic Level Evaluations are criterion-referenced tests designed to provide the necessary diagnostic information for effective speech development and the program of which they are part is also in widespread use (Cole & Mischook, 1985). An adaptation of this test, The Phonetic-Phonologic Speech Evaluation Record was designed by Ling (1991) to permit comparison of pre- and posttraining results with different types of sensory aids and teaching strategies.

TEACHING AND LEARNING: SOME STRATEGIES

INFORMAL AND FORMAL PROCEDURES

Informal speech development procedures can be defined as those that involve activities with children (particularly young ones) that are largely unplanned by adults, that are primarily determined by the children's interests and needs, and that lead to the spontaneous acquisition of spoken language. Informal procedures usually involve parents, caregivers, and/or peers to a greater extent than professionals. Formal procedures are those in which learning and teaching activities are deliberately planned and carried out in accordance with a predetermined program of speech development, usually by teachers or clinicians (Ling, 1988).

The basic techniques, tactics, and tools involved in the teaching and learning of speech communication by children who have hearing impairment are summarized in Table 9–1. The content of this table is illustrative, rather than exhaustive. It simply lists the major elements of effective speech development programs that are discussed in this chapter and details the somewhat sequential nature of the techniques and strategies that can be applied. Note that the tools of greatest importance are sensory aids—primarily hearing aids, but also, cochlear implants or tactile devices for some children. Table 9–1 maps the relationships between material already presented and the discussion that follows.

Whether speech acquisition programs are formal or informal, perception must either precede or accompany production. Speech addressed to, used in the presence of, or produced by children with hearing impairment must be processed through devices that permit the child (as Hirsh, 1940, put it) to detect, discriminate, identify, and comprehend as much as possible of an utterance.

TABLE 9–1. Techniques, Tactics, and Tools Involved in Teaching and Learning Spoken Language

Techniques	Tactics	Tools
Informal learning (enhancement of early childhood experiences and events)	Focus on: Early intervention Early detection Parental involvement Speech reception Speech production Communication Personal-social growth	Appropriate diagnostic technology, sensory aids, everyday objects
Informal teaching (enhancement of care giving practices)	Focus on: Context-based spoken language Perception of message Refinement of dialogue Perception of meaning Clarity of expression Spontaneous discourse Integration of personal-social skills	Tools as above
Formal teaching (initiated only following optimal exposure to informal techniques)	Focus on: Evaluation of sensory aids Systematic programming Development of specific skills Remediation of specific faults Use of anticipatory set Training to automaticity Programming generalization Promoting carryover Developing discourse skills Extending communicative competence	Appropriate and selected materials
Formal learning (school-age through adult life)	Focus on: Conscious and deliberate acquisition of knowledge and skills by an individual	Tools as above

Among the most important cues for the acquisition and maintenance of speech by children who have hearing impairment are the tactile and kinesthetic sensations that are produced as they, themselves, talk. Just as every speech pattern in the language sounds different to a normal listener, so does every such pattern feel different to a normal talker. It is the tactile and kinesthetic codes that are established in the course of speech acquisition that permit older children who lose all of their hearing to maintain most, if not all, of their speech skills. Being sure that children who are (or become) hearing-impaired encode accurate tactile and kinesthetic patterns to guide their speech production must be treated as an essential part of informal or formal learning and teaching (Ling, 1976).

Informal Learning

Informal learning takes place as children receive stimuli from their environments and try to derive meaning from them. Speech is normally addressed to (or used within earshot of) children in the context of activities that permit them to derive meaning from what has been said. The effective use of appropriate sensory aids, supplemented or not by speechreading, provides optimal opportunities for children who have hearing impairment to learn a great deal about speech reception and speech production in much the same way as their normally hearing peers (Wood, Wood, Griffiths, & Howarth, 1986).

Informal Teaching

Informal teaching is usually provided by parents in the course of everyday activities around the home, where repetitive situations such as daily dressing, food preparation, feeding, and housework, as well as caregiving, supervision, and play activities, contribute abundant opportunities for both children and parents to initiate spoken language and for the children to acquire speech perception and speech production skills. With appropriately selected sensory aids, children who have hearing impairment can be encouraged to interact effectively and verbally with parents, caregivers, siblings, and peers. Informal teaching of children by others in the home can be enhanced through parent guidance work and, even with children whose hearing impairment is profound, can at least result in approximations to adult forms of speech that provide the ideal base for more formal teaching.

Informal teaching is not only a part of parent guidance programs. It can also be provided in the course of therapy or education in which the principal purpose of the play or other activity is to promote the acquisition of spoken language through interaction and the encouragement of increasingly complex vocalizations and spontaneous approximations to mature forms of speech. Informal teaching procedures strongly feature the positive reinforcement of involumtary sound patterns, such as those in crying (boo-hoo), laughing (ha-ha), giggling (hee-hee), and babbling. This is done with a view to enhancing awareness and feedback of such sounds through the sensory aid(s) that have been selected. Groundwork can thus be provided for the voluntary production of such sound patterns and their inclusion in speech.

Formal Teaching

Formal teaching involves an adult's planned instruction to a child. The purpose of such instruction is to develop knowledge or skills that the child has not previously acquired (Figure 9–3). Most schoolwork and a great deal of therapy is of this type. Formal teaching of speech may be considered as a remedial procedure that has two major objectives: *first*, helping children to produce particular sounds or sequences of sounds that, even after extensive and appropriate stimulation, have not been acquired through informal procedures, and *second*, the correction of errors. Formal teaching is not appropriate as the first step in promoting children's acquisition of speech skills. Further, if formal teaching of speech is begun before a child is using sentence approximations consisting of at least two or three words to communicate, the development of natural sounding speech may be inhibited. Every opportunity should, therefore, be afforded for children to acquire a wide range of speech patterns spontaneously through the use of suitable sensory aids before formal work is attempted.

The extent to which children acquire speech skills spontaneously depends largely on the degree to which the sensory aids selected for them compensate (with or without speechreading) for their hearing impairment. It follows that when

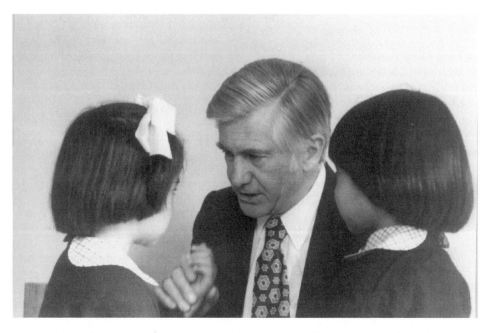

Figure 9–3. Formal teaching is used to develop knowledge or skills the child has not previously acquired).

particular patterns have not emerged (or have emerged in a distorted form) following extensive informal teaching, devices and procedures other than those previously used will be required to elicit the patterns.

Because there are only three sensory modalities through which speech can be perceived—*hearing, vision,* and *touch*—and because the use of hearing and vision (and possibly tactile devices) will already have been promoted in the course of informal teaching, *the direct use of touch* will clearly have to be the basis of much formal speech teaching. Indeed, many tactile strategies are available for guiding speech production. They include having the children feel *vibration* of the chest when vocalizing, the *movement* of the larynx as intonation changes, and the *duration, intensity,* and *temperature* of the breath stream as different vowels, fricatives, and plosives are produced. A *finger tap* on the hand or a *finger drawn* slowly or quickly along

the arm can be used to signal durational cues that a given child can neither hear nor see, such as the difference between /m/ and /b/. Care should, of course, be exercised to ensure that the children receive such cues without feeling that the clinician or teacher is invading their personal space.

Formal Learning

Formal learning is usually undertaken only by quite mature children with a peer or adult to monitor production, because feedback on correctness is an important aspect of formal learning in speech acquisition. If sufficiently accurate feedback is not directly available to a child, then it must be provided through an external source. Analytical feedback provided by a skilled listener is preferable to that derived through instrumental analysis, because whether or not speech patterns are perceived as acceptable or "correct" depends largely on how they interact with other sounds (i.e., coarticulation) in the context in which they are produced.

THE PROCESS OF LEARNING AND TEACHING SPEECH

The most natural and effective process in learning and teaching speech is to ensure that children acquire new patterns as an extension of those that are already mastered. Indeed, all children proceed from one stage of development to the next using previously established skills that, in many instances, are actually prerequisites for new behaviors. For example, control over vocalization has to precede controlled production of prosodic patterns and vowels. The production of vowels, in turn, has to precede the mastery of consonants, because consonants in the dynamic stream of speech are, by and large, merely different ways of initiating, interrupting, or releasing vowels. Encouraging the development of speech through formal teaching based on the recognition of natural ordering has long been advocated (see McDonald, 1964).

THE ANTICIPATORY SET

The use of anticipatory set is a strategy based on both natural ordering and the propensity of human beings to anticipate required future responses on the basis of immediately preceding stimuli. To provide an example of such anticipation, ask literate people to pronounce the two letters (i) and (g) as a syllable and they will say "ig." Then ask them what they call an artificial head of hair and they will say "wig." Finally, ask them to name a large piece of wood broken from a tree and, because anticipatory set is such a compelling force, most will say "twig," even though a response such as "branch" would be more accurate.

Anticipatory set can be applied at all stages of speech development. To apply it to the development of consonants, for instance, first establish

manner of consonant production with an early-occurring speech sound and then through the use of anticipatory set elicit the other consonants, sharing that manner of production one-by-one. Thus, first have a child produce /b/ in repeated syllables such as /ba/, /bi/, and /bu/. This establishes an anticipatory set for manner of production. Then, by reference to /b/, establish /d/. Once this can be easily produced, sufficient anticipatory set is usually established, so that when asked to make a sound like /d/ with a finger placed behind the teeth, children will produce a /g/. Similarly, for unvoiced fricatives, establish the /ə/ first, then have the children draw their tongues back slowly over either their top or bottom teeth and the likelihood is that /s/ will be produced. When the /s/ can be produced with ease, repeating the procedure but taking the tongue back further will usually elicit the /ʃ/. Eliciting sound patterns in this way is, of course, a formal teaching procedure and one that has to be followed up by a generalization program to ensure the necessary transfer of training from lessons to life. Detailed procedures for using anticipatory set in the development of these and numerous other speech patterns are provided by Ling (1988).

One can usually capitalize on the use of residual audition in using and generalizing from early-occurring speech patterns, because most children with impaired hearing have better hearing levels for the lower frequencies—those that carry the most salient cues relating to vocalization, prosodic elements, vowels and diphthongs, and manner of consonant production. In contrast, cues on place of consonant production are carried in the frequency range above 1500 Hz, for which most such children have less, if any, hearing. Because many children with severe and profound hearing impairment are quite unable to hear unvoiced fricatives or cues on place of production, formal teaching that employs both direct touch and the use of anticipatory set is recommended for those who have difficulty with these aspects of speech (Calvert & Silverman, 1983; Ling, 1976, 1988).

Essentially a 7-step program is needed to ensure the effectiveness of formal teaching. These steps are:

1. Ensure the presence of prerequisite behaviors;
2. Decide on the set to be used;
3. Select a child's most appropriate sense modality;
4. Choose the strategies to be used;
5. Achieve production of the targeted speech sound;
6. Provide reinforcement of the behavior; and
7. Generalize production to other contexts, including spoken language.

AUTOMATICITY

The ability to concentrate on *what* one is saying rather than on *how* one is saying it is an essential aspect of spoken language. Speech should, therefore, be developed to be produced automatically—that is, without conscious effort. Speech patterns are acquired by children over at least five distinct stages, with (1) production at first being novel (and difficult), then (2) variable (but easier), (3) controlled, (4) practiced, and finally (5) habitual. Effective formal teaching ensures the development of speech skills through all of these five stages.

To ensure the automaticity of acceptable, coarticulated speech patterns in the variety of contexts in which they occur in spoken language, they must, if taught formally, be developed so that their production meets four basic criteria: (1) accuracy, (2) speed, (3) economy of effort, and (4) flexibility. *Accuracy* is the first requirement, as rehearsal of an inaccurate pattern can lead to a habitual speech problem. The *rate* at which a speech pattern can be repeated or alternated with others is important to a child's ability to integrate it appropriately into the stream of speech. Speech patterns produced with *economy* of effort do not unduly involve extraneous musculature and are not exaggerated.

Thus, they provide a better base for developing further speech patterns and lead to more normal-sounding speech. *Flexibility* in the production of speech has been acquired only when children can produce spoken language patterns appropriately in any context (see Ling, 1976).

GENERALIZATION AND CARRYOVER

When children have learned a skill in one situation and then applied it in another, they are said to have generalized that skill. Generalization and carryover are not serious problems when speech is acquired as a result of informal learning, because most such learning occurs in the context of spoken language communication in everyday situations. The less formal the intervention, the more closely lessons and real life are related. This is not the case when speech is acquired through formal teaching.

Consider the production of a /g/ as described. When it is elicited through formal teaching in one vowel context, such as /a/, children will usually have to be helped to generalize its production to other vowel contexts, particularly those in which the /g/ has to be produced with the high-back and high-front vowels /u/ and /i/. This is because the point of contact between tongue and palate shifts according to vocal tract configuration for the vowels.

To ensure that such generalization occurs, children should repeat several syllables, first with /a/, as in /gagaga/, then repeat the sound with each of the intervening vowels, one-by-one, moving gradually further and further away from the /a/, until /gugugu/ and /gigigi/ can be produced with ease. Production of such syllables may be a necessary speech skill, but unless it is deliberately carried over into real-life usage through integration into words, sentences, and discourse, it will remain far from an effective tool in communication (Calvert & Silverman, 1983; Fey, 1988; Perigoe & Ling, 1986).

PREVENTION AND REMEDIATION OF FAULTS

The most all-embracing statement on deviant speech due to hearing impairment must be that of Black (1971, p. 156) who wrote, "The speech of deaf children differs from normal speech in all regards." The literature since that date indicates that Black's statement still holds true for the majority of children with hearing impairment, in spite of the technological advances that have been made during the past 20 years (Hochberg, Levitt, & Osberger, 1983). Nevertheless, in the writer's experience, the application of current knowledge about speech and language acquisition, present day technology, and up-to-date educational practices would prevent many of the speech faults that are widely reported among children with hearing impairment (Ling, 1984a; Ling & Milne, 1981). In this section, various of the faults that led Black to make his statement are examined and this writer's suggested treatments and expectations for higher level expectations are discussed.

VOCALIZATION AND VOICE PATTERNS

One of the primary requirements for controlled vocalization is adequate breathing. Among speakers with hearing impairment, voice production tends to be begun at, rather than sufficiently above, lung resting level (Forner & Hixon, 1977). Audition is not required for feedback on speech breathing. Sufficient tactile and kinesthetic cues are available for control of breathing patterns in the act of speech production. This fault is not, therefore, an inevitable outcome of hearing impairment. Instead, it appears to be a product of inappropriate speech development procedures. Such faults occur when a great deal of formal teaching of isolated speech patterns or single words is undertaken. The faults are less likely to occur when sufficient approximations to mature forms of speech based on multiword utterances have been developed through informal strategies.

Voices characterized by pharyngeal tension, abnormal pitch and prosody, and hypernasality are commonly associated with hearing impairment (Hochberg et al., 1983; Monsen, 1979). Such problems are, indeed, likely when there is lack of auditory perception and auditory feedback, along with insufficient appropriate teaching or therapy. However, because the harmonics associated with voicing and the nasal murmur are in the low frequency range (250 Hz plus or minus a half-octave), they should be rendered audible in spite of even profound hearing impairment by the use of appropriately fitted hearing aids. These components of speech are also relatively simple to transmit through other forms of sensory aids. It follows that such abnormalities would be reduced or avoided for many children, if more attention were given to the selection and application of suitable devices to improve the reception of these components. Indeed, such abnormalities are less frequently found in the voices of children who have used appropriate sensory aids in the development of spoken language from an early age (Ling, 1988).

VOWEL PRODUCTION

The most common faults with vowel production by children who have hearing impairment are neutralization, prolongation, diphthongization, and exaggeration (Calvert & Silverman, 1983). Residual audition that extends up to at least 2500 Hz is required for the auditory detection of the first two formants of all vowels. On the other hand, the first formants of all vowels can be detected if there is residual audition to about 1000 Hz and most can be identified if speechreading is used. Many fewer vowel errors are likely, if adequate use is made of residual hearing, multichannel cochlear implants, or multichannel tactile aids (Carney & Beachler, 1986) if necessary, in conjunction with speechreading (Ling, 1989). An overstrong focus on speechreading can, however, lead to these faults rather than prevent them, because the problems are mainly from tongue movements that cannot be clearly seen. Neutralization (the predominant use of a central vowel), diphthongization (moving toward a central vowel from other vowels), and prolongation can be from either inadequate feedback, inappropriate teaching, or both. Exaggeration is almost always due to inappropriate teaching of static rather than dynamic strategies.

All four problems can be overcome by focusing remedial speech work on nonvisual feedback, increased tongue and reduced jaw movements, and the rapid alternation of different vowels, as well as syllables and words containing different vowels (Ling, 1976).

CONSONANT PRODUCTION

In addition to normal developmental errors, the major faults in consonant production among children with hearing impairment are reported to be *omission*, *substitution*, and *distortion*, *voiced-voiceless confusions*, and *implosion of stops*. Such problems were reported more than half a century ago by Hudgins and Numbers (1942) and have been reported to persist, but to a much smaller extent, in the phonology of orally taught children today. In the group studied by Abraham (1989), the best levels of correct consonant production were found among the children who had the best hearing levels at 2000 Hz. This finding is, of course, not surprising in view of the fact that place cues are available in, but not below, the octave band centered on 2000 Hz.

The acquisition of acceptably produced consonants can be enhanced through the effective use of hearing aids by those who have useful residual hearing for frequencies over 1500 Hz. It can also be augmented by other sensory aids that provide relevant information, such as cochlear implants (Owens & Kesler, 1988) and tactile devices (Weisenberger, 1989), as well. When sensory aids do not provide sufficient information for the development of certain consonants, systematic formal teaching of the type described by Ling (1976, 1988) can usually lead to their acquisition.

FUTURE TRENDS

PROSTHETIC DEVICES AND PROGRAMS

With advances in technology, new and improved sensory aids that can lead to better perception and production of speech will become available. It follows that one may expect a greater amount of research to be devoted to assessing the potential and the limitations of various sensory aids in the development of speech. One can, on the basis of recent advances in technology, reasonably predict a trend towards greater use of various devices in promoting the acquisition of speech among children with impaired hearing. The extent of that trend will depend not only on how well future sensory aids can be designed to transmit information, but on the number of educational programs committed to the development of spoken language.

There is every reason for the variety of programming that currently exists to be preserved. Paradoxically, however, during recent years, when technology has offered greatly improved opportunities for successful acquisition of spoken language, there has been a trend toward the increased use of sign language and this is likely to continue. Indeed, it has been suggested that American Sign Language programs should now begin to replace both oral and total communication programs (Johnson, Liddell, & Erting, 1989). Such a development would certainly receive widespread support from members of the deaf community (see Sacks, 1989). However, less than 3% of children who have hearing impairment are born to parents who are deaf (Jung, 1989), and the majority of parents will probably continue to press for programs that develop spoken language as the primary mode of communication, so that their children can learn to speak.

The trend towards the use of multichannel as compared with single-channel sensory aids may be expected to continue because, by and large, they appear to yield superior results (Pickett & McFarland, 1985). The thrust in hearing aid design will be toward more digital processing and better hearing aid selection procedures involving children will continue to be made. Accordingly, it is likely that productive strategies for the audiological management of young children will become more widespread and thus permit more children to acquire much of their speech more naturally. Because the means are now at hand, detection and diagnosis of hearing impairment can be carried out at an earlier age. More extensive application of current practices should lead to the expansion, if not proliferation, of parent-infant treatment programs in which children's speech will be more frequently developed within the first few years of life (Cole & Gregory, 1986).

PERSONNEL

In recent years, the focus on training teachers of the deaf in simultaneous communication has reduced the pool of educational personnel who are skilled in developing all aspects of spoken language (Ling, 1984b). At the same time, more audiologists and speech-language pathologists have become involved with spoken language development among children with hearing impairments, either as support personnel or as case managers.

There is a definite need for more personnel who are able to provide auditory-verbal programs and this need is more likely to be met through the recruitment of audiologists and speech-language pathologists to this area of work than through the training of more educators to work with parents and their children. Teacher training programs are more strongly geared to work with school-aged children. Regardless of their children's age and the types of professionals engaged in promoting their speech communication skills, parents will continue to create the strongest demand, and to be the greatest resource, for speech development in children with impaired hearing.

ACKNOWLEDGEMENT

Thanks are due to Richard Seewald and Kevin Munhall, University of Western Ontario, who read and suggested revisions to the first draft of this chapter.

REFERENCES

Abraham, S. (1989). Using a phonological framework to describe speech errors of orally trained, hearing-impaired school-agers. *Journal of Speech and Hearing Disorders, 54*, 600–609

Beasley, D. S. (1984). (Ed.) *Audition in childhood*. San Diego, CA: College-Hill Press.

Bell, A. G. (1916). *The mechanism of speech*. New York, NY: Funk and Wagnalls.

Bess, F. H. (Ed.) (1988). *Hearing impairment in children*. Parkton, MD: York Press.

Black, J. W. (1971). Speech pathology for the deaf. In L. E. Connor (Ed.), *Speech for the deaf child: Knowledge and use* (pp. 154–169). Washington DC: Alexander Graham Bell Association for the Deaf.

Blamey. P. J., & Clark, G. M. (1985). A wearable multiple-electrode electrotactile speech processor for the profoundly deaf. *Journal of the Acoustical Society of America, 77*, 1619–1621.

Boothroyd, A. (1982). *Hearing impairments in young children*. Englewood Cliffs, NJ: Prentice-Hall, Inc.

Calvert, D. R., & Silverman, S. R. (1975). *Speech and deafness*. Washington, DC: Alexander Graham Bell Association for the Deaf.

Calvert, D. R., & Silverman, S. R. (1983). *Speech and deafness*. (2nd ed.) Washington, DC: Alexander Graham Bell Association for the Deaf.

Carney, A. E., & Beachler, C. R. (1986). Vibrotactile perception of suprasegmental features of speech: A comparison of single-channel and multichannel instruments. *Journal of the Acoustical Society of America, 79*, 131–140.

Clark, M. (1989) *Language through living*. Toronto, Canada: Hodder and Stoughton.

Cole, E. B. (1990). *Listening and talking: A guide to promoting spoken language in young, hearing-impaired children.* Washington, DC: Alexander Graham Bell Association for the Deaf.

Cole, E. B., & Gregory, H. (1986). (Eds.). *Auditory learning.* Washington, DC: Alexander Graham Bell Association for the Deaf.

Cole, E. B., & Mischook, M. (1985). Survey and annotated bibliography of curricula used by oral preschool programs. *The Volta Review, 87,* 139–154.

Curtis, J. F. (1987). *An introduction to microcomputers in speech, language, and hearing.* Boston, MA: Little Brown.

DeFilippo, C. L. (1984). Laboratory projects in tactile aids to lipreading. *Ear and Hearing, 5,* 211–227.

DeFilippo, C. L., & Sims, D. G. (Ed.). (1988). *New reflections on speechreading.* Washington, DC: Alexander Graham Bell Association for the Deaf.

Dodd, B., & Campbell, R. (Ed.). (1987). *Hearing by eye: The psychology of lip-reading.* Hillsdale, NJ: Erlbaum.

Doggett, G. (1989) Employers' attitudes toward hearing-impaired people: a comparative study. *The Volta Review, 91,* 269–281.

Erber, N. P. (1972). Auditory, visual and auditory-visual recognition of consonants by children with normal and impaired hearing. *Journal of Speech and Hearing Research, 15,* 413–422.

Estabrooks, W., & Birkenshaw-Fleming, R. (1994). *Hear and listen! Talk and sing!* Toronto, Canada: Arisa Publishing.

Ewing, A. W. C., & Ewing, E. C. (1964). *Teaching deaf children to talk.* Manchester, UK: Manchester University Press.

Fey, M. (1988). Generalization issues facing language interventionists: an introduction. *Language, Speech and Hearing Services in Schools, 19,* 272–281.

Forner, L. L., & Hixon, T. J. (1977). Respiratory kinematics in profoundly hearing-impaired speakers. *Journal of Speech and Hearing Research, 20,* 373–408.

Friedlander, B. Z. (1970). Receptive language development in infancy: issues and problems. *Merrill-Palmer Quarterly of Behavior and Development, 16,* 109–122.

Fry, D. B. (1966). The development of the phonological system in the normal and the deaf child. In F. Smith, & G. A. Miller (Eds.), *The genesis of language.* Cambridge, MA: MIT Press.

Geers, A. E., & Moog, J. S. (1989). Evaluating speech perception skills: Tools for measuring the benefits of cochlear implants, tactile aids and hearing aids. In E. Owens, and D. K. Kessler, (Eds.), *Cochlear implants in young deaf children* (pp. 227–256). Boston, MA: College Hill Press.

Grant, J. (1987). *The hearing-impaired: Birth to six.* Boston: Little Brown.

Hanson, V. L., Liberman, I. Y., & Schankweiler, D. (1984). Linguistic coding by deaf children in relation to beginning reading success. *Journal of Experimental Child Psychology, 37,* 378–393.

Hirsh, I. J. (1940) Acoustical bases of speech perception. *Journal of Sound and Vibration, 27,* 111–122.

Hochberg, I., Levitt, H., & Osberger, M. (Eds.) (1983) *Speech of the hearing-impaired: Research, training and personnel preparation.* Baltimore, MD: University Park Press.

Hudgins, C. V., & Numbers, F. C. (1942). An investigation of the intelligibility of the speech of the deaf. *Genetic Psychology Monographs, 25,* 289–392.

Ijsseldijk, F. J. (1988). Speechreading tests for the deaf. *Journal of the British Association of Teachers of the Deaf, 12,* 3–15.

Jensema, C. J., & Trybus, R. H. (1978). *Communication patterns and educational achievement of hearing-impaired students.* Washington DC.: Office of Demographic Studies.

Jerger, J. (Ed.). (1984). *Pediatric audiology.* San Diego, CA: College-Hill Press.

Johnson, R. E., Liddell. S. K., & Erting, C. J. (1989). *Unlocking the curriculum: Principles for achieving access in deaf education* (Gallaudet Research Institute Working Paper 89–3). Washington, DC: Gallaudet University.

Jung, J. H. (1989). *Genetic syndromes in communication disorders.* Boston, MA: College-Hill Press.

Lauter, J. L. (Ed.). (1985). Proceedings of the Conference on the Planning and Production of Speech in Normal and Hearing-Impaired Individuals: A Seminar in Honor of S. Richard Silverman. *ASHA Reports, 15.*

Lenneberg, E. H. (1967). *Biological foundations of language.* New York: John Wiley and Sons.

Ling, D. (1976). *Speech and the hearing-impaired child: Theory and practice.* Washington, DC: Alexander Graham Bell Association for the Deaf.

Ling, D. (1981). Keep your child within earshot. *Newsounds, 6,* 506.

Ling, D. (Ed.). (1984a). *Early intervention for hearing-impaired children: Oral options.* San Diego, CA: College Hill Press.

Ling D. (Ed.). (l984b). *Early intervention for hearing-impaired children: Total communication options.* San Diego, CA: College-Hill Press.

Ling, D. (1988). *Foundations of spoken language for hearing-impaired children.* Washington, DC: Alexander Graham Bell Association for the Deaf.

Ling, D. (1991). *The phonetic-phonologic speech evaluation record.* Washington, DC: Alexander Graham Bell Association for the Deaf.

Ling, D., & Ling, A. H. (1978). *Aural habilitation: The foundations of verbal learning in hearing-impaired children.* Washington, D.C.: Alexander Graham Bell Association for the Deaf.

Ling, D., & Milne, M. (1981). The development of speech in hearing-impaired children. In F. Bess, B. A. Freeman, & J. S. Sinclair (Eds.), *Amplification in education* (pp. 99–108). Washington, DC: Alexander Graham Bell Association for the Deaf.

McDonald, E. T. (1964). *Articulatory testing and treatment: A sensory-motor approach.* Pittsburgh, PA: Stanwix House.

McGarr, N. S. (Ed.). (1989). *Research on the use of sensory aids for hearing-impaired people.* (Monograph of the *Volta Review, 91* No. 5) Washington, DC: Alexander Graham Bell Association for the Deaf.

Markides, A. (1983). *The speech of hearing-impaired children.* Manchester, UK: Manchester University Press.

Mischook, M., & Cole, E. (1986). Auditory learning and teaching of hearing-impaired infants. *The Volta Review, 88* (5) 67–82.

Monsen, R. B. (1979). Acoustic qualities of phonation in young hearing-impaired children. *Journal of Speech and Hearing Research, 22,* 270–288.

Murry, T., & Murry, J. (Eds.). (1980). *Infant communication.* Houston, TX: College-Hill Press.

Oller, D. K., Eilers, R. E., Bull, D. H., & Carney, A. E. (1985). Prespeech vocalizations of a deaf infant: A comparison with normal metaphonological development. *Journal of Speech and Hearing Research, 28,* 47–63.

Owens, E., & Kessler, D. K. (1988). *Cochlear implants in young deaf children.* Boston, MA: Little, Brown.

Perigoe, C. B., & Ling, D. (1986). Generalization of speech skills in hearing-impaired children. *The Volta Review, 88,* 351–366.

Pickett, J. M., & McFarland, W. (1985). Auditory implants and tactile aids for the profoundly deaf. *Journal of Speech and Hearing Research, 28,* 134–150.

Popelka, G. R. (1981). *Hearing assessment with the acoustic reflex.* New York: Grune and Stratton.

Proctor, A. (1984). Tactile aids for the deaf: a comprehensive bibliography. *American Annals of the Deaf, 129,* 409–416.

Quigley, S. P., & Paul, P. V. (1984). *Language and deafness.* San Diego, CA: College-Hill Press.

Reed, M. (1984). *Educating hearing-impaired children.* Milton Keynes, England: Open University Press.

Sacks, O. (1989) *Seeing voices.* Berkeley, CA: University of California Press.

Silverman, S. R. (1983). Speech training then and now: a critical review. In I. Hochberg, H. Levitt, & M. J. Osberger (Eds.), *Speech of the hearing-impaired* (pp. 1–20). Baltimore, MD: University Park Press.

Stelmachowicz, P. G., & Seewald, R. C. (1990). Probe-tube microphone measures in children. *Seminars in hearing.* New York: Thieme-Stratton.

Stoker, R. G., & Ling, D. (1992). *Speech production in hearing-impaired children and youth: Theory and practice.* Washington, DC: A. G. Bell Association for the Deaf.

Stone, P. (1988). *Blueprint for developing conversational competence.* Washington, DC: Alexander Graham Bell Association for the Deaf.

Studdert-Kennedy, M. (1984). Early development of phonological form. In C. von Euler, H. Forssberg, & H. Lagercrantz (Eds.), *Neurobiology of early infant behavior* (pp. 82–96). New York: Stockton Press.

Subtelny, J. D. (Ed.). (1980). *Speech assessment and speech improvement for the hearing impaired.* Washington, DC: Alexander Graham Bell Association for the Deaf.

Vorce, E. (1974). *Teaching speech to deaf children.* Washington, DC: Alexander Graham Bell Association for the Deaf.

Weisenberger, J. (1989). Tactile aids for speech perception and production by hearing-impaired people. *The Volta Review, 91,* 79–100.

Wilson, W. R., & Thompson, G. (1984). Behavioral audiometry. In J. Jerger (Ed.), *Pediatric audiology* (pp. 1–44). San Diego, CA: College-Hill Press.

Wolk, S., & Schildroth, A. N. (1986) Deaf children and speech intelligibility. In A. N. Schildroth & M. A. Karchmer (Eds.), *Deaf children in America* (pp. 139–156). San Diego, CA: College Hill Press.

Wood, D., Wood H., Griffiths, A., & Howarth, I. (1986). *Teaching and talking with deaf children.* New York: John Wiley and Sons.

END OF CHAPTER EXAMINATION QUESTIONS

CHAPTER 9

1. Fifty years ago speech for those with hearing impairment was generally based on
   a. Speechreading and tactile clues
   b. Sign language
   c. Did not have a focus
   d. Speechreading

2. Which of the following would be considered the most significant hearing loss as it relates to language, learning, and social/emotional behaviors?
   a. Profound
   b. Mild
   c. Severe
   d. Moderate

3. The most efficient use of visual clues in speech understanding also requires
   a. Excellent vision
   b. Even minimal levels of hearing
   c. Good receptive vocabulary
   d. The use of both vision and hearing

4. According to the author of this chapter, what is necessary for a child to produce spoken language patterns appropriately in context?
   a. Economy
   b. Accuracy
   c. Flexibility
   d. Production

END OF CHAPTER ANSWER SHEET

Name   Date

CHAPTER 9

1. Which one(s)?   a   b   c   d

2. Which one(s)?   a   b   c   d

3. Which one(s)?   a   b   c   d

4. Which one(s)?   a   b   c   d

5. _____

_____

_____

_____

_____ .

6. _____

_____

_____

_____ .

7. _____

_____

_____

_____

_____ .

8. _____

_____

_____

_____

_____ .

5. What are the advantages for individuals who have hearing impairment who use both sign and spoken language?

6. Contrast and compare the intrinsic and extrinsic factors that influence acquisition of speech.

7. List or describe the context and the people involved in the formal and informal procedures of teaching and learning.

8. Discuss the advantages and disadvantages of signing. Briefly state your opinion.

Educational Management of Children Who Are Hearing Impaired

■ FREDERICK S. BERG, Ph.D. ■

This chapter describes the education of children who are hearing impaired in the schools. Included are discussions of target populations, educational management, educational methods, bicultural and auditory-verbal and FM radio issues, and acoustical control in classrooms.

TARGET POPULATIONS

In the United States there are millions of school-age children with hearing loss in one or both ears. Perhaps 50,000 of them are deaf. A much greater number are hard of hearing. A still much greater number have marginal hearing impairment, accounting for over 4 million children and young adults ages 3 to 17 years (National Center for Health Statistics, 1994).

Individualized educational plans (IEPs) are written annually for deaf children and for many hard-of-hearing children (Berg, 1987; Ross, 1986). IEPs are also written for thousands of children with marginal hearing losses who have been classified as learning disabled, speech impaired, or mentally retarded (Ray, 1989). These IEPs are provided under Public Law 94-142, initially called the All Handicapped Children's Act, which has become the Individuals with Disabilities Education Act (IDEA, 1997)

IEPs are not written for the great majority of children with marginal hearing losses, although they are at risk educationally (Giolas & Wark, 1967; Quigley & Thomure, 1968; Willeford, personal communication), particularly when enrolled in schools with unfavorable classroom acoustics (Berg, Blair, & Benson, 1996; Crandall & Smaldino, 1995). Most of these children have chronic or recurrent otitis media (Berg, 1987; Bess, 1984; Downs, 1988).

EDUCATIONAL MANAGEMENT

The educational management of children who have hearing impairment is a team effort shared by parents, audiologists, parent advisors, school administrators, and teachers. Parents can learn to help these children develop normal language skills before they go to school, with education following. Parent advisors can help parents and other family members achieve these goals. Audiologists can identify children with hearing loss, evaluate their hearing, and determine and manage amplification and acoustical support for them. School administrators can ensure that classrooms have good room acoustics and that interpreters, transliterators, and FM systems are available when needed. Teachers can keep their classrooms quiet, monitor hearing aid use, and use personal and/or sound field FM systems when needed (Berg, 2000[1]; Blair, 1996; Clarke & Watkins, 1985).

ILLITERACY: EDUCATIONAL PROBLEM OF DEAF CHILDREN

The education problem of deaf children is primarily illiteracy. This is documented in a national report on the education of the deaf (Toward Equality, Education of the Deaf, 1988). This report observes that:

1. The present status of education for persons who are deaf in the United States is unsatisfactory.
2. Most children who are prelingually deaf have serious difficulties and delays in acquiring English language skills.
3. A child without a strong language and communication base faces barriers that often lead to further educational difficulties.

[1]*Literacy and speech for the young deaf child* by F. Berg, 2000, Smithfield, UT: Author. Prepaid copies of this book are available without profit to author from: Fred Berg, 516 E. Summit Creek Dr., Smithfield, Utah 84335, (435) 563-5733, Fredna@cc.usu.edu

4. Learning a language requires interpersonal interaction and ample communication opportunities.
5. As reading ability is highly correlated with prior English language knowledge, many students who are deaf have difficulty becoming proficient readers.
6. The ability to express and comprehend language in written form is closely allied with the ability to express and comprehend language through face-to-face spoken communication.
7. The educational system has not been successful in assisting the majority of students who are deaf to achieve reading skills commensurate with those of their hearing peers.

Three years prior to this report an academic profile of a typical 14-year-old deaf student revealed that he or she typically could read at the third grade level (Gallaudet Institute Newsletter, 1985).

It should be noted that a 14-year-old deaf youngster with a reading level of Grade 3 is not comparable to a hearing peer who may have difficulty reading. The hearing individual enjoys a comfortable mastery of language, even though he or she could be delayed in reading. For the deaf, on the other hand, the reading level is his or her ceiling in linguistic competence. It is inappropriate to designate this latter condition as retardation in reading. It is properly incompetence or deficiency in verbal language, a condition rare among the hearing but almost universal among the deaf (p. 15).

At that time, Orin Cornett, an administrator of the United States Office of Education, came across a similar statement in a report from Gallaudet College, a postsecondary institution for the deaf. It stated that prelingually deaf persons, as a group, were typically very poor readers. His reaction to this sobering finding is described (Cornett & Daisey, 1992):

I was horrified, for I had supposed that deaf people were all bookworms. After all, an adult with normal hearing, if he suffers a severe or profound hearing loss, almost always increases the amount of reading by several times. In fact, reading is the only avenue of access that is undamaged by a loss of hearing. (p. 744)

UNPROVEN METHODS

In the early 1960s there was no method that would enable deaf children to learn English at anywhere near the level achieved by hearing children (Education of the Deaf, 1965). In the early part of the 19th century, the American Sign Language (ASL) and signs with speech (SS) methods had been used to help instruct deaf children. In 1880, these methods were abandoned and replaced by oralism (O) or use of speech without signs. After 1965, SS replaced O as the dominant method in most schools and programs for deaf children. In the 1980s, ASL was reintroduced with strong advocacy from the Deaf Community and some linguists close to the Deaf Culture (Lane, 1984, 1992).

ASL is a visual-spatial gestural language. Its signs consist of handshapes, their locations on or near the body, their orientations, and their movements. It takes many fewer ASL signs than English words to communicate the same information (Lane, 1992). Unlike phonemic-based languages like English, however, ASL has no written form.

SS uses signs from ASL, additional invented signs, and speech in English word order as a communication method for education. This method was used along with ASL in the first schools for the deaf in the United States. When SS replaced O as the dominant method in the 1960s, it was subsumed under an educational philosophy called total communication (TC) (Berg, 2000).

Fingerspelling is used with both SS and ASL to communicate the meaning of any words not conveyed through signs, such as names of persons and places. However, it includes only 26 symbols or letters, whereas English has at least 40 phonemes.

Oralism uses speech and lipreading and/or residual hearing together with written English as a communicative method in deaf education. Prior to 1965, lipreading was emphasized more than residual hearing. With the advent of powerful hearing aids, utilization of residual hearing took precedence over lipreading for oral education. Neither lipreading, nor residual hearing, nor both together, however, provides full access to the phonemes of spoken language (Berg, 2000).

In the United States, the most common method in deaf education today is SS, the next most common O, and the next most common ASL. Each of these methods is provided in more than 50% of schools or programs for the deaf (*American Annals of the Deaf*, 1999). The O method is now called the auditory-oral (AO) method in schools or special classes for hearing impaired children. It is called the auditory-verbal (AV) method when hearing-impaired children are educated alongside normal hearing children, and when unisensory auditory speech stimulation is used instead of multisensory auditory-visual (lipreading) speech stimulation.

In spite of their widespread use, the ASL, SS, and O methods have not proved to be successful for assisting the majority of deaf children to learn the English language (Merrill, 1992). Noever and Andrews (1998) indicate that extensive language teaching strategies have yet to be developed to help the deaf make the "language bridge" from ASL to English. Lane (1984, 1992) states that SS does not help and may even hinder the teaching of English. The oral method does not provide deaf children access to a high enough percentage of English phonemes (Berg, 2000). The AO and AV modifications of O help, but still fall short (Geers, & Moog 1994; Toward Equality, Education of the Deaf, 1988).

A PROVEN METHOD

In 1966 Orin Cornett (1967) developed the Cued Speech (CS) method to enable children who are deaf learn English effectively. With CS, a speaker adds eight hand shapes in four hand locations to the lip shapes and movements visible on his or her lips as he or she says the consonants, vowels, and diphthongs during speech. Each hand shape is a cue for three or four consonants. Each hand location is a cue for two or three vowels. "A sender is able to transmit the cues in real-time synchronously with speech, thus conveying a visual analog of the syllabic-phonemic-rhythmic patterns of spoken language" (Nicholls & Ling, 1982, p. 262). The CS method works because it enables deaf children to perceive a very high percentage of the English phonemes, the building blocks of spoken English which are naturally acquired by hearing children during early childhood (Berg, 2000).

According to Berlin (1995), CS prepares a deaf child for English language comprehension and reading in a most efficient and useful way, independent of amplification success or failure. In 1992 the late Edward C. Merrill, past president of Gallaudet College, stated:

Cued Speech has substantial data showing that it enables deaf children to attain competency in English at the level of hearing students grade by grade. I know of no other system that enables this to happen—not oral, not combined, not AS. (p. vii)

CS is a communicative choice along with other methods for very young deaf and hard of hearing children in many localities of the United States, including the nationwide outreach parent-home services of the SKI-HI Institute (HOPE, 1999). Many of these CS children learn to read at the same age as hearing children and are educated in regular classes. For children educated in schools and programs for the deaf, however, CS is offered only 13% of the time (*American Annals of the Deaf*, 1999). This lack of support for CS by decision makers in deaf education is entirely unwarranted. Deaf children deserve an opportunity to become literate and at an early age (Berg, 2000).

One oral teacher of the deaf who has learned CS is Barbara Lee (1992). After using it for 12 years, she described its effects on herself and her students as **liberating**. Before she began using CS, her teaching success was limited by the handicap of severe language delay. Afterwards, she could teach CS children to their intellect at whatever language level was appropriate, provided cueing was used all day at school and consistently at home. When CS children looked at her, they were more like hearing children than typical deaf kids.

During 1998, Joan Rupert, director of the West Coast Cued Speech Program, stated that only 1 in 10 deaf children in the public schools had learned to read either through the AO or SS methods (personal communication, 1998). With the use of CS, however, 9 of 10 children with hearing loss had learned to read on schedule. More recently she has stated that CS continues to grow in numbers of users and numbers of influential advocates.

When CS was introduced, Powrie Doctor of Gallaudet College stated that it was the first system that showed the syllabification of the spoken language, which is what the deaf had needed from the beginning. However, he predicted its growth would be opposed by advocates of oralism and manualism, which has proved to be the case and continues to be so (Heffernan, 1992). Opposition by oral educators of the deaf has softened in recent years, stemming from a series of supportive research investigations beginning with Gaye Nicholls' study of the use of CS for the reception of spoken language. In her study, 18 children with 97 to 122 dB hearing losses averaged 95% recognition of key words in sentences. Each child had been taught through the use of CS for least 4 years (Nicholls & Ling, 1982).

Beck (1997) summarized other studies supporting CS. One study showed that using CS improved lipreading. Another revealed that children exposed to CS scored higher on language structure than 92% of hearing-impaired children generally. Still another study showed that 30 deaf students who used CS scored as well in reading as a matched group of 30 hearing students. Other groups of deaf students who were trained through O or SS scored lower.

The National Cued Speech Association (NCSA) has endorsed the following statements to promote the importance of literacy among children with hearing loss (Position Statement on Literacy, 1990). These statements pertain to the more than 90% of all deaf children who have hearing parents, who can learn CS and expose their deaf children to it more readily than the fewer numbers of deaf parents of deaf children whose native language is ASL.

1. Literacy is a critical determiner of an individual's life, present and future. Literacy improves career options, employability, economic and social freedom, and self-esteem.
2. Literacy is the original and primary goal of Cued Speech use. The primary goal of Cued Speech use is to enable the person to become literate as he or she would be without a hearing loss. Cued Speech was created to enable deaf children to absorb the same phonemic/phonological language base as hearing children as a foundation for reading.
3. The most efficient route to literacy for a deaf individual is acquisition of the target spoken language (English, French, etc.). The most efficient route to literacy for a deaf individual is to master the vocabulary and syntax of the target spoken language for reading. If a deaf child has hearing parents, the target spoken language should be acquired as his or her first language. This does not rule out bilingualism.
4. Maximum attainment of literacy depends on the conscientious use of Cued Speech by both family and professionals. Cued Speech is best used (1) beginning at identification of hearing loss, and (2) by all professionals directly involved in the child's educational program.
5. Cued Speech can be used in conjunction with aural/oral and/or signing approaches, but improvement in literacy is directly related to increasing exposure to the target spoken language through Cued Speech.

Learning CS is an exciting adventure for families who have children with hearing loss. Learning the basics of CS requires up to a week or so of intensive work. Development of skill sufficient for easy, natural communication takes months to a year of actual use (Rupert, 2000). Fluency typically comes from actual use in communication, but can be obtained by consistent drill. Once a person can cue, even at a slow rate, he or she can begin cueing to the child who is deaf.

There are several formats to teaching or learning CS: (1) group face-to-face workshops, (2) individual face-to-face instruction, (3) audiocassette and/or videocassette instruction, (4) self-instruction, and (5) combinations of these. Family workshops provide opportunities for interaction with beginners and advanced learners. Certified instructors can ensure that learning is correct. The National Cued Speech Association (NCSA) sponsors workshops at several regional service centers throughout the United States (Berg, 2000)

PRIVATE ORAL SCHOOLS

An English learning option for deaf children who have not learned English before attending school is enrollment in one of the private oral schools for the deaf. At the Central Institute for the Deaf (CID) in St. Louis, for example, deaf children attain literacy by the time they graduate from the eighth grade, and sometimes earlier, enabling them to perform well in further schooling. At CID, two related research studies have been conducted. They were designed to answer the questions:

1. Can typical deaf children achieve well above what is generally expected, even approaching the achievement of hearing children with improved teaching? (Geers, 1985)

2. Can hearing aids, tactile speech aids, and cochlear implants facilitate the development of speech perception, speech production, and language development among deaf deaf children at CID? (Geers & Moog, 1994)

To answer the first question, an experiment was designed and implemented at CID, called Experimental Program in Instructional Concentration (EPIC). An experimental group of CID students received concentrated, intense instruction, with a 2:3 student-teacher ratio. A control group received the typical instruction of private oral schools for the deaf, with a higher student-teacher ratio. Pretreatment and posttreatment tests enabled investigators to determine progress in language and vocabulary, speech, reading, and mathematics. All students were taught through an oral-aural approach. The findings showed that both the experimental and control subjects progressed in all areas of tested performance, but the experimental subjects made accelerated gains approaching the performance of normal hearing students (Geers, 1985).

To answer the second question, a 3-year sensory aids study of 39 children enrolled at CID was designed and implemented. At the onset of participation in the study each child (1) had a hearing loss of at least 100 dB, (2) was between 2 and 12 years of age, (3) had been born deaf or become deaf by age 3, (4) had used a hearing aid from an early age, and (5) had received early educational intervention as soon as diagnosed.

The 39 children were divided into three matched groups: 13 used Tactaid tactile aids, 13 Nucleus 22 cochlear implants, and 13 conventional hearing aids. Two years into the study, another group of 13 children were added. They had hearing loss from 90 to 100 dB and used conventional hearing aids.

The children participated in an intensive AO program with daily auditory and speech instruction. At the beginning of the study, all children could detect speech through their hearing aids, but had limited speech discrimination. At the end of the study, the children generally could discriminate speech better. The cochlear implant group outperformed the tactile group and the first (100+ dB) hearing aid group in speech perception, speech production, and language developments, and performed similarly to the second (90–100 dB) hearing aid group (Geers & Moog, 1994).

BICULTURAL ISSUES

Since King Jordan, a deafened man, became president of Gallaudet University, advocates of ASL have solidified their position in deaf education (Christiansen & Barnartt, 1995). These advocates believe ASL should be taught to deaf children as a first language, with English as a second language. Also, they give written language precedence over spoken language (Lane, 1984, 1992). The Learning Center for Deaf Children in Framingham, Massachusetts has also adopted this bicultural approach to deaf education. Their students become aware of multicultural issues and feel they belong to the Deaf community. They also study English to enhance their success in the hearing community. The great majority of these students go on to college, especially the National Institute for the Deaf or Gallaudet University (Goldberg, 1995).

Cornett and Daisey (1992), who have edited the *Cued Speech Resource Book for Parents of Deaf Children*, advocate a different bicultural approach to deaf education. They believe that deaf children of hearing parents should learn English as a first language, with ASL as a second language. A case in point is Debbie Jane Crosby, a deaf fourth grader who has learned English through CS and is also being taught ASL by a native ASL user (Crosby, personal communication, 2000).

CID and other private oral schools have graduates who have become proficient with both speech and signs. A case in point is Heather Whitestone who on September 17, 1994, was named Miss America (Harris, 1995). Heather lost most of her hearing when she was 18 months old and enrolled at CID at age 11. In a special appearance at ASHA's convention in November 1995, Heather said, "I worked very hard to read lips and speak correctly. I really support sign language, and I know sign language. But I believe oral communication has opened more doors for me"(Goldberg, 1995).

Some members of the Deaf Community and some linguists (Lane, Hoffmeister, & Bahan, 1996)

suggest that ASL will not be learned well if delayed beyond early childhood. Yet, many people like the author's brother Tom and his wife Betty have learned ASL after becoming deaf at age 5 or older. Both Tom and Betty, however, prefer SS to ASL for communicating with the deaf, because they think in English. They consider ASL to be used by deaf persons who have not learned English and do not read well (T. Berg, personal communication, 1999).

It is doubtful that many hearing parents of deaf children will learn ASL well enough to become role models in teaching it to their deaf children. It is easier for them to learn CS, which is not a language but simply a code for a language they already know. Ninety percent of parents of deaf children in the United States hear and are native users of spoken English. Only 10% are deaf. Cornett and Daisey (1992) recommend, however, that hearing parents not only learn CS for living in the hearing world but learn enough signs to communicate with deaf peers of their deaf children.

AUDITORY-VERBAL ISSUES

Some educational audiologists and educators state that parents in auditory-verbal programs for deaf children do not have to learn CS or sign language. Flexer (1999, pp. 244–247) expounds this viewpoint:

1. When properly aided, children with hearing impairment can detect most if not all of the speech spectrum.
2. Once all available residual hearing is accessed through amplification technology (e.g., binaural hearing aids and acoustically tuned earmolds, FM units, cochlear implants) to provide maximum detection of the speech spectrum, then a child will have the opportunity to develop language in a natural way through the auditory modality.

3. As verbal language develops through the auditory input of information, reading skills can also develop.
4. Studies show that over 90% of parents do not learn sign language beyond a basic preschool level of competency. Auditory-verbal practice requires that caregivers interact with a child through spoken language and create a listening environment which helps a child to learn.
5. Individuals who have since early childhood been taught through the active use of amplified residual hearing, are indeed independent, speaking, and contributing members of mainstream society.

This viewpoint and some of the evidence supporting it are questionable in specific instances. There are advantages to learning CS and sign language that are not fully compensated for by participation in AV programs. Those include:

1. There are deaf persons, including this author's brother Tom and his wife Betty, who cannot detect any of the speech spectrum. There are others who only detect a part of the speech spectrum (Berg 1986a, Wedenberg 1954). A case in point is Staffan Wedenberg, who could not detect sound above 1500 Hz (Wedenberg & Wedenberg, 1970).
2. In the CID sensory aids study described previously (Geers & Moog, 1994), only 5 of 52 deaf children were able to identify words in open sets after 3 years of intense auditory and speech training. Four of the 5 were among 13 children who used cochlear implants.
3. Evidence is lacking that AV practice for most deaf children receiving it has led to literacy in early childhood to the extent that CS has. For example, Staffan Wedenberg's vocabulary growth between ages 2½ and 3½ was only 25 words through extensive unisensory auditory stimulation and training, whereas Leah Henegar's vocabulary growth for this period through CS was 450 words (Cornett & Daisey, 1992; Wedenberg & Wedenberg, 1970).

4. In open sets of words or sentences, CS offers the advantage of almost 100% speech recognition, which unisensory auditory stimulation or even bisensory (auditory and lipreading) stimulation has not matched (Nicholls & Ling, 1982).
5. Merrill and Daisey (1992) include case histories of children whose parents have shifted them from the AV method to the CS method, with resultant benefits in language development and early development of literacy skills.
6. Both CS and ASL provide more reliability of communication than use of residual hearing and amplification. Flexer (1999), for example, states that more than 50% of hearing aids malfunction on any given day. When hearing aids malfunction, residual hearing becomes dysfunctional and deaf children need a visual mode of communication.
7. Also the expense of purchasing and maintaining hearing aids and especially cochlear implants places these hearing technologies out of reach for families of deaf children with limited resources. This is true for many families in the United States and for most families in underdeveloped countries. For example, in India where this author worked with the National Institute for the Hearing Handicapped, most families could not afford to purchase any hearing technologies. The government provided body-type aids, but they were of low quality.
8. Furthermore, poor acoustical conditions in homes and schools confound hearing aid and cochlear implant use.
   FM systems then must be provided, but these also malfunction or are subject to radio interference at times. To quote Flexer (1999), "the FM unit might be free from interference in the school office, but picks up computer noise in another room of the same building (p. 206)."
9. As deaf children trained through the AV method get older, many of them may desire to learn to communicate with other deaf children who sign or cue and their parents should be

encouaged to learn these methods, also. The use of residual hearing in the education of deaf and hard-of-hearing children, however, has great benefits for listening and speech development that are explained in other chapters of this book. Unlike vision, hearing is multidirectional, like an infinitely wide-angled lens, allowing multi-directional sound input in a quiet environment. Once a child has been trained to listen in quiet situations, the next step is to transfer this skill into school classrooms. Two technologies are used to make the transition to auditory learning in school: (1) control of classroom acoustics and (2) use of FM amplification.

ACOUSTICAL CONTROL

Acoustical control is a direct approach to enhancing auditory learning in school classrooms. It is needed because elementary and secondary school classrooms typically are acoustically hostile listening environments that undermine the learning of children in school. The specific phenomena that need to be controlled are signal, noise, reverberation, echoes, and modes. One or more of these are typically out of control in the schools and sometimes all of them (Berg, 1997).

The effects of classroom acoustics are detailed in Table 10–1, which presents speech recognition scores of school-age children with normal hearing and school-age children with hearing loss under several signal-to-noise (S/N) ratios and reverberation times (RTs) that simulate everyday conditions in American schools. The students with normal hearing had mean speech recognition scores of 95%, and the students with hearing loss had mean scores of 83%, when tested in an audiometric booth with negligible noise and reverberation. The scores in the table suggest that even students with normal hearing cannot listen optimally in a typically noisy classroom, even when the room has little reverberation. The listening scores were obtained at a 12-foot distance, typical of class instruction (Finitzo-Hieber & Tillman, 1978).

Signal is sound that carries information to listeners. This sound is usually speech. In a classroom, speech is transmitted from a teacher to students

TABLE 10–1. Average Speech Discrimination of 12 Normal-hearing and 12 Hard-of-hearing Students Under RTS and S/N Ratios Simulating Various Classroom Conditions.

RT in Seconds	S/N Ratio in dB	Percent Words Repeated Correctly	
		Normal Hearing	Hard of Hearing
0.4	+12	83	60
	+6	71	52
	0	48	28
1.2	+12	70	41
	+6	54	27
	0	30	11

Source: Adapted from Finitzo, T. (1988). Classroom acoustics. In R. J. Roeser & M. P. Downs, (Eds.), *Auditory disorders in school children* (2nd ed., p. 31). New York: Thieme Medical Publishers, Inc. Reprinted with permission.

through a combination of direct and reflected sound. Direct sound is sound that travels outward from its source without being reflected. Reflected sound is sound after it has struck one or more objects or surfaces in a room (Everest, 1989). Direct sound energy predominates close to the teacher and reflected sound away from the teacher (G. Davis & Jones, 1989). When combined appropriately in a quiet classroom, direct sound and reflected sounds enhance classroom communication and enable all students in a classroom to hear the teacher, provided the teacher's voice is strong enough. Some teachers have inherently strong voices and are able to project their voices for long periods of time without tiring. Other teachers have relatively weak voices and struggle or even fail to talk above the classroom noise level (Berg, 1997). Speech-language pathologists who specialize in voice training can provide professional help for teachers with weak voices (Boone, 1991; Cooper, 1990; Johnson, 1991).

Noise is a pervasive problem outside a school, inside a school, and within each classroom. It may be defined as unwanted or unintended sound. If noise is intense enough, it masks or renders inaudible speech communication. The signal or noise level can be measured with a sound-level meter. Classroom noise levels typically are 30–35 dB at night or during a weekend, 40–50 dB when the heating or air conditioning (HVAC) system is turned on, and 55 to 75 dB when a teacher and 25 or more students are occupants. If students are to listen effectively, the noise level for an occupied classroom should not exceed 50 dB. This allows the speech signal, or teacher's raised voice, which has an average intensity of 60 dB, to be 10 dB higher than the noise level. To reduce classroom noise to 50 dB, the many airborne and structure-borne noises outside the school, inside the school, and within classrooms need to be identified, measured, and either isolated or reduced. When feasible, architects, engineers, educational audiologists, and other school personnel should collaborate in this endeavor (Berg, 1997; Berg et al., 1996).

The third acoustical phenomenon to control is *reverberation,* or repeated reflection of sound, from room surfaces. Reverberation is measured with a reverberation analysis device that reads in milliseconds. The reverberation time (RT) is the approximate time required for an intense sound to decay to the point of being inaudible or masked by noise. The RT of a classroom varies with the absorption characteristics of its room surfaces. The less the absorption (or more the reflection) of room surfaces, the higher the RT. The RT time also varies with the frequency of sound, because the absorption of the room surfaces varies with the frequency.

Recommended RTs for school children with normal hearing are about 0.5 second and for school children with hearing impairment, about 0.3 second. The RT of a room should also be fairly uniform across the speech frequency range. The RTs of school classrooms in the United States vary from 0.3 second to 1.5+ seconds for low and high speech frequencies. RTs are also frequently greater at low speech frequencies than at high speech frequencies.The primary effect of excessive reverberation and of greater reverberation at low speech frequencies than at high speech frequencies is that the vowels of speech will mask the less intense and higher frequency consonants and thus degrade speech intelligibility. Reverberation, however, will not be a problem if room surfaces are sufficiently absorbent for both low and high frequency sounds (Berg, 1997; Everest, 1989; Finitzo-Hieber, 1988; Nabalek & Nabalek, 1985).

Echoes are the fourth acoustical problem of concern in classrooms. They may have more adverse effect on speech intelligibility than reverberation. Echoes may be identified as spikes on a time versus intensity display using time energy frequency (TEF) analysis equipment. An echo may be defined as a reflected sound of sufficient amplitude and delay to make it distinct from the sound giving rise to it. Echoes are most noticeable when a sound reflects from a hard, distant surface, such as the back of a large classroom. If a classroom has two hard, opposite surfaces close to each other, *flutter echo* may also be heard. This audible echo sounds like a high-frequency ringing or buzzing. Echoes with short delays must be much stronger to be heard than echoes with longer delays. Echoes are incipient when their presence is recognized, but not perceived as discrete. In classrooms, speech echoes are not usually heard as discrete phenomena, but they influence the apparent level, quality, and intelligibility of sound. Echoes are not a problem if room surfaces are sufficiently absorbent or diffusive. To absorb sound, a surface must be porous, diaphragmatic, or resonant. To diffuse sound, a surface must be irregular, so sound scatters in many directions from it (D'Antonio, 1989; D. Davis & Davis, 1987, 1991).

Brooke (1991) states that most rooms meant for speech activities do not have a lot of need for sound diffusion. He says it is better to focus the available energy as useful reflections and to shift absorbent treatment from the room ceiling to the room floor. He states:

A general rule of thumb for rooms for speech is to make all surface areas that do not provide useful reflections absorbent and, conversely, not to cover any useful reflectors. The latter is widely violated. Almost all classrooms have absorbent ceilings and hard floors, yet the reverse would provide far better room acoustics. Carpet on the floor not only covers a useless reflective surface, it also greatly reduces audience noise. The elimination of footfall and chair- or desk-moving noises are an important contribution to quieter classrooms. (p. 175)

The final acoustical phenomenon of concern in a school classroom is *modes*. A mode is a room resonance. Each classroom has its unique set of modes, resonances, or resonant frequencies at which it will vibrate, if stimulated with sound containing those specific frequencies. The modes of a classroom may be identified with specialized equipment.

Within the 80 to 300 Hz frequency region, modes produce acoustic anomalies that somewhat degrade speech intelligibility. Room modes have a noticeable effect on speech intelligibility when most or all surfaces in a room are hard. For example, when acoustic ceiling tile or floor carpet is installed in a classroom, room modes are still prominent because tile and carpet are poor absorbers of low frequency sound. Speech intelligibility will be affected more by room modes if classrooms are small than if they are large. Room resonances will have little degrading effect on speech intelligibility if room dimensions are not whole number multiples of each other and if room surfaces are sufficiently absorbent for low and high speech frequencies (Everest, 1989).

USING FM AMPLIFICATION

During the last 30 years, FM equipment has been increasingly used with deaf and hard-of-hearing children in schools. Initially, it was used in place of hearing aids. More recently, FM equipment has been used together with hearing aids. Still more recently, FM equipment has been used with entire classes of students (Berg, 1987).

FM is an acronym for frequency modulation. This is a term applied to radio signal transmission. Using FM equipment, a speech or other sound signal is changed into an electrical signal, and is then superimposed on a radio signal, which is transmitted to a receiver. This superimposition modulates the radio signal.

Radio transmission of sound has the effect of bringing the speaker closer to the listener. The effect is noticable when persons listen through loudspeakers and is dramatic when they listen through earphones or a hearing aid coupled to a miniaturized FM receiver. These two radio options are referred to as personal and sound field FM. When the listener uses an earphone or a hearing aid coupled to an FM receiver, listening is personal. When listeners hear through loudspeakers, sound is coming from the near "field."

Basically, a specialized FM system includes a microphone and transmitter, which a teacher wears, and a radio receiver. With personal FM, the listener wears the radio receiver and uses an earphone or, more frequently, a hearing aid. With sound field FM, a common radio receiver, an amplifier, and one or more loudspeakers are used. Both personal FM and sound field FM components can be used in a classroom at the same time.

Teachers using FM transmitters can broadcast their voices from any location up to 200 feet away. Any other sound source, such as a radio or tape recorder, can also be broadcast. The radio receiver is tuned to the broadcast channel of the radio transmitter. FM listening systems can be used in different classrooms, with each system broadcasting a different radio frequency.

The advantage of either a personal FM system or a sound field FM system over a hearing aid is that it increases the S/N ratio. With a personal FM system, room noise and reverberation can be excessive and a deaf or hard-of-hearing child can still hear the signal clearly. With a sound field FM, room noise and reverberation have to be controlled (e.g., ideally reduced to 50 dB noise and 0.3 second RT) for the same child to hear the signal clearly.

Sound field FM systems, however, have advantages over personal FM systems. Three advantages particularly applicable to this discussion are (Anderson, 1989, 1999):

1. Sound field amplification equipment is not subject to student sabotage and is resistant to breakage by the teacher. This results in low maintenance costs and long equipment life.
2. Stigmatization is avoided, because the amplification is beneficial to all students in the classroom.
3. Because the student who has hearing impairment does not wear the amplification system, it is unlikely to be rejected for cosmetic reasons, resulting in longer use and benefit.

The value of sound field FM equipment was originally investigated in a 3-year longitudinal project called Mainstream Amplification Resource Room Study (MARRS) conducted in the Wabash and Ohio Valley schools of southern Illinois (Sarff, Ray, & Bagwell, 1981). The MARRS research compared sound field FM with resource room placement in overcoming educational deficits of fourth-, fifth-, and sixth-grade students with marginal hearing impairments. The findings revealed that both treatments resulted in significant improvements in academic achievement test scores. However, students who received amplification in a mainstreamed classroom achieved gains at a faster rate, to a higher level, and at one-tenth the cost of students taken from the regular classrooms and placed with resource teachers.

Rosenberg et al. (1999) recently completed a sound field FM study in kindergarten, first, and second grade classrooms in the Florida schools. Loudspeakers generally were placed at ear level on bookshelves or mounted on walls using brackets away from classroom traffic, as recommended by Allen (1991). The sound field FM systems provided teachers with an average of +6.94 dBA increase in vocal intensity and a +3.31 dB S/N ratio. Reverberation measures were not obtained. Data on 1,750 students indicated that those in amplified classrooms had significant improvement in listening and learning behavior and skills and progressed at a faster rate than their peers in unamplified classrooms. Younger students demonstrated the greatest improvement. Hearing losses among these children were not reported. In a summary of the study Rosenberg et al. noted:

Because there are no enforceable standards for classroom acoustics at this time, FM sound field amplification may be viewed as at least a part of the solution to improving listening conditions in classrooms. However, audiologists also should advocate for acoustical standards and modifications to enhance the listening environment in addition to recommending the use of sound field amplification. Finally, the vast array of sound field technology and options available as we enter the new millennium should continue to make sound field amplification a very desirable and affordable means to enhance listening and learning in the classroom. (p. 26)

Notwithstanding the benefits of sound field amplification reported, the acoustical data of this study suggest that the acoustical conditions of these classrooms were still detrimental to listening and learning. S/N averages of 3.31 dBA were well below desirable (+10 dBA) or optimal (+20 dBA) levels (Berg, 1997; Blair, 1996). The limited (+6.94 dBA average) increase in vocal intensity with sound field amplification suggests either that (1) these rooms also had undesirable hard surfaces, causing reverberation and echoes, preventing teachers from further increasing the volume controls of the amplifiers, or (2) their noise levels may have averaged 60 dB or even greater. With classroom control, average noise levels in the classrooms can be 50 dB or even lower (Barton, 1989). Coupled with appropriate acoustical treatment, S/N levels in these classrooms might have averaged as high as +20 dBA rather than +3.31 dBA.

The number and placement of loudspeakers in these classrooms may have also adversely affected the S/N ratios and signal levels of the above study. The author believes that a ceiling distributed, 6-unit speaker system will provide more intelligible sound reinforcement coverage than the arrangement used, namely, 3 or 4 speakers placed on bookshelves or mounted on walls of a classroom. To achieve impedance matching and negligible distortion with 6 speakers in a sound field FM system, however, may require individual speaker power units with volume controls attached to each speaker, a mixer/preamplifier in place of a conventional amplifier, and a power booster for a sound field FM system (Berg & Blair, 1998; Lonstein & Washburn, 1993[2]).

The combination of acoustical control of a classroom and a ceiling distributed sound reinforcement system holds promise for enabling sound field FM equipment to be be used effectively not only for children with normal hearing or marginal hearing loss, but with deaf and hard-of-hearing children who use hearing aids. The cost for such audiological adaptation would be less than using a personal sound field FM system. Anderson (1999), however, points out that the practicality of passing a microphone transmitter of either a personal or sound field FM system to every talker, including brief peer conversations and comments, is contraindicated. She states that attention to reverberation and background noise in the classroom is essential, if children who are hard of hearing are to effectively communicate and learn in cooperation with class peers.

HOSTILE ACOUSTICS: EDUCATIONAL PROBLEMS OF HARD OF HEARING CHILDREN

A simple yet flexible listening solution for children who use hearing aids may be to just improve classroom acoustics to where their personal hearing aids can be used effectively. To reduce reverberation and echoes, acoustical materials can be added to classroom walls, particularly the back wall, in addition to being used on the floor and/or ceiling. To reduce classroom noise, a teacher can reward the class for being quiet. He or she can use an inexpensive (e.g. Radio Shack) sound level meter to monitor his or her signal level and the class noise level. If he or she can keep the S/N level at no lower than +10 dB, children with hearing aids will be more likely to adjust the volume upward to hear the teacher and other children.

If steps are not taken to improve classroom acoustics, it is possible hard-of-hearing children will not be able to use their hearing aids effectively in school. Consequently, they will hear poorly and

---

[2]Further information is available from: Molly Lonstein, IMP Systems Inc, 410 West San Marino Drive, Miami Beach, Florida 33139, (800) 710 7786.

their academic growth will be slowed (Quigley & Thomure, 1968). A 1-year loss in the fourth grade, for example, may become a 2-year deficit in the eighth grade, and a 3-year gap in the twelfth grade (Berg, 1986). If such children have moderate to severe bilateral hearing losses, they will speak defectively (DiCarlo, 1968) and there will be unfavorable emotional and social problems (Wright, 1970). These problems will be compounded further by undesirable reactions of parents, teachers, and society at large (Boothroyd, 1982). These deficiencies will also have an adverse impact on preparation for suitable employment and finding the right job (Marshall, 1982).

SUMMARY

Formidable educational problems are faced by children with hearing loss. The primary educational problem of deaf children is illiteracy. The primary educational problem of hard-of-hearing children is hostile room acoustics. These problems currently are not being addressed in American schools. However, methods, technologies, and resources are available to solve or at least alleviate these problems.

REFERENCES

Allen, M. 1991. *A school handbook on classroom amplification equipment.* Elkader, IA: Keystone Area Education Agency.

American Annals of the Deaf (April, 1999, Volume 144). Washington, DC: Gallaudet University.

Anderson, K. (1989). Speech perception and the hard of hearing child. *Monograph of the Educational Audiology Association, 1,* 15–29.

Anderson, K. (1999). Sound field FM use by children with severe hearing loss: two case studies. *Journal of Educational Audiology 7,* 54–57.

Barton, L. (1989). *Sound levels in elementary school classrooms.* Unpublished master's thesis, Utah State University, Logan.

Beck, P. (1997). *Research findings regarding Cued Speech.* Rochester, NY: National Cued Speech Association.

Berg, F. (1986). Characteristics of the target population. In F. Berg, J. Blair, S. Viehweg, & A. Wilson-Vlotman (Eds.), *Educational audiology for the hard of hearing child* (pp. 1–24). Orlando, FL: Grune & Stratton.

Berg, F. (1987). *Facilitating classroom listening.* Boston: College-Hill Press.

Berg, F. (1997). Optimum listening and learning environments. In W. McCracken & S. Laoide-Kemp (Eds.), *Audiology in education* (pp. 348–384). London: Whurr.

Berg, F. (2000). *Literacy and speech for the young deaf child: How parents can take charge.* Smithfield, UT: Author. (Available from Fred Berg, 516 E. Summit Creek Dr., Smithfield, UT 84335.)

Berg, F., & Blair, J. (1998). Sound field FM and hearing loss. Logan, UT: Utah State University.

Berg, F., Blair, J., & Benson, P. (1996). Classroom acoustics: The problem, impact, and solution. *Language, Speech, and Hearing Services in Schools, 27,* 16–20.

Berlin, C. (1985) *Encouraging Audiologists to Recommend Cued Speech.* Presentation Before the Cued Speech Association, Cleveland, Ohio,

Bess, F. (1984). *The hard of hearing child.* Logan, Utah: Institute for Management of the Communicatively Handicapped. Logan, UT: Utah State University.

Blair, J. (1996). Educational audiology. In F. Martin & J. Clark (Eds.), *Hearing care for children* (pp. 316–334). Boston: Allyn and Bacon.

Boone, D. (1991). *Is your voice telling on you? How to find and use your natural voice.* San Diego: Singular Publishing Group.

Boothroyd, A. (1982). *Hearing impairments in young children.* Englewood Cliffs, NJ: Prentice-Hall.

Brooke, R. (1991). Rooms for speech and music. In G. Ballou (Ed.), *Handbook for sound engineers* (pp. 171–201). Indianapolis, IN: Howard W. Sams.

Christiansen, J., & Barnartt C. (1995). *Deaf president now! The 1988 revolution at Gallaudet University.* Washington, DC: Gallaudet University Press.

Clarke, T. & Watkins, S. (1985). *Programming for hearing impaired infants through amplification and home intervention.* Logan, UT: SKI-HI Institute.

Cooper, M. (1990). *Winning with your voice.* Hollywood, FL: Fell.

Cornett, R. O. (1967). Cued Speech. *American Annals of the Deaf, 121,* 513–518.

Cornett, O., & Daisey, M. (1992). *The Cued Speech resource book for parents of deaf children.* Raleigh, NC: National Cued Speech Association.

Crandell, C., & Smaldino, J. (1995). Classroom acoustics. In R. Roeser & M. Downs (Eds.), *Auditory disorders in school children* (pp. 219–234). New York: Thieme Medical Publishers.

D'Antonio, P. (1989). Controlling sound reflections. *Architecture, 109*, 112–137.

Davis, D., & Davis, C. (1987). *Sound system engineering.* Indianapolis, IN: Howard W. Sams.

Davis, D., & Davis, C. (1991). Audio measurements. In G. Ballou (Ed.), *Handbook for sound engineers. The new audio cyclopedia* (pp. 1365–1412). Indianapolis, IN: Howard W. Sams.

Davis, G., & Jones, R. (1989). *The sound reinforcement handbook.* Milwaukee, WI: Hal Leonard.

DiCarlo, L. (1968). Speech, language, and cognitive abilities of the hard of hearing. Proceedings of the Institute on Aural Rehabilitation (pp. 45–66, SRS 212-T-68). Denver, CO: University of Denver.

Downs, M. (1988). Contribution of mild hearing loss to auditory learning problems. In R. Roeser & M. Downs (Eds.), *Auditory disorders in school children* (2nd ed., pp. 186–199). New York: Thieme-Stratton.

Education of the deaf. (1965). *A report to the Secretary of Health, Education, and Welfare by his Advisory Committee on the Education of the Deaf.* Washington, DC: Government Printing Office.

Everest, F. A. (1989). *The master handbook of acoustics.* Blue Ridge Summit, PA: TAB Books.

Finitzo-Hieber, T. (1988). Classroom acoustics. In R. Roeser & M. Downs (Eds.), *Auditory disorders in school children* (2nd ed., pp. 221–233). New York: Thieme Medical.

Finitzo-Hieber, T., & Tillman, T. (1978). Room acoustics effects on monosyllabic word discrimination ability for normal and hearing impaired children. *Journal of Speech and Hearing Research, 21*, 440–458.

Flexer, C. (1999). *Facilitating hearing and listening in young children.* San Diego: Singular Publishing Group.

Furth, H. (1966). A comparision of reading test norms of deaf and hearing children. *American Annals of the Deaf, 111*, 461–462.

Geers, A. (1985). Assessment of hearing impaired children: Determining typical and optimal levels of performance. In F. Powell, T. Finitzo-Hieber, S. Friel-Patti, & D. Henderson (Eds.), *Education of the hearing impaired child* (p. 57–82). San Diego: College-Hill Press.

Geers, A., & Moog, J. (1994). Spoken language results: vocabulary, syntax, and communication. The sensory aids study at Central Institute for the Deaf. *The Volta Review 96*, 131–148.

Goldberg, B. (1995). Families facing choices. *Asha, 37* (5), 39–45.

Harris, R. (1995). Reach for the stars with Miss America, Heather Whitestone, as she shows us that "anything is possible." *SHHH Journal, 16*, 2, 8–10.

Heffernan, C. (1992). Reflections on Cued Speech from "down under." In O. Cornett & M. Daisey (Eds.), *The Cued Speech resource book for parents of deaf children* (pp. 676–684). Raleigh, NC: National Cued Speech Association.

HOPE (Home & family oriented programs essentials). (1999). Logan, Utah: SKI-HI Institute.

Individuals with Disabilities Education Act of 1997, Public Law No. 94-142, 20 U.S.C. §§1400–1485.

Johnson, T. (1991). Prevention of voice disorders. *Seminars in Speech and Language, 12*(1), Preface.

Lane, H. (1984). *When the mind hears: A history of the deaf.* New York: Random House.

Lane, H. (1992). *The mask of benevolence. Disabling the deaf community.* New York: Knopf.

Lane, H., Hoffmeister, R., & Bahan, B. (1996). *A journey into the deaf-world.* San Diego: Dawn Sign Press.

Lee, B. (1992). Thoughts on Cued Speech after 12 years. In O. Cornett & M. Daisey (Eds.), *Cued Speech resource book for parents of deaf children* (pp. 657–660). Raleigh, NC: National Cued Speech Association.

Lonstein, G., & Washburn, D. (1993). Distributed sound systems come of age. *Sound and video contractor.* Overland Park, KS: Intertec Publishing Corporation.

Marshall, K. (1982). The vocational impact of hearing impairment as viewed by the vocational rehabilitation counselor. In R. Hull (Ed.), *Rehabilitative audiology* (pp. 161–169). New York: Grune & Stratton.

Merrill, E. (1992). Forward. In O. Cornett & M. Daisy (Eds.), *The Cued Sspeech resource handbook for parents of deaf children* (pp. vii–viii). Raleigh, NC: National Cued Speech Association.

Nabalek, A., & Nabalek, I. (1985). Room acoustics and speech perception. In J. Katz (Ed.), *Handbook of clinical audiology* (pp. 834–846). Baltimore, MD: Williams & Wilkins.

National Center for Health Statistics (1994). Prevalence and characteristics of persons with hearing trouble. Series 10, No. 188. Data from the National Health Survey. DHHS, PHHS, 5–10.

Nicholls, G., & Ling, D. (1982). Cued Speech and the reception of spoken language. *Journal of Speech and Hearing Research, 25*, 262–269.

Noever, S., & Andrews, J. (1998). *Critical pedagogy in deaf education: Bilingual methodology and staff development.*

(USDLC Star Schools Project Report No. 1). Santa Fe, NM: New Mexico School for the Deaf.

Position statement on literacy (1990). Raleigh, NC: National Cued Speech Association.

Ray, H. (1989, July). *Listening management in the schools.* Presented at Project MARRS, Workshop at Institute for Management of the Communicatively Handicapped. Logan, UT: Utah State University.

Rosenberg, G., Blake-Rahter, P., Heavner, J., Allen, L., Redmond, B., Phillips, J., & Stigers, K. (1999). Improving classroom acoustics (ICA): A three-year FM sound field classroom amplification study. *Journal of Educational Audiology 7*, 8–28.

Ross, M. (1986). A perspective on amplification: Then and now. In D. Luterman (Ed.), *Deafness in perspective* (pp. 35–54). San Diego, CA: College Hill Press.

Rupert, J. (2000). Foreword. In F. Berg *Literacy and speech for the young deaf child.* Smithfield, UT: F. Berg.

Sarff, L., Ray, H., & Bagwell, C. (1981). Why not amplification in every classroom? *Hearing Aid Journal, 34*(10), 11, 44, 47–48, 50, 52.

Toward equality, education of the deaf. (1988). Commission on Education of the Deaf. U. S. Department of Education (1988). *Tenth annual report to Congress on the implementation of P.L. 94-142.* Washington, DC.

Wedenberg, E. (1954). Auditory training of severely hard of hearing preschool children. *Acta Otolaryngologica 54* (Suppl.), 1–129.

Wedenberg, E., & Wedenberg, M. (1970). The advantages of auditory training: A case report, In F. Berg & S. Fletcher (Eds.), *The hard of hearing child: Clinical and educational management* (pp. 319–330). New York: Grune & Stratton.

Wright, W. (1970). Counseling. In F. Berg & S. Fletcher (Eds.), *The hard of hearing child: clinical and educational management* (pp. 155–174). New York and London: Grune & Stratton.

END OF CHAPTER EXAMINATION QUESTIONS

CHAPTER 10

1. In the past, *oral* communication was the choice among educators when teaching children who are nonauditory. In the present, _____ is used in most educational settings; however, there continues to be a controversy about which method is best.

2. Name three reasons why early auditory intervention is advocated for children with severe and profound hearing loss.

3. What is Cued Speech?

4. Name two programs that have been found to be the most cost-effective in upgrading the education of children with hearing impairment.

5. According to the author, _____ and _____ are the lead senses of people and reach out like antennae to bring in the close and distant environment.

6. Reduction of _____ and reverberation is a direct approach at enhancing auditory learning in classroom environments.
   a. amount of students
   b. classroom noise
   c. teacher's voice loudness
   d. furniture

7. Auditory learning in classrooms can be greatly enhanced through _____.

8. (True/False) One of the important things that we can do on behalf of hearing impaired children is to emphasize that classrooms must be designed for enhancing listening skills.

9. What is the AO or OA method of communication?

END OF CHAPTER ANSWER SHEET

Name _____ Date _____

CHAPTER 10

1. _____

2. _____
   _____
   _____

3. _____
   _____
   _____

4. _____
   _____

5. _____
   _____

6. Which one?   a   b   c   d

7. _____

8. Circle one: True   False

9. _____
   _____
   _____

PART III

Aural Rehabilitation: Adults Who Are Hearing Impaired

Introduction to Aural Rehabilitation for Adults

History, Theory, and Application

■ RAYMOND H. HULL, Ph.D. ■

TECHNIQUES FOR IMPROVING COMMUNICATION
FOR ADULTS WHO ARE HEARING IMPAIRED: PAST
AND PRESENT
    Lipreading
    Discussion of Early Approaches

IMPROVING COMMUNICATION SKILLS THROUGH
AURAL REHABILITATION

APPROACHES TO AURAL REHABILITATION

AURAL REHABILITATION APPLICATIONS FOR ADULTS

THE PRINCIPLES OF AURAL REHABILITATION

SUMMARY

One of the basic premises in serving hearing-impaired adults is that some form of rehabilitative activity should accompany the discovery of a hearing loss. The most successful approaches to aural rehabilitation appear to be those that address and incorporate procedures that specifically address the short-term and long-term communicative needs of individual clients. This philosophy is stressed throughout this chapter.

Even though this chapter addresses a number of avenues and approaches to aural rehabilitation, it must be remembered that the complexities observed within hearing impaired adults require a client-oriented approach to treatment. Using a "method" without considering the specific needs of given clients may result in inadequate treatment.

TECHNIQUES FOR IMPROVING COMMUNICATION FOR ADULTS WHO ARE HEARING IMPAIRED: PAST AND PRESENT

Before addressing current issues involved in the process of aural rehabilitation for adults, a review of issues and early approaches is important.

LIPREADING

The visibility of the phonemes of speech has not been found to be sufficient for total communication by most persons. It has been difficult, however, to extinguish the term "lipreading" from its connotations of a vision-alone mode of communication and from the process of aural rehabilitation.

Early definitions of lipreading stressed the eye as literally taking the place of the ear (Bruhn, 1949). She believed that the eye could be trained to distinguish the visible characteristics of the movements of the speech mechanism. Such descriptions of lipreading have been passed on through the years and the term still tends to denote a strict concentration on the visualization of speech.

Other early methods of lipreading stressing the primary use of vision were those of Bunger (1961)—the Jena method, Kinzie (1931), and Nitchie (1950). In the early to middle part of this century, however, it was undoubtedly more necessary to em-phasize the visual mode in communication when providing therapy for hearing-impaired adults. As stated by McCarthy and Alpiner (1978), the visual-only methods stressed in early attempts at aural rehabilitation were necessary because of lack of efficient amplification systems.

A review of those early methods is appropriate, as it is from these that our more current procedures have either evolved or deviated.

The Mueller-Walle Method

Martha Bruhn introduced the Mueller-Walle method in 1902. This method was strictly analytic in its approach. It stressed the development of lipreading skills through kinesthetic awareness of the movements involved in speech production. It involved rapid, rhythmic syllable drills, as it was believed that the syllable is the basic unit of words, that in turn, compose sentences, and should be subconsciously recognized. Bruhn viewed lipreading as training the eye as well as the mind and believed that it involved visual, auditory, and motor memory. Her plans for lipreading lessons were divided into four parts.

1. Definition of the movement(s) of the new sound to be studied, contrasting the movements of the new sound with the ones previously studied;
2. Written work;
3. A story or talk that incorporated the new sound;
4. Group practice, or a period of questions.

Jena Method

Anna Bunger and Bessie Whitaker introduced the Jena method of lipreading. The method was developed by Karl Brauckmann of Germany. Bunger (1944, 1961) outlined Brauckmann's method, which emphasizes the audible, visible, movement, mimetic, and gesture forms of communication, including syllable and rhythm. The movement form was thought of as being complete for all persons, no matter what the level of hearing, as not all movements of the muscular system for speech are completely visible. The mimetic form was viewed as incomplete, but an important component of communication. Brauckmann also believed that the gesture form was not complete, but that it complements all others listed.

Bunger (1961) states that the first aim of persons who desire to learn lipreading is to develop awareness of the movements of speech and to learn how they feel. This was called *kinesthetic awareness*, which was then to become a substitute for audition.

The method included an explanation of the formation and composition of syllables. The consonants were presented and classified under the categories of production, including lips, tongue, and tongue-soft palate. The consonants were combined with words for practice. The consonants were said aloud by the clinician and then the client said them. Clients were asked to concentrate on the manner of articulation for their production and to categorize consonants in accordance with the three areas of production.

The rhythmic component of this method included a basic pattern that was established to accompany the syllable drills, such as hand clapping, tapping, or ball bouncing. The aim of this aspect was to alert the client to the feeling of speech movements as he or she talks and to imitate visible speech movements as another person is speaking.

The materials used included syllable exercises, grammatical forms, and stories and conversations.

The Nitchie Approach

In 1903, Edward Nitchie introduced an approach that was intended to break away from the more analytic approaches. His method advocated a "whole thought" approach to lipreading by emphasizing a working relationship between mind and eye. This mode of thinking paved the way toward a more psychological-synthetic basis for lipreading. Stress was placed on grasping the whole of a message when not all auditory information was available. This was in contrast to the philosophies of Bruhn and Bunger, which stressed working with the analytic components of speech. Elizabeth Nitchie (1950), Edward's wife, later revised his materials and added additional ones. Yet, the integrity of Edward's holistic approach was retained. Ordman and Ralli (1957) utilized Nitchie's approach and, with the aid of Elizabeth Nitchie, developed "lifelike" materials for use in lipreading lessons.

The Kinzie Approach

The Kinzie sisters, Cora and Rose (1931), designed a lipreading approach and materials that evolved from a philosophy that incorporated portions of those by Mueller-Walle and Nitchie, and is considered a synthetic approach. Their method involved a graded sequence of lipreading lessons based on varying levels of lipreading ability for both children and adults. The grading of the lessons was included so that individuals could progress from one level of skill to the next at their own rate.

In the development of their materials, several rules were established:

1. Sentences that were definite should be used.
2. Sentences should be natural in structure.
3. Word selection should also be natural.
4. Sentences should be interesting, pleasing, and rhythmic.
5. All sentences must be dignified.

For their story sections, the Kinzies chose items that were short and humorous. They felt that these held the greatest value for beginners and intermediates. They also chose stories about famous people for these two levels. They felt that higher level literary selections were most appropriate for advanced clients.

As part of their lessons, explanations of articulatory movements for sound production were made, including sample words that contained those sounds, along with contrasting words. Vocabulary lists preceded sentence work. More advanced lessons included stories and accompanying questions. Mirror work in relation to sound production was advocated during lipreading practice. They also stressed the use of voice during lessons to aid clients in the use of their residual hearing. Their materials for adults included 36 lessons on movements of sounds, 36 lessons on stories, and 18 lessons utilizing homophonous words.

DISCUSSION OF EARLY APPROACHES

The methods reviewed above were generally administered to clients in strict, unalterable ways. When clients had progressed through the lessons to the point of completing them or had advanced in their lipreading skills to their apparent maximum, they were dismissed. The actual success rate is still unknown, although many clients apparently felt that they benefitted. And some probably did. In one way or another, they were perhaps better able to understand the speech of others in spite of the fact that they did not have the advantage of advanced amplification devices.

According to Hull (1997), however, strict methods of lipreading that are presented as a structured sequence of lessons are now generally believed to be unsatisfactory for two basic reasons:

1. After the sequence has been completed, clients generally emerge unchanged in their ability to communicate with others. Even though individual clients may thank the audiologist who provided the lipreading sessions by saying, "I

surely learned a lot," or "Thank you, your lessons were *very* interesting," they may have concluded that they did not improve.

2. Those approaches do not lend themselves to a basic need in the process of aural rehabilitation. That is, the programs do not address specific communicative difficulties that clients face on a daily basis or help them to function more efficiently in spite of their auditory deficit.

The strict approaches described, and others like them, are based on the assumption that if the lessons are adhered to and learned, they will help hearing-impaired people to identify the visual clues of speech. In that regard, then, it was felt that clients could likewise be able to communicate better within their everyday worlds. Although the assumption appeared rational to those who advocated the use of those strict and relatively unalterable approaches, it is probably not valid.

The Efficiency of Vision in Communication

The early approaches to aural rehabilitation emphasized the use of vision to take the place of, or at least strongly supplement, impaired hearing in communication. How much does vision enhance communication when hearing is impaired? A number of investigators have studied the efficiency of vision in speech reception. The purpose of the majority of those investigations was to study the reciprocal benefits of vision and audition. However, early studies by Berger (1972), Binnie and Barrager (1969), Binnie, Montgomery, and Jackson (1976), Brannon (1961), DiCarlo and Kataja (1951), Erber (1969), Erber (1979), Franks and Kimble (1972), Heider and Heider (1940), Hull and Alpiner (1976b), Hutton (1959), O'Neill (1954), Utley (1946), and Woodward and Barber (1960), have concluded that vision alone contributes approximately 50% to speech intelligibility when no auditory information is available.

An early study by Erber (1969), for example, confirmed that for essentially inaudible speech, intelligibility scores in vision-alone conditions remain at about 50%. Hull and Alpiner (1976b) reported that among young adults with normal language function, approximately 50% of linguistically and phonemically balanced words within sentences could be identified by vision alone. They also found that only about 30% of sentences could be identified relative to their content when subjects were forced to depend on vision as the only sensory modality.

If hearing impaired adults can, through training, improve in their ability to recognize the phonemes of speech, and then to transfer that ability to improved understanding of conversational speech, continues to be a matter of debate (Walden, Erdman, Montgomery, Schwartz, & Prosek, 1981). However, early studies on the effect of training on the visual recognition of vowels and consonants (Armstrong, 1974; Black, 1957; Black, O'Reilly, & Peck, 1963; Franks, 1976; Hutton, 1959; Walden, Prosek, Montgomery, Scherr, & Jones, 1977, and others) have generally revealed anywhere from subtle to dramatic improvements in phoneme and word recognition. Again, whether this carries over into improved understanding of speech in one's everyday listening situations varies greatly from person to person and is a matter of debate. A lengthy discussion of early research on the complement of vision for the hearing impaired is found in O'Neill and Oyer (1981).

The Complement of Audition to Vision

Erber (1979), as discussed earlier, demonstrated that vision alone under optimal conditions leads to only about 50% intelligibility. For children who possessed a severe sensorineural hearing loss, vision-alone contributed approximately 35% to 41% intelligibility. This study, like others, demonstrated the considerable complement of vision to audition and audition to vision. For example, in utilizing a systematic mechanism for manipulating the amount of visual clarity available to subjects (Plexiglas placed at various distances to simulate visual acuity of from 20/20—normal—to 20/400— severe visual deficit), Erber (1979) found a 44% advantage when clear visual clues were available and combined with audition at a comfortable listening level. This advantage was maintained in spite of a simulated severe high frequency hearing loss (450 Hz low-pass filter with a 35 dB rolloff per octave). Even with the simulated high frequency hearing loss, scores increased from 54% intelligibility for single words in the vision-alone mode at 20/20 vision, to 98% when a distorted auditory mode was also introduced, demonstrating the complement of vision to low frequency hearing when there is a high frequency hearing loss.

Erber (1979) also employed the same procedure for the visual mode with severely hearing-impaired children. Results on the identification of content words within sentences indicated that the benefit of the children's dominant sensory modality (vision) is great under optimal conditions (20/20 vision), but still only allows for approximately 33% intelligibility. When their amplified residual hearing was combined with clear vision, youngsters' intelligibility scores increased to 68%. For profoundly hearing-impaired children, the contribution of the auditory modality was found to be only 6%. However, the combined auditory and visual benefit was 47%. When vision was reduced to replicate a severe loss of vision, scores dropped to 4%. Again, the complement of audition to vision is evident, but proportionate to the degree of auditory impairment. In working with adventitiously hearing-impaired adults, however, the majority are found within the plus or minus moderate hearing loss categories, where the complement of audition to vision and vice versa is very evident.

According to Hull and Alpiner (1976a), the reasons for the lack of definitiveness in the visual-only reception of speech are probably that some phonemes look alike; some phonemes are difficult to identify, because they are not visible by observing the lips (only about one-third of the phonemes of American English are readily recognizable by observing the face of the speaker). Also, there is a general lack of redundancy of the visemes of speech relative to the comprehension of verbal messages. Audition, even at minimal levels, adds greatly to the synthesis and closure required to comprehend speech.

Other earlier studies that confirm the complement of audition to vision include those by Binnie et al. (1976), Erber (1971), Hull and Alpiner (1976), Hutton, Curry, and Armstrong (1969), Miller and Nicely (1955), Montgomery, Walden, Schwartz, and Prosek (1984), O'Neill (1954), Prall (1957), Sumby and Pollack (1954), van Uden (1960), Walden et al. (1977), Walden et al. (1981), and others.

Discussing This Information With Your Client

Although it is important for clients to recognize the benefits of vision in communication, particularly in adverse listening environments, the efficient use of their residual hearing should also be emphasized during aural rehabilitation. They should be made aware not only of the limitations imposed by their impaired hearing, but also of the amount of residual hearing available for use. Both should also be discussed in light of efficient and complementary combined uses of audition and vision in communication.

IMPROVING COMMUNICATION SKILLS THROUGH AURAL REHABILITATION

Up to this point, the discussions in this chapter have centered on early traditional methods used in attempts at improving hearing impaired persons' ability to communicate in their worlds, including the benefits and limitations of the sensory modalities used in verbal communication. As

noted earlier, the approaches to aural rehabilitation for adults that appear to be most effective are those that are holistic in philosophy—that is, they address the specific communicative problems and needs of individual clients. There is more to resolving a communication deficit resulting from an adventitious hearing loss than learning to use one's residual hearing and complementary visual clues. That is not to say, however, that these aspects are not important in the process of aural rehabilitation.

The most critical element in the process of aural rehabilitation is the client. This is where some of the earlier approaches may have lost their validity. Philosophies that stress holistic approaches to aural rehabilitation services for the adult include those by Alpiner & McCarthy (2000), Alpiner (1987), Alpiner and Garstecki (1996), Binnie (1976), Colton (1977), Fleming, Birkle, Kolman, Miltenberger, and Israel (1973), Giolas (1994), Hull (1982), Hull, (1997), Maurer and Schow (1996), and Tannahill and Smoski (1978). Alpiner (1987) states that the goal of therapy for adults is to provide support, to help clients recognize where their communication problems exist and to overcome them to the degree possible.

Hull (1997) stresses the importance of addressing the client's specific needs:

Although the majority of the problems hearing impaired adults encounter revolve around a decreased ability to communicate with others especially in adverse listening environments, each client faces uniquely individual problems as a result of his or her auditory deficit. In order for aural rehabilitation treatment to be appropriate and meaningful for clients, the approach must relate to their specific problems and communicative needs. (p. 182)

In other words, it appears that audiologists are currently adhering to philosophies that address aural rehabilitation as a many-faceted process that goes beyond speechreading and auditory training.

APPROACHES TO AURAL REHABILITATION

More traditional approaches include those of O'Neill and Oyer (1981). In their discussion of visual training, they refer to a number of avenues to train the hearing impaired individual to use vision more fully as a means of communication (Table 11-1).

O'Neill and Oyer suggest that the visual form of training accomplishes two purposes for the lip-reading client. Those are, first, the development of visual concentration, and second, the development of synthetic ability.

O'Neill and Oyer (1981) also present a suggested approach to training clients in the combined use of visual and auditory clues. They state:

The initial stages of aural rehabilitation involve training without voice so that the hard of hearing person can focus his attention upon the visual aspects of speech. If such an approach is not employed from the beginning, the auditory channel will be used exclusively and the subject will not try to make use of the visual cues. Only because of this initial 'sensory' isolation will the individual be alerted to the use of lipreading alone. (pp. 74–75)

Even though their rationale for the visual-only training has merit in some instances for some clients, many audiologists today are avoiding uni-sensory approaches, particularly with adult clients.

The O'Neill and Oyer (1981) approach to the combined use of vision and audition includes beginning with combined practice in environmental noise conditions—in other words, not in an ideal communication environment. They recommend beginning at a 0 dB signal-to-noise ratio. They continue:

1. Progress from words utilizing lip sounds to words with open articulation (vowel) sounds;
2. Enhance auditory discrimination of isolated sounds;

TABLE 11-1. Training Exercises for the Use of Vision in Communication*

Visual Perception
Perceptual field
Peripheral field
Synthetic ability
Figure ground recognition
Attention Span
Tachistoscopic training (speed of reception)
Visual closure (training in the ability to exclude the irrelevant and to organize materials on the basis of observed similarities)
Predictabilities
Sentence completion practice
Word guessing

*Data from O'Neill and Oyer (1981).

3. Work with amplified sound, introduced first at threshold, and then gradually increased to make a smooth transfer from vision to combined vision with audition;
4. Associate gestures and facial expression with quality and rate of speech;
5. Use phrases, sentences, and stories;
6. Promote story retention (thought level rather than words or sentences), assessed by multiple-choice tests.

A summary of the first four weeks of lessons, as described by O'Neill and Oyer is:

1st day: Explanation of purpose of program. Discussion of the value of combined practice. Demonstration of contributions of vision alone, audition alone, and vision and audition together.

2nd day: Fifteen minutes of practice on "speech without auditory cues," followed by fifteen minutes of practice on "speech without visual cues."

3rd day: Initial listening in noise practice.

4th and 5th days: Thirty minutes of practice understanding individual words against interfering noises. Individual monosyllabic words in contrasting pairs are used in the practice.

6th and 7th days: Practice in listening without auditory cues. Paired words differing only in vowel composition. Fifteen minutes of practice with vowel discrimination against a noise background (recordings of various environmental noises).

8th and 9th days: Review of practice with selected consonants and vowels as incorporated in monosyllabic words.

10th day: Discussion of hearing aids and how they assist in lipreading. Discussion of benefits of hearing aids and effects of auditory "sets," plus discussion of critical listening and viewing.

11th day: Practice in speech discrimination. Sentences and phrases. Viewing alone, auditory alone, and combined. Listening against noise backgrounds using phrases.

12th and 13th days: Intelligibility practice with sentences, without voice, with voice, in noise, and in quiet.

14th and 15th days: Practice in rapid response to sentences.

16th day: Demonstration of "whole" approach with magazine covers. Stressed recall of thoughts. Presented description of pictures with no voice, low voice, and conversational voice.

17th day: Work on developing tolerance for noise. Discuss that noise has semantic as well as acoustic aspects.

18th day: Practice on colloquial forms using subject areas: newspapers, automobiles, magazines, and cigarettes. Use of intermittent noise backgrounds with combined approach.

19th day: Situation practice. Discussion of people and objects in the clinic. Go over daily newspaper items, short stories from *Reader's Digest* and *The New Yorker*. Use of white noise as background.

20th day: Start incorporating tachistoscopic practice with 5- and 6-digit numbers presented at 1/50 of a second.

Another traditional approach is presented by Sanders (1993). He believes that what should constitute a tailored management program for a hearing-impaired adult can be facilitated by viewing the task with to a problem-solving model. His involves the following stages:

1. Defining the problem;
2. Assessing the client's needs;
3. Establishing goals;
4. Determining methods for goal achievement; and
5. Evaluating effectiveness of intervention strategies.

Sanders (1993) states that even though formal approaches to lipreading can be utilized for both adults and children, they, "should not detract the teacher from grasping every opportunity to meet the (special) needs . . . both of individual students and of the group" (p. 495). He stresses the importance of viewing aural rehabilitative management from the standpoint of the effects of the disability or handicap that the client is experiencing as a result of the hearing loss. He emphasizes that one's need for aural rehabilitation services becomes evident when: (1) communication abilities are no longer adequate to permit the client to meet the demands encountered in his or her daily life; (2) the psychological cost of meeting daily demands is judged to be too high; (3) the level of communication abilities, although minimally adequate, will limit advancement of the adult.

Sanders (1993) advocates the use of a profile questionnaire approach to probe the difficulties that a client is experiencing, and then to attempt to resolve them to the degree possible. The areas probed include the client's:

1. Home environment;
2. Work environment; and
3. Social environments.

One must recognize that the relative importance of these areas will differ from client to client.

The Committee of Aural Rehabilitation of ASHA (Freeland et al., 1974) as a result of a historic meeting and classic publication on aural rehabilitation, presented an approach that involves more than a formal approach to the use of visual and auditory clues in communication. Even though it is over 25 years old, it emphasizes sound metho-dologies in aural rehabilitation. It includes the following components:

1. Evaluation of peripheral and central auditory disorders;
2. Development or remediation of communication skills through specific training methods;
3. Use of electronic devices to increase sensory input (auditory, vibratory, and others);
4. Counseling regarding the auditory deficit;
5. Periodic reevaluation of auditory function;
6. Assessment of the effectiveness of the procedures used in habilitation.

McCarthy and Culpepper (1987) suggest a "progressive approach" to aural rehabilitation treatment that is based on modifying either the clients' behavior and attitudes, the clients' environment, or a combination of both. In modifying the clients' behavior and attitudes, the emphasis is on developing the willingness to:

1. Admit the hearing loss and its handicapping effects;
2. Admit the hearing loss to others;
3. Take positive action to minimize communication difficulties by asking others to repeat and speak more clearly and requesting selective seating;

According to these authors, the sequence of their approach is:

1. Audiologic and hearing aid evaluation;
2. Assessment of communication function;
3. Identification of problem areas due to hearing loss;

4. Verbal discussion with the group regarding problems;
5. Admission of hearing loss to themselves and to others;
6. Modification of behavior, attitudes, and environment;
7. Willingness to utilize amplification in non-threatening therapy sessions;
8. Reduction of stress in communication situations;
9. Willingness to utilize amplification outside of therapy sessions;
10. More effective communication with normal hearing persons;
11. Termination of therapy. (p. 100)

This approach concentrates on the psychological impact of hearing impairment and a client's response to the deficits experienced in his or her environment. The philosophy seems appropriate for portions of an aural rehabilitation treatment program, and addresses important areas to be covered. It is to be stressed here, however, that not all audiologists are trained as counselors. Those untrained in counseling should not venture into areas where problems (emotional or otherwise) require help by professionals trained to do so.

Hull (1997) presents a holistic approach to aural rehabilitation treatment. It involves (1) counseling, (2) hearing aid orientation, (3) designing a program for increased communicative efficiency that is based on individual clients' prioritized needs, (4) specific treatment procedures, and (5) evaluation of success (or lack of it).

This approach lends itself to both younger and older adult clients. Its premises are that, first, each client has special priority needs that revolve around his or her frequent communicative environments; second, most clients can benefit from specific treatment techniques that are based on language factors that, if brought to a greater level of awareness, aid in communication; and third, the majority of hearing impaired adults complain of difficulty communicating in noisy or otherwise distracting environments. Practice in learning to cope in those environments can be of common benefit to most clients.

McCarthy and Culpepper (1987) stress that aural rehabilitation is a comprehensive process composed of interacting components. They state that the purpose of an aural rehabilitation program is to focus on assisting hearing-impaired persons in realizing their optimal potential (Freeland et al., 1974). The important components of an aural rehabilitation program of hearing impaired adults, according to McCarthy and Culpepper (1987), include:

1. Visual training, including speechreading, interpretation of nonspeech stimuli such as gestures and environmental cues;
2. Auditory training, which involves listening training, or developing auditory attending behaviors;
3. Speech conservation; and
4. Counseling.

Giolas (1994) stresses two major components of aural rehabilitation treatment: (1) optimal use of auditory cues and (2) communication strategies. From those, five subcomponents are derived. Those involve (a) a thorough program of hearing aid orientation, (b) the use of visual cues in communication, (c) the conservative uses of lipreading, (d) the manipulation of one's listening environment, and (e) responses to auditory failure and repair strategies.

AURAL REHABILITATION APPLICATIONS FOR ADULTS

In the end, specific approaches, alone or in combination, rarely fit the needs of all hearing impaired clients. It is best for audiologists to develop a philosophy regarding aural rehabilitation and then, taking that philosophy, extract, remold, and design programs that fit individual client's specific communicative needs.

What, then, is aural rehabilitation for adults? A holistic philosophy that would serve audiologists well was written nearly 40 years ago by Braceland (1963). He states that rehabilitation, in its broadest sense, encompasses a philosophy that a handicapped person has the right to be helped to become a complete person and, not only to be restored as much as possible to usefulness and dignity, but also to be aided in reaching his or her own highest potential.

This is a far-reaching philosophy that should guide all persons who work in helping professions. In aural rehabilitation, however, such a philosophy should guide the audiologist to serve the needs of individual clients. Thus, not every hearing-impaired adult should be placed in long-term aural rehabilitation treatment groups, nor do all require extensive hearing aid orientation, nor do all require special sophisticated amplification devices.

Such a philosophy suggests that, for some, the process of aural rehabilitation may involve:

1. A session or two to discuss difficult listening situations that they experience in their daily lives and develop strategies for dealing successfully with them;
2. A few sessions of hearing aid orientation to adjust satisfactorily to his or her hearing aid, those with whom they communicate, and the places where they communicate;
3. A full program of auditory rehabilitation sessions either in a group or as individual sessions. This author prefers that new clients be involved in individual work at least for several weeks before being introduced into a group setting; or
4. Developing strategies for telephone communication, listening in church, listening in family gatherings, and environmental design to enhance communication in their home, meeting room, or place of worship that may involve no more than several sessions.

THE PRINCIPLES OF AURAL REHABILITATION

There are also principles to guide the planning and execution of efficient aural rehabilitation programs for adult clients. However, they are not intended to supplant the good judgment of a skilled audiologist. In the absence of an extensive body of knowledge surrounding these topics, however, the following are offered as considerations that have guided this author and, as originally discussed in part by Bode, Tweedie, and Hull (1982) and by Hull (1997), which practicing clinicians have reported or demonstrated:

1. **First of all, aural rehabilitation treatment should center on the specific needs of the client.** If a client is having difficulty communicating in a specific environment, then the audiologist must work with him or her to develop strategies to overcome those difficulties to the degree possible.
2. **The clinician should serve as a model of a person who functions as an effective communicator.** Clear, articulate speech without unnatural overarticulation should be the norm. Appropriate intensity levels of speech for maximum intelligibility in varying listening situations should be sought. Unintentional masking of visible speech by hand or head movements should be noted and avoided. By being an example of a good communicator, the audiologist is modeling what hearing-impaired clients can expect among those with whom they can communicate best or, at least, most efficiently.
3. **Clients should not only be informed of the clinician's general and specific objectives, but should also formulate their own goals, some of which should be co-managed with the clinician's, with the remainder being the client's responsibility.** As aural rehabilitation is a learning process, the client must be made aware of his or her part and responsibility. In a learn-

ing or a relearning process, the therapist is only part of the process. The client's degree of active involvement is of paramount importance. Carryover to real life situations cannot and will not be fully accomplished unless the client is totally aware of his or her personal responsibility.

4. **Both individual and group therapy programs should be available to clients. Communication is a dynamic process that must be developed with varying speakers and in varying situations.** The client-therapist model is only one approach and should not be the only one considered. The group situation permits a client to discuss with peers the communication problems which may be common to each member. Each client must be carefully evaluated as to his or her potential for successful entry into the group environment. Many clients should begin treatment on an individual basis before joining group sessions, either because the difficulties they are having in communication contraindicate successful group interaction or the specific communicative difficulties that they are experiencing are not conducive to group discussion. On the other hand, group therapy can be a very powerful source for the development of an awareness of similar difficulties that others are experiencing. Group "problem solving" sessions are extremely beneficial.
5. **Counseling activity should be considered essential to the effectiveness of other components of the therapy relationship.** Audiologists are becoming more and more aware of this, and more training institutions are including formal courses and practica in counseling as part of the curriculum. Counseling is one of the most important activities involved in auditory rehabilitation. In this regard, major attention and effort will need to be directed toward developing counseling skills in graduate students and in practicing audiologists.
6. **Development of assertive influence on the communication environment by the client**

should be an essential component of therapy. Assertiveness without aggression can be an important therapy objective. The client can learn to stage-manage situations and communication events to maximize the probability of successful participation. Reducing background noise levels, decreasing the distance from a talker, optimizing lighting for speechreading cues, requesting that the talker use clearer speech, appropriate gestures, and a microphone, plus manipulating the design of the environment to one's communicative advantage are examples of areas where the client can become assertive and active in improving communicative circumstances.

7. **Clients should be encouraged to establish and maintain a balance between assertiveness and submissiveness during communication.** The client may need counseling directed at emphasizing and demonstrating the give and take of many communication situations. Again, a balance between domination and withdrawal behaviors might be explored during therapy. Acceptance of realistic expectations also should be addressed. Few of us can claim successful communication with even the majority of persons with whom we come in contact. In short, the client may be assuming too much personal responsibility for communication events and communication failures.

8. **Clients should be instructed regarding alternative response criteria appropriate for specific communication events.** Many clients seem to adopt avoidance and/or withdrawal behaviors during situations requiring their participation in the communication act. Therapy planning might include activities that directly involve principles of effective interpersonal communication.

9. **As successful communication is exciting and satisfying, therapy activities also should contain sufficient opportunities for similar positive interactions and experiences.** Interesting but still challenging training activities can be planned. Establishing a relaxed and satisfying communication relationship with clients is an ingredient of successful interaction. Developing and maintaining motivation are important potential effects of a relationship wherein humor, active involvement, and dynamic interaction are part of the therapy program, and not the exception.

10. **Developing technology should be incorporated into therapy activity on an experimental basis and resulting judgments of specific equipment for specific purposes should be shared with other practitioners.** Technological aids, in addition to hearing aids, should be employed throughout the aural rehabilitation program. These include telephone amplifiers, assistive listening devices, prerecorded practice materials for home use, videocassette auditory-visual training systems, and radio transmission devices for specific social or vocational situations. Such technology can be used to enhance communication for clients with special needs.

11. **Innovative avenues for enhancing the peripheral and central auditory and visual systems of the clients should be utilized.** These include enhancement of the speed and efficiency with which clients utilize the auditory and visual information derived from communication. Time-compressed speech and interactive laser video technology are available and useful in this regard. Enhancing central auditory function in older adult clients appears to be an efficient avenue through which speech comprehension can be likewise enhanced. Reactivating the system to regain speed and accuracy of central auditory function is not only beneficial to the clients, but an exciting and challenging process as well. Activities emphasizing speed and accuracy of auditory closure, accuracy of very short-term auditory memory, and speed and accuracy of audito-

ry/visual decision making have all proven beneficial to this author's clients.

12. **Clients should be instructed regarding alternative listening strategies appropriate for specific communication situations.** The clinician should explain to each client why certain communicative situations are more difficult than others. Here a client should be informed, for example, that difficulty is to be expected in certain noisy situations and that an alternative listening approach may be to turn down the hearing aid and rely more on speechreading. Other situations may be so difficult that there is no solution. Such information will add to a client's confidence, by providing knowledge that there are many ways of attempting to overcome difficult communicative environments and that, in some situations, most people have difficulty, not just the one with the hearing loss.

13. **Clinicians should establish an explicit catalog of possible methodologies to achieve specific objectives and then review this information during planning of individual therapy.** Varying approaches to therapy should be gleaned from the literature. Novel approaches developed by colleagues or individual clinics should be evaluated for future use.

14. **Improving the speech habits of the client's family, friends, and others should be included as an important part of aural rehabilitation treatment.** Too often, it seems, clinicians concentrate exclusively on a client, with little or no attention given to significant others who are important to the client. General improvement in the communication expressiveness and effectiveness of these individuals could reduce the client's difficulties as much as, if not more than, therapy activities directed only to a client. This can be an extremely powerful part of therapy on behalf of the client. However, diplomacy is a critical factor here.

SUMMARY

In this chapter, varying philosophies and approaches to aural rehabilitative treatment have been presented. The theme that the author desired to stress throughout is that clinicans must continually remain vigilant to the special needs of individual clients. Some may require specific strategies to address particular problems in communication that are peculiar to them. Others may benefit from speechreading/lipreading instruction to complement their residual hearing. Whatever the assessed needs of clients, the audiologist must be flexible and knowledgeable in offering those services.

REFERENCES

Alpiner, J. G. (1978). (Ed.). *Handbook of adult rehabilitative audiology.* Baltimore, MD: Williams & Wilkins.

Alpiner, J. G. (1987). Rehabilitative audiology: An overview. In J. G. Alpiner & P. McCarthy (Eds.), *Rehabilitative audiology: Children and adults* (pp. 317). Baltimore, MD: Williams & Wilkins.

Alpiner, J., & Garstecki, D. C. (1996). Aural rehabilitation for adults: Assessment and management. In Schow, R. L. & Nerbonne, M.A. (Eds.), *Introduction to audiologic rehabilitation.* (pp. 316–412). Boston, MA: Allyn and Bacon.

Alpiner, J., & McCarthy, P. (Eds.). (2000). *Rehabilitative audiology: Children and adults.* Baltimore, MD: Lippincott, Williams & Wilkins.

Armstrong, M. B. S. (1974). *Visual training in aural rehabilitation.* Unpublished doctoral dissertation, University of Illinois: Champaign-Urbana.

Berger, K. (1972). Visemes and homophenous words. *Teacher of the Deaf, 70,* 396–399.

Binnie, C. A. (1976). Relevant aural rehabilitation. In J. L Northern (Ed.), *Hearing disorders* (pp. 213–227). Boston, MA: Little, Brown.

Binnie, C. A., & Barrager, D. C. (1969, November). *Bisensory established articulation functions for normal hearing and sensorineural hearing loss patients.* Paper presented at the annual convention of the American Speech and Hearing Association, Chicago, IL.

Binnie, C. A., Montgomery, A. A., & Jackson, P. (1976). Auditory and visual contributions to the perception of selected English consonants. *Journal Of Speech and Hearing Disorders, 17,* 619–630.

Black, J. W. (1957). Multiple choice intelligibility tests. *Journal of Speech and Hearing Disorders, 22,* 213–235.

Black, J. W., O'Reilly, P. P., & Peck, L. (1963). Self-administered training in lipreading. *Journal of Speech and Hearing Disorders, 28,* 183–186.

Bode, D., Tweedie, D., & Hull, R. H. (1982). Improving communication through aural rehabilitation. In R. H. Hull (Ed.), *Rehabilitative audiology* (pp. 101–115). New York: Grune & Stratton.

Braceland, F. J. (1963, October). *The restoration of man.* Donald Dabelstein Memorial Lecture presented at the annual conference of the National Rehabilitation Association, Chicago, IL

Brannon, C. (1961). Speechreading of various materials. *Journal of Speech and Hearing Disorders, 26,* 348–354.

Bruhn, M. D. (1949). *The Mueller-Walle method of lip-reading.* Washington, DC: Volta Bureau.

Bunger, A. M. (1944). *Speech reading—Jena method.* Danville, IL: The Interstate Press.

Bunger, A. M. (1961). *Speech reading—Jena method.* Danville, IL: The Interstate Printers and Publishers.

Colton, J. (1977). Student participation in aural rehabilitation programs. *Journal of the Academy of Rehabilitative Audiology, 10,* 31–35.

Costello, M. R., Freeland, E. E., Hill, M. J., Jeffers, J., Matkin, N. D., Stream, R. W., & Tobin, H. (1974). The audiologist: Responsibilities in the habilitation of the auditorily handicapped. *Journal of the American Speech and Hearing Association, 16,* 68–70.

DiCarlo, L. M., & Kataja, R. (1951). An analysis of the Utley lipreading test. *Journal of Speech and Hearing Disorders, 16,* 226–240.

Erber, N. P. (1969). Interaction of audition and vision in the recognition of oral speech stimuli. *Journal of Speech and Hearing Research, 12,* 423–425.

Erber, N. P. (1971). Auditory and audiovisual reception of words in low frequency noise by children with normal hearing and by children with impaired hearing. *Journal of Speech and Hearing Research, 14,* 496–512.

Erber, N. P. (1979). Auditory-visual perception of speech with reduced optical clarity. *Journal of Speech and Hearing Research, 22,* 212–223.

Fleming, M., Birkle, L., Kolman, I., Miltenberger, G., & Israel, R. (1973). Development of workable aural rehabilitation programs. *Journal of the Academy of Rehabilitative Audiology, 6,* 35–36.

Franks, J. R. (1976). The relationship of non-linguistic visual perception to lipreading skill. *Journal of the Academy of Rehabilitative Audiology, 9,* 31–37.

Franks, J. R., & Kimble, J. (1972). The confusion of English consonant clusters in lipreading. *Journal of Speech and Hearing Research, 15,* 474–482.

Freeland, E. E., Hill, M. J., Jeffers, J., Matkin, N. D., Stream, R. W., Tobin, H., & Costello, M. R. (1974). The audiologist: Responsibilities in the habilitation of the auditorily handicapped. *ASHA, 16,* 68–70.

Giolas, T. G. (1994). Aural rehabilitation of adults with hearing impairment. In Katz, J. (Ed.), *Handbook of clinical audiology.* Baltimore, MD: Williams and Wilkins.

Heider, F. K., & Heider, G. M. (1940). A comparison of sentence structure of deaf and hard of hearing children. *Psychological Monographs, 52,* 42–103.

Hull, R. H. (1997). *Rehabilitative audiology.* San Diego: Singular Publishing Group

Hull, R. H. (1997). Techniques for aural rehabilitation for aging adults who are hearing impaired. In Hull, R. H. (Ed.). *Aural rehabilitation* (pp. 367–393). San Diego: Singular Publishing Group.

Hull, R. H., & Alpiner, J. G. (1976a). The effect of syntactic word variations on the predictability of sentence content in speechreading. *Journal of the Academy of Rehabilitative Audiology, 9,* 42–56.

Hull, R. H., & Alpiner, J. G. (1976b). A linguistic approach to the teaching of speechreading: Theoretical and practical concepts. *Journal of the Academy of Rehabilitative Audiology, 9,* 4–19.

Hutton, C. (1959). Combining auditory and visual stimuli in aural rehabilitation. *Volta Review, 61,* 316–319.

Hutton, C., Curry, E. T., & Armstrong, M. B. (1969). Semidiagnostic test materials for aural rehabilitation. *Journal of Speech and Hearing Disorders, 24,* 318–329.

Kinzie, C. E., & Kinzie, R. (1931). *Lip-reading for the deafened adult.* Philadelphia, PA: John C. Winston.

Maurer, J., & Schow, R. L. (1996). Audiologic rehabilitation for elderly adults: Assessment and management. In R. L. Schow & M. A. Nerbonne (Eds.), *Introduction to audiologic rehabilitation.* Boston, MA: Allyn and Bacon.

McCarthy, P. A., & Culpepper, N. B. (1987). The adult remediation process. In J. Alpiner & P. A. McCarthy (Eds.), *Rehabilitative audiology: Children and adults* (pp. 305–342). Baltimore, MD: Williams & WiLkins.

Miller, G. A., & Nicely, P. E. (1955). An analysis of perceptual confusions among some English consonants. *Journal of the Acoustical Society of America, 27,* 338–352.

Montgomery, A., Walden, B., Schwartz, D., & Prosek, R. (1984). Training auditory-visual speech recognition in adults with moderate sensorineural hearing loss. *Ear and Hearing, 5,* 30–36.

Nitchie, E. H. (1950). *New lessons in lip-reading.* Philadelphia, PA: J. B. Lippincott.

O'Neill, J. J. (1954). Contributions of the visual components of oral symbols to speech comprehension. *Journal of Speech and Hearing Disorders, 19,* 429–439.

O'Neill, J. J., & Oyer, H. J. (1981). *Visual communication for the hard of hearing.* Englewood Cliffs, NJ: Prentice-Hall.

Ordman, K. A., & Ralli, M. P. (1957). What people say. Washington, DC: The Volta Bureau.

Prall, J. (1957). Lipreading and hearing aids combine for better comprehension. *Volta Bureau, 59,* 64–65.

Sanders, D. A. (1993). *Management of hearing handicap: Infants to elderly* (3rd ed.).Englewood Cliffs, NJ: Prentice-Hall.

Sumby, W. H., & Pollack, I. (1954). Visual contributions to speech intelligibility in noise. *Journal of the Acoustical Society of America, 26,* 212–215.

Tannahill, J. C., & Smoski, W. J. (1978). Introduction to aural rehabilitation. In J. Katz (Ed.), *Handbook of clinical audiology* (pp. 442–446). Baltimore, MD: Williams & Wilkins.

Utley, J. (1946). Factors involved in the teaching and testing of lipreading through the use of motion pictures. *Volta Review, 38,* 657–659.

van Uden, A. (1960). A sound-perceptive method. In A. W. G. Ewing (Ed.), *The modern educational treatment of deafness* (pp. 3–19). Washington, DC: The Volta Bureau.

Walden, B., Erdman, S., Montgomery, A., Schwartz, D., & Prosek, R. (1981). Some effects of training on speech perception by hearing-impaired adults. *Journal of Speech and Hearing Research, 24,* 207–216.

Walden, B., Prosek, R., Montgomery, A., Scherr, C., & Jones, C. (1977). Effects of training on the visual recognition of consonants. *Journal of Speech and Hearing Research, 20,* 130–145.

Woodward, M. F., & Barber, C. G. (1960). Phoneme perception in lipreading. *Journal of Speech and Hearing Research, 3,* 212–222.

END OF CHAPTER
EXAMINATION QUESTIONS

CHAPTER 11

1. Briefly discuss why strict methods of lipreading presented as a structured sequence of lessons are generally felt to be unsatisfactory.

2. In this chapter, the author presents a philosophical statement by Sanders (1993) that describes three indicators of the need for aural rehabilitation. What are those three indicators?

   a.

   b.

   c.

3. According to the author of this chapter, a holistic philosophy for audiologists to follow is in the provision of aural rehabilitation services. What are some of the services that may be provided?

4. Vision alone contributes approximately _____% to speech intelligibility when no auditory information is available.

   a. 20%

   b. 50%

   c. 31%

   d. 70%

5. The most critical element in the process of aural rehabilitation is _____.

   a. the complement of audition to vision

   b. the degree of auditory impairment

   c. the client

   d. all of the above

END OF CHAPTER
ANSWER SHEET

Name   Date

CHAPTER 11

1. _____

   _____

   _____

   _____

2. a.

   b.

   c.

3. _____

   _____

   _____

   _____

4. a.

   b.

   c.

   d.

5. a.

   b.

   c.

   d.

6. a.

   b.

   c.

   d.

7. _____

   _____

   _____

   _____

8. Circle one: True   False

9. _____

   _____

   _____

   _____

10. a.

    b.

    c.

    d.

6. McCarthy and Alpiner (1987) suggest a "progressive approach" to aural rehabilitation. It concentrates on the _____ of hearing impairment.

   a. psychological impact

   b. physical impact

   c. economic impact

   d. none of the above

7. Hull (1992) presents a holistic approach to aural rehabilitation. It involves _____. (Please list the components)

8. (True/False) According to the author of this chapter, "all aural rehabilitation should center only on the degree of hearing impairment of the client."

9. It is important for clients to recognize the benefits of vision in communication. But, that is not all that should be recognized to help in overcoming the handicap of hearing loss. What else should be involved?

10. List four of the early methods of lipreading.

    a.

    b.

    c.

    d.

Counseling Adults Who Are Hearing Impaired

■ HARRIET F. KAPLAN, Ph.D. ■

The sense of hearing is integrally related to communication and interaction with other people; to a very great extent persons relate to others through verbal language. For the vast majority of people who are deaf and hard-of-hearing, impairment of the sense of hearing means the ability to relate may be impaired as well. Messages may not be interpreted properly, because crucial words are missed or because nuances of meaning conveyed by a rising inflection, a pause, or an emphasis in a particular part of an utterance are not caught. Faulty hearing often leads to misunderstanding and inappropriate behavior. Helping an individual deal with these problems must be considered an integral part of the total process of aural rehabilitation.

The relatively small group of individuals who consider themselves culturally deaf represent a notable exception. Adults who are culturally deaf are those individuals who have chosen to use sign language as their primary means of communication and to associate primarily with others who do likewise. They identify with and obtain most of their social experiences within the deaf community. Such individuals find sign language to be a complete, unambiguous communication system and find a vast array of social and cultural support systems within the signing deaf community (Kannapell & Adams, 1984).

Any type of psychological problem and the degree to which it is seen varies with every individual's lifestyle and personality and the characteristics of a hearing loss. Although there are inevitably individual differences among persons who are hard of hearing or deaf, similar adjustment problems are frequently observed.

EMOTIONAL REACTIONS TO HEARING LOSS

DEPRESSION AND FEELINGS OF INADEQUACY

People who are nonculturally deaf or hard of hearing often feel shut off from the world, not only because of difficulty communicating with others, but also because some or all of the subliminal auditory clues that permit one to maintain contact with the "hearing world" are no longer available. They may react to this depression by withdrawing from social situations and from contact with other people. They may even modify vocational aspirations. An example of this type of behavior is the case of the man who, as a result of a gradually worsening hearing loss, requested a transfer to a lower status, lower-income position requiring minimal communication, even though such a change was clearly not what he really desired.

Depression is frequently complicated by feelings of inadequacy. People who are deaf or hard of hearing may feel that they should be able to cope better with a hearing loss and that the inability to do so indicates weakness. In addition, there may be feelings of shame, because of the rationalization that hearing difficulty is associated with abnormalities such as thinking, learning, remembering, or decision-making disabilities. Such people apologize for not understanding and assume that the "fault" for communication breakdown is always theirs. This is typified by the man who was hard of hearing who took a trip to an area where people spoke a dialect unfamiliar to him. He automatically assumed that his communication problems were his "fault," although he acknowledged that normal hearing people were experiencing the same differences.

Depression and feelings of inadequacy tend to be lesser problems for adults who are culturally deaf because of the many support systems within the deaf community. Many individuals who are culturally deaf, however, desire to function within the hearing community as well. Their communication problems are related to their attempts to become bilingual, bicultural people.

DEFENSE MECHANISMS

Denial

In most cases, the threat to self-esteem is handled by one or more defense mechanisms. A common defense mechanism is denial. People with mild to moderate hearing losses may simply not acknowledge they have a hearing loss, because to them acceptance implies abnormality. Those same individuals would probably have no difficulty accepting the reality of a visual problem, because visual problems tend not to be associated with the general adequacy of the person. Denial increases the problem because it makes it more difficult to seek help or accept the need for a hearing aid, because the visibility of the hearing aid would make the hearing impairment apparent to others. Undoubtedly, we all know people who are hard of hearing who insist that their communication problems would disappear, if only people would speak plainly.

Hostility and Suspicion

Persons who are deaf or hard of hearing may blame others for their difficulties, accusing them of mumbling or of deliberately excluding them from a conversation. They may become suspicious, accusing others of saying unpleasant things or planning unpleasant situations. Laughter may be misinterpreted as ridicule. People who are culturally deaf may react in that manner to people who communicate with each other in their presence, without using sign language. Suspicion or hostility is frequently directed at those who are closest, such as spouses, children, or friends, further complicating adjustment. Persons who are deaf or hard of hearing may react negatively to such service providers as a doctor, an audiologist, or a hearing aid dispenser.

It is very important for the helping professional to realize the true source of this unpleasant behavior and remain objective about it. It is equally important for any professional working with individuals who are culturally deaf to use sign language for communication with those clients or in their presence.

PSYCHOLOGICAL LEVELS OF HEARING

Ramsdell (1978) has described three psychological levels of hearing for the normal hearing person and the problems associated with loss of hearing at each level.

Primitive Level

At the primitive level, sound functions as auditory coupling to the world. Individuals react to the changing background sounds of the world without being aware of it. As Ramsdell (1978) states:

> At this level, we react to such sounds as the tick of a clock, the distant roar of traffic, vague echoes of people moving in other rooms of the house, without being aware that we are hearing them. These incidental noises maintain our feeling of being part of a living world and contribute to our own sense of being alive. (p. 501)

When this primitive function is lost, acute depression may occur. Because the primitive level of hearing is not on a conscious level, the person who is deaf may not be aware of the cause of the depression. Frequently, the depression is attributed to inadequacy in coping with the hearing impairment.

The severity of the depression will be greatest among persons who have a sudden hearing loss, whether it is through trauma, surgery such as acoustic tumor removal, or other causes. Fortunately, hearing loss of sudden onset most frequently affects one ear only, although bilateral losses do occur.

Depression due to the loss of the primitive level will occur in the individual with slowly deteriorating hearing as well. In this case it is more insidious, occurring more slowly, but the resulting depression may be equally great. In some instances, the depression may be more severe because the person may not be aware that hearing is deteriorating. Informing the client of the true cause of the depression will help alleviate some of the problem, although this knowledge will not eliminate it entirely. Often properly fitted amplification (hearings aids or cochlear implants) can restore the primitive level, even if speech understanding is not possible. In some cases if amplification is not possible, such as with CN VIII destruction, a vibrotactile device may serve to couple the deaf individual to the world of sound.

The loss of the primitive level is a problem primarily with severe to profound adventitious losses. Most adults who are culturally deaf have never experienced the world of sound and, therefore, are not aware of the absence of subliminal auditory cues.

Warning or Signal Level of Hearing

At the warning level, sounds convey information about objects or events. The doorbell indicates the presence of a visitor. Footsteps indicate that someone is approaching. A siren indicates an emergency vehicle is near. A fire alarm indicates danger. Because warning sounds are frequently intense, loss of the warning level is generally found among persons with severe to profound losses. Some warning sounds, however, are of low intensity, and may be missed by persons with less severe hearing losses. These are mainly distant sounds, such as the whistle of an approaching train.

PSYCHOLOGICAL IMPACT OF HEARING LOSS

Insecurity

When there is an inability to hear warning sounds such as a smoke alarm, a door knock, or a child in another room, feelings of insecurity are understandable. Such problems are found within all segments of the deaf and severely hard-of-hearing population, including people who are culturally deaf. A vast array of electronic visual systems have been developed to deal with warning level problems. These systems can monitor a doorbell, a person in another room, a smoke alarm, and any other important sound within the home or office. More complete discussions of alerting device systems can be found in Compton, (1993), DiPietro, Williams, and Kaplan (1984), Kaplan (1987), and Chapter 14 of this text.

Annoyance

Feelings of annoyance are caused by disruption of normal patterns of life due to loss of hearing at the warning level. The person who is deaf or hard of hearing who cannot hear the alarm clock may oversleep in the morning and suffer penalties at work as a result. When the ring of the telephone can no longer be heard, social activities may be affected or business opportunities lost. Visual alerting systems can be very useful in overcoming these problems.

Localization

Localization problems may be considered a special type of warning level difficulty. To predict direction of sound, approximately equal sensitivity is needed in both ears; therefore the inability to localize sound is a special problem for persons with unilateral losses. What is not always realized, however, is that localization problems also exist for individuals who have bilateral hearing impairment who are aided monaurally.

In addition to alerting device technology, warning level difficulties can be dealt with by training a person who is hard-of-hearing or deaf to become more visually aware of his or her environment.

Loss of Esthetic Experiences

For many individuals, music provides an esthetic experience. For some people the inability to hear the sounds of nature, such as bird calls, may represent significant esthetic loss. Amplification cannot always restore these sounds to the extent that esthetic experiences are restored.

Symbolic Level of Hearing

At the symbolic level, individuals deal with sound as language and a major channel of communication. Nearly all people who are deaf or hard-of-hearing have difficulty at this level to one degree or another. Many children and adults who have deafness early in childhood experience delayed English language development, which later affects reading and other academic skills. Although adults who are culturally deaf tend to communicate comfortably in sign language and consider English a second language, they may have difficulties with the vocabulary and structure of English. English language deficits create a variety of communication problems for anyone who needs to function within the mainstream community for any reason.

Although adults who are hard-of-hearing or deafened do not generally suffer delayed language development, they do face the problem of communicating under conditions of reduced verbal redundancy imposed by impaired auditory reception. Depending on degree, type, and configuration of loss, such individuals lose linguistic cues inherent in a sentence, prosodic cues such as stress and inflection, and phonemic information. The fewer auditory cues that are available, the more likely a person is to misinterpret what is heard, with consequent embarrassment, frustration, and social penalty. This situation is worsened if the communication environment has background noise, competing speech, or other auditory or visual distractions.

At Home

The home can be a source of tension because of communication difficulties for a number of reasons. First, there is more opportunity for interpersonal communication and, consequently, more opportunity for communication breakdown. Second, the person who is hard-of-hearing or deaf expects the family to be more understanding of the special problems imposed by hearing loss than nonrelatives and is disappointed if that is not the case. Third, households tend to be noisy places. The noise level in a typical kitchen was measured at l00 dB SPL with water running at moderate speed, the refrigerator on, and the radio tuned to a comfortable listening level.

Typical is the problem of a client who complained that he could use his hearing aid comfortably everywhere but at home, because his family showed no consideration for his needs. His children slammed doors when entering the house and played rock music at high intensity levels. At the dinner table everyone talked at once, making it impossible for him to sort out one conversation from another. Worst of all, his wife insisted on talking to him from another room, raising the level of her voice when asked to repeat, but not entering into his line of sight. His solution to these problems was, first, to not use his hearing aid at home and, second, to minimize communication with his family. Several conferences with the entire family, which included discussions of the limitations imposed by hearing loss, improved the situation for the client. Unfortunately, not all families are equally adaptable.

When there are preexisting conflicts already within a family, a hearing loss can accentuate them. The hearing impairment can be used as a weapon either by the person who is hard-of-hearing or by other family members. A supportive family is important to an individual who is deaf or hard-of-hearing; at the same time, the person with the hearing loss must be willing to assume part of the responsibility for successful communication.

An individual who is culturally deaf will not have communication difficulties with the family, if the family is willing and able to use sign language as the primary mode of communication. However, many adults who are culturally deaf have grown up in hearing families. Unless the deaf person can communicate orally with the family or the family can sign to the deaf person, limited communication occurs in the home and the stresses are great.

At Work

Work-related problems are common. The extent and nature of a difficulty depend on the nature of the hearing loss, itself, and the type of job the person holds. The greater the amount of oral communication required and the greater the need for precision of understanding, the more difficulty a client is likely to have. The receptionist who has difficulty understanding speech on the telephone may be in danger of losing the job. The physician who finds it difficult to monitor a patient's heartbeat may find it increasingly difficult to function professionally. Large or small group meetings pose special problems, because of the need to follow rapidly changing conversation, often against background noise or reverberation. If not dealt with, anxiety and frustration created by such demands complicate communication problems caused by the hearing loss.

The majority of individuals who are culturally deaf work in environments where the communication system is spoken English. To function successfully, they must either develop strategies to communicate comfortably with hearing people or constantly use an interpreter. If communication is limited, the person who is deaf may be lonely at work and may face limited opportunities for advancement. The vocational impact of hearing impairment and the role of the vocational counselor is discussed in depth in Chapter 3 of this text.

The Telephone

A special problem at the symbolic level is inability to use the telephone. The telephone message has become an integral part of our lives, affecting communication at home, work, school, and in social environments. The person who cannot understand speech transmitted by telephone or who cannot hear the telephone ring is affected in every aspect of life. Social contacts are reduced because friends and family cannot be easily contacted. Vocational opportunities are limited to the minority of jobs not requiring telephone use. The inability to use the telephone to summon help is threatening, particularly for an individual who lives alone.

Many people who are deaf or hard-of-hearing can learn to use the telephone more effectively by developing appropriate telephone strategies. Telecommunication devices for the deaf (TDDs) are viable options for those who cannot use the voice telephone; proper use of TDDs, however, requires telephone strategies and ability to write understandable messages. Telephone training is discussed in depth by Castle (1980) and Erber (1985).

At School

The adult or adolescent in school often has special problems. Classrooms are rarely quiet places. Ross (1982) reported that the average noise level in 45 classrooms was 60 dBA; an optimal level for students who are hard-of-hearing is 35 dBA. At noise levels of 60 dBA or greater, it is often difficult for a normal hearing individual to correctly understand a teacher. The task is immeasurably more difficult for a student who is deaf or hard-of-hearing, who must function with an auditory system that distorts the incoming speech signal even under favorable conditions.

Not only are many classrooms noisy, but they tend to be reverberant, as well, because of large areas of rigid, smooth surface and few absorbent materials, such as drapes or carpets. Such room conditions further distort speech and add to the burden of a student who is deaf or hard-of-hearing who is trying to function with amplification. These conditions interfere with the efficient use of a hearing aid, which amplifies noise, speech, and distortion caused by reverberation with equal effectiveness.

Teachers are not always aware of the special needs of a student who is deaf or hard-of-hearing and do not always adequately project their voices. Teachers will occasionally speak with their backs to a class while writing at the chalkboard, thus distorting and reducing the intensity of their voices. Speechreading becomes impossible. A barrier to both speechreading and sign language reception in class is the need to take notes; one cannot concentrate on interpreting visual information and write at the same time. All of these problems tend to limit educational opportunities for adults who are hard-of-hearing or deaf, with consequent vocational limitations. Assistive listening systems to minimize effects of noise and reverberation, notetakers, interpreters, and greater awareness by teachers of the needs of students who are deaf and hard-of-hearing are needed.

Social Activities

For many adults, sudden or increasing hearing loss results in a restriction of social activities. The difficulty in understanding speech exposes individuals who are deaf or hard-of-hearing to the danger and embarrassment of misinterpreting what is said. As a result, they may react inappropriately and be exposed to ridicule. It is a rare person who possesses enough ego strength to continually explain the presence of a hearing loss and continually ask people to repeat what has been said. Even well-meaning friends do not always succeed in making a person who is deaf or hard-of-hearing feel comfortable.

Normal hearing people feel uncomfortable when they know a listener is not understanding what is being said. Often they are at a loss as to how to help the listener understand better, particularly when the person who is deaf or hard-of-hearing attempts to "bluff" and does it badly. Both partners in the conversation may attempt to deny a hearing loss, but communication is disrupted and speaker and listener are embarrassed.

When the hearing loss is severe or has been present for a long time, speech may deteriorate. In that case, the person who is deaf or hard-of-hearing may not be clearly understood, adding to the possible social penalties imposed by the hearing loss.

Conversational difficulties increase exponentially in difficult listening situations. Following a conversation alternating between members of a group can be very difficult, particularly with background noise. A dinner party can be extremely anxiety-provoking and a cocktail party impossible.

Social activities are further limited when a person who is deaf or hard-of-hearing can no longer enjoy the theater or lectures. Just as in face-to-face conversation, the person must cope with speakers or actors who may not project adequately, speech that shifts rapidly from one person to another, and poor room acoustics, as well as the loss of sensitivity and distortion imposed by the hearing loss.

More and more, as social activities become restricted, the person who is deaf or hard-of-hearing is isolated and lonely. This condition may ultimately be accepted with resignation, or it may be met with aggression. The individual may deny the reality of the problem and attribute a shrinking social life to the malice of others. Regardless of whether the problem is met with resignation or aggression, the person who is deaf or hard-of-hearing suffers deterioration in the quality of his or her lifestyle.

Individuals who are culturally deaf do not suffer social penalties because of hearing loss so long as their social contacts remain within the deaf community. For many, that is a satisfying and healthy choice. However, those who wish to socialize outside of the deaf culture encounter the same barriers as individuals who are hard-of-hearing and individuals who are not culturally deaf. Generally, successful crosscultural friendships occur when a hearing person can sign comfortably and both parties are good communicators.

Other Problems at the Symbolic Level

Every person who is deaf or hard-of-hearing has had, at one time or another, difficulties in obtaining services. This may involve mailing a package at the post office, purchasing an airline ticket, placing an order at a restaurant, or communicating effectively with a physician. Persons who are deaf or hard-of-hearing are at a definite disadvantage when dealing with the law. In recognition of this, a legal center for the deaf has been established at Gallaudet University. Most hospitals do not make special provisions for communicating with patients who are deaf or hard-of-hearing, nor are personnel aware of their communication problems. Often hearing aids are removed for safekeeping, effectively destroying any possible communication.

Another problem at the symbolic level is the ability to hear and understand television. Many people who are hard-of-hearing increase the volume beyond the tolerance level of hearing family members and neighbors, thereby creating a great deal of tension. Many people who are deaf cannot understand the TV signal, regardless of its intensity. The inability to enjoy television is not only a social loss, but eliminates an important source of information. Assistive device technology can make television accessible to almost everyone (Compton, 1993). In addition, many people who are deaf or hard-of-hearing find the use of closed captioning very useful.

FACILITATING ADJUSTMENT

The professional faces a twofold task in helping the person who is deaf or hard-of-hearing adjust to the problems imposed by hearing impairment. First, through educational and personal adjustment counseling (Sanders, 1988), clients must be helped to accept themselves as people who are deaf or hard-of-hearing and understand the limitations imposed by the hearing loss. Once this is achieved, clients can be helped to manipulate the environment to minimize penalties. Environmental manipulation may involve use of listening aids, modification of communication situations, and education of family, friends, and associates.

DEFINITION OF THE PROBLEM

To provide meaningful assistance to a client who is hard-of-hearing or deaf, it is necessary to obtain information on the specific communicative difficulties encountered in daily activities. Not only is it important to identify specific difficult listening situations, but also to assess coping strategies and attitudes of a client toward communication and toward him- or herself as a person with a hearing loss.

To one degree or another the traditional case history explores areas of communicative difficulty and allows the interviewer to assess an individual's motivation to cope with communicative difficulties. However, a case history interview provides only a general overview of a client's communicative difficulties. It does not provide quantitative information about degree of difficulty in various situations, nor generally does it sufficiently and systematically probe the specific social, vocational, and interpersonal situations creating problems. There are a number of communication scales available to provide more precise evaluation about difficult communication situations, communication strategies used by the client, and attitudes about hearing loss. This information helps an aural rehabilitation specialist to plan a program of therapy and observe progress as it occurs. A review of the more widely used communication scales is presented in Chapter 20 of this book.

Assessing a Client's Need for Amplification

In assessing a client's need for amplification, audiologists customarily examine the degree of hearing loss, the pure-tone configuration, speech recognition in quiet and noise, and the presence of tolerance difficulties. There is another factor that is equally important and must be considered when deciding whether to recommend a hearing aid. That factor is: Does the client really want a hearing aid?

The audiologist and client must objectively discuss the positive and negative aspects of amplification, leaving the decision to the client. Even if the choice is not to use a hearing aid, aural rehabilitation should be recommended. Frequently, after a period of aural rehabilitation, the individual who is deaf or hard-of-hearing begins to feel more positive about amplification. For further discussion of this issue, see Rupp, Higgins, and Maurer (1977) and Sanders (1988).

COUNSELING

After the specific communicative and attitudinal problems of a client have been defined, a specific aural rehabilitation program needs to be developed to meet the identified needs. In addition to speechreading, auditory training, and other skill development activities, personal adjustment and informational counseling must be included in the program as needed.

Personal Adjustment Counseling

Although personal adjustment and informational counseling are artificially separated here for purposes of discussion, they are intertwined in an actual rehabilitative program. The personal adjustment counselor functions as a facilitator to help clients modify maladaptive attitudes about themselves as hearing-impaired persons. Kodman (1967) discusses three facilitative conditions that must be present, if the therapist is to be successful.

ACCURATE EMPATHY. The first condition is **accurate empathy**. This is the understanding by a therapist of the true feelings that underlie statements the client might make. The therapist then responds in such a way that the client's feelings are reflected back, so that his or her difficulties can be viewed objectively. For example, a client might say, "Most people don't speak plainly these days. I'd rather read a book than talk to people." The empathetic clinician might reply, "It must be terribly frustrating not to understand people. Let's talk about some of your experiences." As the client begins to relate difficult listening experiences, the therapist can continue reflecting back upon the client's feelings and perhaps, in the process, lead the client to suggest ways of coping with these situations. This is a *nondirective approach*. The client makes decisions based on increased perception of the situation; decisions are not imposed on the client.

The use of accurate empathy is as important in a group situation as in an individual session. In the group situation, the therapist must reflect the feelings of each member as they are expressed. After a group becomes a cohesive unit, the members may begin to practice accurate empathy toward each other, providing strong positive reinforcement for attitudinal change.

UNCONDITIONAL POSITIVE REGARD. The second condition is **unconditional positive regard**. This involves acceptance of clients as they are, regardless of any hostility, belligerence, or apparent lack of cooperation. It is sometimes difficult for a novice clinician to accept expressions of negativism from a client and not to consider such behavior as a personal attack. However, it is important to realize that unpleasant actions or expressions are simply manifestations of a client's problems. Typical of this type of behavior is the woman who entered into aural rehabilitation with the stipulation that under no conditions would she take a hearing test. Her terms were accepted, although hearing testing was an integral part of the program.

After a semester of group therapy, she apologized for her attitudes, explaining that she had been convinced that a hearing test would be part of an attempt to sell hearing aids. She became one of the most hardworking and motivated members of the group, despite surfacing of other expressions of hostility every now and then. *Perspective taking*, the ability to take another's point of view (Erdmann,

1993), is a combination of accurate empathy and unconditional positive regard. Client management is facilitated if an aural rehabilitation specialist can view experiences from the client's point of view.

GENUINENESS. A third facilitative condition is **genuineness**. This condition implies a relaxed, friendly attitude toward a client, respect for the client's suggestions, ability to accept criticism, and communication with the client in a manner he or she can easily understand. A genuine clinician does not retreat into professional jargon or assume a pose of superiority because of professional stature. An example of a low level of genuineness is:

Client: I don't think this hearing aid will do me a bit of good.

Clinician: You're not correct. The tests show a definite improvement with the hearing aid.

A more genuine type of response might be: "Maybe you're right. Why don't you try the hearing aid at home for a few weeks and if it doesn't help, you can return it and get your money back. Let's talk again in a week."

These facilitative conditions are especially important when working with clients who are culturally deaf. Their language and culture must be understood and respected. American Sign Language (ASL) is not English; idioms and other figurative language vary from English. ASL tends to be a more direct language, with different pragmatic conventions and far fewer euphemisms than English; expression of ideas tends to be more direct. What may appear to be rudeness may simply reflect differences in the languages. To work effectively with a person who is culturally deaf, it is important for a clinician to have a working knowledge of the client's language and be willing to use it. Even if the clinician is not fluent in ASL, he or she should make every effort to maximize communication with the client. Most people who

are culturally deaf will meet hearing clinicians half way communicatively, if convinced of the genuineness of the relationship.

Clients who are culturally deaf sometimes make decisions from a different cultural base than clients who are not culturally deaf or are hard-of-hearing. Some have no desire to mainstream into majority culture; these people enter into therapy with a desire to develop greater communicative independence in those situations where it is advantageous to communicate using English speech or writing. The aural rehabilitation specialist must respect such decisions and work with clients on their own terms.

The qualities of accurate empathy, unconditional positive regard, and genuiness can be developed or enhanced through experience. Audio- or videotaping sessions—with the permission of the client, of course—and later reviewing the client-clinician interchange is an excellent way for the novice clinician to improve skills.

ACCEPTING THE REALITY OF THE HEARING LOSS. One of the most important goals of personal adjustment counseling is to help a client accept the reality of the hearing loss and the need for help. One must not assume that because a client has opted for a clinic evaluation, that acceptance of amplification or therapy is a given. The client may simply be appeasing family or friends or perhaps be taking the first tenuous steps toward seeking help although remaining ambivalent about self-acceptance as a hard-of-hearing person. There is no point in recommending amplification if a client is not ready to accept it.

It is far better to persuade the individual to enroll in an aural rehabilitation program that includes discussion-counseling to help with acceptance of the reality of the hearing problem. If necessary, the group discussions can be supplemented with individual counseling. It must be made clear that participation in aural rehabilitation is not contingent on hearing aid use. It must be emphasized that the audiologist is ready to assist with selection of a hearing aid if and when a client becomes ready.

Recognizing a Client's Fears

When a person feels a loss of self-esteem because of an inability to hear normally, he or she has a tendency to conceal the hearing loss. The fear is often related to the concern that people will view him or her as different. To such an individual, a hearing aid is a visible indication that he or she is an inferior person. Although it may be recognized logically that there is no truth to such fears, a fearful person may not be able to emotionally accept use of a hearing aid. Even when the hearing aid can be completely hidden from view, the problem of acceptance is not solved for some people; they believe that wearing a hearing aid represents tangible evidence of inferiority. These feelings are especially prevalent among adolescents, where peer identification and acceptance are overriding concerns. In addition, many adolescents and adults fear that hearing loss and its visible badge, the hearing aid, will make them less attractive to the opposite sex.

If an individual who is deaf or hard-of-hearing does succeed in working through the emotional objections to amplification, the usual expectation is that the hearing aid will restore good hearing. If the hearing aid user is not properly prepared for the limitations of amplification and the adjustment necessary to use it well, he or she will be disappointed during attempts to use the hearing aid. If the hearing aid is discarded, the person who is deaf or hard-of-hearing may feel even more isolated and depressed, as hopes of solving his or her communication problem with a mechanical prosthesis have not been fulfilled.

Educational, or Informational, Counseling

Educational or informational counseling is the provision of information about hearing loss, its effect on communication, and intervention procedures. Although this type of counseling can be accomplished either in an individual or a group situation, the group situation is often more effective, because experiences can be shared and peer reinforcement can occur. However, group participation requires that individuals identify themselves as persons with hearing problems. If a client is not ready for this level of acceptance, individual therapy is preferable until the goal of ultimate participation in a group can be met.

Topics that should be included in an informational counseling program are:

- The nature of the auditory system and hearing loss, including interpretation of audiograms.
- Effects of hearing loss on communication and impact of background noise and poor listening conditions.
- Importance of visual input, audiovisual integration, and attending behavior.
- Impact of talker differences and social conditions to communication.
- Benefits and limitations of speechreading.
- Benefits and limitations of hearing aids and their use and care.
- Benefits and limitations of assistive devices.
- Use of community resources such as self-help groups.

IDENTIFYING DIFFICULT LISTENING SITUATIONS. An important part of informational counseling is identification of difficult communication situations and development of coping strategies that work. The group format is especially effective for identification of and practice with communication strategies, but such training can be incorporated into individual sessions, if necessary.

Assertiveness Training

Assertiveness training can be easily incorporated into aural rehabilitation sessions. It is important for clients who are deaf or hard-of-hearing to understand that they have a right to understand, that it is acceptable to ask for help in a polite, courteous fashion, and that it is the responsibility of the person with hearing loss to instruct the communication partner in ways of helping. Clients need to learn to distinguish between: (1) aggressive, which involves violation of other people's rights; (2) passive, which involves allowing others to violate their rights; and (3) assertive, in which clients protect their rights without violating those of other people.

The aural rehabilitation specialist might pose the problem: "Suppose you meet two friends on a noisy street who are having a conversation. They greet you and try to include you in their conversation, but you are unable to follow what they are saying. What might you do?" The therapist would then try to elicit some of the following examples of assertive behavior:

1. Ask the people to move away from the source of the noise so that you can understand better.
2. Ask one of the two people to briefly summarize what has been said before you entered the conversation.
3. Admit you do not understand and ask for repetition or rephrasing of an idea.
4. Ask the people to speak louder.

The clients would then be asked to give examples of aggressive behavior, such as verbal or physical abuse of the speakers, and of passive behavior, such as saying nothing about the lack of understanding.

Role playing can be incorporated into assertiveness training sessions very effectively to help clients define appropriate behaviors. Homework assignments involving the use of these behaviors in actual life situations can follow the role playing and be followed up by discussions during subsequent classes.

Once clients are able to function assertively, they are ready to learn the many behaviors that facilitate communication. There are two broad categories of communication strategies: *anticipation* and *repair*.

ANTICIPATORY STRATEGIES. Anticipatory strategies involve thinking about a communication situation in advance and figuring out ways to minimize difficulties. They include such things as educating speakers to keep their faces visible, coming early to a meeting to get a seat close to the speaker, identifying tables in restaurants that provide optimal lighting and minimal noise, and making advance reservations to secure those tables, arranging for note-takers or interpreters in classes or meetings, and obtaining assistive devices. An excellent anticipatory strategy involves predicting vocabulary or dialogue that is likely to occur in a particular situation and practicing such language in advance. Appendixes A and B of this chapter contain lists of anticipatory strategies.

REPAIR STRATEGIES. Repair strategies are behaviors that are used to facilitate communication when it breaks down either because the deaf or hard-of-hearing person did not understand a speaker or produced speech that was not understood. Strategies include: repetition, partial repetition in which only what was not understood is repeated, rephrasing, request for key words such as the topic of the conversation, request for spelling of important words such as names or numbers, repeating numbers as single digits (e.g., 1-7-2 instead of 172), or asking a general or specific question, as appropriate, to clarify misunderstanding. An example of asking a specific question in response to lack of understanding is, "What is that person's name?" All people who are deaf or hard-of-hearing should be taught to use the confirmation or summarizing strategy frequently. The individual states what he or she thought was said to make sure the information is correct. An example of confirmation might be, "I think you said we're meeting at your house tonight at 9 p.m. Right?" The communication partner then confirms the accuracy of the statement or corrects inaccurate information.

Clients need to learn how to use these strategies and when they are appropriate. Detailed discussion of communication strategies and exercises for practice can be found in Kaplan, Bally, and Garretson (1987), Tye-Murray (1991, 1993), and Tye-Murray, Purdy, and Woodworth (1992).

It is important to realize that it is difficult for many people who deaf or hard-of-hearing to be assertive, particularly as they are often rebuffed. Coping with difficult listening situations in the manner suggested requires practice and development of a "thick skin." Clinicians should be sure to make their clients understand that they are aware of the difficulties involved in implementing these suggestions.

Educating Significant Others

Because communication involves not only the person who is deaf or hard-of-hearing but also family members, friends, and others, educational counseling of these people is important to the adjustment of the client. Family members or associates must understand the nature of a client's hearing problem and the specific ways in which communication is affected. After testing it is highly desirable to include spouses, children, parents, or friends in the counseling session for the initial explanation of the hearing loss.

The limitations imposed by some types of hearing loss are baffling to the lay person who finds it difficult to understand why some things can be heard easily and other conversations are handled poorly. The effect of a high-frequency hearing loss on speech perception, the practical effects of a word recognition problem, and the devastating effects of competing noise or competing speech on speech understanding must be carefully explained. For complete understanding, several explanations

at different times may be necessary for both a client and significant others. For that reason, normal hearing family members or friends should be encouraged to enter a rehabilitation group with a client.

EXAMPLES OF PATIENT MANAGEMENT

Mrs. K is a 53-year-old woman who had a mild bilateral hearing loss since age 30. She is bilingual, with Spanish as her native language. She had adjusted well to amplification and was able to function as an English teacher in a local high school until 2 years previously, when her bilateral hearing sensitivity dropped dramatically. The drop in hearing was accompanied by dizziness and persisted after the dizziness had subsided. For 1 month, hearing sensitivity improved to the level of moderate impairment, but dropped again after exposure to a fire siren. Antihistamines and vasodilators were administered by her physician in an attempt to improve the hearing, but were unsuccessful.

Audiological evaluation revealed a severe bilateral sensorineural hearing loss with poor word recognition and a severe tolerance problem. The site of lesion was the cochlea. Although binaural hearing aids were fitted, sufficient gain for her degree of loss could not be used for fear of triggering another episode. Therefore, the hearing aids were not completely satisfactory in transmitting intelligible speech. Because her speech understanding was no longer sufficient to allow her to continue teaching, and because she could no longer tolerate the normal noise levels of a school, she was forced to retire from her teaching position.

Mrs. K's first visit occurred after the second sudden drop in auditory sensitivity. She was undergoing otoneurological tests to determine the source of the problem and had been referred for an audiological evaluation as part of the diagnostic workup. She appeared depressed and anxious, but hopeful that some medical remedy for her problem would be found. The case history interview and results of the Hearing Performance Inventory (Lamb, Owens, & Schubert, 1983) revealed:

1. Communication difficulties in almost all situations.
2. A feeling of worthlessness because she could no longer work.
3. Extreme sensitivity to what she perceived as callousness by anyone with whom she could not communicate.
4. Resentment toward her husband because she felt he was unsympathetic toward her problems.
5. Fear that another attack of dizziness and further deterioration of hearing could occur at any time.

She was eager to try any type of amplification that might improve her communication.

At the conclusion of the audiological evaluation, her hearing loss was briefly explained. Detail was avoided, because the audiologist judged that she could not absorb a lengthy explanation of her hearing status then. It was agreed that she would experiment with different types of amplification and start a speechreading-counseling program concurrent with the otolaryngologist's attempts to treat the situation medically. As she was not receptive to enrollment in a group, individual therapy was arranged on a twice-weekly schedule. It was suggested that she ask her husband to attend sessions with her, but she felt that would not be appropriate.

Each therapy session consisted of speechreading training, educational counseling, and discussion of her problems. Specific problem situations were defined to find strategies that might facilitate communication. Various modifications of her binaural hearing aids were tried during these sessions to find an optimal arrangement for her. A variety of assistive listening devices were also tried. Some

time was spent during each therapy session in hearing aid orientation activities. Goals of therapy were:

1. To improve communication by improving speechreading skills.
2. To teach ways of better handling difficult listening situations.
3. To help her view communication partners, particularly her husband, in a more realistic and less threatening manner.
4. To help her identify warning signs of an impending attack of dizziness, so that she could either leave the situation or take one of the pills her doctor had given her for control. (Her doctors had been able to find a medication that would prevent or minimize attacks.)
5. To find one or more amplification systems that would provide maximal speech intelligibility.
6. To help her seek another source of employment or volunteer work that would restore a sense of self-worth.

During the first semester of therapy, her speechreading skills improved rapidly. That, in combination with strategies designed to help with difficult listening situations, improved her handling of communication sufficiently to allow some increased self-confidence. She also learned to recognize impending symptoms of an attack of dizziness earlier and, thus, became more willing to enter situations where there might be noise.

At the end of the first semester, she felt she was ready to enter group therapy. At first, she was fearful she would not be accepted by the group because her hearing would be far worse than anyone else's. However, it quickly became apparent that others in the group suffered equally great or more severe hearing losses and were managing to cope with them. She found the group a source of support in her attempts to adjust to her own problems and also found that she, in turn, could be of help to other group members. Her ability to assist others enhanced her feelings of worth. Initially she did not ask her husband to participate in the group, but after seeing that other spouses attended, she agreed to invite him. The information that he received from the classes has brought them closer together and has eased tensions at home.

She is still a member of the group. Her speechreading skills continue to improve, along with her ability to handle difficult communication situations. These skills partially compensate for the less than optimal speech understanding provided by her hearing aids. She has purchased a telephone amplifier, a closed-captioned decoder for her television, and an infrared receiver for the theater. She has joined a local self-help group whose purpose is to improve services for people who are hard-of-hearing, and is well on her way to becoming an activist. She has had one attack of dizziness triggered by noise exposure, but with no further deterioration of hearing. Her reaction to this attack was markedly different than previously. She simply attributed it to the fact that she had delayed taking her pill and considered the episode a warning that she must be more vigilant to minimal symptoms in the future. Perhaps most important, she is currently negotiating for a position as an English language tutor to a group of Spanish-speaking adolescents who have hearing impairment.

SUMMARY

The psychological impact of hearing impairment or deafness on adults is real and can be severe. The avenues available to those who serve these persons can be employed in constructive and meaningful ways to restore feelings of self-worth and to assist clients in adjusting to the demands of their world. Only audiologists who are willing to enter into a close working relationship with these adults with hearing impairment should become a part of the process of facilitative counseling.

REFERENCES

Castle, D. L. (1980). *Telephone training for the deaf.* Rochester, NY: National Technical Institute for the Deaf.

Compton, C. L. (1989). Assistive devices. *Seminars in Hearing, 10,* 66–77.

Compton, C. L. (1993). Assistive technology for deaf and hard-of-hearing people. In J. G. Alpiner & P. A. McCarthy (Eds.), *Rehabilitative audiology: Children and adults* (2nd ed., pp. 440–468). Baltimore: Williams & Wilkins.

DiPietro, L., Williams, P., & Kaplan, H. (1984). *Alerting and communication devices for hearing impaired people: What's available now.* Washington, DC: National Information Center on Deafness, Gallaudet University.

Erber, N. P. (1985). *Telephone communication and hearing impairment.* San Diego, CA: College-Hill Press.

Erdmann, S. A. (1993). Counseling hearing-impaired adults. In J. G. Alpiner & P. A. McCarthy. *Rehabilitative audiology: Children and adults* (2nd ed., pp. 374–413). Baltimore: Williams & Wilkins.

Kannapell, B., & Adams, P. (1984). *An orientation to deafness: A handbook and resource guide* (pp. 1–11). Washington, DC: Gallaludet University Press.

Kaplan, H. (1987). Assistive devices. In H. G. Mueller & V. C. Geoffrey (Eds.), *Communication disorders in aging* (pp. 464–493). Washington, DC: Gallaudet University Press.

Kaplan, H., Bally, S. J., & Garretson, C. (1987). *Speechreading, a way to improve understanding* (pp. 18–80). Washington, DC: Gallaudet University Press.

Kodman, F. (1967). Techniques for counseling the hearing aid client. *Maico audiological library series* (Vol. 8, Reports 23–25). Minneapolis, MN: Maico Hearing Instruments.

Lamb, S. H., Owens, E., & Schubert, E. D. (1983). The revised form of the Hearing Performance Inventory. *Ear and Hearing, 4,* 152–159.

Ramsdell, D. A. (1978). The psychology of the hard-of-hearing and the deafened adult. In H. Davis & S. R. Silverman (Eds.), *Hearing and deafness* (pp. 502–523). New York: Holt, Rinehart, and Winston.

Ross, M. (1982). *Hard-of-hearing children in regular schools.* Englewood Cliffs, NJ: Prentice-Hall.

Rupp, R. R., Higgins, J., & Maurer, J. F. (1977). A feasibility scale for predicting hearing aid use (FSPHAU) with older individuals. *Journal of the Academy of Rehabilitative Audiology, l0,* 81–91.

Sanders, D. A. (1988). Hearing aid orientation and counseling. In M.C. Pollack (Ed.), *Amplification for the hearing impaired* (pp. 343–389). New York: Grune and Stratton.

Tye-Murray, N. (l991). Repair strategy usage by hearing-impaired adults and changes following communication therapy. *Journal of Speech and Hearing Research, 34,* 921–928.

Tye-Murray, N. (l993). Aural rehabilitation and patient management. In R. S. Tyler (Ed.), *Cochlear implants: Audiological foundations.* San Diego, CA: Singular Publishing Group.

Tye-Murray, N., Purdy, S. C., & Woodworth, G. G. (l992). Reported use of communication strategies by SHHH members: Client, talker, and situational variables. *Journal of Speech and Hearing Research, 35,* 708–717.

APPENDIX 12A:

HOW TO COPE WITH DIFFICULT LISTENING SITUATIONS

- Ask the speaker to speak in a good light and to face the listener, so that speechreading skills can be used.

- Ask the speaker to speak clearly and naturally, but not to shout or exaggerate articulatory movements.

- If you do not understand what a speaker is saying, ask the speaker to repeat or rephrase the statement.

- If entering a group in the middle of a conversation, ask one person to sum up the gist of the conversation.

- If someone is speaking at a distance, that person should be asked to stand closer.

- If the speaker turns his or her head away, ask him or her to face you to permit optimal speech-reading and listening.

- If you are attempting to understand speech in the presence of noise, try to move yourself and the speaker away from the source of the noise.

- When in a communication situation requiring exact information, such as asking directions or obtaining schedules for a trip, request that the speaker write the crucial information.

- If the speaker is talking while eating, smoking, or chewing, request that he or she not do so, because it makes speechreading difficult.

- A person who has a unilateral loss should be sure to keep the good ear facing the speaker at all times.

- If possible, avoid rooms with poor acoustics. If meetings are held in such rooms, request that they be transferred to rooms with less reverberation.

- If a speaker at a meeting cannot be heard, request that he or she use a microphone.

- Arrive early for meetings, so that you can sit close to the speaker. Avoid taking a seat near a wall to minimize the possibility of reverberation. This is particularly important for those who use hearing aids.

- If you are going to a movie or to the theater, read the reviews in advance to familiarize yourself with the plot.

- In an extremely noisy situation, limit conversation to before the noise has started or after the noise has subsided. Normal hearing people do this all the time. For example, if a plane goes overhead and a conversation is going on, most people will halt their conversations and wait until the plane has passed.

APPENDIX 12B:

HELPING THE STUDENT WHO IS DEAF OR HARD-OF-HEARING

- Preferential seating is important for anyone with a hearing problem. The adult who is deaf or hard-of-hearing will usually know which place in a classroom is best. However, as the focus of attention may change during a lecture, the student should be assured that any change of seat will not be considered disruptive.

- The teacher should be careful to speak only when a student who is deaf or hard-of-hearing can see his or her lips. The following situations should be avoided if possible:
  — Talking with one's back to the class, as when writing on the chalkboard.
  — Standing in front of a window or a bright light. The light should be shining on the speaker's face, not in the student's eyes.
  — Teaching from the back of the room, where the student cannot see.
  — Walking around the classroom while talking.

- The teacher should:
  — Speak in a careful yet natural manner. Avoid exaggerated lip movements.
  — Restate or rephrase statements when the student fails to understand.
  — Not cover the face with a hand or a book while reading.
  — Not stand too close to a student who must lipread. He or she might have to tilt the head back to see the speaker's face, causing unnecessary strain and fatigue.
- Students who are deaf or hard-of-hearing rely heavily on written material to obtain information. It is helpful to inform them in advance what material will be covered on a particular day, so that pertinent material can be read in advance.

- It is not possible for a student who is deaf or hard-of-hearing to use visual cues in class and take notes simultaneously. The teacher can either prepare special lecture notes or request that a fellow student share notes with a student who is deaf or hard-of-hearing.

- The teacher should use the chalkboard or the overhead projector as much as possible. If the written material must be copied by the student, lecturing should not occur at the same time.

- Oral tests should never be given to a student who is deaf or hard-of-hearing.

- The teacher should be available for extra tutoring. A student who is deaf or hard-of-hearing should be encouraged to meet with the teacher after class for explanation of material not understood.

END OF CHAPTER EXAMINATION QUESTIONS

CHAPTER 12

1. Compare and contrast the terms "nonculturally deaf" and "culturally deaf."

2. According to the author, in contrast with persons who possess normal hearing, adults who have hearing impairment generally have feelings of inadequacy and assume that the "fault" for communication breakdowns is always _____ .

3. Name and describe the three psychological levels of hearing presented in this chapter.
   a.
   b.
   c.

4. According to the author, _____ is one of the most important goals of personal adjustment counseling for those with hearing impairment.

5. When persons feel a loss of self-esteem because of an inability to hear normally, they:
   a. are usually open about their disability and discuss their problems without hesitation.
   b. have a tendency to conceal their hearing loss from others.
   c. seek professional help to work through their problems without referral.

6. The term "educational, or informational, counseling" refers to:
   a. the provision of information about hearing loss.
   b. the effect of a hearing loss on communication.
   c. discussions of intervention procedures.
   d. all of the above.

END OF CHAPTER ANSWER SHEET

Name _____ Date _____

CHAPTER 12

1. Culturally deaf _____

   _____

   _____

   _____ .

   Nonculturally deaf _____

   _____

   _____

   _____ .

2. _____

   _____ .

3. a.

   b.

   c.

4. _____

   _____ .

5. Which one(s)?   a   b   c

6. Which one(s)?   a   b   c   d

7. Which one(s)?   a   b   c

8. Which one(s)?   a   b   c   d

9. Which one(s)?   a   b   c

7. List three coping strategies that can assist hearing-impaired adults, as described by the author.
   a.
   b.
   c.

8. What steps should teachers take to assist students who have sufficient hearing loss to be able to function with greater efficiency in the classroom. *List four.*
   a.
   b.
   c.
   d.

9. According to the author of this chapter, the home of a deaf or hearing-impaired person is:
   a. Their "safe place" where they stay a majority of the time.
   b. A quiet place for them to return to after being out in the "real world."

   c. A place for interpersonal communication and consequently more opportunity for communication breakdowns.

Hearing Aid Orientation for Adults Who Are Hearing Impaired

■ RAYMOND H. HULL, Ph.D. ■
and
■ ROBERT M. McLAUCHLIN, Ph.D. ■

CONSIDERATIONS FOR THE ORIENTATION TO HEARING AIDS FOR ADULTS WHO ARE HEARING IMPAIRED

HEARING AID ORIENTATION IN RETROSPECT

INDIVIDUALIZED PLANNING IN THE PROCESS OF HEARING AID ORIENTATION
    Involvement of Family and Friends
    User Evaluation Scales and Single-Subject Tracking

ESSENTIAL HEARING AID ORIENTATION SERVICES
    Understanding the Component Parts and Controls of
        Hearing Aids

(continued)

One of the very important areas of expertise of audiologists is the fitting and dispensing of hearing aids and non-hearing aid assistive listening devices. This has become such an integral component of the scope of practice of audiologists that "audiology" and "dispensing of prosthetic listening devices" go hand-in-hand both in the preparation of future professionals in audiology, and in the practice of audiology. Other than the accurate fitting of the most appropriate hearing aid(s) for individual clients, probably the other single most important element in the successful fitting and dispensing of hearing aids and other assistive listening devices is a good program of hearing aid orientation and hearing aid counseling. This chapter provides an historical and practical look at considerations in the orientation to and uses of hearing aids by adults who have hearing impairment.

CONSIDERATIONS FOR THE ORIENTATION TO HEARING AIDS FOR ADULTS WHO ARE HEARING IMPAIRED

No matter what type of hearing aid has been fit for adult clients, audiologists usually express the need for hearing aid orientation (HAO) services, and many claim they are offering them. Problems, however, have occurred in effective and efficient provision of those services. The American Speech-Language-Hearing Association's (ASHA's) early "Guidelines on the Responsibilities of Audiologists in the Rehabilitation of the Auditorily Handicapped" (Freeland et al. 1974) emphasized that hearing aid users and their families should be provided with information about the use of amplification. These guidelines also mentioned the need for periodic reassessment of an amplification device and a client's adjustment to it. These admonishments by ASHA and the American Academy of Audiology have continued and are assumed to be critical in the fitting and dispensing of hearing aids.

It is assumed that most hearing aid users need hearing aid orientation or, at least, more comprehensive and realistic orientation services than some apparently receive. In a review of 377 Army clients, Scherr, Schwartz, and Montgomery (1983) found 32.6% of them required some follow-up orientation in the use of their hearing aid(s). These clients were experiencing minor problems, such as feedback and earmold discomfort, and most needed at least some counseling on using amplification.

According to Eggen (1988), the major complaints of hearing aid users reported by 60 Michigan audiologists and hearing aid dealers were:

1. Background noise;
2. Sound quality of client's voice;
3. Insertion of the hearing aid;
4. Feeling of a fullness in the ear;
5. Sounds too loud;
6. Adjusting the volume control; and
7. Comfort of the hearing aid.

All of these complaints can be addressed through ongoing hearing aid orientation. Madell, Pfeffer, Ross, and Chellappa (1991) surveyed 92 clients who had returned dispensed hearing aids at the New York League for the Hard of Hearing. The most frequent reasons for returning hearing aids were (a) less benefit than expected, (b) discomfort, and (c) problems hearing in noise. Thus, the audiology profession and clinical services surveys substantiate the essential need for effective hearing aid orientation before and after hearing aid fitting.

HEARING AID ORIENTATION IN RETROSPECT

Hearing aid orientation has been an extensive and integral part of aural rehabilitation, even at the inception of the audiology profession. Carhart (1946) described the hearing aid selection procedures used with military personnel during World War II that included activities designed to familiarize adults with hearing aid use. These activities were all carried out prior to the final selection of an individual's hearing aid. The major emphasis on HAO in that hearing aid selection program is apparent when reviewing the military's three goals to (a) obtain a hearing aid with optimal efficiency in everyday situations for each client; (b) provide each client with an understanding of hearing aids, establish habits of efficient use, and initiate auric-

ular training; and (c) help the person foster a full psychological acceptance of hearing aids (Carhart, 1946).

Preliminary to the actual hearing aid selection in Carhart's protocol, orientation activities included an explanation about the person's hearing impairment and handicapping conditions, what to expect and what not to expect from wearing a hearing aid, any special problems that might occur, and group instructions about hearing aid selection procedures.

As a part of the Carhart (1946) protocol, in an effort to select hearing aids from the total available stock of about 200 instruments. For manageable assessment with each individual, the hearing aid selection began with an informal trial of instruments during an interview. Audiometric and case history information also was used in narrowing the selection to 7–10 hearing aids. Certainly, this trial also served as an orientation to hearing aids.

The second stage of the Carhart (1946) process involved a 24-hour trial of each preselected aid with a listening hour following every trial. Frequently, 25 to 30 persons participated in a single listening hour. Individuals rated 13 different kinds of controlled sounds on a 5-point rating scale for each of the preselected hearing aids. The sounds included six musical, three speech, and five environmental selections. A similar rating was done for each person's ability to localize sound, listen on the telephone, and experience a 24-hour trial. Finally, a sound discrimination test was administered. Prospective hearing aid users were allowed to adjust their aids for comfort during all of these listening experiences. These ratings, with a weighted score for the discrimination test, were combined and used in eliminating all but three aids for potential selection. The final selection was made from the three remaining hearing aids, based on controlled comparisons of these instruments for speech reception threshold, speech discrimination, tolerance, comfort level, and signal-to-noise ratio tests.

Granted, comprehensive HAO activities in the Carhart process were possible with these prospective hearing aid users because they were a captive audience, as their full-time assignment was to be rehabilitated for return to civilian life or active duty. Moreover, the cost of such a program in its entirety for full-time employed civilians might be prohibitive. Despite these limitations for the general adult population, many aspects of this early HAO program have been adapted for use in familiarizing prospective adult hearing aid users to wearable amplification (Hardick, 1977; Hawkins, 1985).

This lengthy review of the early Carhart hearing aid selection procedures is a tribute to one of the founders of the audiology profession. It is worthy to note that from the inception of this profession, hearing aid orientation was an integral part of audiological services, *and these early orientation procedures were as comprehensive (and lengthy) as they were novel.*

INDIVIDUALIZED PLANNING IN THE PROCESS OF HEARING AID ORIENTATION

As is the case with all rehabilitative procedures, hearing aid orientation cannot be packaged for uniform use with all persons who are hearing handicapped. As early as 1967, Panel IV participants at an ASHA conference on hearing aid evaluation procedures (Castle, 1967) recognized that a single HAO program is not adaptable for all persons. The range and extent of HAO services should vary depending on individual factors, including:

1. Age of onset and progression of hearing impairment,
2. Severity of impairment,
3. Present age,
4. Experience with and understanding of hearing aids,
5. Attitude of hearing aid wearer about the use of amplification,
6. Attitudes of family members and associates concerning the hearing aid wearer and hearing aid use,
8. Personal interests,
9. Intelligence and language abilities,
10. Complexity of the hearing aid system being used,
11. Intended use of the hearing aid,
12. Amount and success of previously received rehabilitation; and
13. Presence of concomitant impairments, such as blindness, mental retardation, psychiatric disorders, or arthritis in the hands.

An excellent model of individualized planning for persons who have disability is in the federal regulation to educate all handicapped children (U.S. Office of Education, 1977). Although the model is titled Individualized Education Program (IEP) and is intended specifically for children, the major aspects of this model are applicable for planning HAO and other rehabilitative services for adults, according to individual needs. An IEP includes a written statement indicating what services are needed and appropriate: (a) present levels of performance, (b) long-range goals and short-term objectives, (c) projected dates for initiation and duration of services, (d) services to be provided, (e) appropriate objective criteria and assessment procedures, and (f) timelines for determining whether short-term objectives are being achieved.

Individualized planning is not a new concept for professionals in communication sciences and disorders. In fact, what is required in an individualized rehabilitation program is no more extensive than what has long been considered professionally appropriate practice in audiology and speech-language pathology.

INVOLVEMENT OF FAMILY AND FRIENDS

Why is it important to involve family members and friends of hearing aid users in HAO programs? There are several reasons, but perhaps the most important is because communication is social interaction between persons who interchangeably speak and listen. As the sophistication of the persons who interact with a hearing aid user increases relative to hearing impairment and amplification, substantial improvements in communication can be anticipated. For example, a wife may require orientation because she has had to raise the level of her voice for the previous 10 years when speaking to her husband to accommodate his unaided moderate bilateral hearing loss. Without some advice and possibly direct orientation, the wife may continue to speak to her husband in her habitually loud voice and will be perceived by him as speaking too loudly when he wears his hearing aid. This situation could contribute to a deterioration in their social interaction and satisfactory hearing aid use. An inappropriate solution is for the husband to turn the gain of the hearing aid down when listening to his wife. Resolving the situation in this way might lead to frequent adjustments of the gain control between conversing with his wife and others. It also could perpetuate any irritation the family members and friends might have been experiencing in listening to the wife's loud voice. Therefore, both the husband and wife must be advised and, preferably, shown during orientation sessions how to share in the responsibility of helping each other adjust to hearing aid use and achieving improved social interaction.

As another example, satisfactory adjustment to hearing aid use can be jeopardized by family members and friends who have unrealistic expectations about wearable amplification. This problem can happen even when the hearing aid user clearly understands the limitations of amplification for his or her type of hearing impairment and attempts to explain those limitations to family members and friends. These limitations often have to be explained and demonstrated to family members and friends before they can understand. More importantly, people who communicate frequently with the hearing aid user should understand how they can help to compensate for residual communicative problems that continue, even with the use of amplification.

Family members need to understand the dynamics for improving or hindering the perception of a spoken message by a hearing aid user. To illustrate, assume that a wife has a moderate bilateral loss in hearing sensitivity and a moderate-to-severe impairment in speech discrimination ability and is wearing hearing aids in both ears. The husband can appreciably improve her ability to perceive a spoken message correctly by (a) initially gaining her visual as well as auditory attention, (b) moving closer to her, (c) initially identifying the topic of conversation, (d) reducing the background noise or improving the speech-to-noise ratio, (e) increasing the environmental light or moving away from a window when the sun is at his back, and (f) removing the pipe from his mouth when he talks.

There are other reasons for participation of family members and close associates in HAO programs. There will be less confusion about information provided in HAO sessions with additional listeners who have normal hearing and, thus, have less chance of incorrectly perceiving spoken information. Moreover, participation in planning and understanding orientation activities outside of a clinical setting helps in successfully accomplishing these activities.

The ultimate HAO occurs in the daily communication activities of the hearing aid user. Therefore, a successful rehabilitation program involves orientation directly or indirectly for all significant participants in the user's communication activities. Eggen (1988) found 94% of a sample of 60 Michigan audiologists and hearing aid dealers routinely include family members and significant others. It is hoped that this sample is reflective of all specialists providing HAOs.

USER EVALUATION SCALES AND SINGLE-SUBJECT TRACKING

Routine employment of user evaluation scales and tracking procedures is strongly recommended in assessing HAO success. If designed appropriately, a rating scale may serve as a daily or weekly schedule for the hearing aid user to complete during the first few weeks or months of hearing aid use. For example, the user can be asked to take 5 minutes each day to check the appropriate responses to several questions and record any comments or questions. Such a scale is useful in determining the appropriateness of the hearing aid selection and success of HAO. Moreover, the scaled data and comments provide information that is helpful in modifying future HAO programs and hearing aid selection procedures to better serve adults who have hearing impairment.

Rating scales developed for assessing communication handicap (Alpiner, 1987; Cox, Gilmore, & Alexander, 1991; Cox & Rivera, 1992; Demorest & Erdman, 1987; Harless & McConnell, 1982; Lamb, Owens, & Schubert, 1983; Sanders, 1993) are useful in determining difficult listening situations for prospective or current hearing aid users and in determining users' and their associates' attitudes toward their hearing impairments. Gauger (1978) developed a series of rating scales and other materials for orienting deaf college students to hearing aid use. The Gauger materials can be adapted easily for use with other adult hearing aid users. Walden, Demorest, and Hepler (1984) also developed a hearing aid performance inventory—making it more directly applicable to hearing aid orientation.

Smaldino and Smaldino (1988) combined the use of a hearing handicap scale and a cognitive learning style instrument to investigate the effects of HAO and cognitive style on the perception of hearing handicap by first-time hearing aid users.

Newman, Jacobson, Hug, Weinstein, and Malinoff (1991) found the short form of the Hearing Handicapped Inventory for the Elderly to be an expedient tool for quantifying hearing aid benefit. According to Hawkins (1985), it will be difficult to validate hearing aid selection and assessment procedures without employing user evaluation scales. Unfortunately, in 1989, only 12% of a sample of 465 responding audiologists used a hearing handicap measure (Martin & Morris, 1989). One trusts more are using these tools today.

Single-subject research designs can be adapted easily for use in tracking treatment effects (McReynolds & Thompson, 1986), specifically for adults who have hearing impairment (Lesner, Lynn, & Brainard, 1988). Many of the attitudes, experiences, knowledge, and performances associated with hearing aids described in subsequent sections of this chapter could be evaluated more objectively with user evaluation scales and single-subject designs (Chmiel & Jerger, 1993).

ESSENTIAL HEARING AID ORIENTATION SERVICES

Some HOA services are essential to all hearing aid orientation programs. The user should receive:

1. Understanding of the function of the component parts and adjustments of hearing aids;
2. Practice in fitting, adjusting, and maintaining amplification;
3. Understanding of the limitations of amplification;
4. Knowledge of why the particular aid was selected;
5. How to begin using a newly selected hearing aid;
6. How to troubleshoot hearing aid problems; and
7. How to exercise a hearing aid user's legal rights.

HAO need not be restricted to a limited time frame following the selection and fitting of hearing aids. Orientation may continue for several weeks or many months until a person achieves his or her fullest understanding of hearing aid use and maximum potential performance in operating and communicating through amplifying devices. Certain aspects of HAO, such as explaining the component parts and adjustments of hearing aids and the anticipated limitations and benefits to be derived from amplification, might be presented before performing a hearing aid selection. Miller and Schein (1987) subscribe to providing HAO before fitting hearing aids. Thus, this chapter's author suggests that HAO not be limited to any specific rehabilitative services or time frame. Moreover, some aspects of HAO can be presented efficiently in a group and the sharing of common experiences results in valuable rehabilitation.

UNDERSTANDING THE COMPONENT PARTS AND CONTROLS OF HEARING AIDS

It is disheartening to evaluate an intelligent adult who purchased a hearing aid a year earlier, but is unable to tell the audiologist the location of the hearing aid microphone or the purpose of the component. Adult hearing aid users should be able to name, locate, and describe the functions of the major hearing aid components, including the microphone, amplifier, battery, receiver, tubing (if it is a behind-the-ear [BTE]), ear hook, or "goose neck" (if it is a BTE hearing aid), and earmold (if it is not an in-the-canal [ITC] hearing aid). Similarly, hearing aid users should be able to locate and explain the function of the controls on their hearing aids, such as the gain-control and on-off, tone, and telephone switches.

An effective HAO must go beyond providing information, however. It must assess user understanding and performance to see if goals in these areas are accomplished. This author suggests employing a user performance checklist or rating scale to record whether users can satisfactorily can name, locate, and describe the functions of the component parts and controls of their hearing aids. (Byrne, 1992).

Objectives, as always, will have to be tailored to individual needs and capabilities. For example, this author has explained the ANSI standards for evaluating the electroacoustic characteristics of hearing aids in substantial detail to an engineer for whom a hearing aid was selected.

Videotapes can be prepared by service facilities or purchased commercially (Orton, 1989) to illustrate the component parts of hearing aids and how to fit, adjust, and maintain different models of hearing aids. These tapes can be shown to individuals or used efficiently with groups of individuals who have hearing impairment and their family members and friends. They also can be shown in a room for family members and friends while the client is being seen for services. Only 5% of a sample of 60 Michigan audiologists and hearing aid dealers were using videotapes for HAO (Eggen, 1988). With current technology, a computerized interactive video program could be developed to assess knowledge and performance related to hearing aids.

Given the current hearing aid sales statistics, most of these video programs need to emphasize in-the-ear (ITE), but not exclude BTE aids. In 1999, approximately 80% of fittings were ITE aids, and 20% were BTE aids.

PRACTICE IN FITTING, ADJUSTING, AND MAINTAINING AMPLIFICATION

A hearing aid user, particularly a new user, needs more than a description and demonstration of how to fit, operate, and maintain a newly selected hearing aid. To determine if orientation has been successful, an assessment of a user's ability to perform these tasks is essential. Preferably, this assessment should be done when the aid is fitted and repeated at a follow-up appointment within a month. A simple user-performance checklist or rating scale can be used to record a user's ability to perform the many fitting, adjustment, and maintenance functions associated with the user's hearing aid. For example, audiologists should rate a hearing aid user's ability to connect and disconnect tubing and earmolds to a BTE hearing aid, insert and remove the earmold or ITE hearing aid from the ear, operate the hearing aid controls, and change a battery.

Some clients will need to learn how to program their digital hearing aids. This performance-based assessment should be used for all hearing aid users. Do not assume a person is adequately oriented to hearing aid use just because he or she has previously worn a hearing aid.

The hearing aid user should be given a list of maintenance suggestions and be provided an opportunity to demonstrate basic maintenance skills. The following suggestions are some examples of what might be included on a maintenance list:

1. Protect hearing aids against exposure to excessive heat from sources such as hair dryers, radiators, heaters, and closed cars on a hot sunny day;
2. Avoid exposing hearing aids to excessive humidity of rain, saunas, steam baths, or when aids have been placed in a pants pocket and sent to the laundry;
3. Place hearing aids in a container with silica gel at night to remove any moisture, particularly for persons who perspire heavily;
4. Prevent hair sprays, insecticides, and other sprays from being directed at the aids;
5. Clean earmolds and tubing periodically with mild soap and water or commercially available cleaning solutions;
6. Keep hearing aids away from dogs and small children when not wearing them; and
7. Remove hearing aids from the ear and handle them over a soft surface, so, if dropped, potential damage is reduced.

LIMITATIONS OF AMPLIFICATION

Prospective hearing aid users, as well as their family members and friends, frequently have unrealistic expectations about the benefits of wearable amplification. (Kricos Lesner, & Sandridge, 1991). These expectations range from total lack of benefit to the expectation of "normal" hearing. These perceptions must be explored, if audiologists hope to successfully acquaint hearing aid users and the persons with whom they communicate with amplification. A very positive, although straightforward, approach may be required with an acquaintance or family member who is extremely skeptical about the benefits of amplification. Conversely, a guarded and realistic approach may be needed for an individual who expects a hearing aid to resolve all hearing problems, especially if speech discrimination ability is significantly reduced. Two other potential limitations include restricted dynamic range and tolerance problems, and monaural fitting when binaural hearing aids were appropriate (Hurley, 1993).

WHY WAS A PARTICULAR HEARING AID SELECTED?

Hearing aid users, if capable of understanding, should be told why:

1. A particular type of hearing aid, such as an in-the-ear instrument, was selected,
2. The aid is a particular make,
3. A monaural aid for the right or left ear or binaural instruments were chosen,
4. The particular external controls were chosen and how they should be set,
5. The type of earmold was selected, and
6. Special features were selected.

The inability of a new hearing aid user to tell a close friend why she or he is using the aid in the right ear can result in feelings of insecurity and inadequacy. Conversely, telling the friend why he or she has insufficient hearing or why the clarity of speech is so poor in the left ear as to warrant amplification may impair the user's understanding of the impairment and a feeling of adequacy. Moreover, if the hearing aid user enlists the friend's help by asking him or her to walk or sit on the user's right side, this demonstrates the user's willingness to discuss and cope with the handicapping condition with friends. A thorough knowledge about one's impairment and hearing aid, combined with an open approach to using the hearing aid, can contribute appreciably to successful hearing aid use.

USING NEWLY SELECTED HEARING AIDS

The length of time necessary for satisfactory adjustment to newly selected hearing aids will vary substantially from person to person, depending on the amount and type of impairment; whether amplification has been used previously; the extent of concomitant handicapping conditions such as mental impairment, spasticity, or visual impairment; the age of onset and progression of hearing impairment; and the person's daily activities. An intelligent, long-time, successful hearing aid user who has just procured a replacement instrument might immediately begin wearing the new hearing aid during all of his or her waking hours without needing any formalized HAO beyond an explanation of any new or different hearing aid controls. Conversely, a developmentally disabled adult who has a long-standing hearing impairment and has never tried amplification may require many months of HAO. Typically, a satisfactory HAO can be com-pleted for most adults who have hearing impairment within 2 to 6 weeks and include all essential services for successful hearing aid use.

New hearing aid users generally are encouraged to begin employing their aids in easy listening situations and progress to more difficult listening experiences. An easy listening situation would involve listening:

1. To a single known speaker,
2. In a quiet environment,
3. To a familiar topic,
4. While watching the speaker,
5. With good lighting on the speaker's face, and
6. With minimal visual or auditory distractions.

After new users adjust to easy listening situations, the conditions may be varied to increase the difficulty of listening situations. HAO is not complete until clients have adjusted to using their new hearing aids in a variety of daily listening activities, particularly in those situations where they want and need to communicate for social, vocational, or educational purposes.

HOW TO TROUBLESHOOT HEARING AID PROBLEMS

If hearing aid users sufficiently understand the functions of the component parts and controls of hearing aids, they intuitively may be able to solve many of their own hearing aid problems. However, troubleshooting ability should not be left to chance. Quite the contrary—hearing aid users should be told about possible problems that can occur, how to locate the problems, and how to seek a resolution. A set of used hearing aids with a variety of problems is very helpful in demonstrating troubleshooting techniques. Moreover, a chart listing problems, possible causes, and remedies should be provided to hearing aid users. The clinician can ask users to study their charts and be prepared to answer questions about malfunctioning aids. At a later appointment clients should be able to demonstrate their understanding of the material by locating problems and remedying them with a stock of used aids. Hearing aid users should be encouraged to keep the troubleshooting chart with important papers for immediate reference, if hearing aid problems arise. The chart might cover these problems:

1. Squealing (whistling);
2. No amplification;

3. Reduced amplification;
4. Intermittent amplification or scratchy, frying, crashing sound;
5. Sharp sound (as though through a barrel);
6. "Tinny," or "thin," sound;
7. Sound too noisy;
8. Reduced clarity of speech;
9. Ear canal hurts; or
10. Problem not describable, but change noticed.

Additionally, the chart should list possible causes, how to locate the problems, and the remedies. It would be helpful for clients to know that common problems with BTE hearing aids involve receivers, microphones, and wires; whereas with ITE and canal-type instruments, breakdowns involve wax-clogged receivers and volume controls (Mahon, 1989a). The chart should indicate clearly which causes can be remedied by the user and which ones should be fixed by a hearing aid dispenser. The hearing aid user should be encouraged to call the specialist who selected the hearing instrument, if problems arise that the user is unable to resolve. The specialist's address and phone number should be printed prominently on the chart.

These charts are available commercially through a variety of sources. Hearing aid manufacturers frequently include these charts in the "User Instructional Brochure" that is required to accompany hearing aids by the U.S. Food and Drug Administration (FDA) (1994). Other HAO booklets and pamphlets are available from a variety of sources (Armbruster & Miller, 1986; Gauger, 1978; Gendel, 1984; Krames Communications, 1987; Madell, 1986; Self Help for Hard of Hearing People, 1986, 1987; and Williams & Jacobs-Condit, 1985).

CONSUMER RIGHTS OF HEARING AID USERS

Individuals should be informed of their legal rights and options as owners or users of wearable amplification. The cost of aids and most expenses associated with hearing impairment, for example, are allowed as medical expenses in computing federal income tax. Many prospective purchasers of hearing aids may qualify for public or private funds to cover the cost, such as funds available through Medicaid, Rehabilitation Services Administration, Veterans Administration, or employee health benefits. They should also be informed of their legal rights and restrictions under the Labeling and Conditions for Sale Regulation promulgated by the FDA. Certain information must be provided to prospective hearing aid users in the form of a User Instructional Brochure, as mandated by the FDA. Although many hearing aid manufacturers provided brochures with their instruments prior to this regulation, the extent and uniformity of information varied substantially. This was particularly true concerning electroacoustic characteristics of hearing aids.

Since August 15, 1977, the effective date of the FDA regulation, all hearing aids are to be accompanied by a User Instructional Brochure containing the categories of information:

1. Illustration of the hearing aid showing controls, adjustments, and battery compartment;
2. Printed material on the operation of all controls designed for user adjustment;
3. Description of possible accompanying accessories;
4. Instructions on how to use, maintain, and care for as well as replace or recharge batteries;
5. How to and where to procure repair services;
6. Conditions to be avoided in preventing damage to hearing aids, such as dropping or exposing to excessive heat or humidity;
7. Warning to seek medical advice when encountering any side effects such as skin irritation or increased accumulation of cerumen;
8. Statement that a hearing aid will not restore normal hearing or prevent or improve a hearing impairment caused by organic conditions;

9. Statement that with most persons, infrequent use of wearable amplification will not allow them to attain full benefit from hearing aid use;

10. Statement that hearing aid use is only one aspect of hearing rehabilitation and may need to be augmented by auditory training and lip-reading instruction;

11. Warning statement to hearing aid dispensers to advise prospective hearing aid users to see a licensed physician before dispensing hearing aids if any of eight medical conditions exist (see any User Instructional Brochure for these conditions);

12. Notice to prospective hearing aid users indicating, among other things, that hearing aids cannot be sold to individuals until they have obtained a medical evaluation from a licensed physician (preferably one who specializes in diseases of the ear); however a fully informed adult may waive the medical evaluation.

13. Electroacoustical data obtained in accordance with the Acoustical Society of America (1987) *Standard for Specification of Hearing Aid Characteristics* (this information may be included on separate labeling that accompanies the hearing aid).

Other information may be included in the User Instructional Brochure if it is not false, misleading, or prohibited by this regulation or by Federal Trade Commission (FTC) regulations. Audiologists, hearing aid sales personnel, and physicians specializing in diseases of the ear should have a reference copy of this important FDA regulation.

In addition to the seven services discussed in this chapter, an individualized rehabilitation plan for a client might require counseling, auditory training, situational training, speechreading, motivational training, and speech production training. Although some or all of these additional five rehabilitative services might be required, they are not essential for all clients. Moreover, these latter ser-vices are discussed in more detail in other chapters of this textbook.

SUMMARY

Because of the limited survey and research data on adult HAO services, these authors challenge all specialists working with the hearing impaired to make significant clinical and research contributions to improving HAOs. The prospects for improvement are great given the current rapid rate of informational and technological change. Only a commitment to positive change is needed to fulfill this challenge.

REFERENCES

Acoustical Society of America. (1987). *Standard for specification of hearing aid characteristics.* ANSI 3.22. New York.

Alpiner, J. (1987). Evaluation of adult communication function. In J. Alpiner & P. McCarthy (Eds.), *Rehabilitative audiology: Children and adults* (pp. 44–114). Baltimore: Williams & Wilkins.

American Speech-Language-Hearing Association (1984b). Position statement: Definition of competencies for aural rehabilitation. *Asha, 26,* 37–41.

American Speech-Language-Hearing Association (1990). Scope of practice, speech-language pathology and audiology. *Asha* (Suppl., April), 1–2.

Armbruster, J., & Miller, M. (1986). *How to get the most out of your hearing aid.* Washington, DC: Alexander Graham Bell Association for the Deaf.

Carhart, R. (1946). Selection of hearing aids. *Archives of Otolaryngology, 44,* 1–18.

Castle, W. E. (Ed.). (1967). A conference on hearing aid evaluation procedures. *ASHA Reports 2,* 21–38.

Chmiel, R., & Jerger, J. (1993). Some factors affecting assessment of hearing handicap in the elderly. *Journal of the American Academy of Audiology, 4,* 249–257.

Cox, R. M., Gilmore, C., & Alexander, G. C. (1991). Comparison of two questionnaires for patient-assessed hearing aid benefit. *Journal of the American Academy of Audiology, 2,* 134–145.

Cox, R. M., & Rivera, I. M. (1992). Predictability and reliability of hearing aid benefit measured using the PHAB. *Journal of the American Academy of Audiology, 3*, 242–254.

Demorest, M., & Erdman, S. (1987). Development of the communication profile for the hearing impaired. *Journal of Speech and Hearing Disorders, 52*, 129–143.

Eggen, R. E. (1988). *A survey of hearing aid orientation process in the state of Michigan.* Unpublished master's independent study, Central Michigan University, Mt. Pleasant.

FDA Holds Hearings On Hearing Aid Performance Claims. (1994). *Audiology Today*, Sept./Oct., 26.

Freeland, E. E., Hill, M.J., Jeffers, J., Matkin, N.D., Stream, R. W., Tobin, H., & Costello, M.R. (1974). The audiologist: Responsibilities in the habilitation of the auditorily handicapped. *Journal of the American Speech and Hearing Association, 16*, 68–70.

Gatehouse, S. (1993). Role of perceptual acclimatization in the selection of frequency response for hearing aids. *Journal of the American Academy of Audiology, 4*, 296–306.

Gauger, J. S. (1978). *Orientation to hearing aids.* Rochester, NY: National Technical Institute for the Deaf.

Gendel, J. (1984). *Questions most often asked about earmolds.* New York: New York League for the Hard of Hearing.

Hardick, E. J. (1977). Aural rehabilitation programs for the aged can be successful. *Journal of the Academy of Rehabilitative Audiology, 10*, 51–67.

Harless, E. L., & McConnell, F. (1982). Effects of hearing aid use on self concept in older persons. *Journal of Speech and Hearing Disorders, 47*, 305–309.

Hawkins, D. B. (1985). Reflections on amplification: Validation of performance. *Journal of the Academy of Rehabilitative Audiology, 18*, 42–54.

Hurley, R. M. (1993). Monaural hearing aid effect: Case presentations. *Journal of the American Academy of Audiology. 4*, 285–294.

Krames Communications (1987). *Hearing aids: A guide to their wear and care:* Daly City, CA: Author.

Kricos, P. B., Lesner, S. A., & Sandridge, S. A. (1991). Expectations of older adults regarding the use of hearing aids. *Journal of the American Academy of Audiology, 2*, 129–133.

Lamb, S., Owens, E., & Schubert, E. (1983). The revised form of the Hearing Performance Inventory. *Ear and Hearing, 4*, 152–157.

Lesner, S. A., Lynn, J. M., & Brainard, J. (1988). Feasibility of using a single-subject design for continuous discourse tracking measurement. *Journal of the Academy of Rehabilitative Audiology, 21*, 83–89.

Madell, J. (1986). *You and your hearing aid.* New York: New York League for the Hard of Hearing.

Madell, J., Pfeffer, E., Ross, M., & Chellappa, M. (1991). Hearing aid returns at a community hearing and speech agency. *The Hearing Journal, 44*, 18–23.

Mahon, W. J. (1989a). A close look at hearing aid repair. *The Hearing Aid Journal 42*, 9–12.

Mahon, W. J. (1989b). 1989 U.S. hearing aid sale summary. *The Hearing Aid Journal, 42*, 9–14.

Martin, F. N., & Morris, L. J. (1989). Current audiologic practices in the United States. *The Hearing Aid Journal, 42*, 25–44.

McReynolds, L.V., & Thompson, C.K. (1986). Flexibility of single-subject experimental designs. Part I: Review of the basics of single-subject designs. *Journal of Speech and Hearing Disorders, 51*, 194–203.

Miller, M. H., & Schein, J. D. (1987). Improving consumer acceptance of hearing aids. *The Hearing Journal, 40*, 25-30.

Newman, C. W., Jacobson, G. P., Hug, G. A., Weinstein, B. E., & Malinoff, R. L. (1991). Practical method for quantifying hearing aid benefit in older adults. *Journal of the American Academy of Audiology, 2*, 70–75.

Orton, C. (1989). *Help with your hearing aids.* (Videotape). Stinson Beach, CA: Orton-Palmer & Associates.

Palmer, C. V. (1992). Assistive devices in the audiology practice. *American Journal of Audiology, 1*, 37–57.

Sanders, D. A. (1993). Profile questionnaire for rating communicative performance in a home environment, occupational environment, social environment. In M. Pollack (Ed.), *Amplification for the hearing impaired* (pp. 385–395). Orlando, FL: Grune & Stratton.

Scherr, C. K., Schwartz, D. M., & Montgomery, A. A. (1983). Follow-up survey of new hearing aid users. *Journal of Academy of Rehabilitative Audiology, 1*, 202–209.

Schow, R. L., Balsara, N. R., Smedley, T. C., & Whitcomb, C. J. (1993). Aural rehabilitation by ASHA audiologists: 1980–1990. *American Journal of Audiology, 2*, 28–37.

Self-Help for Hard of Hearing People. (1986). *I think I have a problem. What do I do?* Bethesda, MD: Author.

Self-Help for Hard of Hearing People. (1987). *ABCs of hearing aids.* Bethesda, MD: Author.

Sinclair, J. S., & Goldstein, J. L. (1991). Long-term benefit, satisfaction, and use of amplification among military retirees. *Journal of the Academy of Rehabilitative Audiology, 24*, 55–64.

Smaldino, S. E., & Smaldino, J. J. (1988). The influence of aural rehabilitation and cognitive style disclosure on the perception of hearing handicap. *Journal of the Academy of Rehabilitative Audiology, 21,* 57–64.

Tyler, R. S. (1994). The use of speech-perception tests in audiological rehabilitation: Current and future research needs. *Journal of the Academy of Rehabilitative Audiology, 27,* 67–92.

U.S. Food and Drug Administration. (1994). Hearing aid devices, professional and patient labeling and conditions for sale. *Federal Register, 42,* 9286–9296.

U.S. Office of Education, Bureau of Education for Handicapped Children. (1977). Implementation of Part B of the Education of the Handicapped Act. *Federal Register, 42,* 42474–42518.

Walden, B., Demorest, M., & Hepler, E. (1984). Self-report approach to assessing benefit derived from amplification. *Journal of Speech and Hearing Research, 27,* 49–56.

Williams, P., & Jacobs-Condit, L. (1985). *Hearing aids, what are they?* Washington, DC: National Information Center on Deafness, Gallaudet University.

END OF CHAPTER EXAMINATION QUESTIONS

CHAPTER 13

1. Hearing aid users may complain about certain aspects of hearing aid use. Name at least four of the seven major complaints of hearing aid users.
   a.
   b.
   c.
   d.

2. According to the author, what are the most frequent reasons for hearing aid returns?

3. What are some of the reasons that hearing aid orientation (HAO) programs may have to be modified to fit the needs of individual clients?

4. Why is it important to involve family members and friends of hearing aid users in HAO programs?

5. Hearing aid orientation must be an extensive and integral part of the _____ program.

6. All hearing aid orientation programs should contain the same basic elements. List five of the most essential elements of hearing aid orientation.
   a.
   b.
   c.
   d.
   e.

END OF CHAPTER ANSWER SHEET

Name _____ Date

CHAPTER 13

1. a.

   b.

   c.

   d.

2. _____

   _____

   _____

   _____

3. _____

   _____

   _____

   _____

4. _____

   _____

   _____

   _____

5. _____

_____

_____

_____

6. a.

b.

c.

d.

e.

7. Which one(s)?   a   b   c   d

8. Which one(s)?   a   b   c   d

9. Which one(s)?   a   b   c   d

7. New hearing aid users generally are encouraged to begin using their hearing aids in easy listening situations and then progress to more difficult listening experiences. An easy listening situation would involve listening to
   a. flute playing
   b. a group of people at a party
   c. a single speaker who is known to the listener
   d. a familiar radio station

8. The most common hearing aid problem that may arise is
   a. a dead battery
   b. acoustic feedback
   c. uncomfortable earmold
   d. all of the above

9. In addition to the seven hearing aid orientation services discussed in this chapter, _____ _____ is always welcomed by a hearing-impaired client.
   a. a follow-up call by the audiologist
   b. a grant for funds
   c. rescheduling of appointments
   d. an individualized rehabilitation plan

Assistive Listening Devices and Systems for Adults Who Are Hearing Impaired

■   ROBERT KIRK LIGHTFOOT, M.S.   ■

Historically, society has concentrated on the education of children who are deaf or profoundly hard of hearing. Only recently have efforts been made to address the problems of adults who have hearing impairment to varying degrees. Hearing impairment seriously hampers educational achievement for younger adults and can interfere with vocational performance in older adults. Optimal health care and rewarding family and social relationships can become seriously affected for most persons who have hearing impairment. These areas of communication are of special concern to older adults.

To address multiple listening and talking problems associated with hearing loss, a comprehensive aural rehabilitation program should consider assistive listening devices and systems (ALDS) as alternative and companion devices for use with the traditional types of personal hearing aids. ALDS can bring listeners and talkers improved personal, social, educational, vocational, cultural, and recreational relationships.

LISTENER AND TALKER RIGHTS

Both listeners and talkers have the right, as well as the need, to participate in interpersonal communication. Most modern environments are so pervaded by noise, distance and reverberation that aural and oral communication is often highly unsatisfactory. Table 14–1 sets forth a Bill of Rights for Listeners and Talkers (Vaughn, 1986).

SPEECH SIGNAL DELIVERY

Although great improvements have been made in hearing aids, few hearing aid users find speech easily understandable when it is masked by noise, distance, and reverberation. The background noise of cocktail parties, restaurants, and other group gatherings is likely to cause problems for most persons who have hearing impairment. Difficulties for listeners are increased whenever poor lighting and distance interfere with speechreading.

To achieve the goals of Table 14–1, assistive listening devices and systems (ALDS) are designed to deliver a sound from its source directly to the ears of the listener. The "lips-to-ears" speech delivery of ALDS is illustrated in Figure 14-1.

SELECTION OF ASSISTIVE LISTENING DEVICES AND SYSTEMS

The successful selection of ALDS for a person who has hearing impairment usually depends on four considerations:

1. The cost of the ALDS,
2. The degree of the client's hearing loss,
3. The acceptance of the ALDS by the client and significant others, and
4. The client's lifestyle.

When selecting a personal hearing aid for a client, audiologists consider the client's degree of loss and his or her acceptance of amplification. When dispensing ALDS, audiologists must follow the same selection protocol. In addition, however, they need to make a careful analysis of the client's lifestyle. The successful selection of an ALDS depends not only on the satisfaction of the listener, but also that of the talkers who wish to communicate with him or her. Figure 14–2 is a flowchart that can be useful during the selection of an ALDS (Vaughn & Lightfoot, 1989).

Assistive listening devices should be portable, affordable, commercially available, and not require any architectural modification. Table 14–2 presents an ALDS checklist for listening and talking situations (Vaughn & Lightfoot, 1983). The answers to this checklist can serve as the basis for the recommendation of one or more ALDS.

TABLE 14–1. Bill of Rights for Listeners and Talkers

Personal Rights	Communication Rights
Entitlement to quality care	in receiving areas, hospitals, nursing homes, outpatient waiting rooms, reception areas, physician's offices, and rehabilitative settings.
Opportunity for equal employment	during job interviews, telephone usage, and employment in professions, offices, industries, and fine arts.
Protection of legal rights	through availability of ALDS in police stations, courtrooms, and jails.
Admittance to legislative and diplomatic action	town meetings, state legislatures, Congress, and international organizations.
Participation in business activities	in negotiations, conferences, meetings, and contacts with bank tellers, telephone operators, receptionists, and managers.
Access to protection	by fire departments, emergency services, and police.
Assurance of safety	in industry, home, public and private buildings, hotels, airports, and places for public assembly.
Recognition of dignity as listener and talker	in interpersonal communication with family and friends in restaurants, social gatherings, automobiles, and over the telephone.
Freedom of religion	in worship services, counseling sessions, and confessionals.
Opportunity to travel	through accessibility to translation services, lectures by guides, recorded information at historical sites, and verbal exchange with group members.
Understanding of information	through graphic displays of ALDS in conjunction with public address systems, public telephones, radio, and television.
Obtaining of basic and continuing education	through amplification systems during tutoring, teleconferencing, and video and audio recordings.
Appreciation of entertainment	in concert halls, theaters, and movies.
Participation in recreational activities	indoor and outdoor games, active and spectator sports, and table and group games.

Source: From Vaughn, G. R. (1986). Bill of rights for listeners and talkers. *Hearing Instruments, 37*, 7. Reprinted with permission.

ALDS ADAPTIVE PROCEDURES

There are special adaptive procedures that can be used with ALDS. These self-administered procedures permit the users of hardwire and frequency modulation (FM) ALDS to place all of the components of the ALDS on their own bodies. The amplifier of a hardwire ALDS can be put in a listener's pocket for easy access to the volume control; the microphone can be clipped to the listener's lapel; and the earphones can be placed on the listener's ears. The transmitter and receiver of an FM ALDS can be placed in the listener's pockets or pocketbook allowing the listeners to "wire themselves."

Self-wiring permits a person to carry his or her own listening/talking system into various listen-

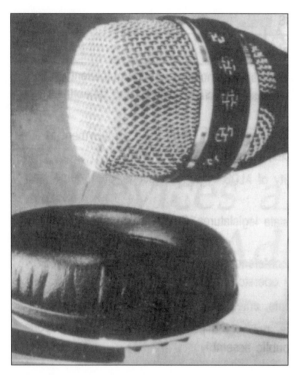

Figure 14–1. Delivery of speech sounds from the lips of the talker to the ears of the listener. (Courtesy of Sennheiser)

ing environments. Depending on the background noise levels and the loudness of the talker's voice, self-wiring can provide an easy and satisfactory solution to listening difficulties.

For talking in restaurants, around conference tables, in small groups at home, or in social gatherings, an ALDS microphone can be placed in a wind-screen. The windscreen can then be located in the center of the table, or it can be suspended above the group. The windscreen is a foam cover that protects the microphone from wind noise and vibrations.

CATEGORIES OF ALDS

Assistive listening devices are generally categorized as:

1. Hardwire,
2. Infrared,
3. Frequency modulation (FM),
4. Audio induction loop,
5. Vibrotactile systems, and
6. Sensory and alerting devices.

Television and telephone aids are found among many of these categories.

HARDWIRE DEVICES

Hardwire devices are extremely popular because of their easy procurement, quality of sound, simple technology, and, most of all, their low cost. The basic components of a hardwire ALDS are: (a) an amplifier, (b) a microphone, and (c) an earphone. Additional components may be purchased to accommodate such special needs as television or telephone listening. The name hardwire is used because the listener and the sound source are physically connected by a wire. The listener usually puts the hardwire amplifier in a pocket so that the volume control and on/off switch are accessible. He or she puts the earphones on his or her ears and places the microphone on or near the sound source. For television viewing, for example, the listener may simply plug his or her earphones into the output jack of the television set for a direct-wire system.

Early Hardwire ALDS

Earlier generations of hardwire systems were used in houses of worship and other public meeting places. These systems were permanently installed in designated pews or seats, usually at the front of the seating area. The earphone jacks were connected to the public address system. Users who had hearing impairment had to plug in their own earphones or they had to use some that were installed by the facility. As a result, listeners who had hearing impairment were sometimes unable to sit with their family members or friends.

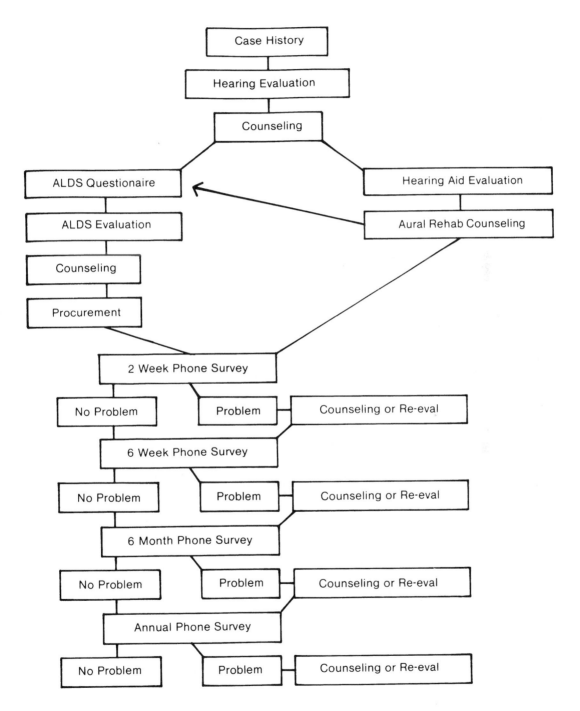

Figure 14–2. Assistive Listening Device flow chart.

TABLE 14–2. ALDS Checklist for Listening and Talking Problems

Some of the information that would help in making suggestions concerning assistive listening devices is listed below. Please check the items that pertain to your listening and talking problems.

Problem Listening and Talking Situations

I have difficulty understanding:

☐ in an automobile

☐ television or radio

☐ over the telephone

☐ one person at mealtime or around the home

☐ a physician, nurse, religious counselor, employer

☐ other (please list) _____

☐ in a restaurant or dining room

☐ at a conference table

☐ in medium-sized conference rooms

☐ at a party

☐ in a small family group

☐ when walking down the street

☐ in the theater (play)

☐ in the movies

☐ in a house of worship

☐ in a classroom

☐ in a dayroom or recreation room

☐ in a conference or lecture hall

☐ on the job

Amplification Devices

☐ I do not have a new hearing aid.

☐ I am pleased with my hearing aid.

☐ I do not wish to use a regular hearing aid.

☐ My hearing aid has a telephone switch.

☐ I can afford an alternative system that costs:

  ☐ $100 ☐ $300 ☐ $500 ☐ $700

Large Area Sound Systems

My community has the following sound systems:

☐ Hardwire (☐ church ☐ theater ☐ movie ☐ other)

☐ Infrared (☐ church ☐ theater ☐ movie ☐ other)

☐ FM (☐ church ☐ theater ☐ movie ☐ other)

☐ Loop (☐ church ☐ theater ☐ movie ☐ other)

Special Sensory Devices

I use some of the following special sensory devices and rate their effectiveness as:

	Poor	Fair	Good	Excellent
Telecaptioning	☐	☐	☐	☐
Teletypewriter	☐	☐	☐	☐
Gongs, bells	☐	☐	☐	☐
Lights	☐	☐	☐	☐
Vibrators	☐	☐	☐	☐
Hearing dog	☐	☐	☐	☐
_____ (other)	☐	☐	☐	☐
None ☐	☐	☐	☐	☐

Source: Adapted from Lightfoot, R. K., & Vaughn, G. R. (1989). Resource materials. In R. L. Schow & M. A. Nerbonne (Eds.), *Introduction to aural rehabilitation* (2nd ed., pp. 586–605). Austin, TX: Pro-Ed.

Present Hardwire ALDS

Hardwire devices are currently marketed by several distributors. As prepackaged devices, they can be procured from several manufacturers. A hardwire ALDS package usually includes: (a) an amplifier, (b) a microphone, (c) an earpiece, (d) a battery, (e) the instructions for using an ALDS, and (f) a carrying case. An extension cord may also be required by a listener. The length of the extension cord depends on the distance between the listener and the sound source. Other accessories may include (a) a neckloop that transmits to a telecoil (T-coil) in the listener's personal hearing aid, and (b) a battery charger for use with rechargeable batteries. For an innovative consumer, the individual components for a hardwire ALDS may be obtained from radio and television repair and parts stores. Care must be taken when personally assembling a hardwire ALDS that the output does not exceed safe listening levels and that the impedance between components is not mismatched.

Hardwire Devices and Special Needs

Hardwire ALDS are also useful for people who only need a bit of "hearing help" in certain situations. For example, listeners who have difficulties in noisy public offices, at teller windows, in automobiles, in restaurants, when using public telephones, or when they and others are viewing television or listening to the radio, often find ALDS are excellent problem solvers.

HEALTH CARE. Hardwire devices are becoming a necessary piece of equipment for all types of health clinics, hospitals, nursing homes, and emergency rooms. Hardwire ALDS should be available to receptionists, bank tellers, and others who greet the public. Audiologists, speech pathologists, physicians, nurses, social workers, dentists, pharmacists, chaplains, counselors, and other members of the health care field should keep hardwire ALDS or other amplification devices available to assist persons who have hearing impairment.

One of the commercially available hardwire ALDS is the PockeTalker by Williams Sound. Figure 14–3 demonstrates how a hardwire ALDS can enhance communication between a patient who is hard-of-hearing and a member of the health care system.

AUTOMOBILES. To overcome the excessive ambient noise level in an automobile, a person who has hearing impairment can wear the earpiece of an ALDS and place the microphone in one of the following positions: (a) on the talker's lapel or (b) on the back of the front seat (if he or she is in the front), thus, giving him or her access to the talkers in back. The listener may wish to pass the microphone from talker to talker, if the above suggestions do not provide a satisfactory signal-to-noise ratio. Figure 14–4 illustrates the use of a hardwire ALDS in an automobile.

RESTAURANT. Restaurant noise causes problems for most hearing-impaired listeners. One way to carry on a satisfactory conversation with one companion at a table is to pass an ALDS microphone under the table and clip it to the lapel of the talker. The microphone may also be placed in the center of the table or suspended above. This last placement improves effective communication for the listener who has hearing impairment when one or more talkers are present. Figure 14–5 demonstrates the use of a hardwire ALDS in a restaurant.

PARTIES. The hardwire microphone can be passed from talker to talker at parties if the noise level is too high for self-wiring. Otherwise, the listener can self-wire him or herself and stand in an advantageous position within a small group.

Television and Radio

When one member of a family is hard-of-hearing, television and radio listening levels can become a source of concern. The family members complain that the person who has hearing impairment turns

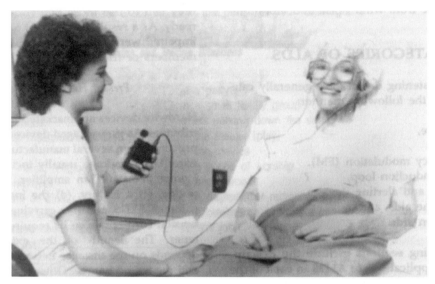

Figure 14–3. A hardwire ALS enhances communication between a patient and a member of the health care team. (Courtesy of Williams Sound)

the volume up so high that it is uncomfortable for them, the normally hearing listeners. As a result, the normally hearing listeners often move to a separate room, leaving the person who has hearing impairment to listen alone.

There are several ways to address the problem of the volume control for the television and radio. One simple way is to clip or tape a microphone to the grille of the television or radio. If an extension cord is used, care must be taken that cords do not pose a hazard that could be tripped on. This permits the person who has hearing impairment to independently adjust the loudness to meet his or her own needs. At the same time, normally hearing listeners are able to adjust the loudness of the television set by using the volume control on the set. Thus, both normally hearing listeners and listeners who have hearing impairment can enjoy listening in the same room to the same television or radio program.

With the ALDS technology that is available today, infrared or FM systems provide an effective means through which adults who have impaired hearing can enjoy television or radio. Both system types are readily available through audiology clinics and provide excellent fidelity and acoustic gain for even those who have a severe hearing loss.

DIRECT WIRING. Hardwire devices do not necessarily have to include a separate microphone and amplifier. An inexpensive approach to television and radio listening is direct wiring. This is achieved by using a direct wire between the television or radio and an earplug or earphones. The television or radio must have a listening jack to use a direct wire. Some televisions have two external jacks, one for exclusive private listening use. When the private listening jack is used, the internal speaker of the set is disconnected and private listening is available to the person wearing the earphones. If the other jack is used, both the internal speaker and the private listening jack are operational. The volume for both jacks is adjusted by the volume control of the television set.

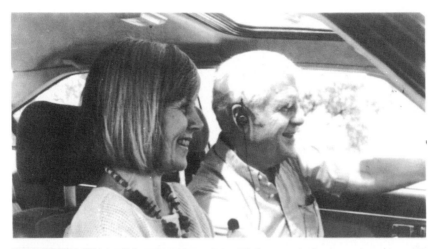

Figure 14–4. A hardwire ALS can provide good, amplified communication in a noisy environment. (Courtesy of Williams Sound)

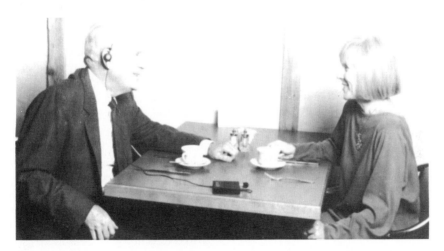

Figure 14–5. When a hardwire ALS microphone is placed on the table, it can provide good communication to a person who is hearing impaired in a noisy restaurant. (Courtesy of Birmingham VA Medical Center)

At times, listeners who have hearing impairment find it necessary to increase the distance between themselves and a television or radio. This distancing can be achieved by adding an extension cord with the appropriate connectors between the set and the earphones.

Hardwire Devices For Telephone Amplification

The telephone can present a great problem for listeners who have hearing impairment. Hardwire devices often can alleviate this problem by replacing the microphone of the ALDS with a magnetic telephone pickup. This pickup is attached to the listening end of the telephone handset. Some manufacturers produce modular couplers that allow a telephone to be connected to a free-standing amplifier or to an ALDS.

Dexterity and Hardwire Systems

Hardwire devices also have proven to be convenient for persons who have hearing impairment who are unable to adjust traditional hearing aids because of their small controls. The volume controls of hardwire ALDS are usually large enough for persons with dexterity problems caused by arthritis or other conditions to make the necessary adjustments. The under-the-chin stenographer type of earphone also has been very useful for persons with decreased dexterity. For persons who do not have any difficulty in adjusting or positioning an ALDS, the more up-to-date "earbuds" usually are preferred because they are less conspicuous and are lightweight. Persons who have visual impairment also find that the manipulation of hardwire devices is simple.

Cost

Hardwire ALDS usually cost between $50 and $200. The price makes them accessible and attractive to people on fixed incomes.

INFRARED LISTENING SYSTEMS

Infrared light technology has made remarkable contributions to the field of electronics. Televisions, stereos, and VCRs employ the use of infrared light for their remote control options. Infrared light beams are now used to carry audio signals from the special light emitting diodes (LEDs) of the transmitters to the infrared receivers worn by normally hearing listeners and listeners who have hearing impairment. Although varying amounts of infrared light are in all sources of light, technology has reduced the problems of infrared interference from incandescent and fluorescent lighting. The natural infrared light from the sun is so great that the use of infrared systems is not possible when the eye of a receiver is in direct sunlight. As a result, an infrared system is usually confined to indoor use, and depending on specific needs, various sizes and signal strengths are available for home, small meeting areas, or large areas such as auditoriums and church sanctuarys.

One difficulty with infrared is that the receiver must be in line-of-sight with the transmitter. It is possible for the receiver to respond to a signal that has bounced off of a surface such as a smooth ceiling or wall, tile floor, glossy painted wall, or other reflective surface. When considering the placement of transmitters in a facility, care must be taken that the signal is not obstructed by supporting structures or by the heads of the persons who are seated or standing between the listeners and the transmitter.

One great advantage of infrared light transmission is that it does not pass through walls or curtains, thus infrared ALDS provide transmission privacy. Some of the locations in which this privacy is desirable include courtrooms, boardrooms, or theaters. Infrared prevents the illegal recording of a performance outside places such as those listed above or the "listening in" to proceedings in a courtroom. A second advantage of an infrared ALDS is that it is usually not affected by FM or AM transmissions or by electromagnetic interference, unless the master system (amplifier) that it is wired to is not well grounded.

Infrared listening systems have been installed in many theaters and churches for patrons who have hearing impairment, as well as for normally hearing persons who enjoy the quality of infrared reception. The frequency spectrum allows for high quality reproduction.

Large Area Listening

Infrared listening systems are appropriate for all situations in which a listener is in a fixed position.

These situations include the large area infrared transmitter systems for houses of worship, theaters, and concert halls. The entire listening area must be "bathed" with infrared light; the possibility of head shadows must be eliminated. Figure 14–6 shows an infrared transmitter that can cover a large area.

Small Area Infrared Listening

For small area usage, such as home television viewing or small group meetings, a smaller transmitter provides adequate IR coverage. This small transmitter makes infrared listening relatively inexpensive. Figure 14–7 illustrates the use of a small infrared system.

Reception of any infrared signal can be accomplished by several means. The most common is by the use of an "under-the-chin" receiver that receives the infrared signal, converts it to acoustic energy, and delivers it to the ear of the listener. Figure 14–8 shows an infrared receiver. Note the volume control pictured on the left and the "eye" shown on the right. A second type of receiver is a body receiver that is worn with a cord that delivers the signal electronically to (a) an earplug or earphone, (b) a magnetic induction silhouette worn behind the ear or against the T-coil of a hearing aid, (c) a magnetic neck loop, or (d) a personal hearing aid with direct audio input.

A listener who is interested in using an Infrared ALDS should experiment with the various receivers, since all of the previously mentioned modes of infrared reception are excellent.

FREQUENCY MODULATION DEVICES

Frequency modulation (FM) systems employ frequency modulation radio waves to transmit a signal from the talker or sound source to listeners. The FM transmitter may be thought of as a miniature radio station that transmits to FM receivers, similar in concept to the radios used by the general public. The FM transmitter and FM receiver must be "tuned" to each other—that is, transmission and reception must be on the same waveband.

FM systems have been used for many years in classrooms for children who have hearing impairment. These systems commonly are known as auditory trainers. The choice of FM receivers is based on the auditory need of each student. The teacher speaks into the microphone of an FM transmitter. Using this system, regular classroom activities as well as special language, speechreading, and articulation classes can be conducted through this wireless system. In the past, the receivers were collected from the students before they left a classroom. The transmitters and receivers were placed on "charge," ensuring that the battery would be ready for use the next day. As a result, the students were unable to avail themselves of the extensive language exposure on the playground, in the cafeteria, and at home with normally hearing siblings and parents.

In many situations in the past, students with only traditional hearing aids did not function well. This was especially true in large areas, such as houses of worship, theaters, auditoriums, or other

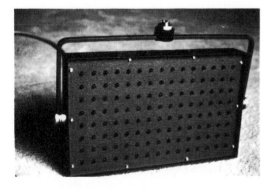

Figure 14–6. An infrared transmitter provides quality ALDS listening in a large area. (Courtesy of Siemens)

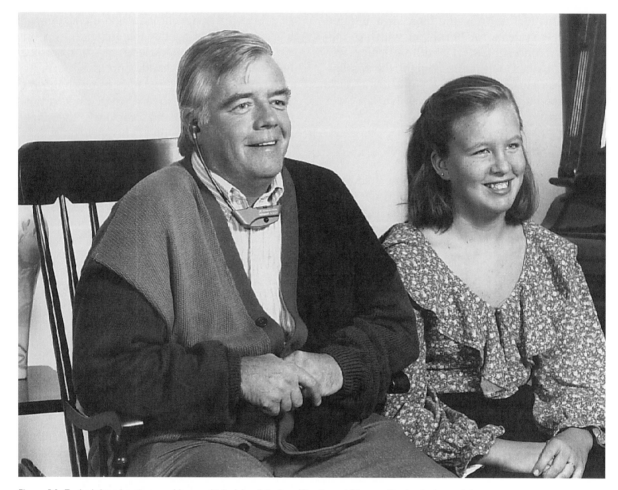

Figure 14–7. An infrared system provides good television listening. (Courtesy of Siemens Hearing Instruments)

settings in which distance, noise, and reverberation interfered with important auditory signals. Despite these difficulties, FM systems were restricted to educational settings.

In 1991, the Federal Communications Commission (FCC) was finally convinced that the special needs of persons who have hearing impairment justified the approval of FM systems in settings other than educational. The new rules allowed the use of 72 MHz to 76 MHz wavebands for general use. At present, 32 narrowband and 8 wideband channels are available for personal, social, vocational, recreational, and religious activities. During educational activities, narrowband channels are predominantly used in classrooms. The simultaneous broadcast of FM signals in adjacent classrooms requires that different frequencies be used in separate rooms.

FM receivers interface with a variety of monaural and binaural modes to deliver a signal at ear-

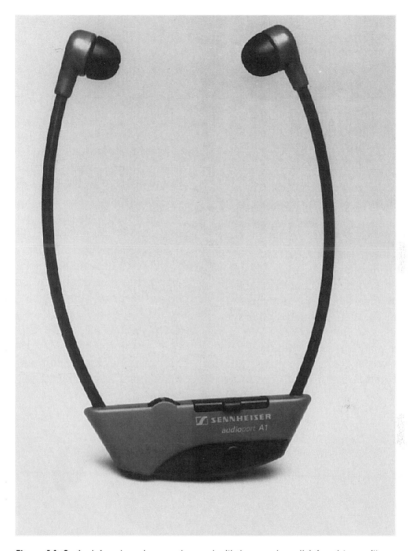

Figure 14–8. An infrared receiver can be used with large and small infrared transmitters. (Courtesy of Siemens)

level. Probably the most common is the "walkman" type of earphones (or earplugs). Other modes include: (a) a snap-in earmold and transducer, (b) direct audio input to an ear level or body hearing aid, (c) an induction neck loop or silhouette used with the telecoil (T-coil) of a personal hearing aid, or (d) a bone conduction vibrator. Tape recorders also can be paired with FM receivers for simultaneous recording and listening in classroom situations.

Large Area FM Transmission

Wideband FM channels are primarily used in large areas, since the signal-to-noise ratio is greater than that of narrowband channels, and clarity is enhanced. Another advantage of wideband FM channels is that they provide a more natural range for speech and music. Presently, the use of only one open transmitter per channel is possible. However, any number of receivers on the same channel can be used in a listening area. When using narrow or wideband channels, the frequencies of all FM channels used in a certain listening area must be specified before additional FM systems are introduced.

FM transmission range is usually 300 to 500 feet from a transmitter, thus making a system ideal for use in large areas and outdoor recreational activities. FM ALDS provide listener freedom in seat selection. However, as an FM signal will travel through walls, floors, and other barriers, FM is not the system of choice when privacy is required. The FM signal has been known to carry for miles, if the FM transmission signal and the FM receivers are in line-of-sight.

FM ALDS And Special Needs

FM FOR ONE-TO-ONE COMMUNICATION. FM systems are excellent for nearly all problem listening environments. In one-to-one communication, the microphone and transmitter can be handheld by the talker or they can be permanently positioned on the corner of a desk or table for interviewing and counseling situations. Figure 14–9 demonstrates the FM transmitter that is sending the signal of the talker's voice to an FM receiver worn by the listener. In this figure, the listener is wearing an ear-level hearing aid and an FM receiver, with a neckloop plugged into the receiver. This, in turn, provides an electromagnetic field from which the T-coil of the patient's hearing aid picks up the signal. The latter is then converted into acoustic signals by the personal hearing aid.

FM FOR AUTOMOBILES. For use in automobiles or other transportation modes, the microphone of an FM transmitter can be clipped to the front or back of a car seat to be as close to as many talkers as possible.

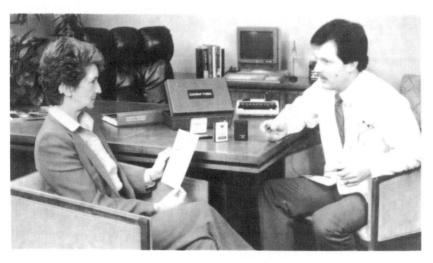

Figure 14–9. The FM transmitter (white) sends the physician's voice to an FM receiver worn by the patient. (Courtesy of Comtek)

FM FOR RESTAURANTS. Restaurant noise can be overcome by placing an FM microphone as close to the sound source as possible by: (a) clipping it to the talker's lapel, (b) placing it in the center of the table, or (c) hanging it from the ceiling or light fixture above the table. Figure 14–10 shows an FM ALDS placed in the center of the table. These configurations can be used for table games and boardroom tables.

FM FOR GROUPS. Comtek has developed a "sound collector" for FM transmission that is called the Conference Mate. The Conference Mate houses an FM transmitter that broadcasts a talker's message to the FM receivers of listeners who have hearing impairment. Figure 14–11 shows the Conference Mate positioned on a table during a group session.

FM FOR TELEVISION AND RADIO. Television and radio reception can be improved by positioning a microphone in front of the internal speaker of the television or radio. The volume level on the set should be adjusted so that it is at a listening level that is comfortable for the normally hearing listeners in the area. Figure 14–12 displays an FM transmitter on top of a television set. The microphone is shown clipped near the internal speaker of the set. The listener who has hearing impairment holds the receiver and adjusts the volume to a comfortable level.

FM AND GLASS BARRIERS. One of the most difficult situations for persons who have hearing impairment is caused by the glass barriers used at bank teller windows and in office reception areas. Figure 14–13 demonstrates the use of a self-wired

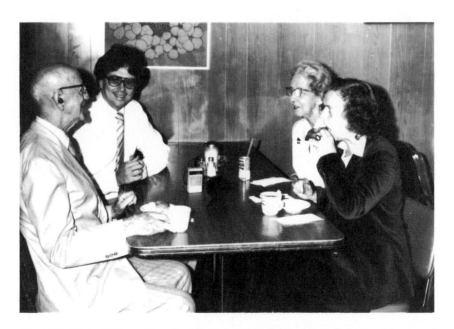

Figure 14–10. An FM transmitter with microphone windscreen is placed in the center of a restaurant table. The gentleman is wearing an FM receiver in his pocket and an earbud in his ear. (Courtesy of Birmingham VA Medical Center)

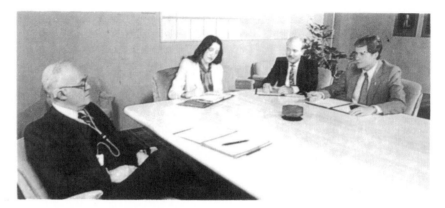

Figure 14–11. The FM receiver "collects the sounds" from the talkers around the table and transmits them to members of the group who are hearing impaired. (Courtesy of Comtek)

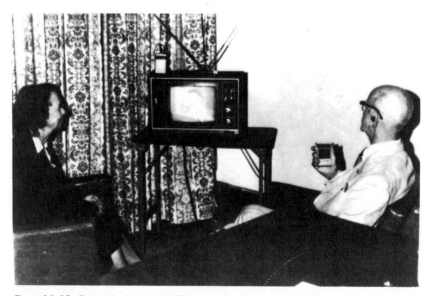

Figure 14–12. For quality listening, an FM transmitter is placed on top of the television set with the microphone located in front of the internal speaker. The gentleman is holding an FM receiver. (Courtesy of Birmingham VA Medical Center)

FM ALDS system. He is wearing both the FM transmitter and FM receiver. If there is an opening in the glass barrier, he has the option of passing the microphone through the opening for the best speech signal.

LARGE AREA FM APPLICATIONS. The problems encountered in large area listening can be overcome by giving the microphone to the talker or by placing it at the sound source. FM transmission is highly satisfactory for activities such as religious

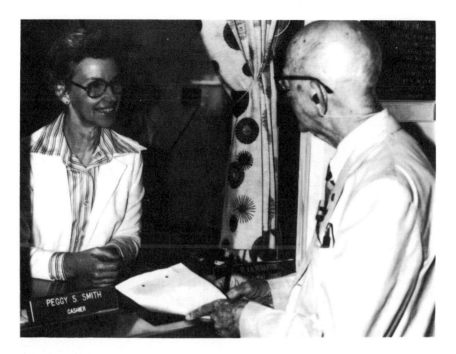

Figure 14–13. Glass barriers can be overcome by the placement of an FM microphone held close to the opening in the glass panel. The listener wears the receiver and earpiece. (Courtesy of Birmingham VA Medical Center)

gatherings, lectures, group meetings, classrooms, or even movie theaters. As a courtesy, permission should be given by the talker or the management of a facility prior to the placement of a transmitter. This will avoid any misunderstanding about the legality of the recording. Figure 14–14 shows a minister using an FM transmitter to deliver his sermon. The congregation includes persons with hearing impairment who are using FM receivers.

FM AND OUTDOOR ACTIVITIES. Outdoor instructional activities such as horseback riding, bicycling, snow skiing, and golfing can be enhanced by FM technology.

FM AND MOBILITY TRAINING FOR THE BLIND. Rehabilitation specialists for the blind have

included FM devices as an important tool for mobility training and other activities in which the blind person is at a distance from the instructor.

FM ADVANTAGES. Advantages of the FM ALDS include: (a) portability, (b) ease of use, (c) wireless distance between transmitter and receiver, (d) low maintenance, and (3) lack of interference from electrical and magnetic sources.

Cost

In the past, the initial cost of the FM system was one of the major disadvantages for potential users of ALDS. Today, however, the cost is not prohibitive. In fact, even large-area FM systems are within a modest price range.

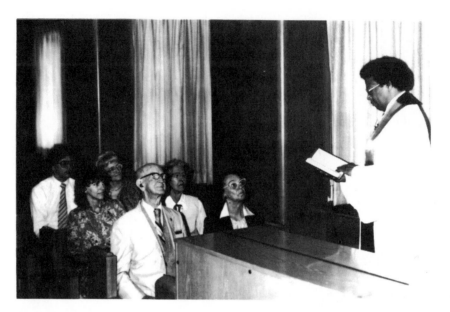

Figure 14–14. An FM transmitter with microphone sends the signal from the minister to members of the congregation who have FM receivers and earplugs. (Courtesy of Birmingham VA Medical Center)

AUDIO INDUCTION LOOP SYSTEMS

The audio induction loop system is one of the oldest assistive listening devices. In Europe, loops have been used widely in conjunction with personal hearing aids. They are found in most public buildings. In several countries, the law requires the installation of this technology in churches and other public areas. The popularity of this system in Europe resulted from the widespread use of hearing aid T-coils. The use of loops spread to the United States in the 1950s. The basic components of an audio loop system include: (a) a microphone, (b) an amplifier, and (c) a coil of wire that is looped around a room or a personal listening area. The wire generates an electromagnetic field in and around the loop of wire. This electromagnetic field is received by the telephone pickup coil in personal hearing aids.

Although the size of the loop can vary, it is best suited for medium and small listening areas. The loop has a number of applications: (a) it can be placed around a group of chairs in an auditorium, (b) it can encircle a single chair in a living room for television viewing, (c) it can be worn around the neck, or (d) it can take the form of a small silhouette induction loop that can be placed next to the ear level or body hearing aid with a T-coil. Figure 14–15 illustrates the use of a loop ALDS and the television.

The major disadvantages of loop technology include interference from electric wiring, fluorescent lights, and transformers. Distance from the loop and improper head positioning can cause a reduction in the signal. Consumers report the greatest advantage to loop technology is that no special receiver is required for users who have personal hearing aids with working T-coils. Loop system

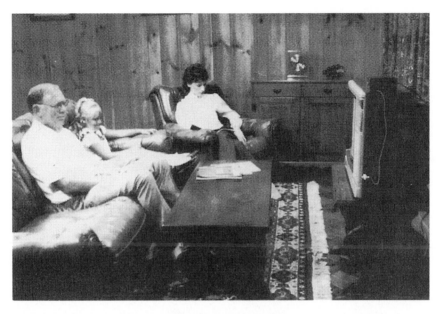

Figure 14–15. A Loop ALDS encircles a chair for enhanced television listening. The listener wears his hearing aid with a T-coil. (Courtesy of Oticon)

ALDS are easy to install and the technology is simple and easily understood.

In the late 1970s and early 1980s, a major movement by consumer groups and health care professionals interested in the improvement of T-coil technology for personal hearing aids resulted in more efficient and sensitive T-coils in hearing aids. As a result, there has been an expanded application of loop ALDS in the United States.

VIBROTACTILE SYSTEMS

Vibrotactile stimulators translate sounds into vibrations on the skin. According to Martin (1994) small vibrators are worn on the chest, neck, wrist, or back of the hand and are connected to separate channels to the input unit (amplifier and microphone) which can be worn in a carrying case or pocket. The microphone is clipped to the wearer's clothing. Tactaid, by Audiological Engineering Corporation, incorporates seven channels of vibrotactile stimulation and provides a wearer with a wide range of information regarding the characteristics of speech, including voicing/unvoicing, inflection, time cues, intensity, and others. See Figure 14–16 for a seven-channel vibrotactile unit (Courtesy of Tactaid).

SENSORY AND ALERTING DEVICES

Persons who are profoundly hard-of-hearing or deaf have used alerting and signaling devices for many years. These devices also are useful for persons who are hearing impaired with high frequency losses. Sensory and alerting devices use visual, auditory, and tactile avenues. Some of these devices are discussed in the following paragraphs.

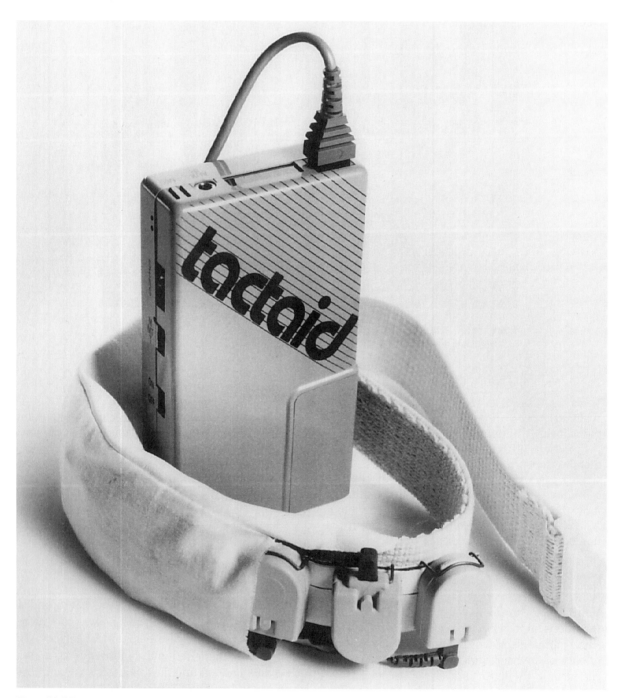

Figure 14–16. A Tactaid seven-channel vibrotactile device. (Courtesy of Audiological Engineering Corporation)

AUDITORY, VISUAL, AND TACTILE ALERTING DEVICES

AUDITORY AND VISUAL

Telephones can be purchased with bell ringers that greatly increase the volume of the sound. Horns, sirens, and warehouse bells can also be added. Signals from telephones and doorbells can be increased by attaching magnetic pickup suction cups that are connected to loudspeakers. The same stimuli work with door knocks, doorbells, doormats, voices, crying babies, barking dogs, smoke detectors, and burglar alarms. Flashing lights in various forms are available. Remote lamps also can be installed to alert a person to a telephone that is ringing in another location. Other visual devices that can assist persons who have hearing impairment include the use of convex mirrors and peepholes.

Sounds with special patterns, such as the ringing of the telephone, are easily identified through visual and auditory signals. Security alarms for driveways and gateways can provide intruder alerts for persons with hearing impairment. Telephone dialing for emergency and special police numbers can be activated by some of the alerting systems.

Microphones can be installed near the source of a sound. The arrangement works as an alerting system for the various needs just listed. The sensitivity of the microphone must be adjusted to pick up an immediate signal to cut back on unwanted responses to sounds in the area.

A master control unit acts as the central receiver for remote sensors such as: smoke detectors, doorbells, telephones, baby cries, and security systems. A master unit usually is connected to some form of flashing light or vibrator. A remote lamp also can be made to act as an alerting system.

These systems also are useful for monitoring clothes dryers, washing machines, ovens, and night sounds around a house. They also serve as warning systems to indicate equipment maintenance problems.

TACTILE DEVICES

Alarm clocks can use vibration as an alerting signal. Beds can be made to vibrate, as can portable timers and wrist watches. One tactile device includes a wrist-worn receiver with many sensor-transmitters. Each sensor-transmitter identifies a specific sound and sends a coded radio signal to a wrist-worn receiver. The wearer is alerted by the vibration of the wrist-worn receiver. The sound source is identified by a coded light on the receiver. The range of transmission is approximately 100 feet. Fans can also serve as alerting systems when attached to timers.

Figure 14–17 provides a display of a variety of auditory, visual and tactile alerting devices. Many others are on the market and provide for a sense of security and attachment for persons with moderate-to-severe hearing impairments.

SUMMARY

If quality care involving ALDS is to be made available, audiologists, hearing aid dispensers, speech-language pathologists, and other members of the hearing health care team need to be familiar with ALDS options and applications. They should also be familiar with the philosophy and practical considerations involved in the selection and utilization of these devices. Figure 14–18 shows the Decision Circles that were designed by Vaughn, Lightfoot, and Teter (1988). These circles present the ALDS options that are appropriate for different listening and talking situations.

Professionals, persons who have hearing impairment, and significant others can refer to the assistive listening devices and systems (ALDS) decision circles for examples of how the various

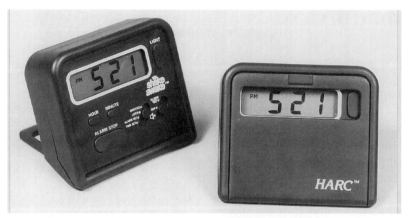

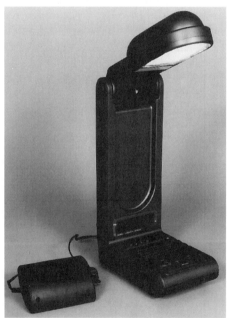

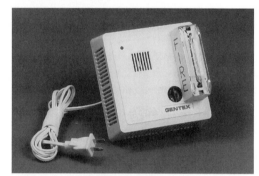

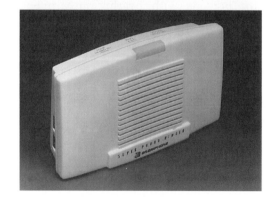

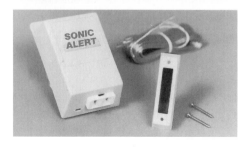

Figure 14–17. Examples of various alerting devices that are available for adults who are hearing impaired. (Courtesy of William Sound Corporation)

Assistive Listening Devices and Systems (ALDS)
Decision Circles

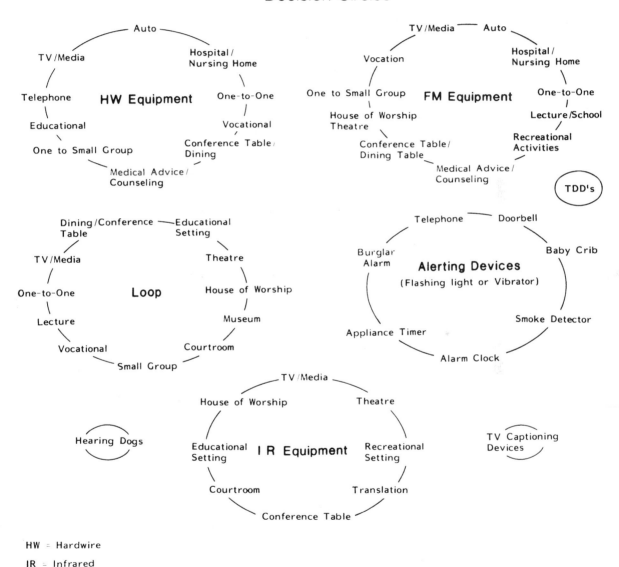

HW = Hardwire

IR = Infrared

Figure 14–18. Assistive Listening Devices and Systems (ALDS) Decision Circles suggest applications for users of ALDS. (From Vaughn, G. R., Lightfoot, R. K., & Teter, D. L. [1988]. Assistive listening devices and systems [ALDS] enhance the lifestyles of hearing-impaired persons. *The American Journal of Otology, 9* [Suppl.], 101–106. Reprinted with permission.)

ALDS can be used. The examples are not all-inclusive, but provide a sampling of the most popular applications. When clients are counseled about their special needs for hearing help, professionals can use the decision circles to narrow the selection. Sometimes a single piece of equipment is sufficient; but sometimes a lifestyle demands a "hearing help plan" that involves the future procurement of ALDS.

REFERENCES

Federal Communications Commission (1991). 47 CFR Parts 0 and 64: *Federal Register, 56* (148, August), 36729–36733.

Martin, F. N. (1994). Management of hearing impairment. In F. N. Martin (Ed.), *Introduction to audiology* (pp. 443–444). Englewood Cliffs, NJ: Prentice Hall.

Vaughn, G. R. (1986). Bill of rights for listeners and talkers. *Hearing Instruments, 37,* 8.

Vaughn, G. R., & Lightfoot, R. K. (1983). Lifestyles and assistive listening devices and systems. *Hearing Instruments, 3,* 128–134.

Vaughn, G. R., & Lightfoot, R. K. (1989). Resource materials. In R. L. Schow & M. A. Nerbonne (Eds.), *Introduction to aural rehabilitation* (pp. 586–605). Austin, TX: Pro-Ed.

Vaughn, G. R., Lightfoot, R. K., & Teter, D. L. (1988). Assistive listening devices and systems (ALDS) enhance the lifestyles of hearing-impaired persons. *American Journal of Otology, 9* (Suppl.), 101–106.

END OF CHAPTER EXAMINATION QUESTIONS

CHAPTER 14

1. What factors influence the selection of an ALDS:
   a. the life-style of the client
   b. the cost of the ALDS
   c. the hearing loss of the client
   d. the willingness of the client and significant others of the ALDS
   e. all of the above

2. (True/False) According to Public Law, it is the responsibility of the person who is hearing impaired to provide his/her own ALDS for use in public places.

3. List at least three (3) situations in which an ALDS is useful for the typical hearing impaired adult.
   a.
   b.
   c.

4. (True/False) The hardwire devices available today are generally the most difficult devices for people with dexterity problems to operate.

5. Name two advantages and two disadvantages of infrared listening devices as compared to other assistive listening systems.

END OF CHAPTER ANSWER SHEET

Name   Date

CHAPTER 14

1. Which one(s)?   a   b   c   d   e

2. Circle one: True   False

3. a.

   b.

   c.

4. Circle one: True   False

5. Advantages:

   a.

   b.

   Disadvantages:

   a.

   b.

6. a.

   b.

   c.

   d.

7. _____

   _____

   _____

   _____

   _____ .

8. a.

   b.

   c.

   d.

9. a.

   b.

   c.

10. _____

    _____

    _____

    _____

    _____

    _____ .

6. According to the author, the careful selection of ALDS for a person who is hearing impaired usually depends on four considerations. Those are:

   a.

   b.

   c.

   d.

7. _____FM channels are primarily used in large areas, why?

8. What are four advantages of the FM ALDS over other forms of assistive listening systems?

   a.

   b.

   c.

   d.

9. What are the three basic components of a loop listening system?

   a.

   b.

   c.

10. Vibrotactile devices have gained popularity in the United States over the past decade. Generally, what characteristics of speech do vibrotactile devices transmit to the "listener"?

Speech Conservation for Adults Who Are Hearing Impaired

■ PAMELA L. JACKSON, PH.D. ■

Speech characteristics and therapy techniques for clients who have prelingual hearing impairment are well documented in the literature. The degree of auditory impairment and the extent of a resulting handicap for this population have drawn the attention of researchers and clinicians, alike. Their efforts have resulted in a documented body of literature that is the basis for communication training programs throughout the United States.

There is, however, another subgroup of the population with hearing impairment that is often overlooked in these descriptions of speech behaviors. That group is the *adventitiously* hearing impaired, who have losses after speech and language skills had developed normally. With the onset of the hearing loss, speech monitoring ability may diminish and, in time, there can be changes in speech production. The task facing clinicians who deal with this clientele is one of conservation of existing skills rather than the development of new ones. **Maintenance of intelligibility is the goal**.

FACTORS INFLUENCING SPEECH DETERIORATION

A description of the typical characteristics of this population is nearly impossible, because there is no typical case. Many factors and their interaction are responsible for the amount of deterioration after a hearing impairment develops. These factors are discussed in the following paragraphs.

DEGREE OF HEARING LOSS

If the hearing loss allows at least partial monitoring of speech, the problem will be less severe than if no speech monitoring is possible. In the majority of cases of adventitious hearing loss, the onset is gradual and the degree is mild enough that no change in speech production is noticed.

CONFIGURATION OF THE HEARING LOSS

Configuration and degree of hearing loss interact to impose a certain amount of distortion on an incoming auditory signal. For example, a precipitous high-frequency hearing loss will either nullify or distort sibilant or high-frequency voiceless consonants and may remove the higher frequency second formant information that is needed for vowel identification. The configuration will be a prime determiner of speech monitoring ability, with the amount of high frequency residual hearing, especially at 2000 Hz and above, being critical.

AGE OF ONSET

In general, the more years of normal hearing a client has, the better will be his or her oral speech skills. Yet, the relationship between age of onset and speech intelligibility is complex. Binnie, Daniloff, and Buckingham (1982) reported on the case of a child with a profound bilateral hearing loss as a result of spinal meningitis when he was 5 years old. Prior to his hospitalization, he reportedly showed no indications of speech or language problems. Approximately 6 weeks after his illness began, the child was seen for auditory management, which included periodic tape recording of his spontaneous speech, as well as his responses to the screening portion of the Templin-Darley Tests of Articulation (Templin, 1969). Testing was conducted at 2-week intervals for 9 months. Phonetic, spectrographic, and perceptual analyses of the tapes were conducted and revealed: (1) increases in word duration, (2) increases in duration variability, (3) a rise in fundamental frequency (F_o), (4) less variation in pitch inflection, (5) syllabification of final consonants, and (6) significantly depressed speech intelligibility scores. Within a 9-month period, the speech of this 5-year-old had changed markedly.

The age factor must be considered a critical determiner of speech deterioration when other, older clients are compared to this 5-year-old. For example, consider a client who had a sudden, profound hearing loss at age 21 due to antibiotic treatment for a kidney infection. Several years following the onset, speech intelligibility remained intact, with only minor sibilant distortion being noted. Prosodic features remained unaffected. Cases of similar etiology have been reported, however, in which speech deterioration was much more extensive and intelligibility was noticeably affected.

The influence of age of onset of hearing loss on speech intelligibility has never been systematically explored. The need for such an investigation is supported by the concluding statements made by Kent (1976) following his survey of acoustic studies of speech development. He concluded that the variability of speech motor control progressively diminishes, beginning by 3 years of age and continuing until a child is 8 to 12 years of age, when adult stability is achieved. This development of precise motor control occurs, therefore, after the majority of speech sounds have already reached the point where they are phonetically acceptable. This statement implies that 8 to 12 years of age may be a critical dividing line for predicting speech deterioration following the onset of a hearing loss.

HEARING AID HISTORY

Ideally, amplification is employed shortly after a hearing loss is discovered to maintain speech monitoring ability. The timing of initiating amplification and the early success in restoring speech understanding ability influences the severity of speech deterioration.

ACCOMPANYING PROBLEMS

Mental retardation, learning disabilities, neuromuscular problems, and similar disorders possibly will affect speech skills in the adventitiously hearing-impaired population, just as in the congenitally hearing-impaired population.

NEED TO USE SPEECH

As with those with congenital hearing impairment, speech skills are largely dependent on the need for ongoing oral communication. This continued use may need to be reinforced and monitored to ensure that skills are maintained.

SPEECH CHARACTERISTICS OF THE ADULT HEARING-IMPAIRED POPULATION

The type of speech problem that occurs with acquired hearing loss varies widely and, as a result, each case must be evaluated for individual patterns. Error patterns may involve a combination of three different components, including articulation, voice and resonance, and rhythm and timing.

ARTICULATION

The phoneme production errors involved in the speech of the deaf have been thoroughly described in the classic study by Hudgins and Numbers (1942) and are summarized in Table 15-1.

Errors appearing in the speech of each person with adventitious hearing impairment depends on the factors mentioned earlier. Based on a knowledge of speech acoustics, certain predictions can be made as to which speech sounds may deteriorate from a particular hearing loss. Based on that information and, according to Calvert and Silverman (1975), common errors include omissions and distortions of the sibilants, especially /s/, described previously. These errors can be explained, in part, by comparing them with the acoustic characteristics of the speech signal. In general, speech sounds that are more difficult to hear are more often in error. Each sound contains energy at several frequencies, which means that a given audiometric configuration may remove only part of the identifying information and result in a distortion. The sound may be detected based on lower fre-

TABLE 15–1. Phoneme Production Errors

Consonant Errors

Failure to distinguish between voiced and voiceless consonants

Consonant substitutions

Excessive nasality

Misarticulation of consonant clusters
Two types of errors may occur: (1) one of the sounds may be dropped from the cluster, or (2) the sounds may be produced so slowly that additional syllables are added when /ə/ is inserted between the cluster elements.

Misarticulation of abutting consonants in different syllables with /ə/ being inserted between the final consonant of one syllable and the initial consonant of the next.

Omission of initial consonants

Omission of final consonants

Vowel Errors

Vowel substitution

Misarticulation of diphthongs

Two types of errors may occur: (1) the diphthong may be produced as two separate vowels, or (2) one component of the diphthong, usually the second, may be omitted.

Diphthongization of simple vowels

Neutralization of vowels so that the production approaches /ə/

Nasalization of vowels

---

quency cues, but may no longer be understood, thus resulting in faulty auditory monitoring and possible distorted output.

VOICE AND RESONANCE

The disorders of voice and resonance that can occur in a hearing impaired population have been listed by Magner (1971) and can be seen in Table 15-2.

The specific characteristics of voice and resonance that occur in an individual also vary greatly. It has been shown, however, that subtle quality and resonance differences occur early in the speech deterioration process of adults who have adventitious hearing impairment. These changes may be due, at

least in part, to a speaker's attempts to replace the decrease in auditory monitoring ability with an increase in tactile-kinesthetic feedback.

RHYTHM AND TIMING

Hudgins and Numbers (1942) reported three types of rhythm patterns in the speech of the deaf: correct rhythm, abnormal rhythm, and nonrhythm. They also emphasized the importance of speech rhythm on overall intelligibility by indicating that its contribution is equal to that of consonant articulation.

The relationship between rhythm and intelligibility was also supported by Hood and Dixon (1969) in their study of the physical characteristics

TABLE 15–2. Voice and Resonance Disorders in the Hearing Impaired

Strength	Resonance	Placement	Inflection
Lacking voice	Hypernasality	High pitch	Lacking variation
Lacking control of volume	Hyponasality	Low pitch	Erratic variation
Weakness		Glutteral voice	
Harshness		Erratic changes	
Breathiness			

of speech rhythm of speakers who were deaf. For the purpose of their investigation, they defined speech rhythm as composed of intonation changes, loudness changes, and two temporal factors—relative syllable duration in a sentence and rate of utterance of a sentence. They concluded that deaf speakers showed less fundamental frequency and intensity variation and greater duration of both syllables and total utterances than did normal hearing speakers. They also found that ratings of rhythm proficiency were highly correlated with the two duration measures and slightly related to intensity variation. No relationship existed between rhythm proficiency ratings and fundamental frequency variation.

A great deal of research concerning the timing and rhythm patterns of deaf speech was reviewed by Nickerson (1975). He concluded:

1. Speakers who are deaf use a slower speaking rate than normal speakers;
2. Speakers who are deaf do not make a large enough duration difference between stressed and unstressed syllables;
3. Pauses of speakers who are deaf are more numerous, longer, and/or inserted in inappropriate places;
4. Speakers who are deaf use inappropriate rhythm or syllable grouping; and
5. Speakers who are deaf demonstrate some timing problems related to speech sound production.

As with articulation and voice/resonance problems, the speech rhythm characteristics of a person who has adventitious hearing impairment will vary considerably, depending on the factors summarized earlier. It appears, however, that once speech rhythm patterns are well established, they are maintained more consistently than articulation and voice or resonance patterns. In view of their importance in speech intelligibility, however, rhythm and timing must not be overlooked.

DIAGNOSTICS FOR SPEECH CONSERVATION

RECEPTIVE SKILLS

To obtain a complete evaluation of the communication problems created by a hearing loss, both receptive and expressive skills must be explored. The initial receptive evaluation should include the items listed in Table 15-3. These data should give the audiologist information to help in medical diagnosis, to serve as a guide for aural rehabilitation recommendations, and to predict communication difficulties.

Based on the results of the initial testing, aural rehabilitation may be recommended. The receptive portion of the diagnostic evaluation would continue with a hearing aid evaluation and addi-

TABLE 15–3. The Initial Receptive Communication Evaluation

Pure tone air and bone conduction testing

Speech audiometry

    A sensitivity measure such as a speech recognition threshold (SRT) or a speech detection threshold (SDT)

    A discrimination measure such as the CID W-22 word lists

Immittance testing

Site of lesion testing

---

tional communication evaluation to assess skills with the recommended hearing aids. Additional tests or areas of exploration may include:

1. Speech recognition threshold (SRT)/speech detection threshold (SDT);
2. Speech recognition in quiet and in noise using materials with different levels of redundancy. Examples of materials are word tests, such as the Central Institute for the Deaf (CID) Auditory Test W-22, the Word Intelligibility by Picture Identification (WIPI) test, and the Monosyllable-Trochee-Spondee (MTS) test; phoneme tests (i.e., consonant and/or vowel confusion tests); and sentence tests such as the CID Everyday Speech Sentences; and
3. Prosodic feature tests, such as measures of stress pattern recognition in words and/or sentences.

SPEECH RECEPTION

The key point that must be remembered in performing an evaluation of receptive skills is that the examiner is seeking the *starting point* for auditory training, as well as attempting to obtain a measure of communication difficulty in normal listening situations. These goals may be met, at least in part, through recognition testing using the standard W-22 word lists in quiet. But, in many cases, this procedure may be inappropriate.

In some instances, the use of the W-22 word lists may result in scores near 100%, even though the client reports communication difficulty. The listen-

ing task must be made difficult enough to find the fine dividing line between success and failure. This may mean increasing the difficulty of the listening task by increasing the complexity of the material (i.e., a sentence test such as the CID Everyday Speech Sentences), by reducing the redundancy of the materials (i.e., a phoneme recognition task), or by increasing the level of background noise.

In other cases, the W-22 word lists are too difficult and the errors are so numerous and random that no patterns emerge that can be systematically incorporated into auditory training. In these instances, the task must be made easier, and this usually means selecting a closed-response set of materials. In many cases, a test such as the WIPI (Ross & Lerman, 1971) is appropriate even though the standardized norms do not apply, as the task can also be performed by adults with more severe losses. Written multiple-choice response forms can be created for adults to eliminate the picture-pointing response features. The point is that in the evaluation of receptive skills for communication purposes, the audiologist must look for a level of task difficulty where some success is achieved and yet systematic errors are made. This will be the starting level for auditory training.

The final area of auditory diagnostics involves an assessment of prosodic feature perception. The importance of this area should be fairly obvious in light of the documented importance of prosodic features in the intelligibility of speech of the deaf (Hudgins & Numbers, 1942). At present, few tests probe the area of prosodic feature perception in those with hearing impairment. One is the CID-CAT or MTS test (Erber & Alencewicz, 1976) or the expanded version of the same concept, the CID-MONSTR. The MTS consists of 4 words in each of three different stress pattern categories (monosyllable, trochee, and spondee), with the MONSTR consisting of 10 words in each of the three categories. In either case, the concept is the same. The test is scored in two ways: *first* by percentage of words recognized correctly and *second* by percentage of stress pattern recognition. In other words, if a monosyllable is presented and a monosyllable is the response, it is counted as correct in the prosodic feature scoring, even if the exact word is incorrect. In many cases of severe-to-profound hearing loss, a client is unable to receive enough phonetic information through the auditory channel to recognize the words and yet he or she can perform the stress recognition task because he or she can at least feel the patterns. In such a case, auditory training may need to start at a prosodic feature level to prevent speech deterioration in the stress and rhythm areas.

PROSODIC FEATURE PERCEPTION

A second test that is available to probe prosodic feature perception is the Stress Pattern Recognition in Sentence test (SPRIS) (Jackson & Kelly-Ballweber, 1979). This 48-sentence test consists of four repetitions of each of 12 simple sentences. Each sentence consists of 4 monosyllabic words. For each repetition of a sentence, a different word is stressed, thus giving a slightly different connotative meaning to the utterance. The subject's responses are scored in the same way the MTS is scored, first by percentage of correct sentence identification and second, by percentage of correct sentence stress pattern identification. This test has also been shown to be appropriate for an adult hearing-impaired population.

When the receptive diagnostic information is pulled together, the aural rehabilitation specialist has an indication of how much distortion the hearing loss is imposing on the incoming speech signal. This indication is derived from the audiogram, which is a frequency-by-intensity plot of hearing sensitivity across the frequency range. The speech results are an indication of how well the client is using his or her residual hearing. The areas of auditory perception that have become more difficult for the person with adventitious hearing impairment become the core of auditory training to maintain the client's speech monitoring ability. It is this speech monitoring ability that is the key to speech conservation.

EXPRESSIVE SKILLS

Articulation

Evaluation of the expressive speech skills of the population with adventitious hearing impairment follows the same basic principles as any speech evaluation. A client's articulation characteristics are evaluated with various types of materials under various conditions. The clinician is interested in obtaining information concerning usual speech sound production, error contexts and consistency, and stimulability of error sounds.

EVALUATION OF SPEECH SOUND PRODUCTION: WORD LEVEL. Several tests are commercially available to probe phoneme production at the word level, but the general thrust of the materials is toward consonant production in a younger population, using pictures to elicit responses. Any of these materials can serve the same purpose for an adult population, if written word lists rather than pictures are used as the stimulus items.

Although vowel articulation may not be of primary importance in the typical normally hearing client, it is of major concern in the speech productions of the hearing-impaired population. Errors in vowel production are common in a client with congenital hearing impairment and, as mentioned earlier, vowel errors in the form of resonance changes may be among the first to appear in the speech of those with adventitious hearing impairment. For this reason, it is critical that a test of articulation ability be selected that will probe vowel as well as consonant productions.

For the evaluation of the speech skills for those with hearing impairment, Berg (1976) recommends the Templin-Darley Tests of Articulation (Templin & Darley, 1969) or his own shortened version of this test. The Templin-Darley Tests of Articulation were designed as a basic tool of the speech pathologist to assess speech production skills at the word level of children age 3 to 8 years. The stimulus materials consist of 57 cards, each with two to four pictures used to elicit responses.

There are also printed lists of words and sentences for use with older clients for whom pictures may be inappropriate. This results in 141 items in the Templin-Darley Revised Diagnostic Test. To increase the versatility of the test, the items are combined into two specific tests and also into several groupings of sounds to meet specific purposes in testing articulation. Various units in the test are presented in Table 15-4.

Berg's shortened version of the Templin-Darley test consists of 67 items chosen to sample all vowels and diphthongs; all single consonants in the prevocalic position of words; the voiced stops /b/, /d/, and /g/; the sibilants /s/, /z/, /ʃ/, /ʒ/, /tʃ/ and /dʒ/, and the glides /r/ and /l/ in the postvocalic position; and several blends involving /s/, /r/, and /l/ with other phonemes. His suggested recording form and list of stimulus words are in Table 15-5.

Each item in this table contains the phoneme to be tested and the stimulus word that is to be used in eliciting the production. Berg also presents pic-tures that can be used with children to elicit a verbal response. In the case of the young adult who has hearing impairment, a word list to be read by the client may be substituted. The position of the phoneme within the word is specified by the *i* (initial or prevocalic), *m* (medial or intervocalic), or *f* (final or postvocalic) beside the word.

The recording form provides a blank for scoring the acceptability of each production. Any scoring code can be used, but a suggested system is to mark an omission with "om," a substitution with the phonetic symbol of the error sound, and an addition with the phonetic symbols. If the clinician's ear is trained to pick up fine production differences, a scaling system may be used to differentiate various levels of distortion. An example of one such system is:

1 = Correct production. The sound is produced correctly with no distortion.
2 = Mild distortion. The distortion would be noticeable only to the trained listener.

TABLE 15–4. Various Units in the Templin-Darley Tests of Articulation

The 50-item Screening Test

A 42-item Grouping of Consonant Singles, composed of 22 initial and 20 final consonants, which probes the client's mastery of consonant production.

The 43-item Iowa Pressure Articulation Test, which explores the adequacy of velopharyngeal closure by assessing the adequacy of oral pressure for speech sound production (Morris, Spriestersbach, & Darley, 1961).

Groupings of Consonant Clusters intended to determine the consistency of the speech sound production in various phonetic contexts.

    A 31-item /r/ and /ɝ/ Cluster Grouping made up of two- and three-phoneme clusters

    An 18-item /l/ and /ḷ/ Cluster Grouping made up of two- and three-phoneme clusters

    A 17-item /s/ Cluster Grouping made up of two- and three-phoneme clusters

    A 9-item Miscellaneous Consonant Cluster Grouping

Groupings of Vowels and Diphthongs

An 11-item Vowel Grouping

A 6-item Diphthong Grouping made up of five diphthongs and one consonant-vowel combination.

TABLE 15–5. Recording Form for Berg's Shortened Version of the Templin-Darley Test of Articulation.

1.	p (i)	pencil	35.	śm–	smoke
2.	t (i)	two	36.	skr–	scratch
3.	k (i)	cat	37.	–ks	socks
4.	b (i)	bicycle	38.	z (m)	scissors
5.	d (i)	door	39.	z (i)	zipper
6.	g (i)	girl	40.	z (f)	ties
7.	m (i)	mittens	41.	–lz	nails
8.	n (i)	nose	42.	ʃ (i)	shoe
9.	ŋ (f)	ring	43.	ʃ (m)	dishes
10.	f (i)	fence	44.	ʃ (f)	fish
11.	θ (i)	thumb	45.	ʃr–	shred
12.	v (i)	valentine	46.	ʒ (i)	Zhivago
13.	ð (i)	there	47.	ʒ (m)	television
14.	w (i)	window	48.	ʒ (f)	mirage
15.	tw–	twins	49.	tʃ (i)	chair
16.	b (f)	tub	50.	tʃ (m)	matches
17.	d (f)	slide	51.	tʃ (f)	watch
18.	g (f)	dog	52.	dʒ (i)	jump
19.	i (m)	feet	53.	dʒ (m)	engine
20.	ɪ (m)	pin	54.	dʒ (f)	cage
21.	ɛ (m)	bed	55.	ə dʒ	large
22.	æ (m)	bat	56.	ɝ	bird
23.	ʌ (m)	gun	57.	r (i)	red
24.	ɚ	car	58.	r (m)	arrow
25.	a (m)	clock	59.	pr–	presents
26.	ʊ (m)	book	60.	dr–	drum
27.	u (f)	blue	61.	str–	string
28.	o (m)	cone	62	mə	hammer
29.	aʊ (m)	house	63.	l (i)	leaf
30.	e (m)	cake	64.	l (f)	bell
31.	aɪ (f)	pie	65.	gl–	glasses
32.	ɔɪ (f)	boy	66.	–tl	bottle
33.	e (i)	sun	67.	–lt	belt
34.	s (f)	mouse			

Source: From Berg, F. S. (1976). *Educational audiology: Hearing and speech management,* p. 168. New York: Grune & Stratton. Reprinted with permission.

3 = Distortion. The distortion would be noticeable to the layman, but would not affect intelligibility.

4 = Marked distortion. The distortion would distract the average listener from the speech content.

5 = Severe distortion. The distortion is so severe that the sound is not recognizable.

The importance of such a system must be stressed. A distortion of an articulation may occur in varying degrees, and the severity of the problem may be determined by the severity of the distortions in addition to the number of phonemes involved. The clinician must be careful to judge an articulation as a distortion even if it only mildly deviates from accepted standards. The productions of persons with hearing impairment must be judged relative to normal hearing articulation and not judged as acceptable as long as it is intelligible. Intelligible speech may very well be distorted speech.

Additional commercially available tests to probe articulation skills at the word level include the Fisher-Logemann Test of Articulation Competence (Fisher & Logemann, 1971) and the Goldman-Fristoe Test of Articulation (Goldman & Fristoe, 1969). The Fisher-Logemann Test of Articulation Competence consists of 109 picture stimuli on 35 bound cards for use with adults as well as children. Eleven of the cards may be used as a screening test. The test explores the production of all English phonemes, both vowels and consonants, and provides for errors to be analyzed in terms of distinctive features.

The Goldman-Fristoe Test of Articulation was developed mainly to assess consonant articulation ability. The test materials consist of 35 pictures of objects or activities. The client names the pictures or answers questions to provide a total of 44 responses. Even though vowels are not specifically probed, the Sounds-in-Words Subtest contains all of the vowels and diphthongs except /U/, /ɑ/, and /ɔI/ and, therefore, could be used for that purpose.

EVALUATION OF SPEECH SOUND PRODUCTION: SENTENCE LEVEL. When attention is focused on a particular phoneme in a word articulation test, it may be possible for a client to produce it correctly. Yet when the same sound occurs in conversation, it is omitted, distorted, or erroneously produced in some way. For this reason, it is important to explore the ability of a person with adventitious hearing impairment to produce speech sounds in sentences or in conversation as well as in isolated words.

Several tests are also available to probe articulation ability at the sentence level. One is the Templin-Darley Tests of Articulation mentioned earlier. The sentence portion of this test consists of 141 items constructed and organized to evaluate the same speech sounds as in the word portion.

A second test is the sentence form of the Fisher-Logemann Test of Articulation Competence. It consists of 15 sentences printed on a single card and is designed to test all English speech sounds. The sounds within the sentences are arranged so that each voiced-voiceless cognate pair of consonants is tested in the same sentence. Consonants having no cognate are grouped into sentences according to manner of production. The last four sentences probe productions with the sounds being arranged in terms of place of articulation. A third test for sentence articulation is the Sounds-in-Sentences Subtest of the Goldman-Fristoe Test of Articulation. This subtest was developed to systematically assess speech sound production in a context similar to conversational speech. The material consists of two stories that are read by the examiner while the client watches sets of four or five pictures. The subject then repeats the story in his or her own words, using the pictures to guide the narrative and, thus, the words in the speech sample. The result is content-controlled speech that approximates conversational speech.

EVALUATION OF ERROR CONTEXTS AND CONSISTENCY. It is possible that the misarticulations that occur in a specific phonetic context do not occur in others. This inconsistency of production creates a need to examine speech sound articulation in more than one context. This type of evaluation is possible with the Templin-Darley Tests of Articulation, as certain consonants occur in a number of different clusters. The results may reveal one or more contexts in which a speech sound is correctly produced. This information, in turn, will serve as an aid in the remediation process.

Berg (1976) recommends the Deep Test of Articulation by McDonald (1964) to explore error contexts in the speech of children who have hearing impairment. This test would also be appropriate for use with adults having adventitious hearing impairment. The materials consist of both a picture and a sentence version, with the items being designed to test the articulation of the 13 speech sounds in several phonemic contexts: /s/, /z/, /r/, /l/, /ʃ/, /tʃ/, /dʒ/, /θ/, /ð/, /k/, /g/, /f/, and /v/.

The information obtained from such a probe may reveal one or more contexts in which speech is produced correctly. This, in turn, allows selection of appropriate materials for training when kinesthetic and visual feedback mechanisms are being used to lead to correct production in all contexts.

EVALUATION OF STIMULABILITY OF ERROR SOUNDS. In planning a speech conservation program, it is helpful if information is available concerning the susceptibility of a particular sound to remediation. Although Snow and Milisen (1954) indicate that prognostic information can be obtained by comparing productions obtained from pictorial and oral articulation tests, it is not known whether this information can be applied to an adventitiously hearing-impaired population in which articulation skills are deteriorating rather than developing. It is known, however, that those sounds that are most susceptible to correction are the easiest to incorporate into a kinesthetic feedback program, as the target is already closely approximated.

The suggested procedure for stimulability testing (Milisen, 1954) involves having the client watch and listen carefully while the examiner produces the sound two or three times. Then the client is to imitate the production. This procedure is carried out using all sounds that were misarticulated on the previous test and should place the sounds in speech of varying complexity (i.e., in

isolation, in nonsense syllables, and in words). The task is repeated twice and the best response is recorded.

Specific materials for probing error stimulability include some of the tests already discussed. The Templin-Darley Tests of Articulation include directions for determining how well the client can produce the error sounds when furnished with optimal auditory-visual stimulation. The directions indicate that each sound is to be presented in isolation, in a syllable, and in a word as well as in a consonant cluster within a word. The Goldman-Fristoe Test of Articulation also includes a Stimulability Subtest where the simplest level of production is the syllable followed by words and simple sentences.

Two tests have been designed specifically to probe stimulability of error sounds. The first is the Carter-Buck Prognostic Articulation Test (Carter & Back, 1958) which consists of a spontaneous word portion and an imitated nonsense syllable portion. The second is the Van Riper-Erickson Predictive Screening Test of Articulation (Van Riper & Erickson, 1968), which consists of nine imitation tasks, placing sounds in isolation, syllables, words, and sentences. Because both of these instruments were developed to predict which children will master articulation errors without therapy, it is uncertain if these materials could be applied to persons with adventitious hearing impairment. However, even though the normative scores will not apply, the concept may still be applicable.

Voice and Resonance

Evaluation of the voice and resonance characteristics of a client who has hearing impairment could be conducted on several levels. One might be by *direct observation* of the laryngeal and velar mechanisms to investigate any physical change in structure. This should always be done in cases of vocal deviation to rule out any underlying pathological cause.

A second level for voice and resonance evaluation is at the *listening level*, where the clinician's ear is used to make a value judgment concerning the acceptability of the production. Because intelligibility is seldom affected by voice or resonance changes only, the clinician must decide if a deviant production is inappropriate based on age, sex, regional, and physical considerations.

The third level of evaluation is the *acoustic level*. This involves direct measurement of the various parameters of the voice or resonance, such as fundamental frequency, fundamental frequency variation, intensity, periodicity, or degree of nasal resonance. Several instruments are available for such measurement as well as for feedback in therapy and are reviewed in Appendix-15.

The typical voice and resonance evaluation involves systematically obtaining a representative sample of a client's communication skills. Ideally, this sample is tape-recorded for future reference. The verbal behavior should include a sample of conversational speech; impromptu speech such as telling a story, oral reading, or singing; and automatic speech such as counting or naming the days of the week. The sample should be listened to carefully for deviations in laryngeal function (tension, breathiness, harshness), pitch level and variability, intensity, and resonance, with acoustic measures being made whenever possible. This information describes the client's typical vocal behavior.

A second part of the voice/resonance evaluation involves additional probes aimed at further assessing capabilities. Procedures designed to evaluate laryngeal function include:

- Ask the client to produce an /ɑ/ with a gradual soft onset (i.e., /hɑ/). Listen for an abrupt onset of voicing at both loud and soft intensities.
- Listen specifically for how voice is initiated in the various speech samples. That is, listen to whether it occurs within a hard or a soft glottal attack.
- Time three sustained productions of /ɑ/ using normal air intake. Listen for efficient use of air. A client with normal breath support should be able to produce the sustained vowel for 12 to 13 seconds.
- Observe what happens to vocal quality with changes in intensity.
- Stand behind the client and place your finger on the thyroid cartilage. Feel for the presence of laryngeal tension during phonation.
- Have the client clear his or her throat and listen for a potential change in clarity.

Procedures aimed at evaluating pitch level and variability include:

- Ask the client to produce a clear /ɑ/ at the lowest pitch level possible and then to slide through the scale to the highest level he or she can reach without going into falsetto phonation. This will give an indication of the client's pitch range.
- Ask the client to produce a vocalized sigh. This should occur near his or her habitual pitch level.
- Compare the client's pitch level during oral reading with that of a sustained vowel.
- Compare the client's pitch level at various intensities. Look for the direction, frequency, and extent of pitch breaks.

Procedures for the evaluation of intensity include:

- Observe what changes occur in intensity level with changes in pitch.
- Have the client vary his or her pitch at a given intensity and observe the control that can be achieved.
- Observe the client's intensity at various rates.
- Note whether the client is using clavicular or diaphragmatic breathing during phonation.

Finally, procedures for the evaluation of resonance include:

- Observe velopharyngeal mobility on vocalization.
- Listen for variation of nasality with different vowels.

- Listen for changes in nasality with increased loudness.

Because of the difficulty involved in making subjective judgments of nasality, acoustical measures of this parameter may assist the clinician in making difficult clinical decisions. The degree of nasal resonance in an individual's speech can be quantified using the Kay Elemetrics Model 6200 Nasometer. With this device, oral and nasal components of a subject's speech are sensed by microphones on either side of a sound separator that rests on the subject's upper lip. The signal from each microphone is filtered and digitized by custom electronic modules. The data are then processed by a computer and accompanying software. The resultant signal is a ratio of nasal to nasal-plus-oral acoustic energy. This ratio is multiplied by 100 and expressed as a "nasalance" score. Therefore, the Nasometer provides a numeric output indicating the relative amount of nasal acoustic energy in an individual's speech. This nasalance value has been shown to provide useful information about the speech of normal speakers (Seaver, Dalston, Leeper, & Adams, 1991), patients with velopharyngeal impairments (Dalston, Warren, & Dalston, 1991), and patients with severe-to-profound hearing impairments (Cain, Seaver, Jackson, & Sandridge, 1989). In addition, data have been presented about the use of nasometry in monitoring changes in acoustical energy associated with changes in velopharyngeal activity among normal speakers (Dalston, 1989; Dalston & Seaver, 1990; Seaver & Dalston, 1990).

Following the overall voice and resonance evaluation, specific problems in laryngeal function, pitch, intensity, and resonance are identified in various contexts. As in articulation testing, the next step is to evaluate the stimulability of the various errors. Again, this information will influence decisions for therapy and will be beneficial when tactual-kinesthetic feedback is being stressed for an individual who has hearing impairment.

Rhythm and Timing

The diagnostic evaluation of the rhythm and timing characteristics of the speech of a person with adventitious hearing impairment involves analysis of the same type of speech sample that was collected for the evaluation of voice and resonance. In this case, the clinician judges the utterances for the following rhythm characteristics: overall rate (i.e., too fast, too slow, monotonous), uncontrolled variability, patterned rate, phrasing, variation in syllable duration, and variation in pause duration. Physical measurements need to be made to support listener judgments.

TECHNIQUES FOR SPEECH CONSERVATION—GENERAL THERAPY PROCEDURES

In the 1974 report from the ASHA Committee on Rehabilitative Audiology, Freeland and associates stated that the single most important component of the aural rehabilitation program was the selection and fitting of a hearing aid. The earlier the use of amplification is initiated and the more success in restoring usable hearing, the less chance there is that the ability to monitor speech will deteriorate. However, in cases in which auditory self-monitoring is lacking, auditory training and speechreading training need to be integral parts of the speech conservation program. If the auditory skills that are achieved with amplification are insufficient to allow auditory monitoring, kinesthetic monitoring must be substituted and may be reinforced with visual and/or vibrotactile training aids.

Speech conservation training may include several areas of emphasis depending on which expressive skills are affected by the hearing loss. These areas include articulation, voice and resonance, and rhythm training.

A comprehensive speech perception and production diagnostic evaluation will uncover specific problems that potentially may develop or that have already started to develop with a decrease in auditory feedback. The goals in a speech conservation program, therefore, are, first, to maintain existing production skills that are in danger of deteriorating, and second, to correct any errors that have developed as a result of the adventitious hearing loss.

Several methodologies are available for speech production training and each varies somewhat in principle and procedures. In general, however, the majority of techniques involve presentation of a *model production* by the clinician followed by an imitated response from the client. The role of the clinician in this paradigm is one of orienting the client to the task, stimulating the production, listening carefully to the response and judging its acceptability, offering immediate feedback and reinforcement, and providing continuous evaluation of progress. The procedures are designed to shape an articulation, voice, or rhythm error into a correct production. Changes in behavior across time can be charted using procedures such as precision therapy described by Waters, Bill, and Lowell (1977).

Van Riper (1972) has provided a comprehensive outline of his classic stages of articulation therapy that includes numerous suggestions for training that are appropriate for use in therapy on behalf of adults with hearing impairment. Although ear training techniques receive a major emphasis in his program, Van Riper stresses that the clinician is free to choose other techniques to stimulate correct production. Production is considered at four specific operational levels, with progression from one to the next suggested but not required. Therapy can be initiated at whatever level seems appropriate. These four successive levels are:

1. The isolated sound level
2. The syllable level
3. The word level
4. The sentence level

From this last step, carryover into controlled conversation and finally into everyday speech is initiated.

Within this framework, Van Riper outlines four steps to be used in training the error sounds at each of the four levels. These steps are:

1. **Have the client identify the error and the standard of production for the specific sound.** This stage normally involves ear training aimed at drawing attention to the specific characteristics of the sound in question, so that the client will begin to discriminate it from incorrect productions. Obviously, this task may be difficult for the client who has adventitious hearing impairment, so some modification is needed.

   With a hearing-impaired population, this stage can be considered the one in which a client learns the characteristics of the sounds that may potentially degrade or that have begun to deteriorate. This involves auditory training and speechreading training, both being integral components of the speech conservation program. It also includes vocabulary building of terms such as those listed by Fisher (1975) that will be used in the correction process. This might include terms such as *harsh, hoarse, glottal attack, denasal, voiced,* and others. It must be remembered that this stage involves no production by client. It involves only structured input and comparison.

2. **Have the client scan and compare his or her own utterance with the standard.** This step also involves ear training, but now it is intended that the client carefully listen to his or her own productions rather than to the speech of others. It is assumed at this stage that the client clearly understands the characteristics of the target to which comparisons are made with his or her own approximations.

   Again, at this stage, modification is needed for an adult hearing impaired population. What really is involved at this level is self-monitoring through whatever perceptual channel is needed. Hopefully, residual hearing will play a major role, especially with amplification. Visual, tactual, and kinesthetic feedback information is used to supplement the auditory channel.

Van Riper stresses that this monitoring ability will occur at various times for each production as therapy progresses. Initially, the error will be recognized after it occurs, next while it is happening, and finally, it can be identified and hopefully corrected before the production.

3. **Have the client vary his or her production until the correct sound is achieved.** At this stage, the new sound is being taught to the client. Van Riper (1972) explains that this must occur at all levels mentioned earlier (isolation, syllable, word, sentence, and conversation) through a process in which the client is taught to vary his or her utterance. Five methods are outlined for approaching this task: progressive approximation, auditory stimulation, phonetic placement, modification of sounds that are produced correctly, and key words.

The first method, progressive approximation, is Van Riper's method of choice. It involves shaping the response and rewarding productions that are progressively approaching the target.

The second method, auditory stimulation, involves ear training followed by imitation of the correct production. With the adult client who has hearing impairment, the approach should be termed auditory-visual stimulation, stressing the inclusion of speechreading cues that must be emphasized. The success of this method will vary depending on the amount of residual hearing and the success of amplification.

The third method, phonetic placement, involves the clinician instructing the client in the specific placement and movement of the articulators for the production of each sound. The position is analyzed, and changes in positioning are suggested. Application of this approach involves the use of a mirror, diagrams, models to guide placement, and visual speech aids for additional feedback.

The fourth method, modification of correct sounds, involves having the client produce a sound which he or she can do correctly and then gradually vary the production to approximate the target for the error sound. For example, the client may be instructed to slide the tongue forward from an /ʃ/ production to approximate the /s/ that normally is in error.

The fifth method, key words, requires utilization of words in which the defective sound can be produced correctly and thereby makes use of information obtained from the evaluation of error contexts described earlier. Emphasis is placed on the sound within the contexts where success is achieved and the production is then introduced in isolation and in other words. Kinesthetic and auditory monitoring from one area to the next is stressed.

Another method for obtaining correct sound production is the *motokinesthetic method* described over 40 years ago by Young and Stinchfield-Hawk (1955). This method has application with a hearing-impaired population, as auditory stimulation is supplemented by tactile stimulation. This method is based on the assumption that by manipulation of the client's articulators, the clinician can establish tactile and kinesthetic feedback patterns. The client, therefore, passively produces the sound as the clinician manipulates the articulators until the movement pattern is established.

4. **Have the client stabilize the correct sound production so that it becomes automatic.** This stage involves activities at each level of complexity designed to strengthen a new sound production so that it occurs automatically without any conscious effort. To achieve this goal, Van Riper (1972) suggests such activities as simultaneous writing and talking, babbling, unison speech, and negative practice. It is important that this stage be concentrated on until the production has stabilized in all contexts and has become a natural part of the client's speech repertoire.

Within the framework just outlined, the clinician is free to deal with the speech production errors that have been identified. Specific techniques within the areas of articulation, voice and resonance, and rhythm are needed to accomplish various remediation goals. Several sources are now commercially available that delineate remediation techniques for individual speech sounds and various voice, resonance, and rhythm disorders. The reader is urged to refer to these sources for specifics. They include texts by Calvert and Silverman (1975), Fisher (1975), Haycock (1942), Ling (1976), Magner (1971), and Vorce (1974).

ARTICULATION TRAINING

In articulation training, the ability to imitate a correct sound depends to a large degree on the ability to perceive the model. In cases of adventitious hearing loss, this means using visual and tactile stimulation in addition to auditory stimulation. Several of the references, therefore, stress the need for the use of a mirror and somewhat slower speech to emphasize the positioning of the articulators.

Tactile cues are also outlined and described by the various authors to be used to improve feedback during stimulation. As an example, production features can be cued in the following ways:

1. Voicing (vowels and /b, d, g, v, ð, z, ʒ, dʒ, m, n, ŋ, l, r, w, j/) can be cued by feeling the vibration at the side of the throat and then contrasting it with voiceless productions.
2. Nasality (/m, n, ŋ/) can be cued by feeling the vibration at the side of the nose.
3. Plosives (/p, t, k, b, d, g/) can be cued by the pulse of air that can be demonstrated by holding a strip of paper or the back of a hand in front of the mouth.
4. Fricatives (f, θ, s, ʃ, tʃ, v, ð, z, ʒ, dʒ/) can be cued by the flow of air that can be demonstrated by holding a strip of paper or the back of a hand in front of the mouth.

These tactile cues can be used in the initial shaping of the sound, but should soon be faded as more emphasis is placed on kinesthetic feedback. They are appropriate in isolation, syllables, or words but may not be successful at the sentence level.

VOICE AND RESONANCE TRAINING

Remedial treatment of voice and resonance disorders involves establishing new habits or preventing bad habits from forming. The same basic therapy outline is used. First the problem must be identified and then analyzed in terms of its specific defect. Next, the voice or resonance pattern must be varied in some way, and eventually the new voice or resonance level must be located through successive approximation. Stabilization of the new pattern in communication is then stressed.

The texts mentioned earlier also offer suggestions for the remediation of voice and resonance disorders. A few examples are summarized in Table 15-6.

RHYTHM AND TIMING TRAINING

With an adventitiously hearing-impaired population, errors in rhythm and timing can be prevented or corrected, for the most part, by reviewing the importance of stress and rhythm and by reviewing some already established rules. This may be accomplished by employing some form of prosodic notation in the therapy session to stress phrasing, stress, and inflection rules.

Several such notation systems are available, but one that appears fairly straightforward is presented by Calvert and Silverman (1975). They suggest a system that indicates pitch changes with a curving line, loudness by the height of a horizontal line above a syllable, and duration by the length of the line. Slash marks are used to indicate phrasing. They present the illustration:

TABLE 15–6. Suggestions for the Remediation of Voice Disorders

To correct excessive harshness:

    Conduct exercises to reduce laryngeal tension such as head rotation and alternate tension and relaxation

    Improve speech breathing

    Emphasize easy vocalization through the use of aspirated voice onset

To correct excessive breathiness:

    Improve speech breathing

    Have the client count and increase the number he or she reaches on one inhalation

    Increase the loudness somewhat

    Have the client grip his or her chair or hold a book at shoulder height and count while the increased laryngeal tension is felt

To correct pitch problems:

    Work on sustaining vowels at an even, optimum pitch level

    Write *high* at the top and *low* at the bottom of a blackboard to give visual feedback as pitch is lowered and raised

    Use a resonating object such as a balloon, a cardboard tube, or metal, and have the client feel the high and low vibrations

To correct intensity problems:

    Improve speech breathing

    Again, use a resonating object to demonstrate intensity changes

To correct resonance disorders:

    Lower vocal pitch or increase vocal intensity slightly to reduce general nasality

    Alternate productions of /n/ and /a/, first slowly and then more rapidly stressing kinesthetic awareness

    Combine alternate /m/ and /n/ productions, again emphasizing the feeling of the nasal resonance

"Yesterday was a beautiful day/but

today//it's terrible."

These markings can then be incorporated into activities that draw attention to the importance of stress, rhythm, and timing in speech perception and production.

SUMMARY

Even though specific programs of receptive training and speech conservation are being conducted, the client who has adventitious hearing impairment is still faced with the problem of maintaining a healthy attitude toward communication. It is all too easy to withdraw socially and admit defeat in difficult listening or speaking situations. If this happens, a vicious circle is formed, for it is only through continuous practice that speech skills can be maintained, if a hearing loss is severe. Because of this, the need often arises for assertiveness training and counseling to change attitudes toward a hearing impairment. This assertiveness training can be an integral part of the aural rehabilitation program, along with hearing aid orientation, speechreading, auditory training, and speech conservation.

Communication assertiveness involves, first of all, motivation. This motivation is obvious for the client, but it should also involve family members. Their role in the maintenance of speech skills is critical, so it is important that they also understand the consequences of an auditory impairment. Next, specific problem communication areas must be identified and the client must be desensitized so that he or she no longer avoids difficult situations. At this point, the client becomes involved in receptive training and speech conservation work, so that a client learns to vary his or her behavior gradually and in positive ways to approximate more correct productions or improved speech monitoring skills. These newly learned skills are then stabilized in general communication situations.

Speech conservation, therefore, involves not only training in specific monitoring and production skills, but also support for communication, in general. The clinician must be aware that a hearing loss will affect many phases of a client's life and all these phases need to be considered in an aural rehabilitation program.

REFERENCES

Berg, F. S. (1976). *Educational audiology: Hearing and speech management*. New York: Grune and Stratton.

Binnie, C. A., Daniloff, R. G., & Buckingham, H. W., Jr. (1982). Phonetic disintegration in a five-year-old following sudden hearing loss. *Journal of Speech and Hearing Disorders, 47*, 181–189.

Cain, M. E., Seaver, E. J., Jackson, P. L., & Sandridge, S. A. (1989, November). *Aerodynamic and nasometric assessment of velopharyngeal functioning in hearing-impaired speakers*. Paper presented at the annual meeting of the American Speech-Language-Hearing Association, St. Louis, MO.

Calvert, D. R., & Silverman, S. R. (1975). *Speech and deafness*. Washington, DC: Alexander Graham Bell Association for the Deaf.

Carter, E. T., & Buck, Mc K. (1958). Prognostic testing for functional articulation disorders among children in the first grade. *Journal of Speech and Hearing Disorders, 23*, 124–133.

Dalston, R. M. (1989). Using simultaneous photodetection and nasometry to monitor velopharyngeal behavior during speech. *Journal of Speech and Hearing Research, 32*, 195–202.

Dalston, R. M. & Seaver, E. J. (1990). Nasometric and phototransductive measurements of reaction times among normal adult speakers. *Cleft Palate Journal, 27*, 61–67.

Dalston, R. M., Warren, D., & Dalston, E. (1991). Use of nasometry as a diagnostic tool for identifying patients with velopharyngeal impairment. *Cleft Palate-Craniofacial Journal, 28*, 184–188.

Erber, N. P., & Alencewicz, C. M. (1976). Audiologic evaluation of deaf children. *Journal of Speech and Hearing Disorders, 41*, 257–267.

Fisher, H. B. (1975). *Improving voice and articulation* (2nd ed.) Boston: Houghton Mifflin.

Fisher, H. B., & Logemann, J. A. (1971). *The Fisher-Logemann Test of Articulation Competence*. Boston: Houghton Mifflin.

Freeland, E. E., Hill, M. J., Stream, R. W., Tobin, H., & Costello, M. R. (1974). The audiologist: Responsibilities in the habilitation of the auditorily handicapped. Report of the Committee on Rehabilitative Audiology. *Asha, 16*, 68–70.

Goldman, R., & Fristoe, M. (1969). *Goldman-Fristoe Test of Articulation*. Circle Pines, MN: American Guidance Service, Inc.

Haycock, G. S. (1942). *The teaching of speech*. Washington, D.C.: Alexander Graham Bell Association for the Deaf.

Hood, R. B., & Dixon, R. F. (1969). Physical characteristics of speech rhythm of deaf and normal-hearing speakers. *Journal of Communication Disorders, 2*, 20–28.

Hudgins, C. V., & Numbers, F. C. (1942). An investigation of the intelligibility of the speech of the deaf. *Genetic Psychology Monographs, 25*, 289–392.

Jackson, P. L., & Kelly-Ballweber, D. (1979, November). *Auditory stress pattern recognition in sentences*. Paper presented at the annual meeting of the American Speech-Language-Hearing Association, Atlanta, GA.

Kent, R. D. (1976). Anatomical and neuromuscular maturation of the speech mechanism: Evidence from acoustic studies. *Journal of Speech and Hearing Research, 19*, 421–447.

Ling, D. (1976). *Speech and the hearing-impaired child: Theory and practice.* Washington, DC: Alexander Graham Bell Association for the Deaf.

Magner, M. (1971). *Speech development.* Northampton, MA: Clarke School for the Deaf.

McDonald, E. T. (1964). *A Deep Test of Articulation.* Pittsburgh: Stanwix House, Inc.

Milisen, R. (1954). A rationale for articulation disorders. The disorder of articulation: A systematic clinical and experimental approach [Monograph]. *Journal of Speech and Hearing Disorders, 9,* (Suppl. 4), 5–17.

Morris, H. L., Spriestersbach, D. C., & Darley, F. L. (1961). An articulation test for assessing competency of velopharyngeal closure. *Journal of Speech and Hearing Research, 4,* 48–55.

Nickerson, R. S. (1975). Characteristics of the speech of deaf persons. *Volta Review, 77,* 342–362.

Ross, M., & Lerman, J. (1971). *Word Intelligibility by Picture Identification.* Pittsburgh, PA: Stanwix House, Inc.

Seaver, E. J. & Dalston, R. M. (1990). Using simultaneous nasometry and standard audio recordings to detect acoustic onsets and offsets of speech. *Journal of Speech and Hearing Research, 33,* 358–362.

Seaver, E. J., Dalston, R. M., Leeper, H. A., & Adams, L. E. (1991). A study of nasometric values for normal nasal resonance. *Journal of Speech and Hearing Research, 34,* 715–721.

Snow, K., & Milisen, R. (1954). Spontaneous improvement in articulation as related to differential responses to oral and picture articulation tests. The disorder of articulation: A systematic clinical and experimental approach. [Monograph]. *Journal of Speech and Hearing Disorders, 9,* (Suppl. 4), 45–49.

Templin, M. C., & Darley, F. L. (1969). *The Templin-Darley Tests of Articulation* (2nd ed.). Iowa City: University of Iowa.

Van Riper, C. (1972). *Speech correction: Principles and methods* (5th ed.). Englewood Cliffs, NJ: Prentice-Hall.

Van Riper, C., & Erickson, R. L. (1968). *Predictive Screening Test of Articulation.* Kalamazoo, MI: Western Michigan University.

Vorce, E. (1974). *Teaching speech to deaf children.* Washington, DC: Alexander Graham Bell Association for the Deaf.

Waters, B. J., Bill, M. D., & Lowell, E. L. (1977). Precision therapy—An interpretation. *Language, Speech and Hearing Services in Schools, 8,* 234–244.

Young, E. H., & Stinchfield-Hawk, S. (1955). *Moto-kinesthetic speech training.* Palo Alto, CA: Stanford University Press.

APPENDIX-15:

VISUAL AND VIBROTACTILE SPEECH TRAINING AIDS

One of the central concepts in speech conservation with adults having adventitious hearing impairment is the effective use of amplification and auditory training to make maximum use of residual hearing. There are several cases, however, in which additional sensory cues are needed to provide monitoring in speech conservation programs. Several devices are commercially available that provide visual and/or vibrotactile information. A few of these are described here.

KAY SONAGRAPH

This instrument provides visual cues for consonant and vowel articulation, duration, voice, pitch, and nasality. The cues are in the form of a sonagram, which is a time-by-frequency-by-intensity representation of the acoustic parameters of speech. A printout of this sonagram is available to become a permanent record.

Contact: Kay Elemetrics
12 Maple Avenue
Pine Brook, NJ 07058-9798

SERIES 700 SOUND SPECTROGRAPH

This instrument provides visual cues for consonant and vowel articulation, duration, voice, and pitch. The cues are in the form of a printed spectrogram, which becomes a permanent record.

Contact: Voice Identification, Incorporated
P.O. Box 714
Somerville, NJ 08876

LUCIA SPECTRUM INDICATOR

This instrument provides visual cues designed to give feedback in vowel and voiced-voiceless fricative training. The instrument displays frequency by intensity spectral information in light displays. Intensity is represented in 10 levels of 3.5 dB each, and frequency information covers a range of 180–6800 Hz. There is also a mirror attached to the front of the unit for speechreading cues.

Contact: SI America
1900 Rittenhouse Square
Philadelphia, PA 19103

VISIBLE SPEECH APPARATUS

This instrument provides visual cues for the training of fricative and plosive consonants, vowels, and pitch. The display is a light indication system, which provides spectra of speech sounds. Frequency is displayed with 16 bandpass filters and covers a range of 90–8000 Hz. The intensity of each column is in 10 dB steps. Color coding on the display indicates fundamental frequency and first and second formants.

Contact: Precision Acoustics Corporation
501 5th Avenue, Room 704
New York, NY 10017

VISIPITCH

This device displays fundamental frequency and amplitude information from the speech signal in real time on the screen for biofeedback information. On-screen cursors allow precise measurements of a speech sample to be made and stored for later use. A hardcopy printout is also available.

Contact: Kay Elemetrics Corporation
12 Maple Avenue
Pine Brook, NY 07058-9798

PM SERIES OF PITCH INSTRUMENTS

This system consists of a microphone, a 12-inch video monitor, and an electronics module with keyboard that houses up to four separate programs. The available programs include (1) PM100—split screen speech "modeling"; (2) PM201—split screen—pitch on the upper half, loudness on the lower half; (3) PM300 long duration (up to 23 minutes) pitch analysis; (4) PM301—long duration analysis of pitch, loudness, and pause time; and (5) PM302—perturbation ("jitter") analysis. A hardcopy printout is available.

Contact: Voice Identification, Inc.
P.O. Box 714
Somerville, NJ 08876

VOCAL-2

This instrument provides visual cues for word stress patterns, fundamental frequency, and /s/ phoneme production. The visual display is on a split screen with an example placed on the top and client trials on the bottom. It displays intensity by time patterns, frequency by time patterns, or /s/ information.

Contact: Madsen Electronics
908 Niagara Falls Blvd.
North Tonawanda, NY 14120-2060

S-INDICATOR

This instrument provides visual and tactile information to train /s/ as well as other voiceless fricatives. The visual cues are from a display panel with a meter and a light to indicate the quality of the /s/ production. There is an optional vibrator, which also signals a correct /s/.

Contact: SI America
1900 Rittenhouse Square
Philadelphia, PA 19103

F_O-INDICATOR

This instrument provides visual cues to train pitch level, intonation, phonation, voiced versus voiceless articulation, and breath control. The visual cues are from a meter and from red and green lights that monitor the limits of the frequency range. A contact microphone is held against the throat and the rate of vocal fold vibration is measured within a range of 50 to 550 Hz.

Contact: SI America
1900 Rittenhouse Square
Philadelphia, PA 19103

NASOMETER

This device is a microcomputer-based instrument designed for use in both the assessment and treatment of nasality problems. It measures the ratio of acoustic energy from the nasal and oral cavities in real-time and displays the resulting nasalance value on the screen of the computer monitor. This allows the device to be used as a biofeedback tool to modify abnormal nasal resonance.

Contact: Kay Elemetrics Corporation
12 Maple Avenue
Pine Brook, NY 07058-9798

N-INDICATOR

This instrument provides visual cues for training nasalization, denasalization, and phonation. A contact microphone is held against the nose and the intensity of nasal vibration is shown on a meter. The panel has a green and a red light to signal when the production is below or above a 50% deflection point.

Contact: SI America
1900 Rittenhouse Square
Philadelphia, PA 19103

VOICE LITE

This instrument provides visual and tactile cues for use in training phonation, loudness, duration, stress and rhythm, voiced versus voiceless articulation, nasality, and breath control. The visual cues are provided by a translucent dome with a light that reacts to sound. Brightness of the light is intensity related. The unit has an optional microphone that indicates nasality, and it also has an optional tactile stimulator.

Contact: Behavioral Controls, Incorporated
3818 West Mitchell
Milwaukee, WI 53215

MONO-FONATOR AND POLY-FONATOR

The mono-fonator is designed for individual use, with the poly-fonator designed for use by one to four clients. This instrument provides tactile information for use in training stress, duration, phonation, and some phonetic features. The clinician or client speaks into the microphone and the vibrational cues are produced by a vibrator placed on the hand. Earphones are included for auditory information.

Contact: Siemens Hearing Instruments
10 Constitution Ave., P.O. Box 1397
Piscataway, NJ 08855-1397

TACTAID II AND TACTAID 7

The Tactaid II is a wearable, two-channel vibrotactile aid that makes use of two vibrators. It is worn in its own pouch or on a belt, and has an input jack for direct hookup to FM systems along with a built-in T-coil for telephone and audio system use. The Tactaid 7 uses seven channels and seven vibrators to produce a unique tactile pattern for every phoneme.

Contact: Audiological Engineering Corporation
35 Medford Street
Somerville, MA 02143

END OF CHAPTER EXAMINATION QUESTIONS

CHAPTER 15

1. What is the critical age for predicting speech deterioration following the onset of significant hearing loss?

2. What can be done to prevent further deterioration of speech following the onset of hearing loss? What is the process?

3. The first speech sounds to deteriorate with the onset of permanent hearing loss are

4. What are the typical characteristic timing and rhythm patterns of "deaf speech"?

5. The negative influence of a precipitous high-frequency sensorineural hearing loss on speech involves

6. According to the author, the primary goal of speech conservation is

7. Also, according to the author, to obtain a complete evaluation of the communication problems created by a hearing loss, both _____ and _____ skills must be explored.

8. What two primary tests of articulation are available that probe the stimulability of error sounds?

9. How are the voice and resonance characteristics of hearing-impaired adults evaluated? What measures are used?

10. According to the author of this chapter, the goals of a speech conservation program on behalf of hearing-impaired adults are to _____ and _____.

END OF CHAPTER ANSWER SHEET

Name _____ Date _____

CHAPTER 15

1. _____

   _____ .

2. _____

   _____

   _____

   _____ .

3. _____

   _____ .

4. _____

   _____

   _____

   _____ .

5. _____

   _____ .

6. _____

   _____ .

7. _____and

_____ .

8. _____and

_____ .

9. _____

_____

_____

_____ .

10. _____and

_____ .

PART IV

Considerations For the Older Adult Client

Who are These Aging Persons?

■ JUDAH L. RONCH, PH.D. ■

In working with speech, language, and hearing problems, older persons inevitably constitute a significant portion of the clients seen. As ours is a youth-oriented society in which myths, stereotypes, and half-truths about aging abound, practitioners must confront and overcome any personal biases about aging. Not to do so dilutes the strength of the therapeutic endeavor and disempowers older clients.

This chapter is presented to help service providers appreciate the realities of aging—both positive and negative and to, thereby, better understand and serve older persons with the problems discussed elsewhere in this book. Answers to the question, Who are these aging persons? often are based on idealizations, personal experiences, or ignorance of the realities of aging in the United States. Attitudes toward the aged can be discerned from the words people use to designate this segment of society and by the psychological devices younger persons use to differentiate and distance themselves from "them."

For many years, the old have occupied a position of respect and, throughout history, society's vocabulary has reflected this attitude. Terms such as senator, alderman, guru, presbyter, and veteran all have their roots in the words of various languages for "old," and denote a position of honor and privilege by the aged. The current public vocabulary about aging includes expressions such as "golden age" and "senior citizen," but the aged more often are referred to in private by words denoting negative attitudes about being old and fears about aging. Older people are often seen as—and easily can feel—obsolete in a rapidly changing, youth-oriented technological society. Twenty-five years ago Butler (1975) termed aging people "the neglected stepchildren in the human life-cycle." Despite more social awareness about the anticipated cohort of aging "Baby Boomers," to be old is still not "OK."

Currently, the aged constitute about 15% of the U.S. population, or about 1 in every 8 Americans.

The percentage of people 65 and older has tripled since 1900, with the largest gains being made in the number of people beyond the age of 85. Americans beyond the age of 65 numbered almost 40 million in 1996. By the year 2031, when the baby boom population peak reaches age 70, there will be about 76 million older persons in the United States.

To answer the question posed by this chapter's title, emphasis is placed on integrating data about aging with examples of the diverse people who make up the aged group. The author hopes that those who work with the aged may begin to develop a realistic understanding of the diverse nature of the aging process, in general, as well as appreciate the diversity of aged persons as individuals. As the coming "Age Wave" (Dychtwald & Flower, 1989) leads to greater numbers and heterogeneity of older persons, service providers will have to keep finding new, more accurate answers to the question: Who are these aging persons?

DIMENSIONS OF AGING: IS THERE A TYPICAL AGING PERSON?

There are as many experiences of aging as there are aged persons. However, some characteristics of the aging population merit attention, so that the overall circumstances of the aged may be better understood.

Gerontologists have found it useful to divide the aged into the "young-old" (ages 45–64), the "old" (ages 65–74), and the "old-old" (people more than 75 years of age) (Shanas & Maddox, 1976). There are significant differences in the life tasks, abilities, resources, health, and other factors between 50- or 55-year-olds and people age 75 and a greater likelihood (although not a certainty) of similarities among a cohort of 65-year-olds. Still, all persons of the same age do not experience aging in the same way, and physiological, psychological, and social changes do not unfold solely as determined by chronological age.

Biological aging refers to the length of life in years, *psychological aging* to the adaptation capacity of the organism, and *social aging* to the performance of a person relative to his or her culture and social group (Birren & Renner, 1977). Rather than look solely at a person's chronological age to explain what we see, greater insight can be derived by looking at the multiple spheres in which a person grows, develops, and gains experience and satisfaction. People of the same biological age are quite diverse in their adaptational capacity and social accomplishments. It is, therefore, important to realize that each aged person must be appreciated both in terms of his or her similarity to other elders and the lifelong patterns of individuality brought into the later stage of life.

THE INTERDISCIPLINARY PERSPECTIVE

Because an elderly person is really a complex organism attempting to interact with an equally complicated environment in a dynamic, mutually demanding way, it is necessary to understand the many factors that make up the world of an older adult. It has been said that no single discipline, whether it be psychiatry, sociology, biology, or economics, can claim to offer a comprehensive explanation of how aged people act, think, and feel or what the multiple determinants of their behavior are (Busse & Pfeiffer, 1977).

If a practitioner is to obtain maximum understanding of the whys and hows of behavior in the aged, knowledge must be gathered and integrated into an interdisciplinary perspective to develop the most accurate, parsimonious, and factually powerful explanation available. In this light, it becomes apparent why a psychologist must know that depression in an old woman who barely survives on a monthly Social Security check cannot

be alleviated by psychotherapy alone. Treatment of the woman's social and economic realities takes primacy over delving into her childhood experiences. The process means that psychotic behavior in an old man can appropriately be alleviated by having a physician adjust his insulin dose rather than give him an antipsychotic drug or write him off as "senile." Similarly, professionals who are trained along the traditional lines of disciplinary focus must be willing and able to understand the need to know as much as possible about all of the factors outside of their primary discipline that must be in harmony, if an aged client is to function well and enjoy life.

QUALITY OF LIFE ISSUES: STRESS AND ITS SOURCES

Older age is a stage of life in which people have multiple stresses, with a dwindling number of internal and external resources available to reduce the stress and promote comfort. Eisdorfer and Wilkie (1977) define a stressful stimulus as one that is "perceived in some way as potentially harmful, threatening, damaging, unpleasant, or overwhelming to the organism's adaptive capacity" (p. 252). Different events will be variably stressful depending on the time of life they are experienced (Neugarten, 1973) and the experience of the person with such stimuli. Many sources of stress can be consequences of the objective reality of the aging process, and the biological, psychological, and social changes that may occur (Lawton, 1977). These changes induce further stress, depending on an individual's personality and characteristic response to change and resultant success, helplessness, or loss of control. The period of life beginning in the fifth decade and continuing for the rest of one's life is a time when many aspects of a person's world undergo change. Typically, there are significant, stressful changes in these areas (among others):

- The family of origin: parents, brothers, and sisters become ill or die and children relocate or die.
- Marital relationship: death or illness of spouse, estrangement due to empty-nest syndrome, pressures caused by retirement.
- Peer group: friends die or become separated by geographical relocation for health, family, or retirement.
- Occupation: retirement and loss of work-role identity.
- Recreation: opportunities may become scarce because of physical limitations or unavailability from lack of interest or opportunity or few resources.
- Economic: income reduced by retirement; limited income tapped by inflation or medical costs not covered by insurance.
- Physical condition: loss of youth with concomitant biological decline of body function, causing risk of poor health and its emotional consequences.
- Emotional/sexual life: loss of significant others through death, separation, and reduction in sexual activity because of societal expectations, personal preference, or death of partners.

DEGREE OF STRESS

Old age is a difficult and stressful time because two things occur in a complementary and simultaneous manner. The various domains of life, as suggested previously, are prone to stresses in greater numbers. At the same time, each domain is the source of a greater degree of stress than in the past. When experienced in combination with the all-too-often limited biological, psychological, and societal resources available to alleviate stress quickly and efficiently, the organism's ability to adapt is compromised. In other words, older persons may experience more stress in increasing domains of life (with fewer internal and societal supports available to them to promote a comfortable readaptation) that they are likely to become disor-

ganized and feel incapable of coping. It then becomes imperative that stress be reduced as much as possible, if an older person is to successfully negotiate the potentially treacherous old age using their retained strengths and continue to derive pleasure from living.

If treatment is to be appropriate, effective, and dignified, it must be borne in mind that rarely can a person of any age (and surely not an aging person) benefit from a helping relationship that does not recognize the total life situation of the client. It is only when the *total person* is addressed and understood that discrete problems may be most beneficially remediated and stress effectively reduced.

THE PSYCHOLOGICAL EXPERIENCES OF AGING

Aging is a biopsychosocial experience and, as such, requires understanding aging as a series of mutually interactive processes rather than as discrete events (Cohen, 1988). The changes of physical aging, for example, produce both a discrete decrement in organ efficiency (e.g., heart output, visual ability, hearing acuity, gastrointestinal motility) as well as a subjective emotional reaction to the resulting functional losses. Thus, it is not how much physical, psychological, or social loss a person experiences, but what that particular loss means to that individual that is the key to understanding the personal, subjective impact of the loss. An avid reader whose vision is failing from macular degeneration, a social gadabout who cannot hear well, and a housekeeper who can no longer dust when she gets anxious because she fractured a hip and cannot walk are three of the many possible individual examples of persons at risk for strong emotional reactions, including anxiety and depressions.

The many physical changes that accompany aging have a psychosocial impact not only on a person's subjective sense of well-being and self-esteem (i.e., they must potentially confront the evidence of their "agedness"), but on service providers as well. The service providers' usual techniques, common habits, style of helping, and ability to provide services in their usual settings may have to be modified to assist some older persons. This may prompt providers to think about (consciously or unconsciously) their feelings about aging and youth, control and power, emotions about aging persons they care about, and other psychosocial issues relevant to the providers' personal experiences.

PSYCHOLOGICAL CHANGES: MYTH AND REALITIES

The myth that cognitive and emotional regression are inevitable with advancing years still persists with surprising tenacity, despite a growing body of evidence to the contrary. Sadly, many health care professionals and the lay public adamantly hold on to the old stereotypes about "normal senility" and a "second childhood" characterized by selfishness, childlike dependency and stubbornness, or passivity in older persons. These nihilistic notions not only lower the self-esteem of older persons who believe these to be the cause—rather than the result—of psychosocial and/or physical problems, but often contribute to the exclusion of older persons from sources of potential help for their difficulties.

COGNITIVE ABILITIES

Normal aging does include an inevitable, clearly demonstrable decline in cognitive abilities that compromises normal function. Measures of cognitive performance used to investigate age differences in memory, learning, and intelligence are complicated by the intervening effects of sociocultural factors, for example, educational experience, ethnicity, test motivation, and overall physical

health of individuals participating in the studies. Changes in learning capacity, intelligence (as reflected on a standardized test performance), or memory ability that are purely a function of chronological aging have been difficult to demonstrate. It is even less clear how any changes found by investigations reflect actual changes in everyday functional abilities experienced by older persons in the general population.

Anyone working with an older person would probably find it beneficial to ascertain each older client's ability to attend to, remember, and integrate new information in an appropriate and consistent way as they work together. A client's sensory difficulties, comfort about being in a helping relationship, fear of failure, embarrassment at receiving assistance or having a problem, or personality variables (see the following paragraphs) will frequently have a more profound effect on his or her ability to change behavioral patterns than will any change in cognitive ability. A factor such as cognitive style (how one attempts to understand, analyze, and solve problems) is usually an important dimension that has more relevance to how older persons adapt to new demands than do intelligence, memory capacity, or learning ability in a cognitively intact older person.

EMOTIONS AND AGING

The emotional life of older persons is the outcome of how life-long personality traits and tendencies are affected by the experiences one has while aging. Longitudinal stability of personality, interests, sources of emotional gratification, comfort with emotional expression, and characteristic defenses used against anxiety appear to be consistent over time (see Britton & Britton, 1977; Butler & Lewis, 1982; Neugarten, 1973). Thus, the myth that older people develop rigid, cantankerous, infantile, or controlling personalities *because they have grown old* is not substantiated, and it may reflect observations of older people who are unhappy, powerless, ill, debilitated, or responding emotionally to their life circumstances.

Rather than aging leading to a personality change, negativities are more likely either an exacerbation of lifelong personality traits or a response to stress and helplessness not exclusive to later life in any particular older person or the aging population as a whole. (How many times do younger persons react similarly when angry, depressed, helpless, or sick?) People at any age will react to unpleasant or upsetting circumstances in their own characteristic fashion. It is negative stereotyping of the aged to conclude that because a particular response is seen in an older person that it is a universal, age-related reaction.

Oberleder (1966) observed many years ago that emotional characteristics of older persons seem to fall into four basic categories:

1. The psychological characteristics that result from societal expectations about old age, to which the aged adhere to expedite conformity and acceptance (social aging).
2. The psychological reactions to the losses and deficits incurred as a result of the aging process.
3. Those characteristics that are independent of age and arise from poor health.
4. The psychological characteristics that are basic to a elderly person and have been so throughout the individual's life span.

Later life is like other phases of the life span, in that a person has much developmental work to do to attain a sense of well-being. Some developmental tasks of later life include (Butler & Lewis, 1982):

1. The desire to leave a legacy and develop a feeling of continuity (through money, land, ideas, children, or students).
2. The need to serve an "elder" function and to share their knowledge and experience (a task made difficult by the information explosion and rapid obsolescence of old knowledge by new technology).

3. An attachment to familiar objects (as in the case of Mr. W., who wanted to leave his awful rooming house, but feared losing his books, clothes, and other treasured possessions if he couldn't find a new room of adequate size).
4. A change in the sense of time, resulting in a sense of immediacy, with emphasis on the "here and now."
5. A sense of the finite life cycle and a need for completion, resulting in a renewed emphasis on spirituality, religion, and culture. (In Japan, old men frequently begin to write poetry as a way of expressing their relationship to life.)
6. A sense of consummation and fulfillment, described by Erikson (1959) as the drive toward ego-integrity. Some authors (Butler & Lewis, 1982; Lieberman & Tobin, 1983) have observed that it is common for the elderly to seek to escape their identities through the continuous process by which people "create the self" (Scheibe, 1989), using distortion and other devices that help a person look better in his or her own eyes.

The continuity of emotional development in later life has been described as occurring along multiple lines of development rather than on a unitary dimension (Colarusso & Nemiroff, 1981). This provides a more accurate notion of the complexity of emotional issues faced by aging persons and allows clinicians to help clients focus on specific issues that, either alone or interactively, are producing emotional distress. Domains such as: (1) intimacy, love, and sex; (2) the body; (3) time and death; (4) relationship to children; (5) relationship to parents; (6) work; (7) finances; and (8) play are dimensions that are operative throughout the adult years. These require a person's ongoing psychological work, if he or she is to attain mastery and well-being. An individual's ability to meet the many, often taxing demands made by the realities of aging are central in determining an older person's emotional satisfaction and personal development.

AFFECTIONAL AND SEXUAL NEEDS

It is widely believed that sexuality in the aged is (or ought to be) nonexistent and that if it does exist, it is surely a sign of aberrant, senile, "second childhood" regression. This belief is based on many subjective feelings, such as that old people are physically unattractive or that any sexuality in older persons is wrong and shameful (a notion probably rooted in the anxieties young people have about the sexual activity of their parents).

Actually, sex is a matter of great concern in later life and is the source of many satisfactions, as well as emotional problems. Masters and Johnson (1966) found that sexual response in old age diminished in speed and activity, but not in the capacity to achieve orgasm. They also found that like most aspects of the behavior of older persons, levels of sexual activity tended to be stable over a person's lifetime. Consistent with the cultural values of this cohort, older men may be more active sexually than are women. However, the preponderance of women and the lack of sexual partners among the older population, as well as older people's belief in their asexuality, are strong influences working against sexual satisfaction in the aged.

PSYCHOLOGICAL DYSFUNCTION IN LATER LIFE

It is noteworthy that although generalizations about aging may be becoming more accurate as a result of recent methodologically sophisticated research, there is no universal aging experience. Although psychological problems are not inevitable or universal in older persons, there are certain realities that predispose older persons to being particularly vulnerable to mental dysfunction. Notable among these is the likelihood that physical problems influence mental functioning and vice versa in a dynamic fashion. Cohen (1988) illustrates four paradigms of effect:

1. **Severe psychological stress leads to compromised physical health.** For example, depression leads to dehydration, which can cause electrolyte imbalance and a resulting dementia may be misdiagnosed as Alzheimer's disease.
2. **Physical disorder leads to psychiatric disturbance.** For example, hearing loss leads to delusions (and possibly late-life paraphrenia).
3. **Coexisting mental and physical disorders** develop a mutual, dynamic influence on the clinical course of each. For example, congestive heart failure leads to depression, with indirect suicidal behavior, specifically, failure to take medication properly. Further deterioration of cardiac status may result in deepened depression.
4. **Psychosocial factors** affect the course of physical health problems. For example, elderly persons with diabetes living in isolation are at risk for complications as a result of inadequate monitoring of diet and medication. Physical sequelae (e.g., infection of an extremity) may result, exposing the patient to the risk of amputation and further functional dependence.

Thus, it becomes prudent to consider a "multifactorial basis" for emotional and physical disorders in the elderly (Cohen, 1988), and to engage in coordinated interdisciplinary treatment modalities and procedures when emotional difficulties surface. Older persons faced with psychosocial, physical, economic, existential, and other stressors are at risk of developing anxiety disorders, depression, and other serious, but treatable, psychological disturbances.

DRUGS AND OLDER PERSONS

As more medications are used by the elderly than by any other age group (Lamy, 1980), it is likely that service providers who treat the older person will frequently encounter potential or actual negative side effects of the many drugs older people take. Medication for cardiovascular problems and psychotropic prescriptions are the most frequently prescribed and have a high potential for harmful side effects in older persons (Salzman, 1984). Psychotropics include antidepressants, antianxiety drugs, antipsychotics (neuroleptics), sleeping medications, and lithium (for bipolar disorder).

The dynamics of drug action in an older person's body mean that psychotropic drugs are particularly likely to take longer to work, stay in the body for a longer period of time, and are more potent than they would be in a younger person's body (Cohen, 1988). Older persons are also at risk for drug-drug and drug-food interactions. With the great numbers and variety of drugs used by older persons, it is not rare that an older person experiences confusion, depression, and other changes in psychological functioning because of the mind-altering effects of medication mixtures. This picture is further compounded when older persons use drugs differently than as they are prescribed. Sensory problems (a person is unable to read the small print on the bottle), difficult-to-open containers, "informal" prescriptions given out by neighbors, self-medication (if the doctor says one pill works, two will work more quickly), and other factors lead to medication usage errors that have been found to be rather significant in older persons (Vestal, 1985).

Too frequently, drugs are used to achieve the impossible in the lives of older persons. The risk-to-benefit ratio of using each drug must be considered. Drugs will not erase the effects of aging. They will not make a person suddenly pleasant or amiable or get them to change their life-long personality traits. And they will most certainly not make aging free of discomfort and travail.

SOCIAL PATHOLOGIES: ISOLATION, POVERTY, HOMELESSNESS

Social isolation may be the most significant cause of mental illness in the aged. It may occur as a result of multiple friend and family losses and from the lack of opportunity to form new relationships. This problem is especially severe for women beyond the age of 65, nearly half of whom are widows, and who, by the age of 75, outnumber men nearly 2 to 1. Both men and women frequently sense the loss of their role in society, their sense of being needed, and a concomitant loss of self-esteem.

Contrary to popular opinion, the aged usually are not abandoned by family and friends. In 1987, according to the U.S. Bureau of the Census, 67% of older noninstitutionalized elders lived in a family setting. These living arrangements, however, may be undesirable and family conflicts may arise under the pressure of new stresses or unresolved family issues. As the number of frail elderly in our society increases, so can the strain on family relationships, health, and resources.

Economic conditions under which the majority of aged must survive further compound the stresses of old age. The major source of income for older families continues to be Social Security, which does not compensate for present increases in the cost of living. According to the U.S. Bureau of the Census, in 1987 the median income for men over the age of 65 was $11,854 and $6,734 for women. About 3.5 million elderly persons were below the poverty level. Poverty brings with it an increased risk of chronic disease, dental problems, poor vision, and hearing impairments, along with poorer medical care.

Thus, isolation, poverty, and other social pathologies may contribute significantly to psychological dysfunction in later life. For half of America's older persons, poverty does not become reality until after they reach age 65. Although each cohort of aged persons is coming to later life with more financial resources, better education, increased longevity, and better prospects for a longer and healthier retirement, many older persons find that retirement and the accompanying loss of income (about 50%) exposes them to the harrowing effects of poverty or near-poverty conditions.

RETIREMENT

The primary factor in producing a drastic change in economic status for the aged is retirement. Although this is an event that is sometimes eagerly sought, it is more regarded as an achievement in principle but dreaded as a crisis when it actually occurs. There are many reasons for this, particularly in our work-oriented society. One is that retirement is actually a two-pronged process, wherein a person "retires" both economically and socially and loses a work role, a source of identification, and frequently the social contacts and relationships the work situation provided (Back, 1977). In addition, retirement in a society like that in the United States involves withdrawal from productive activities and the transfer of control over resources to others. With the latter, power is yielded to the next generation, and the formerly powerful must cope with a new degree of powerlessness.

The newer, more youthful cohorts of older persons increasingly have discovered that one must retire *to* something, be it leisure or a second career (or third) (often lasting 20 years). Not all people feel that unstructured leisure time is satisfying. With increased longevity, growth in numbers, and rising pension incomes, more middle- and working-class elders are finding that they retain a greater proportion of their power than did the generations before them. Thus, older persons are increasingly better prepared for an active retirement phase of life by virtue of improved economic, political, and educational opportunities. Recent economic boom-times have not distributed our nation's wealth equally throughout all social classes, however, and the number of older people retiring with limited means is not declining, despite prosperity for some.

ETHNICITY AND AGING

To be old and poor is bad enough. To be old, poor, and a member of a racial or ethnic minority (particularly if one is a woman), places the aged person in "multiple jeopardy" (Butler, 1975). African-Americans, Latinos, Native-Americans, Asians, and other minority groups are over-represented among the old poor and under-represented among the nation's elderly. African-Americans, for example, compose 10% of the population but only 8% of the elderly population and they are disproportionately represented among the poor aged, especially if they are women.

The situation is worse for elderly Latinos who compose only 4% of the total population. There are about 11.2 million Latinos elderly in the continental United States, including persons of Cuban, Mexican, Puerto Rican, and South American origin, and this number does not include the almost 8 million undocumented aliens of Latin origin. Wherever they live, their life expectancy is significantly lower than their White counterparts. In Colorado, for example, the average White resident lives to be about 67.5 years old, while an Hispanic lives an average of only about 56.7 years (Butler & Lewis, 1982).

Native-Americans get to be old much less frequently than any other group in the U.S. In 1970, there were estimated to be almost 800,000 Native-American elderly, nearly half of whom lived in the western United States, although there are no reliable estimates of the number of elderly among the group. One is shocked to discover that their average life expectancy is only 47 years. Those few Native-Americans who do grow old are left impoverished and cut off from traditional family supports (Butler & Lewis, 1982).

ETHNICITY

African-Americans, Asians, Latinos, Native-Americans, and other minorities continue to be outnumbered by White elderly, but the minority population has been growing and by the year 2025 it will compose 15% of the elderly population. Assistance with health care costs is of special concern to minority elderly, because of social discrimination that has resulted in poverty, malnutrition, and resulting health problems. Cultural and language differences, as well as lack of cultural sensitivity among health care providers often keep the minority elderly from using available public programs. Quality of life for these elderly is, therefore, bleak because of lack of educational opportunities, low level of employment with few health benefits and small pensions, and poor health care.

Many minority elderly speak English as their second language. As they age, they may find it difficult to adjust to the differences in language and culture between themselves and the rest of society. For many, English fluency may decrease as they begin to experience difficulty in the way that their central nervous system processes their second language. This can be compounded in persons with hearing loss and/or dementia whose anxiety approaches panic and terror as they are less and less able to understand what they hear and increasingly revert to their native language in an attempt to make order out of linguistic-cognitive chaos.

THE AGED AND THE FAMILY

The family life of older persons does not escape change as people age and, as in other aspects of life, there is a high likelihood of loss. Stresses may take their toll on marital relationships, for example, when one spouse becomes ill and thereby creates a "disequilibrium" in the marriage and the inherent caregiving balance of old role relationships. Whether it be a physical or emotional illness that is the problem, the "patient" can come to be resented for all of the demands for care (realistic or exaggerated) he or she makes on the healthier spouse. The latter, in turn, may become depressed and angry and also develop physical and/or psychiatric symptoms. Typically, the woman becomes the one "in charge" and is confronted with her own feelings about being a caregiver and decision maker. In some relationships, however, men play this role, or two friends of the same sex who share a household may assign roles based on the realities of need and not gender. Thankfully, there is a increasing recognition of the opportunities for personal growth available when someone becomes a caregiver (e.g. to give back, to have one's nurturing side emerge), and caregiving is no longer seen only as a burden.

When a spouse is not available or capable of providing needed supports, the next most sought resource is a child. Four-fifths of older persons have living children (Butler & Lewis, 1982), and about 83% of these aged live less than an hour's distance away from one child (Sussman, 1986). Almost 30% of the elderly reside with their children, a phenomenon reported to be on the increase in rural areas (Sussman, 1976). Usually it is a daughter to whom older persons turn in times of crisis (Brody, 1981), a choice usually based on long-standing family dynamics and gender role expectations. The one chosen may be the one who lives closest, is the wealthiest, was the most- or least-favored as a child, who wishes to increase his or her favor with the parents, or who historically could be prevailed on by the siblings to do almost anything.

Many older persons are now developing alternative living arrangements, which involve cohabitation of unmarried men and women (because either their children or Social Security regulations discourage marriage), moving in with a friend of the same sex to allow for companionship and reduced expenses, or entering communal residences where tasks are shared by all residents. The advent of assisted living has revolutionized elder care and created a viable but not yet universally affordable option.

Relationships between aged parents and their children (who are usually in "middle age," that is, caught in the middle of their parents and their children) do not necessarily deteriorate, nor do all marriages. Although some families are able to be involved positively and happily with each other no matter what stresses arise, others may be fraught with tension, guilt, anxiety, and multigenerational unhappiness. In most cases, the outcome is influenced significantly by the nature of the family relationship as it had been for years and not as a result of the aging process of some of its members.

FEELINGS OF CAREGIVERS ABOUT AGING PERSONS

Butler (1975) coined the term "ageism" to denote the "systematic stereotyping of and discrimination against people because they are old, just as racism and sexism accomplish this with skin color and gender" (p. 12). Much of this bigotry functions to provide a temporary distance between younger generations and their own eventual aging, although long-lived ageists stand to become objects of their own prejudice (Butler & Lewis, 1982). Comfort (1977) points out that "even Archie Bunker confines his bigotry to groups he will never join." People with negative attitudes about the aged also tend to have more negative attitudes toward people who are physically or mentally disabled and ethnic minorities, especially Blacks (Kogan, 1961). The vulnerability for elderly persons with such "multiple jeopardies" is significant.

Professionals in many fields have been found to have definite prejudices against treating elderly patients (Butler & Lewis, 1982). Some of the reasons for this may be that the aged stimulate the anxiety and conflicts professionals have about their own aging and aging relatives, the belief that old people cannot be helped so professional expertise and time is wasted on "senile" or soon-to-be-dead patients, that it is a waste of their good training, or that they are uncomfortable "giving" to an emotionally demanding older person in what is unconsciously perceived as an incongruous role reversal (Group for the Advancement of Psychiatry, 1971).

On a realistic level, many professionals find it difficult to give as much of themselves as the aged client or patient demands of their nurturing or social interaction. An older person often will want to talk about his or her children, tell old stories, or do anything to hold the attention of the often overworked professional. When one does not have an audience or a responsive and regular conversation partner, the "ticket of admission" often can be a physical complaint. This may be evident as hypochondriasis, a depressive equivalent, but the complaint of physical illness or other symptom really can be understood as a safe way of saying "I want to be taken care of" (Pfeiffer, 1973). These complaints usually are about a physical problem, as psychological or emotional problems are too stigmatic or too threatening to talk about.

Just as all older persons are not sick or needy, it is equally unrealistic to perceive aged persons as all being "lovely," "wonderful," and otherwise without human faults. Such stereotyping usually hides fears about one's own aging and an inability to see older persons as people first. The tendency to idealize and romanticize aging and aged persons projects a wish for one's own future and projections about how lovely it would be to be treated as faultless and ideal. It is essentially demeaning and infantilizing—hence dehumanizing.

SUMMARY

An aged person, although undergoing changes in almost every aspect of life, is fundamentally no less like him- or herself than in the earlier part of life. In the later, as in every other life stage, individual differences are maintained, with no reduction in the dimensions or magnitude of variation. Despite myths, stereotypes, and prejudicial distortions to the contrary, people retain their essential personalities and continue to manifest most of their essential abilities to adapt and change as they become old. Major sources of inability to cope or adequately adapt come mainly from the severe stresses and limited resources that the elderly experience in a variety of ways, depending on genetics, life experiences, past and present environment, and traditional ways of dealing with life.

Knowing older persons as people who possess characteristic individuality and a lifetime of experience enables the most productive possible relationship with them. In addition, it aids in establishing fertile ground for the development of their trust and thus encourages an older person to assume an optimistic, strength-based, growth-oriented approach toward treatment as well as toward life. Nothing is worse than for older persons to perceive the negative, impatient attitude of those who purport to help them, but who have, in fact, given up hope of providing appropriate aid simply because the person in need is old. In many cases, calming reassurance and objective listening do wonders in reducing anxiety and encouraging older persons to mobilize their own resources to help produce improved functioning.

Who, then, are these aging persons? The question might be rephrased to ask not only who, but what are they like, and why are they so. The answers are crucial not only to the achievement of a full understanding of the aged, but on a most personal level, to ourselves, for we are all, ultimately, aging persons.

REFERENCES

Back, K. W. (1977). The ambiguity of retirement. In E. W. Bussee & E. Pfeiffer (Eds.), *Behavior and adaptation in late life* (pp. 78–98). Boston: Little, Brown.

Birren, J. E., & Renner, V. (1977). Research on the psychology of aging. In J. E. Birren & K. W. Schaie (Eds.), *Handbook of the psychology of aging* (pp. 3–21) New York: Van Nostrand Reinhold.

Britton, J. H., & Britton, J. O. (1972). *Personality changes in aging.* New York: Springer.

Brody, E. (1981). "Women in the middle" and family help to older people. *The Gerontologist, 21,* 471–480.

Busse, E. W., & Pfeiffer, E. (1977). Functional psychiatric disorders in old age. In E. W. Busse & E. Pfeiffer (Eds.), *Behavior and adaptation in later life* (pp. 158–211). Boston: Little, Brown.

Butler, R. N. (1975). *Why survive? Being old in America.* New York: Harper & Row.

Butler, R. N., & Lewis, M. (1982) *Aging and mental health* (3rd ed.). St. Louis, MO: C.V. Mosby.

Cohen, G. (1988). *The brain and human aging.* New York: Springer.

Colarusso, C., & Nemiroff, R. (1981). *Adult development.* New York: Plenum.

Comfort, A. (1977, April 17). Review of *Growing old in America* by D. H. Fischer. *New York Times Book Review,* pp. 6–11.

Dychtwald, K. & Flower, J., (1989). *Age wave.* Los Angeles, CA: Jeremy P. Tarcher.

Eisdorfer, C., & Wilkie, F. (1977). Stress, disease, aging and behavior. In J. E. Birren & K. W. Schaie (Eds.), *Handbook of the psychology of aging* (pp. 251–275). New York: Van Nostrand Reinhold.

Erikson, E. (1959). The problem of age identity, in Identity and the life cycle. *Psychological Issues, 1,* 101–164.

Group for the Advancement of Psychiatry. (1971). *Aging and mental health: A guide to program development* (Vol. 8). New York: Author.

Kogan, N. (1961). Attitudes toward old people: The development of a scale and an examination of correlates. *Journal of Abnormal Psychology, 62,* 616–626.

Lamy, P. (1980). *Prescribing for the elderly.* Littleton, MA: PSG Publishing.

Lawton, M.P. (1977). Impact of the environment on aging and behavior. In J. E. Birren & K. W. Schaie (Eds.), *Handbook of the psychology of aging* (pp. 276–301). New York: Van Nostrand Reinhold.

Lieberman, M., & Tobin, S. (1983). *The experience of old age.* New York: Basic Books.

Masters, W. H., & Johnson, V. E. (1966). *Human sexual response.* Boston: Little, Brown.

Neugarten, B.L. (1973). Personality changes in late life: A developmental perspective. In C. Eisdorfer & M. P. Lawton (Eds.), *The psychology of adult development and aging* (pp. 311–335). Washington, DC: American Psychological Association.

Oberleder, M. (1966, November). *Psychological characteristics of old age.* Paper presented at the U.S. Department of Public Health Geriatric Training Conference, Philadelphia.

Pfeiffer, E. (1973). Interacting with older patients. In E. W. Busse & E. Pfeiffer (Eds.), *Mental illness in later life* (pp. 5–18). Boston: Little, Brown.

Salzman, C. (Ed.). (1984). *Clinical geriatric psychopharmacology*. New York: McGraw-Hill.

Scheibe, K. (1989). Memory: Identity, history and the understanding of dementia. In L. E. Thomas (Ed.), *Research on adulthood and aging: The human science approach*. Albany, NY: SUNY Press.

Shanas, E., & Maddox, G. L. (1976). Aging, health and the organization of health resources. In R. H. Bin-

stock & E. Shanas (Eds.), *Handbook of aging and the social sciences* (pp. 592–618). New York: Van Nostrand Rienhold.

Sussman, M. B. (1986). The family life of old people. In R. H. Binstock & E. Shanas (Eds.), *Handbook of aging and the social sciences* (pp. 229–252). New York: Van Nostrand Reinhold.

U.S. Bureau of the Census. (1988). [Data published in *A profile of older Americans.*] Long Beach, CA: American Association of Retired Persons.

Vestal, R. (1985). Clinical pharmacology. In R. Andres, E. Bierman, & W. R. Hazzard (Eds.), *Principles of geriatric medicine.* (pp. 85–109) New York: McGraw-Hill.

END OF CHAPTER EXAMINATION QUESTIONS

CHAPTER 16

1. Currently, the aged constitute _____ % of the United States population, and by the year 2000, those more than age 65 years were more than _____ million strong.

2. Describe and explain the difference between biological aging and social aging.

3. List five different life events that might be stressful to an elderly person.
   a.
   b.
   c.
   d.
   e.

4. Who are the "young-old," the "old," and the "old-old"?

5. Oberleder, as presented by the author, describes four categories of emotional characteristics of older persons. What are they?
   a.
   b.
   c.
   d.

6. Explain the four realities listed by the author that predispose older persons to being particularly vulnerable to mental dysfunction.
   a.
   b.
   c.
   d.

7. What are two risk factors involved with older persons taking drugs/medications?
   a.
   b.

END OF CHAPTER ANSWER SHEET

Name _____ Date

CHAPTER 16

1. _____ percent _____ people

2. _____

_____

_____

_____

_____

_____

_____

3. a.

   b.

   c.

   d.

   e.

4. "young-old" _____

_____

"old" _____

_____

"old-old" _____

_____

5. a.

b.

c.

d.

6. a.

b.

c.

d.

7. a.

b.

8. a.

b.

9. _____

_____

_____

_____

_____

_____

_____

8. What are two prejudices that some professionals are found to possess that may negatively influence their treatment on behalf of older adults?

a.

b.

9. Describe the "multifactorial basis" for emotional and physical disorders in the elderly as presented by the author of this chapter.

Hearing Loss in Older Adulthood

■ RAYMOND H. HULL, Ph.D. ■

It is a common observation that a reduction in auditory acuity, accompanied by a frustrating decline in speech understanding, frequently accompanies advancing age. If we are to provide meaningful diagnostic and aural rehabilitative services to older persons with this disorder, it is important to understand the nature of the auditory problem that accompanies aging to the extent that past and current literature provides.

INCIDENCE OF HEARING LOSS IN OLDER ADULTHOOD

There are almost as many estimates of the amount of hearing loss among older adults as there are professionals assessing or treating those who possess it. Because of the complexity of presbycusis (hearing loss that accompanies aging), incidence studies such as the Public Health Service National Health Surveys have resulted in data of questionable reliability. Much of this questionable data appears to result from a lack of reliable criteria for describing hearing impairment in older age.

The inability to arrive at a consistent criteria appears related to the definitions used to describe "hearing impairment" by those establishing failure criteria. We do know that older persons are more likely to have a hearing impairment than younger people. For example, according to the National Center for Health Statistics (1994a), only 5% of people between 3 and 17 years old have some degree of hearing impairment. The same study suggests that between ages 18 and 44 years, 23% possess hearing impairment. Between ages 45 and 64 years, the estimated incidence rises to 29%. At age 65 and above, the incidence is estimated at 43%. Among the latter 43%, approximately one-half are found among the 65–74 year age group, and one-half are among those 75 years and older (National Center for Health Statistics, 1994b).

It is interesting to note that since the 1971 Health Interview Survey (National Center for Health Statistics, 1975), the number of persons with hearing impairment is estimated to be 53.4% greater than the 13.2 million persons reported to have hearing loss in 1971. According to the National Health Interview Survey (NHIS) report (National Center for Health Statistics, 1994a), a significant proportion of this increase is due to the increase in the aging population during that 23-year period. According to the National Center for Health Statistics (1994a), in 1971 there were 69 persons per 1,000 population with hearing impairment and, in 1991, the incidence was 86.1 per 1,000. And, the NHIS (1994) report stresses the relationship between aging and hearing loss (National Center for Health Statistics, 1994a). Table 17-1 presents comparative data on the number of persons with impaired hearing between 1971 and 1991.

Among nursing home (health care facility) populations, Schow and Nerbonne (1980) found the incidence of hearing loss to be more than 80%, with an earlier study (Chafee, 1967) finding the incidence to be nearly 90%. Persons who reside in health care or nursing home environments are also generally a more frail elderly population and, of course, the incidence of various disorders will certainly vary from nursing home to nursing home, depending on the type and purpose of the nursing home and the characteristics of the residents.

Historically, there has been some controversy about the estimates of hearing loss among older adults. The figures have varied as much as 30% among surveys. The problem appears to revolve around the complexities common to presbycusis that make this disorder a difficult one to diagnose accurately. For example, some elderly individuals with significant difficulties in understanding speech (a common symptom in presbycusis) also may be found to not have a hearing loss indicative of such a severe impairment in speech understanding.

Conflicting viewpoints regarding the symptoms of presbycusis and conflicting audiometric data may have contributed to inconsistent inci-

TABLE 17–1. Population, Prevalence, Crude and Age-Adjusted Prevalence Rates, and Change Since 1971 for Persons 3 Years and Over With Reported Hearing Loss: United States 1971, 1977, and 1990–1991 Average Annual.

Item	1971	1977	1990–1991
All persons 3 years of age and over (in thousands)	191,602	202,936	235,688
Prevalence of hearing trouble (in thousands)	13,228	14,240	20,295
Percent increase in prevalence since 1971	—	7.7	53.4
Number with hearing trouble per 1,000 persons	69.0	70.2	86.1
Percent increase in prevalence rate since 1971	—	1.7	24.8
Age-adjusted number with hearing trouble per 1,000 persons[1]	75.3	73.6	86.1
Percent change in age-adjusted prevalence rate since 1971	—	−2.5	14.0

[1]The 1971 and 1977 prevalence rates are age-adjusted to the average 1990–1991 population.

Reprinted with permission from the *National Center For Health Statistics, U.S. Department of Health and Human Services*, March, 1994.

dence figures over the years. However, even though some current survey figures regarding presbycusis appear to be rather realistic, estimates reported by practicing audiologists would indicate that the incidence of hearing impairment that can interfere with communication among the approximate 33 million persons aged 65 years and beyond may be greater than anticipated—as high as 60% (Hull, 1992c), although earlier estimates indicate that the percentage may be as high as 80% (Brock, 1975).

WHAT IS PRESBYCUSIS?

Of all the handicaps that affect the aged, the inability to communicate with others due to hearing impairment can be one of the most frustrating and can result in other sociopsychological problems. The loss of auditory sensitivity that is the result of aging is *presbycusis*. This term has for many years been used to describe the defective hearing of old people" (Schaie, Warner, & Strother, 1964, p. 453).

Over four decades ago the term was accurately used to describe a multidimensional disorder

that includes the pathology associated with aging, impaired auditory sensitivity, temporal discrimination, auditory judgment, and associated social and psychological difficulties (Hinchcliffe, 1959). Hinchcliffe (1962) in his early studies defined the pathology of presbycusis as (1) an impairment of auditory-threshold sensitivity, frequency discrimination, temporal discrimination, sound discrimination, auditory judgment, and speech discrimination; (2) a lowering of the higher frequency limit; and (3) decreases in the interpretation of distorted speech and the ability to recall long sentences.

MORE THAN JUST A HEARING LOSS

Although there are many physical reasons why a person's hearing may deteriorate, it is important to consider that the impairment of auditory acuity per se is not the only component of presbycusis. It also appears to involve the central auditory system, the system that allows for interpretation of what a person hears. Therefore, the difficulties in understanding what is being said that are uniquely experienced by elderly persons with presbycusis are oftentimes disproportionately greater than one would expect in light of their measured level of auditory acuity.

The literature reveals that a decline in the function of the central auditory system, including the brainstem and auditory cortex, appears to be involved in the disproportionate decline in speech understanding that is observed among many elderly adults. Authors continue to confirm an age-related central auditory decline that results in a mixed type of receptive and perceptual impairment, involving both the peripheral and central auditory systems (Bergman, 1980; Bezold, 1894; Hull, 1982, 1988a & b; Jerger, Oliver, & Pirozzolo, 1990; Jerger, Oliver, & Pirozzolo, 1990; Rodriguez, DiSarno, & Hardiman, 1990; Stach, Spretnjak, & Jerger, 1990; Townsend & Bess, 1980; L. W. Welsh, Welsh, & Healy, 1985; Working Group on Speech Understanding and Aging, 1988; and many others). Twenty years ago Kasten (1980) and McCroskey & Kasten (1981) described the auditory behaviors of older adults with central auditory decline as similar to the perceptual and comprehension difficulties observed among children with central auditory processing problems, particularly in auditorily or visually distracting communicative environments.

RESEARCH ON PRESBYCUSIS

According to Schaie et al. (1964), scientific research into changes in threshold for hearing began as early as 1894 with studies by Bezold (1894) and Zwaardemaker (1891). Most early studies consisted of observations relating to changes of hearing level in accordance with increasing age. With advances in electron microscopy, more detailed histopathological studies of the deterioration of bodily function associated with aging have been made possible. During recent years, much scientifically based research has been conducted in rela-

tion to the degeneration of the hearing mechanism. The areas of interest have been the cochlea, the spiral ganglion, the brainstem auditory pathways, and the auditory cortex, although the primary area of concentration through the years has involved research on the aging cochlea (inner ear).

STRUCTURAL CHANGES OF THE AUDITORY SYSTEM IN AGING

THE PINNA

As one views the pinna of an older individual, it is generally noted that it has increased in size and appears more flaccid than that of a younger person. Johnson and Hadley (1964) described the changes reflected in the pinna as involving a fine scaliness accompanied by dryness, inelasticity, and loss of rebound seen in younger epithelium. They further describe a general increase in hair growth within the folds of the pinna, especially among males. Pigmentation spots appear, wrinkling of skin accumulates, and the skin appears to be more thin and translucent (Weg, 1975).

Although there are obvious changes in the appearance of the outer ear, they do not appear to influence the auditory acuity of the older person.

THE EXTERNAL AUDITORY MEATUS

In a review by Zafar (1994), studies by Babbit (1947) and Rosenwasser (1964) are cited in which atrophic alterations of the tissues lining the external auditory meatus (EAM) with aging were confirmed.

Magladery (1959) describes a narrowing of the EAM. It was suggested that this may be due to a sagging of the skin lining of the EAM as a result of degeneration of cartilage of the wall of the canal.

Other observations made during studies over the years by Anderson and Meyerhoff (1982) Rosenwasser (1964), and Senturia (1957) include a general thinning of the epithelial lining of the EAM, which must be kept in mind by audiologists who conduct impedance audiometry or engage in cerumen management. Other findings included diminished elasticity of the tissues of the EAM, with drying and cracking, and excessive cerumen in many ears of aged persons, although in others, less than normal cerumen was observed.

THE MIDDLE EAR

It is interesting to consider the results of an early study by Rosenwasser (1964), which revealed what he thought to be ossicular atrophy predominantly in the joint of the stapes and the cudal joint of the malleus. He also felt that he had discovered atrophy of the middle ear muscle tendons in the region of the tympanic membrane. This is one of a number of early studies that attempted to include the middle ear system in the total picture of presbycusis.

An early study by Leake (1963) also brought focus to the muscles and tendons of the middle ear in aging. He discovered through research on middle ear muscle function among aging cats that a reduction of attentiveness and elasticity of the muscles in older middle ears appears to be the norm. He stated that this may contribute to reduced signal analysis for sound transmitted through the middle ear.

An earlier study by Glorig and Davis (1961) revealed that auditory acuity in aging persons may be affected by conductive factors due to the loss of elasticity of the incudo-malleolar and incudo-stapedial joints of the middle ear and a loss of elasticity of the tympanic membrane. They felt that these factors could be responsible for the consistent air-bone gap observed at 4kHz among older persons. They termed this phenomenon "conductive presbycusis." Earlier studies by Békésy (1949) and Davies (1948) noted an increase in the rigidity of the ossicular chain among older persons. Studies by Klotz and Kilbane (1962) and Crabbe (1963) also suggested an increase in rigidity of the

ossicular chain among older adults, along with some arthritic changes. They attributed it to changes in the bones due to age (Zafar, 1994).

THE COCHLEA

There are approximately 15,000 receptor cells in each cochlea, which when stimulated, send electrically coded signals to the auditory portion of the brain by way of the auditory pathways of the brainstem. If nerve fibers within the cochlea, spiral ganglion, or cranial nerve VII are destroyed, neural function does not regenerate.

HISTOLOGIC STUDIES

An early study by Crowe, Guild, and Polvogt (1934) involved a histological study on the ears of 74 subjects who had experienced a high-frequency hearing loss during their life. This study provided early histologic evidence of neural degeneration at the basal turn of the cochlea and, in some cases, partial atrophy of the cochlear branch of the CN VIII. These findings have been substantiated in numerous studies over the years (Zafar, 1994).

Jorgensen (1961), while conducting postmortem studies of the effect of aging on the ear, found a loss of ganglion cells in the basal portion of the cochlea along with thickenings of the capillary walls in the stria vascularis. This pathology was believed to be the result of arteriosclerosis. It was suggested that the thickenings could affect not only the oxygen level of the cochlear duct, but also the electrical potentials in the same area.

Kirikae, Sato, and Shitara (1964) also attempted to discover the primary site of lesion of presbycusis. They proposed that the cause of presbycusis principally involves lesions of the inner ear, particularly within the organ of Corti of the cochlea and the spiral ganglion cells. They described two specific types of changes: (1) atrophy of the spiral ganglion and (2) angiosclerotic degeneration of the inner ear. In an investigation by those authors that involved 20 subjects (10 subjects from 50 to 70 years of age and 10 control subjects from 20 to 30 years of age, all with normal hearing within the speech range), auditory discrimination for distorted speech was consistently found to be poorer in the older subjects, even when pure-tone thresholds were equal in both groups.

The authors felt that the poor auditory discrimination scores among the older subjects were due to senile changes of the auditory nervous system. It was also surmised that the elevation of pure-tone thresholds, especially at the higher frequencies, the lowered speech discrimination scores, and the diminished sense of binaural hearing were also due to senile changes of the auditory nervous system, including reduction and atrophy of ganglion cells from the level of the spiral ganglion to the auditory cortex.

Proctor (1961) felt that the predisposing factors for presbycusis may include arteriosclerosis and high blood cholesterol. He postulated that the progressive hearing impairment seen in aging may be due to atrophy of CN VIII, but that the causative mechanism in presbycusis is atrophy at the basal end of the cochlea.

Johnsson and Hawkins (1972) concluded that it is difficult to differentiate between the effects of ototoxic drugs, noise exposure, and the actual effects of aging when attempting to determine the effects of aging on hearing. In postmortem studies, they discovered cochlear hair cell degeneration in newborns only a few hours old. They also found definite nerve degeneration secondary to hair cell damage within the extreme basal turn of the cochlea in teenagers. They feel that the degeneration progresses steadily with aging. Hawkins (1973, p. 139), in comparing the effects of those factors on the aging cochlea, stated:

The processes involved in ototoxic injury by aminoglycosides (ototoxic substances) and in the degenerative changes leading to presbycusis are so similar that one may serve as a model for the other. The ototoxic process resembles nothing so much as an accelerated aging of the inner ear, a sort of "galloping presbycusis."

Unlike Dr. Oliver Wendell Holmes' New England deacon who built the wonderful one-horse shay, the Architect of the cochlea did not design it to give perfect service for "a hundred years to a day" or even for the traditional three-score-and-ten. Cochlear condition in old age, however, seldom represents the effects of aging alone, but rather the cumulative, combined assaults of noise and drugs, as well as time (Hawkins, 1973).

We must also consider the compounding effects of noise and drugs on the aging ear that probably begin at birth. Schuknecht (1974) supports the concept of additive factors involved in the structural pathology of presbycusis that occur throughout life, stating, "This is deafness of aging, not of the aged."

Schuknecht (1964), in his early studies, described four distinct types of presbycusis that he had identified:

1. **Sensory presbycusis.** He felt that this type is caused by atrophy of the organ of Corti and degeneration of hair cells, beginning at the basal end of the cochlea and moving toward the apex. The profile is usually seen at 8000 Hz and above in the average adult who has an abrupt high-frequency hearing loss in audiometric testing. It is the most common of the four types.
2. **Neural presbycusis.** This type results from the loss of neurons in the auditory pathways and cochlea. It usually becomes noticeable when 30% to 40% of the neurons are lost or damaged. There is a relatively more severe speech discrimination problem than with the first type. Although 90% of the cochlear nerves can be destroyed without affecting pure-tone thresholds, speech discrimination is affected much more quickly. Amplification frequently does not benefit persons affected.
3. **Stria vascularis atrophy, or metabolic, presbycusis.** This type is often seen when there is a family history of hearing loss and an insidious onset in the third or fourth decade of life. Degeneration takes place in the apical area of

the cochlea and causes a flat pure-tone hearing loss to about 50 dB, at which point speech discrimination is affected. Schuknecht feels this is probably a genetically determined condition. Amplification is often found to benefit persons with this problem.

4. **Inner ear conductive-type presbycusis** (somewhat theoretical). Although there are no evident histological changes, Schuknecht feels that an increase in the stiffness of the supportive structures of the cochlear duct may result in a reduction of membrane movement and, therefore, a "mechanically based" sensorineural hearing loss.

According to the Working Group on Speech Understanding and Aging of the Committee on Hearing, Bioacoustics and Biomechanics (1988), the four types of presbycusis described by Schuknecht (1964) have not been substantiated with any degree of certainty, except for the sensory category. The metabolic type, according to the Working Group, appears to be highly genetically determined, pure neural types are infrequently observed, with the mechanical form still speculative or, at least, hypothetical.

A study by Suga and Lindsay (1976) reported findings from temporal bone sections from 17 patients with presbycusic audiometric histories. They did not find the multiple sites of cochlear pathology reported by Schuknecht, nor likewise the similarities between the histologic and audiologic manifestations.

However, in 1993, Schuknecht and Gacek disclosed the results of more histologic studies from the temporal bone collection at the Massachusetts Eye and Ear Infirmary. They, in contrast to the Working Group On Speech Understanding and Aging (1988) and Suga and Lindsay (1976), stated that they have confirmed the existence of the four types of presbycusis proposed by Schuknecht in 1964. They state that (1) an abrupt high-frequency hearing loss signals the *sensory type*; (2) a loss of word discrimination is characteristic of *neural pres-*

bycusis; (3) *conductive presbycusis* has no pathologic tissue correlate, but is characterized by a gradually decreasing linear distribution pattern on the audiometric scale; and (4) a flat threshold pattern is indicative of *strial presbycusis*. They further state that about 25% of all cases of presbycusis show none of the listed characteristics and are classified as indeterminate presbycusis.

Another histologic study by Ramadan and Schuknecht (1989) revealed what they feel is confirmation of the fourth type of presbycusis discussed by Schuknecht in 1964—that is, the *conductive* form of presbycusis. The authors found what they feel to be an alteration in cochlear motion mechanics along the basilar membrane of the cochlea that they feel explains, in part, the gradual high-frequency hearing loss found frequently among older adults.

ARTERIOSCLEROSIS

There has been some speculation over the years about a direct relationship between presbycusis and arteriosclerosis. As the cochlea and the central auditory system are extremely sensitive to oxygen/metabolic change, such a theoretical relationship is a natural one. Fisch, Bobozi, and Greig (1972) studied degenerative factors of the internal auditory artery and found enough decline in blood supply to negatively affect the function of the cochlea. Makishima (1978) found a positive correlation between the extent of the narrowing of the internal auditory artery with atrophy of the spiral ganglion and degree of hearing loss, with Johnsson and Hawkins (1972) finding a positive relationship between stria vascularis atrophy with concomitant reduction in blood supply, accompanied by degenerative changes along the basilar membrane of the cochlea. Suga and Lindsay (1976), on the other hand, reported arteriosclerosis in a number of the histologic studies they conducted, although they did not find a relationship between arteriosclerosis and degeneration of the cochlear tissue. Gatehouse and Lowe (1990) attribute deficiencies in blood supply to a decline in cochlear function with age, not only in terms of blood availability, but also as it relates to bulk rheological properties and the properties of individual red cells. All of the studies, except for that by Suga and Lindsay (1976), support a blood supply-related cause for a decline in electrosensory function of the cochlea.

THE BRAINSTEM AND AUDITORY CORTEX

A discussion of the site of lesion of presbycusis should not be restricted to the cochlea. As presbycusis presents itself as a disproportionate inability to understand what others are saying as compared to the individual's level of auditory acuity, one cannot exclude the possibility of pathology beyond the cochlea and CN VIII—that is, within the brainstem and the auditory cortex.

A common audiologic picture of presbycusis includes obvious cochlear pathology as represented by a sloping sensorineural hearing loss, accompanied by a corresponding impairment in speech perception. As the audiologist views the results of the pure-tone audiometric evaluation, it often appears that the individual should be able to function adequately, even in light of the evident peripheral hearing loss. However, when speech recognition abilities are assessed (the ability to correctly identify the acoustical/phonemic elements of speech), a different picture becomes apparent. A greater than expected impairment in speech understanding is frequently observed. The common complaint of the aging person with presbycusis is that he or she can hear people talk, but cannot understand what they are saying. The client complains that speech sounds "jumbled" or that people seem to "mumble," nowadays. The greatest difficulty is generally experienced in auditorily distracting environments—those that are noisy or reverberant.

The problem appears to involve the sorting and synthesis of the auditory-phonemic elements of speech and cannot be truly explained by the auditory acuity of an individual or by the shape of the audiogram. This significant characteristic of presbycusis is termed "phonemic regression," as earlier described by Gaeth (1948). It represents speech recognition scores that may be significantly poorer than might be expected when observing an individual's threshold for pure tones and speech. According to Gaeth in his early study (1948), this is due to a "generalized deterioration of centers within the CNS concerned with sound transmission and reception. Further, this deterioration can exist with a relatively intact end organ (cochlea)."

Later, Hinchcliffe (1962) described the auditory features of presbycusis and discussed the possible histological changes that cause them. He concluded that "although a number of degenerative changes throughout the auditory mechanism must contribute to the development of presbycusis, it seems more likely that changes in the brain are primarily responsible for the overall audiologic picture of presbycusis" (p. 306). Earlier, Pestalozza and Shore (1955) included in their findings lesions located in the organ of Corti as well as in spiral ganglion cells, the eighth cranial nerve, and the central pathways.

In 1964, Kirikae et al. (1964) reported neuron loss in the cochlear nuclei and the medial geniculate bodies. They discussed the possibilities of a relationship between lowered speech discrimination and senile changes of the central auditory system, including reduction and atrophy of nerve cells and their attachments from the eighth cranial nerve through the brainstem and including the auditory cortex.

Hansen and Reske-Nielsen (1965) described neuron loss in the cochlear nuclei, the inferior colliculus, and Heschel's gyrus. On the other hand, Konigsmark and Murphy (1972) made cell counts on the central cochlear nucleus and concluded that there was no cell loss as related to aging. In 1982, Casey and Feldman reported their studies on rat brainstem auditory nuclei. Their findings reported no cell loss in the medial nucleus of the trapezoid body, although there appeared to be some general structural degeneration within the nuclei.

Ferraro and Minckler (1977) reported cell counts and studies of glial density and cellular configuration in human brainstems, specifically the lateral lemniscus, from birth to age 90 years. Hull (1972) studied the same brainstems, but only looked at the inferior colliculi. The conclusions of both studies were that there is a general decrease in cell size and dendritic number, but across nine decades there is little cell loss. However, a general observation was that with the decrease in cell size, the state of health of the cells and the neural glia appeared to decline.

NEUROCHEMICAL-NEUROTRANSMITTER CHANGES

Studies published within the past half decade have reached a general consensus that the brainstem and auditory cortex of older adults do play a role in reduced speech recognition and speech comprehension. For example, a study by Caspary, Raza, Lawhorn-Armour, Pippin, and Arneric (1990) confirmed substantial age-related loss of the putative inhibitory neurotransmitter GABA in the central nucleus of the inferior colliculus. They state that this confirmed age-related impairment of neurotransmission can account for or, at least, contribute to abnormal auditory perception and processing that is observed in presbycusis. This is in light of brainstem auditory nuclei that otherwise appear structurally within normal limits.

A study by Briner and Willott (1989) focused on changes in the brainstem, concentrating on the cochlear nucleus, including the anteroventral cochlear nucleus and its dorsal component. Both the physical and neurochemical changes observed in this aspect of the brainstem were significant enough for them to conclude that they can play roles in reduced function of this portion of the central auditory system that provides early interpretation of auditory information.

Although studies such as those cited above would tend to support changes in the brainstem that could lead to central auditory system (CNS) decline as a function of age, there is still no conclusive evidence that there are marked age-related neuroanatomic changes in the central auditory system. This does not, however, deny the behavioral changes that are noted among many persons in advanced age as it relates to speech understanding, including a decline in auditory processing, auditory synthesis, and auditory/linguistic processing that interferes with one's daily communicative function, as is discussed later in this chapter.

A comprehensive study by Stach et al. (1990) revealed that the prevalence of CNS involvement in presbycusis increases with age and that among the population beyond 80 years old, 95% possess a central auditory decline. In fact, Rodriguez et al. (1990) found central auditory processing disorders among older adults without concomitant peripheral involvement.

It is probable that, if a basis for those changes in auditory processing is to be discovered, it will be found as a general decline in the health state of the peripheral and CNS auditory system, along with a reduction in neurochemical/neurotransmitter function that is primarily focused on the brainstem auditory nuclei and their pathways, the auditory cortex, and the association areas of the brain.

SUMMARY OF AUDITORY SYSTEM CHANGES IN AGING

Presbycusis, as is currently understood, then, involves: (1) the structural pathology of the aging ear, including one or more causes ranging from previous noise exposure, biochemical factors, heredity, metabolic changes, and others; (2) the CNS-based auditory processing/comprehension problems seen among many aging persons; and (3) the myriad of social/psychological problems facing elderly individuals with presbycusis. Schuknecht (1974) has stated that aging is apparently caused by a complex integration of inherited defects, injuries, environmental exposure, and accumulation of DNA errors (which results in a reduction of the body's capability of mitosis for repair), the person's genetic makeup, accumulation of pigment, and chemical changes in individual body cells.

From reviewing the literature, one can observe trends in thought resulting from scientific investigation on presbycusis. Most emphasis has been placed in the area of the cochlea, deterioration of ganglion cells in the organ of Corti and spiral ganglion, and degeneration of the eighth cranial nerve. There is also strong evidence that presbycusis is a disorder of hearing that involves processing difficulties of the central auditory system, the cause of which may be at least partially neurochemical in nature, which is compounded by a sensorineural hearing loss that principally involves the higher frequencies.

THE EFFECTS OF PRESBYCUSIS ON HEARING

HEARING FOR PURE TONES

Békésy (1957) stated:

In childhood some of us can hear well at frequencies as high as 40,000 cycles per second. But with age our acuteness of hearing in the high-frequency range steadily falls. Normally, the drop is almost as regular as clockwork. Testing several persons in their 40s with tones at a fixed level of intensity, we find that over a period of five years, their upper limit dropped about 80 cycles per second every six months. (p. 2)

Two major manifestations of presbycusis are generally seen by an audiologist. First, a progressive bilateral reduction in sensitivity for pure tones is observed, particularly in the high fre-

quencies and, second, decreased auditory discrimination when speech is presented loudly enough for the person to hear, even though pure-tone loss may be minimal. This observation was substantiated more than two decades ago by Jerger (1973), who stated: "The aging process produces systematic changes in each of the two critical dimensions of hearing impairment—loss in threshold sensitivity and loss in the ability to understand suprathreshold speech" (p. 124). The aging person's threshold for hearing, then, reveals a typical loss of acuity for the higher frequencies, generally first seen at around 4000 Hz and then gradually involving the lower frequencies. The most observable and debilitating aspect of presbycusis, however, is a general decline in speech understanding.

THE SENSORINEURAL ASPECTS OF PRESBYCUSIS

The loss of sensitivity for pure tones observed in presbycusis reveals a gradually sloping pattern, with the greatest loss centering in the high frequencies around 4000 Hz. An early study by Glorig, Wheeler, Quiggle, Grings, and Summerfield (1957) surveyed the hearing of large numbers of people, ranging in age from 10 to 79 years of age. As can be seen in Figure 17-1, the greatest degree of impairment in auditory acuity for pure tones is seen in the higher frequencies for subjects of all ages, even beginning to some degree in subjects from 10 to 19 years of age. In the age range from 50 years to 79 years, a decline in auditory acuity also includes the lower frequencies.

The loss of hearing acuity in the higher frequencies in aging has been documented by many persons, including Békésy (1957), Brant and Fozard (1990), Corso (1963), Corso (1976), Corso (1981), Hinchcliffe (1962), Jerger (1973), Miller and Ort (1965), Rosen, Bergman, Pleste, El-Mofty, and Satti (1962), Rosenwasser (1964), Schock et al. (1984), Schuknecht (1964), Schuknecht and Woellner (1955), Traynor and Hull (1974), and many others.

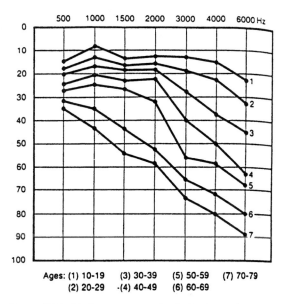

Figure 17-1. Median pure-tone thresholds for males ages 10–79. Data are converted to ANSI-1969 reference. (Adapted from Glorig et al. (1957).)

The phenomenon was reported earlier by Bunch and Railford (1931) and Beasley (1938) and much earlier by Galton in 1884 (as cited in Birren & Clayton, 1975). Figure 17-2 presents data on longitudinal changes in thresholds for pure tones for 813 male subjects (Brant & Fozard, 1990).

An early study by Traynor and Hull (1974) established mean auditory thresholds for 120 elderly individuals ranging in age from 65 to 90 confined to health care facilities. These means were then compared with the results of a similar investigation by Miller and Ort (1965). The compared results of the two studies are presented in Figure 17-3. As can be seen, the results are quite similar. The general pure-tone audiometric configuration is revealed as a relatively flat sensorineural hearing loss sloping gently into the higher frequencies. Speech-reception thresholds are generally equal to and reflected by a best two- or three-frequency pure-tone average.

In an attempt to obtain as reliable a picture as possible of "true" presbycusic changes in hearing, Glorig and Nixon (1960) attempted to control for such contaminating factors as disease and noise (environmental exposure) by selecting 328 men out of 2,000 who had not been unduly exposed to noise or other elements that can result in hearing loss. These 328 men had no evidence or history of otological disease and no history of having been exposed to gunfire or noise levels high enough to make conversation difficult. Figure 17-4 shows the effect of age on hearing levels for several different frequencies within that study. The aging process reveals itself by changes in auditory sensitivity at 1000 Hz beginning at age 30. On the basis of these data, the rate of decrease in auditory sensitivity for 1000 Hz is about 3 dB for every 10 years of age through 70 years. For 6000 Hz, the decrease is approximately 10 dB for every 10 years through 70 years.

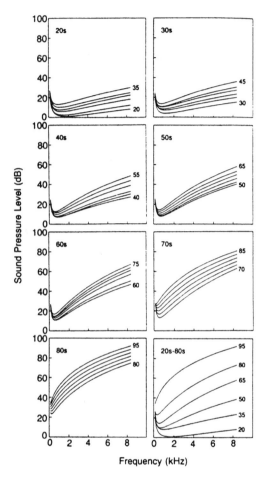

Figure 17-2. Longitudinal changes in thresholds for continuously presented pure tones from 0.125 to 8.0 kHz in 813 males. The six idealized functions in each panel characterize the thresholds for men in each age group measured at 3-year intervals from the youngest to the oldest age represented in the panel. The right-hand panel at the bottom of the figure is a composite of the other data. Figure is constructed from data by Brant and Fozard (1987) by Fozard (1990), and reprinted by permission.

Much of the research on the effects of aging on hearing has been motivated by a need for identifying the presbycusic component in noise-induced hearing loss (Corso, 1976). In an effort to describe

the presbycusic effect on auditory sensitivity for pure-tones, Spoor (1967) analyzed the results of eight studies on pure-tone thresholds as a function of age including those by the Z24-X-2 report of the American Standards Association (1954), Beasley (1938); Corso (1963), Glorig and Nixon (1960), Glorig et al. (1957) report of the 1954 Wisconsin State Fair, Hinchcliffe (1959), Jatho and Heck (1959), and Johansen (1943).

Because these studies reported hearing levels based on reference threshold levels (SPL) in effect prior to American National Standards Institute 1969, Lebo and Reddell (1972) applied corrections to Spoor's (1967) data to show presbycusic curves relative to the ANSI 1969 standard (American National Standards Institute, 1970). These curves are shown in Figure 17-5 for males and Figure 17-6 for females. The curves show that the reduction of auditory sensitivity as a function of age is frequency dependent. Pure-tone sensitivity for 250, 500, and 1000 Hz is approximately equivalent for males and females across decade-age groups, although females reveal a slightly greater loss for the lower frequencies. On the other hand, males experience a more rapid decline in sensitivity than females for frequencies 2000 Hz and higher.

A study by Jerger, Chmiel, Stach, and Spretnjak (1993) supported a gender affect as it relates to threshold change among aging adults. They found that above 1k Hz, males show greater average losses for pure tones. However, below 1k Hz, females show a greater average loss than males. According to these authors, the difference in audiometric configuration occurs whether or not a person is aware of a hearing loss and it occurs even when subjects who have a history of noise exposure are excluded. They conclude that a possible explanation for the audiometric differences may be a greater likelihood of cardiovascular disease in elderly females.

A study by Brant and Fozard (1990) that involved seven age groups over a 20-year time

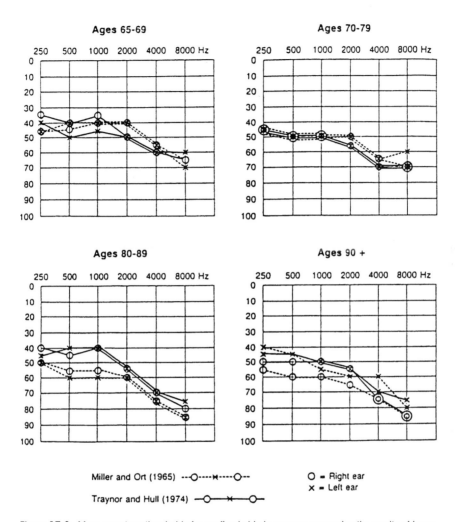

Figure 17-3. Mean pure-tone thresholds for confined elderly persons, comparing the results of investigations by Traynor & Hull (1974) and Miller and Ort (1965). (All threshold levels have been converted where necessary to ANSI-1969 reference.)

frame essentially confirms all of the previous studies on auditory acuity and aging. Over time, acuity for pure tones declines at an average rate of approximately 1 dB per year, particularly for the higher frequencies. This study also affirmed significant individual differences within all age groups, including the oldest (the 80s decade).

SPEECH RECOGNITION

It becomes quite disturbing to aging persons when they feel that they can hear people talk, but have difficulty "making sense" out of it. That is, in essence, the disorder of speech recognition so commonly observed in presbycusis. An auditory

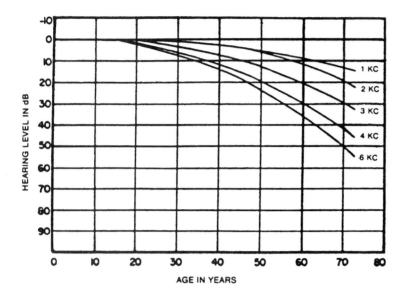

Figure 17-4. Average hearing levels as a function of age of 328 males who reported negative otologic history, and no exposure to high-level noise. (Reproduced with permission from Glorig, A., & Nixon, J. (1969). Distribution of hearing loss in various populations. *Annals of Otology, Rhinology and Laryngology, 69*, 502.)

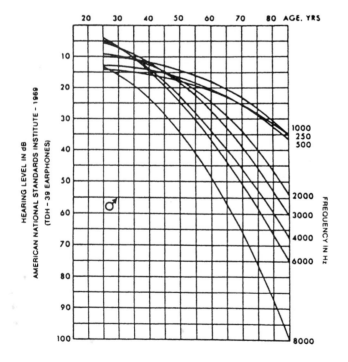

Figure 17-5. Spoor's composite male presbycusic curves modified to conform to the ANSI 1969 standard. (Reproduced with permission from Lebo, C. P., & Reddell, R. C. (1972). The presbycusis component in occupational hearing loss. *Laryngoscope, 82*, 1402.)

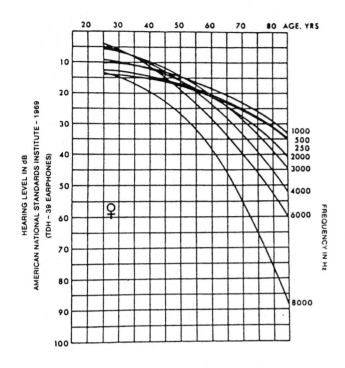

Figure 17-6. Spoor's composite female presbycusic curves modified to conform to the ANSI 1969 standard. (Reproduced with permission from Lebo, C. P., & Reddell, R. C. (1972). The presbycusis component in occupational hearing loss. *Laryngoscope, 82,* 1402.)

communicative symptom of this phenomenon, then, is a frequent inability of an older person to understand what others are saying when auditory acuity appears adequate for purposes of communication. A typical statement made by an elderly person is, "I can hear you, but I cannot understand what you are saying." When this statement is made, it can generally be assumed that the elderly person is describing the problem accurately.

It should be noted that the loss of hearing sensitivity in the higher frequencies, itself, generally results in some difficulties in understanding the speech of others, especially in auditorily distracting environments. However, the difficulties are variable and depend on the extent of hearing loss for higher and other frequencies, plus the ability of the individual to compensate for the loss of acuity for certain phonemes of speech and to communicate in certain communicative environments.

The cause of the most severe disability of speech recognition and comprehension among the elderly, however, cannot be restricted simply to a hearing loss for the high frequencies. The disorder exemplified in presbycusis, which appears to involve difficulties in auditory comprehension, auditory synthesis, and the sorting of both the phonemic and linguistic features of speech, occurs at levels beyond the cochlea and eighth cranial nerve.

To the lay person, the auditory confusions observed in aging persons may, unfortunately, appear to take on the characteristics of confusion and "senility." It should be understood, however, that an aging person, faced with the embarrassment of such comprehension confusion, may also have considered this possibility. As the older person is embarrassed by his or her confusion of auditory verbal messages, there may be withdrawal and a self-imposed isolation from other possible communication situations. Although a person may be alert and intelligent, he or she is faced with a frustrating auditory discrimination problem.

Jerger (1973), in an early investigation cited earlier, systematically studied changes in speech understanding observed among aging persons. He subjected 18 elderly persons to a number of tests for speech recognition. Five younger subjects were controls. All subjects demonstrated equal sensorineural hearing loss with similar pure-tone configuration. The tests for auditory discrimination included: (1) PB max, (2) PB scores at 5 dB sensation level, (3) sentences in competition, and (4) time-compressed speech. Mean scores are presented in Figure 17-7. Jerger found that the sensorineural hearing impairment resulted in lowered auditory discrimination scores that are not strictly related to the age of the subject. Elderly subjects did, however, demonstrate slightly depressed scores as compared to younger subjects.

Jerger (1973) concluded that for the relatively easy task of repeating back PB words at a level well above threshold (PB max), there is little difference among the three groups. When the task is made somewhat more difficult, however, by simply presenting the words at a very faint level (5 dB SL), the presbycusic group had more difficulty than either the normal or the control groups. Sentence identification in the presence of ipsilateral competing message (SSI-ICM) shows an even more pronounced effect. Younger hearing impaired subjects had greater difficulty than normals, but those with presbycusis showed an even greater loss in sentence identification.

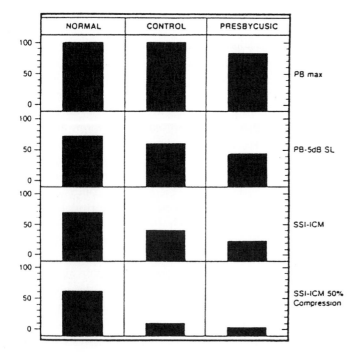

Figure 17-7. Average scores for four auditory discrimination tasks for three subject groups. (Reprinted with permission from Jerger, J. (1973). Audiological findings in aging. *Advances in Oto-rhino Laryngology, 20*, 115–124.)

Finally, subjecting the SSI sentences to time compression accentuated the effect even more. Both the control and presbycusic groups showed a severe breakdown in comparison with the normal group. The presbycusic group showed a slightly greater effect than the younger hearing-impaired control group.

In a later study, Jerger (1992) compared subjects' performance on four speech audiometric measures, including the SSI. He found that a decline in performance on the SSI was statistically significant when compared across the age range of 50–90 years. He concluded that the age-related decline in performance on the SSI cannot be explained by peripheral hearing loss, nor can it be explained by a decline in cognitive function. However, a decline in performance on tasks that require precision in speech perception appears to be an age-related phenomenon and is observed frequently enough to be expected.

There is, indeed, a disproportionate loss in speech understanding among older adults that is beyond what can be accounted for by a loss in threshold sensitivity. When hearing loss is held constant across age, the progressive effect of aging on speech intelligibility loss is easily documented. Available evidence supports a central rather than peripheral interpretation of the phenomenon.

In other words, as Jerger (1973) has stated: if cochlear disorders make up the majority of sensorineural loss in young adults, then one must look beyond the cochlea to explain the loss of speech understanding unique to the elderly.

Bergman (1980) and Bergman et al. (1976) conducted a 10-year investigation that permitted a thorough description of the decline in speech recognition found among aging persons. Two hundred and eighty-two adults, ranging in age from 20 to 80 years, were assessed, utilizing a variety of suprathreshold tasks requiring the discrimination of speech. Follow-up studies on the same subjects were conducted at 3 years and 7 years. The tests of degraded speech were:

1. Control test of 10 Central Institute for the Deaf (CID) Everyday Sentences that were undistorted.
2. Similar sentence lists interrupted electronically 8 times per second.
3. Other sentences spoken at a rate 2 ½ times faster than the normal rate of 120 words per minute.
4. Other sentences filtered so that one ear heard them through a low-pass filter extending from 500 to 800 Hz, while the other ear heard them simultaneously through a frequency band from 1800 to 2400 Hz.
5. Two-part words (spondaic words) such as *upstairs* and *downtown* presented to each ear so that the second syllable of one overlapped the first syllable of the second and thereby competed for the listener's attention.
6. A test requiring the listener to attend to a message and understand it through competing speakers' voices (selective listening).
7. Simulated listening in a "lecture" hall with unfavorable acoustics (reverberated speech).

The results revealed some interesting findings relating to the phenomenon of presbycusis. For example, the original subjects, ranging in age from 20 to 29, had definite decreases in speech understanding between the initial testing and the follow-up tests 7 years later. The greatest differences were found in the reverberated speech, speeded speech, selective listening task, and interrupted speech tasks. All subjects in age groups from ages 20 to 29 to ages 60 to 69 demonstrated the poorest scores for the electronically interrupted speech. In fact, there appeared to be a linear relationship between the age of the subjects and the scores on all listening tasks.

All subjects performed best on the control test of 10 undistorted sentences presented at a comfortable listening level. The poorest scores on all listening tasks were found among the age group of 60 to 69 years. The next higher scores were those within the group ranging in age from 50 to 59 years, although their scores were generally significantly better than those among the 60 to 69 year group.

According to Bergman (1980), this study indicates "that the perception of everyday speech declines significantly with aging for conditions other than those which are optimal. . . .This change is noted as early as the fifth decade, with a sharp acceleration occurring in the seventh decade of life" (p. 151).

In a much earlier study by Gaeth (1948), the same phenomenon was described. Gaeth termed it "phonemic regression." He founded his observation on the premise that "certain patients show much greater difficulty in discriminating the phonemic elements of speech than would be expected on the basis of their pure-tone scores" (Willeford, 1971, p. 254). Willeford (1971) presented the characteristics involved in the phenomenon as described by Gaeth (1948):

1. Otological and audiological findings indicate a sensorineural type hearing loss that is either mild or moderate in severity.
2. The threshold shift in hearing for connected speech agrees with the shift for pure tones.
3. There is a greater difficulty in understanding speech as revealed by appropriate discrimination tests than the type and severity of loss would lead one to suspect.
4. The patient does not appear to evidence a general decay in mental capabilities paralleling his or her deterioration in phonemic perception.
5. The patient lacks insight into the quality of his or her discrimination problem, but tends to blame all these troubles on the deficiency in auditory acuity, or on those who are speaking to him or her.
6. These symptoms appear more frequently in adults over 50 years of age than in those younger, but a substantial number of the older individuals with hearing losses do not display the difficulty. Therefore, age alone must be ruled out as the causative factor.

The studies by Bergman (1980), Bergman et al. (1976), Jerger (1973, 1992), and others have generally not supported the final statement by Gaeth (1948). They have continued to specify a relationship between the lack of ability to understand the speech of others, the age of a client, and a decline in CNS auditory function that accompanies the process of aging.

SPEED OF FREQUENCY SELECTIVITY AND SPEECH UNDERSTANDING IN AGING

As described previously, one of the most frequently observed phenomena in presbycusis is that the difficulties in speech understanding experienced by many hearing-impaired older adults are usually disproportionately greater than one would expect by examining their measured loss of hearing acuity (Bergman, 1980; Cranford & Stream, 1991; Gaeth, 1948; Hull, 1994; and others).

One of the elements that appears to contribute to the speech understanding problems encountered by many hearing-impaired older adults involves the speed at which speech is produced and the ability of the aging central nervous system to interpret the coded speech signal accurately with the speed and accuracy necessary for encoding to occur. For example, according to Cranford and Stream (1991), because normal recognition of speech requires integration and perception of rapid changes in temporal dimensions of speech sounds, it would appear that age-related changes in temporal processing may interfere with speech understanding. Many of the words and phrases that are critical for speech understanding are of very short duration, in the range from 7 to 15 milliseconds. The phonemes of speech may be found in the range of 2 to 4 milliseconds. If a decline in the speed of processing of the acoustic elements of speech is, indeed, involved in the disproportionate decline in speech understanding among older hearing-impaired adults, then this must be considered when designing aural rehabilitation programs for these persons.

Earlier studies of temporal factors in speech understanding have revealed a relationship between the integrity of the CNS and the sensitivity of subjects' central auditory system to frequency difference limens (DLFs) (Gengle, 1973). For example, patients with temporal lobe lesions required a greater length of signal presentation to identify subtle differences in frequency, as compared to normal subjects (Cranford, Stream, Rye, & Slade, 1982).

If the ability to make fine discriminations relative to the frequency of brief tones is sensitive to lesions of the temporal lobe, then perhaps these same tests may provide clues to the nature of speech recognition problems exhibited by elderly adults. As early as 1957, Konig (1957) postulated that frequency discrimination may be a sensitive measure in determining differences between younger and older persons in auditory function. This is particularly important as it relates to the central auditory system's ability to make critical decisions about the frequency of a signal in spite of its speed, as speed of the CNS's decision-making power may be an important element in speech understanding in aging.

RECOGNITION OF DEGRADED SPEECH

According to the Working Group On Speech Understanding and Aging (1988), the major problem in interpreting the literature on how aging listeners understand degraded speech is that we do not know how to separate the influence of what is degrading the speech signal from the influence of a hearing loss that produces a nondegraded speech-understanding score that is lower than 100%. We do, however, know that many older listeners tend to perform poorer than younger listeners on degraded speech tasks and that the differences can be consistently demonstrated.

Studies on the performance of older versus younger subjects on degraded speech tasks have concentrated on types of degraded speech that hearing-impaired persons face during their activities of daily living. Those include, among others: (1) competing noise, (2) competing messages, (3) frequency filtering, and (4) the rate of speech production.

SPEECH PERCEPTION IN NOISE

Most older adults have difficulty understanding speech in noisy everyday environments. This also occurs in controlled environments for research in which a masker is employed to determine its effect on speech understanding. Bergman (1980); Dubno, Dirks, and Morgan (1982), Jokinen (1973); Kalikow, Stevens, and Elliott (1977); Levitt, Mayer, and Bergman (1975); Mayer (1975); Smith and Prather (1971), and others have revealed that older listeners perform poorer on tasks requiring speech recognition in noise. The Working Group on Speech Understanding and Aging (1988), however, has stated that the problem in separating out the effects of noise on speech understanding among older listeners stems from the difficulty in separating the influence of the masker from the influence of the hearing loss.

COMPETING MESSAGES

Bergman (1980) in his classic treatise on the effects of age on speech understanding discovered a decline in sentence interpretation in the presence of two competing talkers beginning at around age 40 years when the signal-to-noise ratio was −5 dB. The Levitt et al. (1975) study revealed a decline in speech recognition in subjects in their mid-twenties when subway and traffic noise maskers were utilized. Jokinen (1973) found that by the time subjects were 60 years old, even signal-to-noise ratios of +12 dB and +2 dB resulted in significantly lower performance on speech recognition tasks.

Orchik and Burgess (1977) conducted a study that utilized SSI stimuli at five message-to-competition ratios. The synthetic sentences were presented at a sensation level of 40 dB SL. The older listeners consistently performed at poorer levels than did the younger listeners, as has been consistently shown through research for the past four decades. In other words, most research on speech recognition in aging over the years has consistently revealed results that confirm that older listeners have difficulty performing on speech recognition tasks in the presence of competing noise and competing messages.

FREQUENCY FILTERING

According to the Working Group On Speech Understanding and Aging (1988), most experiments on speech recognition and aging that use filtered speech were designed to study binaural synthesis. A standard research protocol consisted of presenting a low-frequency band of speech to one ear and a high-frequency band to the other. The Working Group On Speech Understanding and Aging (1988), along with other authors including Bergman et al. (1976); Harbert, Young, and Menduke (1966); Kelly-Ballweber and Dobie (1984); Palva and Jokinen (1970); and O. L. Welsh, Luterman, and Bell (1969) found that older adults performed at poorer levels than did younger subjects on speech recognition tasks under these conditions. However, according to those authors, it has been difficult to separate the frequency filtering of the sensorineural hearing loss that elderly subjects exhibit and the artificial filtering utilized in the studies.

Other early studies by such authors as Frager (1968); Kirikae et al. (1964); Korsan-Bengsten (1968); and Marston and Goetzinger (1972) have revealed the following, as summarized by Kopra (1982): (1) older listeners perform significantly poorer than younger listeners under low-pass filter conditions; (2) when a low-band pass signal is delivered to one ear and a higher-band pass signal is fed to the other ear, deterioration in binaural synthesizing ability is evident by the fourth decade of life; (3) listeners who have experienced sensorineural hearing loss early in life perform better on binaural integration tasks than their older counterparts; and (4) elderly listeners with presbycusis perform more variably on filtered speech tasks than young listeners.

CHANGES IN RATE OF SPEECH

Studies employing speeded speech and time-compressed speech have concluded that older subjects generally have difficulty understanding rapid speech. For example, studies by Gordon-Salant & Fitzgibbons (1995); Kirk, Pisoni, & Miyamoto (1997); Letowski & Poch (1995); Schmitt and Carroll (1985); Schmitt and Moore (1989); Vaughan & Letowski (1997); Wingfield, Poon, Lombardi & Lowe (1985); and others have consistently revealed a decline in speech understanding by older subjects when time compression reaches as much as 60%.

The expansion of speech has also been shown to have little positive influence on speech understanding among older subjects. Studies by Korabic, Freeman, and Church (1978); Luterman, Welsh, and Melrose (1966); Schmitt and Carroll (1985); Schmitt and Moore (1989); and others have shown little positive affect of electronic speech expansion on speech understanding in aging. In fact, a study by Korabic et al. (1978) revealed a slight decline in speech understanding when speech was electronically expanded. A study by Schmitt (1983) found that speech expansion aided speech understanding slightly among "young-old" (70+) subjects, but interfered with speech understanding among "old-old" (80+) subjects. This does not mean, however, that speaking slower does not assist hearing-impaired older adults. The influence of electronically, rather than acoustically, slowed speech may have been a negative one.

As is noted in Chapter 20 of this book, Hull (1992c) has utilized time-compressed speech as a part of the aural rehabilitation process with older hearing-impaired adults. It is being utilized experimentally by this author in a project to retrain the aging central auditory system to function with greater efficiency in auditory synthesis and in speed of auditory closure.

DICHOTIC LISTENING

Jerger, Alford, Lew, Rivera, and Chmiel (1995) and Jerger and Chmiel (1997) suggest that the age-related asymmetries in dichotic listening, according to Mehta (1999), are probably related to loss of efficiency of interhemispheric transfer of auditory information through the corpus callosum, because of callosal dysfunction. This, in turn, can lead to increased divergence of processing abilities for right and left ear inputs. According to Mehta (1999), older adults in the Jerger et al. (1995) and Jerger & Chmiel (1997) studies showed an increasing left ear deficit on verbal tasks and an increasing right ear deficit on nonverbal tasks, even after peripheral asymmetries in hearing sensitivity were accounted for (Jerger et al., 1995; Jerger & Chmiel, 1997). The patterns of results obtained in elders with dichotic deficits was similar in pattern to the results of individuals with corpus callosal lesions.

ELECTROPHYSIOLOGIC MEASURES

According to Martin and Cranford (1989), in contrast to behavioral testing procedures, evoked potentials may provide a more objective means of identifying and defining the effects of age-related changes in hearing—that is, to differentiate more objectively between peripheral and central auditory factors. The reason they believed that evoked potential testing may be more reliable is that performance on behavioral measures can be compromised by peripheral hearing impairment, language or cognitive dysfunctions, or motor speech disorders, as well as by psychological characteristics such as low motivation or conservative responses.

It is further postulated by Martin and Cranford (1989) that past studies of evoked-potential measures with elderly subjects have revealed observable indications of age-related changes in all three evoked-response time domains, including ABR (auditory brainstem), MLR (middle latency), and LLR (late latency evoked potentials), although the indications are rather subtle.

According to Hall (1992), the effect of age on ABR responses is clearly not as robust as the gender effect and is not uniformly demonstrated for both males and females (Beagley & Sheldrake, 1978; Rosenhamer, Lindstrom, & Lundborg (1980); Thomsen, Terkeldsen, & Osterhammel, 1978). The ABR wave I-V, according to Hall (1992) appears to increase significantly over the age range of 60–86 years (Allison, Wood, & Goff, 1983; Maurizi, Altissimi, Ottaviani, Paludetti, & Bambini, 1982; Patterson, Michalewski, Thompson, Bowman, & Litzelman, 1981; Rowe, 1978), although inconsistencies related to ABR latencies are revealed throughout the literature. However, according to Hall (1992), age and gender effects appear to contribute substantially to the variability of ABR latency, especially for amplitude measures (Psatta & Matei, 1988). According to Hall (1992), if each of these measures changes over time and differs between sexes, then both of these sources of variability must be included with ABR data for groups of males and females distributed across an age range.

A study by Jerger and Johnson (1988) presented data on the factors of age, gender, and sensorineural hearing loss and the ABR. With increased age, they found that females showed little wave V latency change with increasing hearing loss, but the wave V latency in males lengthened by approximately 0.1 msec for every 20 dB decrease in the effective click level of the stimulus. This study confirms that age and gender appear to interact with hearing loss in affecting ABR latency (Hall, 1992).

The effects of aging on the P300 response have been frequently reported in the literature. Studies by Michalewski, Thompson, Patterson, Bowman, and Litzelman (1980); Pfefferbaum, Wenegrat, Ford, Roth, and Kopell (1984); Puce, Donnan, and Bladin (1989); and others have shown that average P300 latency among subjects ranging in age from 10 to 90 years increases steadily from about 300 ms to 450 ms, with amplitude decreasing at an average rate of 0.2 volt per year. According to Hall (1992), there also appears to be an interaction between age and scalp topography in P300 measurement. Young adults have a pronounced parietal distribution, whereas P300 becomes distributed from the parietal region to the frontal region as a function of advancing age (Pfefferbaum, Ford, Roth, & Kopell, 1980; Pfefferbaum, Ford, Roth, Hopkins, & Kopell, 1979).

CENTRAL AUDITORY FUNCTION AND AGING

According to to the definition of central auditory processing disorders by the ASHA Task Force (1996), and Katz and Kusnierczyk (1993), according to Mehta, 1999, older adults exhibit many, if not all the signs of a central auditory processing disorder seen in younger learning disabled persons, such as difficulties with sound localization, auditory discrimination and pattern recognition, temporal aspects of audition, and decrements in auditory performance for degraded and competing acoustic stimuli. According to Mehta (1999), the bulk of research now supports the hypothesis that the pathogenesis of auditory dysfunction typically observed in older adults once considered to be entirely peripheral, may have a central auditory component.

Jerger (1973, 1979, 1985, 1992), through comparative investigations, has exhaustively studied the possibility of central involvement in presbycusis. The results of his research and that of others, including Rizzo and Gutnick (1991), indicate differences between young and elderly subjects with equal auditory thresholds that are significant enough to conclude that, "We must look beyond the cochlea to explain the loss in speech discrimination unique to the elderly." (Jerger, 1973, p. 124).

Jerger et al. (1990) studied the impact of a central auditory processing disorder on older adults. They found that persons with central auditory processing disorders (CAPD) consistently rated themselves as significantly more handicapped than non-CAPD subjects. Even among subjects without significant peripheral hearing loss, their self-ratings indicated a more significant handicap.

Those findings are supported by Rodriguez et al. (1990) who also found that central auditory involvement in aging can occur without a concomitant decline in peripheral hearing. They further found that the synthetic sentence index test with an ipsilateral competing message influence (SSI-ICM) appears to be the most sensitive measure for central auditory processing involvement.

Stach et al. (1990) have confirmed that among older hearing-impaired persons, the prevalence of central auditory involvement increases with age, until by age 80 years, 95% have a CNS auditory overlay. Their results also showed that even when degree of hearing loss and ability to perform speech audiometric tasks were equated, the prevalence of central presbycusis increased systematically with age.

According to Hull (1988a, 1988b), the premise for a decline in speech comprehension with increasing age is that the complementary intrinsic redundancies inherent in the central auditory system tend to decline as a function of aging. And, as the once natural filtering, tuning, and coding of the peripheral auditory system also declines with increased age and as the older adult is forced to listen in a world of people and environments that degrade the extrinsic redundancies that may have otherwise facilitated auditory function, the older hearing-impaired adult is placed in double jeopardy. Thus, they may exhibit a disproportionate degree of auditory/communicative impairment.

OBSERVATIONS OF LISTENER BEHAVIORS

This author has surveyed older hearing-impaired listeners for 20 years as it relates to their descriptions of difficulties that they experience in speech understanding, including experiences in both nondistracting and auditorily distracting environments and how the listeners cope. Generally, their descriptions and their comparisons with their "recalled" listening skills of earlier years center on changes that reflect an apparent decline in central auditory function within specific areas.

SPEECH VERSUS NONSPEECH

First, older listeners with hearing impairment describe difficulties in attending, sometimes referred to by this author as auditory vigilance, or alerting behaviors, that are important in achieving an auditory "set," or readiness by the auditory system or the person to attend to an auditory/linguistic message. This occurs at either a cognitive or a reflexive level.

SHORT-TERM STORAGE OF INFORMATION

Older hearing-impaired persons describe difficulties in memory, particularly as it relates to short-term storage of linguistic information, from the beginning of a message (or story) to the end. In other words, they retain the last part of a multiple-word message, but under stress to remember, lose

the first or middle part in the transition. Hull (1988a, 1988b) referred to this short-term storage phenomenon as "transitional storage," or "short-term storage-for-analysis and synthesis," or a momentary holding of information, as perhaps a more descriptive term than that of short-term, or working, memory.

EARLY REFINEMENT/PREANALYSIS

Another area of difficulty described by older adults is, for lack of a better descriptor, related to preanalysis, or early refinement, of auditory/linguistic information after it is received. The difficulty may be related to the speed at which speech arrives at the auditory system. For example, if the peripheral and central auditory systems are not provided the time necessary for preanalysis and presynthesis of acoustic/linguistic information, then the coding of a signal both in terms of its electrical-acoustical properties and the synthesis of linguistic/semantic content for translation may become lost in the process.

For the sake of brevity, the factors described by older hearing-impaired listeners, as presented can, at least tentatively, be categorized as those of:

1. Sorting behaviors.
2. Attending behaviors—auditory vigilance.
3. Transitional (working) memory—short-term
4. Alerting, preanalysis, and refinement of the acoustic/linguistic/semantic message content.
5. Phase locking—searching-"locking on" the common acoustical characteristics of a signal for analysis.
6. Speed and accuracy of processing auditory/linguistic information.

These are all critical elements in the integrity of central auditory function, and all perform at the brainstem and cortical levels.

RESEARCH ON CNS AUDITORY FUNCTION AND SPEECH UNDERSTANDING

Research that involves the study of central auditory decline in older age generally centers on the use of various forms of degraded speech, manipulation of nonspeech acoustic signals, or the listening environment. Most involve reducing the redundancy of the auditory stimulus by manipulation of the physical and/or linguistic characteristics of the speech signal to make a listening task more difficult. Most also involve comparisons of performance on the listening task when it is made more difficult. Most also involve comparisons of performance on the listening tasks between younger and older listeners.

DEGRADED SPEECH

The results of various studies involving older subjects have revealed similar findings that older subjects generally have greater difficulty on degraded speech tasks than do younger subjects, even when auditory acuity is essentially normal. For example, Bergman (1980) concluded by stating that,"the understanding of speech in daily life undergoes gradual change with increasing age because of a combination of peripheral and central alterations, even in the absence of a significant hearing loss, and such alterations significantly affect the understanding of speech that is heard under less-than-optimal conditions" (p. 147). He continues his conclusion by stating that part of this phenomenon is a gradual delay in the ability to process rapid speech and, thus, to understand it.

According to L. W. Welsh et al. (1985), the increased difficulty in handling complex auditory tasks that is experienced by older adults is, in all probability, the result of a decline in function of the central auditory system, including factors of:

1. Central competence.
2. Bilateral simultaneous hearing; in other words, a delay in simultaneous binaural routing of signals at the brain stem.
3. Auditory memory.
4. Failure of central fusion when there is incomplete auditory information.
5. Degeneration of neural association (e.g., between hemispheres).
6. Degeneration of neural processing at the brainstem and auditory cortex.
7. Decline in speed of processing within the central nervous system.
8. Neural distortion within the central nervous system.

Early studies by such authors as Bergman (1980); Bilger, Steigel, and Stenson (1976), Jokinen (1973); Smith and Prather (1971); Townsend and Bess (1980); L. W. Welsh et al. (1985); and others have found that, in general, older subjects fare less favorably in signal-to-noise ratios that degrade the speech signal or in situations where there are competing messages.

Studies in which speech stimuli are distorted through filtering also reveal a general decline in performance with increasing age. However, studies by Bergman (1980); Bergman et al. (1976); Harbert et al. (1966); and Palva and Jokinen (1970), do not confirm a significant decline that could not be explained, at least in part, by the peripheral impairment. On the other hand, the study by L. W. Welsh et al. (1985) revealed a general decline in speech understanding with increased age through low-pass filtered speech, even among those with essentially normal hearing.

Studies on the effects of time compression on speech understanding as a factor of age have generally confirmed a decline in tolerance for compression with increased age. These include studies by Hull (1983), Konkle, Beasley, and Less (1977), Schmitt and McCroskey (1981), and others. Schmitt and McCroskey (1981) found fairly great tolerance among older subjects for up to 60% compression. On the other hand, Hull (1982) found a significant decline in speech understanding above 40% compression. In further studies, Hull (1982) discovered that older hearing-impaired subjects could increase speech understanding scores after concentrated practice with time compression, gradually increasing their tolerance to time compressed speech toward the 50% level. This finding has prompted this author to investigate the use of time compression as a therapy tool with hearing-impaired older adults in an attempt to increase the efficiency of the older listener's central auditory system in making auditory/linguistic closure with greater speed and accuracy.

Studies in the literature consistently point to a gradual age-related decline in the auditory system's ability to utilize a speech signal when it is altered either through its temporal (McCroskey & Kasten, 1981) or acoustical characteristics. The primary locus for the decline appears to be the central auditory system, including both the brainstem and auditory cortex. The difficulty experienced by the listener is compounded when there is an accompanying peripheral impairment of a high-frequency nature.

OTHER AUDITORY MANIFESTATIONS OF PRESBYCUSIS

LOUDNESS RECRUITMENT

Loudness is a person's own perception of the relative intensity of sound. *Recruitment*, defined as an abnormally rapid growth of loudness as intensity increases (Carver, 1972), is often observed among clients with a cochlear impairment. It is theorized that the phenomenon of recruitment is the result of damage to the nerve receptors within the cochlea. The abnormal growth of loudness is observed as a perception by the listener that a signal presented appears louder than would ordinarily be observed in an individual with a normal cochlea.

Tests for recruitment have been developed to differentiate between cochlear and retrocochlear auditory impairments. They compare, for example, loudness growth between an impaired frequency in one ear and the same unimpaired frequency in the opposite ear of a person who demonstrates what appears to be a unilateral sensorineural hearing loss. Or, for persons who appear to have a bilateral sensorineural hearing loss, an impaired frequency is compared for abnormal loudness growth with a less impaired or normal frequency in the same ear.

In elderly clients who possess a hearing loss, varying results have been observed regarding recruitment, even though they appear to demonstrate sensorineural hearing impairment. If the presence of recruitment is usually indicative of cochlear pathology, then one would expect to discover it in clients with purely sensorineural involvement.

Pestalozza & Shore (1955) studied the phenomenon of recruitment in 24 elderly subjects with presbycusis. The results of their study indicated that 50% of the subjects did not demonstrate the presence of recruitment, with 50% varying from complete to partial recruitment. Hinchcliffe (1962) has stated that, "the recruitment phenomenon in presbycusis shows that the presence of this phenomenon is not characteristic of presbycusis" (p. 308). As stated earlier, Hinchcliffe does not feel that the hearing loss found in presbycusis is caused wholly by the pathological changes in the cochlea, but by degeneration into the higher auditory pathways. Jerger (1960) supported these findings. He believed that the presence or absence of recruitment is not necessarily related to the phenomenon of presbycusis. Goetzinger, Proud, Dirks, and Embrey (1961), however, found recruitment to be present in 68 out of 80 ears of elderly clients with presbycusis. So the controversy continued at that time. Most of the literature, however, supports the concept that recruitment may or may not be found among the elderly with presbycusis. This further substantiates the presence of pathology beyond the cochlea in presbycusis among elderly clients who possess what appears to be a solely sensorineural hearing impairment.

IMPACT OF REVERBERATION

Communicative environments that are reverberant can play havoc with the older auditory system, whether an person is fit with amplification or not (Bergman, 1980; Humes & Roberts, 1990; Nabelek, 1988; Nabelek & Robinson, 1982). Even for those

with hearing that should be usable for communication, reverberant environments are problematic and can dramatically reduce speech understanding. The cause of the problem is probably the compounding effects of a central auditory deficit (Hull, 1992bc; Nabelek & Robinson, 1982) that is accompanied by a high frequency sensorineural hearing loss. According to Helfer (1991), results from speech understanding tests obtained during routine hearing evaluations in a sound-treated room might be misleading if they are generalized to a person's real-world environments of meeting rooms, church sanctuarys, and other reverberant places. Figure 17-8 presents the results of studies

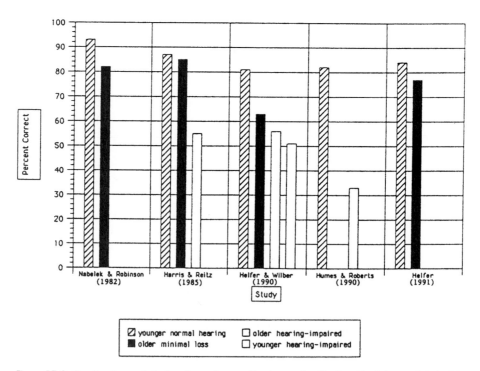

Figure 17-8. Results of several studies of speech perception in reverberation by older listeners. Data in this chart represent performance at the highest level of reverberation in each study (Nabelek & Robinson: T = 1.2 s, Humes & Roberts: T = 3 s, Helfer: T = 0.9 s). Reproduced from Helfer, K. S. (1991). Everyday speech understanding by older listeners. *Journal of the Academy of Rehabilitative Audiology, 24*, 17-34.

dealing with speech understanding by older listeners in reverberant environments as found in Helfer (1991).

It is important that older hearing-impaired clients understand the difficulties that they can expect in reverberant listening environments. Environmental design modifications can often be employed to reduce reverberation and, thus, reduce that barrior to communication, or the client per se can make adjustments in the communicative environment to accommodate his or her needs. Suggestions for these modifications are presented in Chapter 20.

SUMMARY

When one sifts through the many consistencies and inconsistencies in the results of investigations regarding the relationship between the auditory/functional characteristics of presbycusis and the site(s) of lesion of this disorder, there appears to be some commonality of information.

First of all, we seem to be dealing with a compounded disorder that involves the effects of (1) a sensorineural hearing loss that gradually slopes into the higher frequencies, which most certainly would disturb the ability to receive all essential phonemes of oral speech; and (2) a disorder of the higher auditory system (the brainstem and auditory cortex), where the sorting and processing of auditory information takes place. A decrease in the speed and accuracy of processing the auditory code into sets of meaningful linguistic sequences would seem to represent at least a portion of the compounding difficulties seen in presbycusis. When a younger person with an equal sensorineural impairment is found to be only minimally disabled, but the aged person is disabled to the point of embarrassment and withdrawal, the functional pathology involved in presbycusis cannot be restricted to the cochlea and eighth cranial nerve. The central pathways and association areas of the brain must be involved, along, of course,

with many of the social-psychological and physical factors involved in aging.

REFERENCES

Allison, T., Wood, C. C., & Goff, W. R. (1983). Brainstem auditory, pattern-reversal visual and short latency somatosensory evoked potentials; Latencies in relation to age, sex, and brain and body size. *Electroencephalography and Clinical Neurophysiology*, 55, 619–636.

American National Standards Institute. (1970). *American national standard specifications for audiometers, ANSI 3.6-1969*. New York: American National Standards Institute.

American National Standards Institute (1973). *American national standard psychoacoustical terminology, ANSI 3.20-1973*. New York: American National Standards Institute.

American Speech-Language-Hearing Association Task Force on Central Auditory Processing Consensus Development (1996). Central auditory processing: current status of research, and implications for clinical practice. *American Journal of Audiology*, 5, 41–53.

American Standards Association. (1954). Exploratory subcommittee Z24-X-2; *The relations of hearing loss to noise exposure*. New York: American Standards Association.

American Standards Association. (1970). *American standard specification for audiometers for general diagnostic purposes, Z24.5-1951*. New York: American Standards Association.

Anderson, R. G., & Meyerhoff, W. L. (1982). Otologic manifestations of aging. *Otolaryngologic Clinics of North America*, 15, 353–370.

Arenberg, D., Costa, P. T. Jr., Lakatta, E. G., & Tobin, J. D. (1984). *Normal human aging: The Baltimore longitudinal study of aging* (NIH Publication No. 84–2450). Baltimore: U.S. Government Printing Office.

Babbit, J. (1947). The endaural surgery of chronic suppurations. In S. Kapetzky (Ed.), *Looseleaf surgery of the ear*. New York: Nelson and Sons.

Barr, R. A., & Giambra-Leonard, L. M. (1990). Age-related decrement in auditory-selective attention. *Psychology and Aging*, 5, 597–599.

Bayles, K. A. (1987). *Communication and cognition in normal aging and dementia.* San Diego, CA: College-Hill Press.

Beagley, H. A., & Sheldrake, J. B. (1978). Differences in brainstem response latency with age and sex. *British Journal of Audiology, 12,* 69–77.

Beasley, W. C. (1938). *Hearing Study Series Bulletin, No. 7.* National Health Survey. National Institute of Health, United States Public Health Service.

Békésy, G. V. (1957). The ear. *Scientific American, 44,* 1–12.

Békésy, G. V. (1949). The structure of the middle ear and the hearing of one's own voice by bone conduction. *Journal of the Acoustical Society of America, 21,* 217–232.

Békésy, G. V. (1947). A new audiometer. *Acta Otolaryngologica, 35,* 411–422.

Bergman, M. (1980). *Aging and the perception of speech.* Baltimore: University Park Press.

Bergman, M., Blumenfeld, V., Cascardo, D., Dash, B., Levitt, H., & Margulies, M. (1976). Age-related decrement in hearing for speech. *Journal of Geronotology, 31,* 533–538.

Bezold, F. (1894). Investigations concerning the average hearing power of the aged. *Archives of Otology, 23,* 214–227.

Bilger, R. C., Steigel, M. S., & Stenson, N. (1976). Effects of sensorineural loss on hearing speech in noise. *Transactions of the American Academy of Ophthalmology and Otolaryngology, 82,* 363–365.

Birren, J. (1974). Translations in gerontology—from lab to life: Psychophysiology and speed of response. *American Psychologist, 29,* 808–815.

Birren, J., & Clayton, P. (1975) History of gerontology. New York: D. Van Nostrand.

Bowles, N., & Poon, L. (1981). The effect of age on speed of lexical access. *Experiments In Aging Research, 7,* 417–425.

Brant, K. J., & Fozard, J. L. (1990). Age changes in pure-tone thresholds in a longitudinal study of normal aging. *Journal of the Acoustical Society of America, 88,* 813–820.

Briner, W. & Willott, J. F. (1989). Ultrastructural features of neurons in the C57BL/6J mouse anteroventral cochlear nucleus: young mice versus old mice with chronic presbycusis. *Neurobiology of Aging, 10,* 259–303.

Brock, W. (1975, May 20). *Congressional Record IV.,* 81.

Bromley, D. (1958). Some effects of age on short-term learning and remembering. *Journal of Gerontology, 13,* 398–406.

Bunch, C. C., & Railford, T. S. (1931). Race and sex variations in auditory acuity. *Archives of Otolaryngology, 13,* 423–434.

Canestrari, R. Jr. (1963). Paced and self-paced learning in young and elderly adults. *Journal of Gerontology, 18,* 165–168.

Carhart, R. (1957). Clinical determination of abnormal auditory adaptation. *Archives of Otolaryngology, 65,* 32–39.

Carver, W. (1972). Differential diagnostic evaluation: Cochlear vs retrocochlear. In J. Katz (Ed.), *Handbook of clinical audiology* (pp. 485–496). Baltimore: Williams and Wilkins.

Casey, M. A., & Feldman, M. L. (1982). Aging in the rat medial nucleus of the trapezoid body: I. Light microscopy. *Neurobiology of Aging, 3,* 187–195.

Caspary, D. M., Raza, A., Lawhorn-Armour, B. A., Pippin, J., & Arneric, S. P. (1990). Immunocytochemical and neurochemical evidence for age-related loss of GABA in the inferior colliculus: implications for neural presbycusis. *Journal of Neuroscience, 10,* 2363–2372.

Cerella, J., Poon, L., & Fozard, J. (1981). Mental rotation and age reconsidered. *Journal of Gerontology, 36,* 620–624.

Chafee, C. (1967). Rehabilitation needs of nursing home patients: a report of a survey. *Rehabilitation Literature, 18,* 377–389.

Corso, J. F. (1963). Age and sex differences in pure-tone thresholds. *Archives of Otolaryngology, 77,* 385–405.

Corso, J. F. (1976). Presbycusis as a complicating factor in evaluating noise-induced hearing loss. In D. Henderson, R. P. Hamernik, D. S. Dasanjh, & J. H. Mills (Eds.), *Effects of noise on hearing* (pp. 497–524). New York: Raven Press.

Corso, J. F. (1981). *Aging sensory systems and perception.* New York: Praeger.

Crabbe, F. (1963). Presbycusis. *Acta Otolaryngologica, 183* (Suppl.), 24–26.

Craik, F. I. M. (1968). Two components of free recall. *Journal of Verbal Learning and Verbal Behavior, 7,* 996–1004.

Craik, F. I. M. (1977). Age differences in human memory. In J. Birren, & K. Schaie (Eds.), *Handbook of the psychology of aging* (pp. 117–132). New York: Van Nostrand Reinhold.

Cranford, J. L., & Stream, R. (1991). Discrimination of short duration tones by elderly subjects. *Journal of Gerontology, 46,* 37–41.

Cranford, J. L., Stream, R., Rye, C., & Slade, T. (1982). Detection versus discrimination of brief duration tones: Findings in patients with temporal lobe damage. *Archives of Otolaryngology, 108,* 350–356.

Crowe, S. J., Guild, S. R., & Polvogt, L. M. (1934). Observation on the pathology of high tone deafness. *Bulletin of the Johns Hopkins Hospital, 54,* 315–380.

Crowder, R. (1980). Echoic memory and the study of aging memory systems. In Poon, L., Fozard, L., Cermak, D., Arenberg, D., and Thompson, L. (Ed.), *New directions in memory and aging.* Hillsdale, NJ: Lawrence Erlbaum.

Davies, D. V. (1948). A note on the articulations of the auditory ossicles and related structures. *Journal Of Laryngology, 62,* 533–535.

Dirks, D., & Bower, D. (1970). Effect of forward and backward masking on speech intelligibility. *Journal of the Acoustical Society of America, 47,* 1003–1008.

Drachman, D., & Leavitt, J. (1972). Memory impairment in the aged: Storage versus retrieval deficit. *Journal of Experimental Psychology, 93,* 302–308.

Dubno, J. R., Dirks, D. D., & Morgan, D. E. (1982). Effects of mild hearing loss and age on speech recogniton in noise. *Journal of the Acoustical Society of America, 72,* 534–535.

Ferraro, J. A., & Minckler, J. (1977). The human lateral lemniscus and its nuclei. *Brain and Language, 4,* 277–294.

Fisch, U., Bobozi, M., & Greig, D. (1972). Degenerative changes of the arterial vessels of the internal auditory meatus during the process of aging. *Acta Otolaryngologica, 73,* 259–266.

Frager, R. (1968). Manifestations of hearing loss in aging. Unpublished masters thesis, Fort Collins, CO: Colorado State University.

Fullerton, A. M., & Smith, A. D. (1980). Age-related differences in the use of redundancy. *Journal of Gerontology, 35,* 729–735.

Gaeth, J. (1948). *A study of phonemic regression associated with hearing loss.* Unpublished doctoral dissertation, Chicago: Northwestern University. (Cited in Willeford, 1971.)

Galton, F. (1884). Data collected at the international health exhibition, London, England. Cited in Birren & Clayton (1975). *History of gerontology.* New York: D. Van Nostrand.

Gatehouse, S., & Lowe, G. D. (1990). Whole blood viscosity and red cell filterability as factors in sensorineural hearing impairment in the elderly. *Acta-Otolaryngologica, 476*(Suppl.), 37–43.

Gengel, R. W. (1973). Temporal effects in frequency discrimination by hearing-impaired listeners. *Journal of the Acoustical Society of America, 54,* 11–15.

Glorig, A., & Davis, H. (1961). Age, noise, and hearing loss. *Annals of Otology, Rhinology, and Laryngology, 70,* 556–571.

Glorig, A., & Nixon, J. (1960). Distributions of hearing loss in various populations. *Annals of Otology, Rhinology, and Laryngology, 69,* 497–516.

Glorig, A., Wheeler, D., Quiggle, R., Grings, W., & Summerfield, A. (1957; 1954). *Wisconsin state fair hearing survey* [Monograph]. Philadelphia: American Academy of Ophthalmology and Otolaryngology.

Goetzinger, C., Proud, G., Dirks, D., & Embrey, J. (1961). A study of hearing in advanced age. *Archives of Otolaryngology, 73,* 662–674.

Gordon-Salant, S., & Fitzgibbons, P.J. (1995). Recognition of multiply degraded speech by young and elderly listeners. *Journal of Speech-Language and Hearing Research, 38,* 1150–1156.

Hall, J. W. (1992). *Handbook of auditory evoked responses.* Boston: Allyn and Bacon.

Hallpike, C., & Hood, J. (1951). Some recent work on auditory adaptation and its relation to the loudness recruitment phenomenon. *Journal of the Acoustical Society of America, 23,* 270–274.

Hansen, C. C., & Reske-Nielsen, E. (1965). Pathological studies in presbycusis. *Archives of Otolaryngology, 82,* 115–132.

Harbert, F., Young, I., & Menduke, H. (1966). Audiological findings in presbycusis. *Journal of Auditory Research, 6,* 297–312.

Hawkins, J. (1973). Comparative otopathology: Aging, noise, and ototoxic drugs. *Advances in Otorhinolaryngology, 20, 125–141.*

Helfer, K. S. (1991). Everyday speech understanding by older listeners. *Journal of the Academy of Rehabilitative Audiology, 24,* 17–34.

Hinchcliffe, R. (1959). The threshold of hearing as a function of age. *Acoustics, 9,* 303–308.

Hinchcliffe, R. (1962). The anatomical locus of presbycusis. *Journal of Speech and Hearing Disorders, 27,* 301–310.

Hirsh, I. J., Palva, T., & Goodman, A. (1954). Difference limen and recruitment. *Archives of Otolaryngology, 60,* 525–540.

Howard, D. V. (1983). *Cognitive psychology: Memory, language, and thought.* New York: Macmillan.

Howard, D., Shaw, R., & Heisey, J. (1986). Aging and the time course of semantic activation. *Journal of Gerontology, 41,* 195–203.

Hull, R. H. (1972). *Serial study of the inferior colliculus in humans.* Unpublished doctoral study, Denver, CO: University of Denver.

Hull, R. H. (1982). Techniques of aural rehabilitation treatment. In Hull, R. H. (Ed.). *Rehabilitative audiology.* Philadelphia: Grune and Stratton.

Hull, R. H. (1983). Central auditory manifestations in presbycusis. *Journal Internationale d'Audiophonologie, 15,* 61–71.

Hull, R. H. (1988a). *Central auditory processing and aging.* Paper presented at the Research Symposium on Communication Sciences and Disorders and Aging, American Speech-Language-Hearing Association annual meeting, Washington, DC.

Hull, R. H. (1988b). Taking charge: Research on a procedure in geriatric aural rehabilitation. Presentation before the International Congress of the Hard of Hearing. Montreux, Switzerland.

Hull, R. H. (1992a). WSU Communication Appraisal and Priorities Profile. In R. H. Hull (Ed.), *Aural rehabilitation* (pp. 483–485). San Diego, CA: Singular Publishing Group.

Hull, R. H. (1992b). Hearing loss in older adulthood. In R. H. Hull (Ed.), *Aural rehabilitation* (pp.215–234). San Diego, CA: Singular Publishing Group.

Hull, R. H. (1992c). Techniques of aural rehabilitation for older adults. In R.H. Hull (Ed.), *Aural rehabilitation* (pp.278–292). San Diego, CA: Singular Publishing Group.

Hull, R. H. (1994). *Frequency selectivity in aging.* Research supported by the Wichita State University Office of Research Administration. For copies contact the author at Wichita State University, P. O. Box 75, Wichita, KS 67260

Hultsch, D. F., & Dixon, R. A. (1983). The role of preexperimental knowledge in text processing in adulthood. *Experiments in Aging Research, 9,* 17–22.

Hultsch, D. F., & Dixon, R. A. (1984). Memory for text materials in adulthood. In P. B. Baltes & O. G. Brim, J. (Eds.), *Life-span development and behavior.* New York: Academic Press.

Humes, L. E., & Roberts, L. (1990). Speech-recognition difficulties of the hearing-impaired elderly: the contributions of audibility. *Journal of Speech and Hearing Research, 33,* 726–735.

Jatho, K., & Heck, K. H. (1959). Schwellen audiometrisch Untersuchungen uber die Progredienz und Charakteristik der Alterschwerhörigkeit in den verschiedenen Lebensabschnitten. *Zeitschrift für Laryngologie, Rhinologie, Otologie und ihre Grenzgebiete, 1959, 38,* 72. (Cited in Spoor, A. (1967). Presbycusis values in relation to noise induced hearing loss. *International Audiology, 6,* 48–57).

Jerger, J. (1992). Can age-related decline in speech understanding be explained by peripheral hearing loss? *Journal of the American Academy of Audiology, 3,* 33–38.

Jerger, J. (1985). *The locus of presbycusis.* Presentation before The Working Group on Hearing Loss In Aging. Bethesda, MD: National Institutes of Health, Public Health Service.

Jerger, J. (1979). *Studies in central auditory processing and aging.* Presentation before the Working Group On Hearing Loss In Aging. Bethesda: National Institutes of Health, U.S. Public Health Service.

Jerger, J. (1973). Audiological findings in aging. *Advances In Otorhinolaryngology, 20,* 115–24.

Jerger, J. (1960). Békésy audiometry in analysis of auditory disorders. *Journal of Speech and Hearing Research, 3,* 275–287.

Jerger, J., Alford, B., Lew, H., Rivera, V., & Chmiel, R. (1995). Dichotic listening, event-related potentials, and interhemispheric transfer in the elderly. *Ear and Hearing, 16,* 482–498.

Jerger, J., & Chmiel, R. (1997). Factor analytic structure of auditory impairment in elderly persons. *Journal of the American Academy of Audiology, 8,* 269–276.

Jerger, J., Chmiel, R., Stach, B., & Spretnjak, M. (1993). Gender affects audiometric shape in presbyacusis. *Journal of the American Academy of Audiology, 4,* 42–49.

Jerger, J., & Hayes, D. (1977). Diagnostic speech audiometry. *Archives of Otolaryngology, 103,* 216–222.

Jerger, J., & Johnson, K. (1988). Interactions of age, gender, and sensorineural hearing loss on ABR latency. *Ear and Hearing, 9,* 168–176.

Jerger, J., Oliver, T. A., & Pirozzolo, F. (1990). Impact of central auditory processing disorder and cognitive deficit on the self-assessment of hearing handicap in the elderly. *Journal of the American Academy of Audiology*, *1*, 75–80.

Jerger, J., Shedd, J., & Harford, E. (1959). On the detection of extremely small changes of sound intensity. *Archives of Otolaryngology*, *69*, 200–211.

Johansen, H. (1943). *Den Aldersbetingede Tunghorhed*. Copenhagen: Munksgaard. (Cited in Spoor, A. (1967). Presbycusis values in relation to noise-induced hearing loss. *International Audiology*, *6*, 48–57.

Johnson, J., & Hadley, R. (1964). The pinna. In J. Converse (Ed.), *Reconstructive and plastic surgery* (pp. 243–260). Philadelphia: W.B. Saunders.

Johnsson, L., & Hawkins, J. (1972). Sensory and neural degeneration with aging as seen in microdissections of the human inner ear. *Annals of Otology, Rhinology, and Laryngology*, *81*, 179–193.

Jokinen, K. (1973). Presbyacusis VI. Masking of speech. *Acta Otolaryngologica*, *76*, 426–430.

Jorgensen, M. (1961). Changes of aging in the inner ear. *Archives of Otolaryngology*, *74*, 161–170.

Kalikow, D. N., Stevens, K. N., & Elliott, L. L. (1977). Development of a test of speech intelligibility in noise using sentence materials with controlled word predictability. *Journal of the Acoustical Society of America*, *61*, 1337–1351.

Kasten, R. (1982). The impact of aging on auditory perception. In R. H. Hull (Ed.), *The communicatively disordered elderly* (pp. 265–277). New York: Grune and Stratton.

Kasten, R. (1980). Speed of processing as a factor of aging. Paper presented before the *Aspen Symposium on Aging*, Aspen, CO.

Katz, J. & Kusnierczyk, K. (1993). Central auditory processing: The auditory contribution. *Seminars In Hearing*. *14*. 191–199.

Kausler, D. H. (1982). *Experimental psychology and human aging*. New York: Wiley.

Kelly-Ballweber, D., & Dobie, R. A. (1984). Binaural interaction measured behaviorally and electrophysiologically in young and old adults. *Audiology*, *23*, 181–194.

Konkle, D., Beasley, D. S., & Bess, F. (1977). Intelligibility of time-altered speech in relation to chronological aging. *Journal of Speech and Hearing Research*, *20*, 108–115.

Kirikae, I., Sato, T., & Shitara, T. (1964). Study of hearing in advanced age. *Laryngoscope*, *74*, 205–221.

Kirk, K. I., Pisoni, D. B., & Miyzmoto, R. C. (1997). Effects of stimulus variability on speech perception in listeners with hearing impairment. *Journal of Speech-Language-Hearing Research*, *40*, 1395–1405.

Klotz, R., & Kilbane, M. (1962). Hearing in the aging population. *New England Journal of Medicine, 266*, 277–280.

Konig, E. (1957). Pitch discrimination and age. *Acta Otolaryngologica*, *48*, 473–489.

Konigsmark, B. W., & Murphy, E. A. (1972). Volume of the ventral cochlear nucleus in man: Its relationship to neuronal population and age. *Journal of Neuropathology and Experimental Neurology*, *31*, 304–316.

Kopra, L. L. (1982). Auditory-communicative manifestations of presbycusis. In R. H. Hull (Ed.), *Rehabilitative audiology* (pp. 212–235). New York: Grune and Stratton.

Korabic, E. W., Freeman, B. A., & Church, G. T. (1978). Intelligibility of time-expanded speech with normally hearing and elderly subjects. *Audiology*, *17*, 159–164.

Korsan-Bengtsen, M. (1968). The diagnosis of hearing loss in old people. In G. Lidén (Ed.), *Geriatric audiology*. Stockholm: Almquist and Wiksell.

Landis, B. (1958). Recruitment measured by automatic audiometry. *Archives of Otolaryngology*, *68*, 685–696.

Leake, C. (1963). Study of the components of deafness. *Geriatrics*, *18*, 506–509.

Lebo, C. P., & Reddell, R. C. (1972). The presbycusis component in occupational hearing loss. *Laryngoscope*, *82*, 1399–1409.

Letowski, T., & Poch, N. (1995). Understanding time-compressed speech by older adults: Effects of discard internal. *Journal of the American Academy of Audiology*, *6*, 433–439.

Levitt, H., Mayer, C., & Bergman, M. (1980). Criteria for ambient noise zone quality standards. In Bergman, M. (Eds.), *Aging and the perception of speech* (pp. 27–42). Baltimore: University Park Press.

Liberman, A., Cooper, F., Shankweiler, D., & Studdert-Kennedy, M. (1967). Perception of the speech code. *Psychological Reivew*, *74*, 431–461.

Luterman, D. M., Welsh, O. L., & Melrose, J. (1966). Responses of aged males to time-altered speech stimuli. *Journal of Speech and Hearing Research*, *9*, 226–230.

Magladery, J. (1959). Neurophysiology of aging. In J. Birren (Ed.), *Handbook of aging and the individual: Psychological and biological aspects* (pp. 220–231). Chicago: University of Chicago Press.

Madden, D. (1985). Age-related slowing in the retrieval of information from long-term memory. *Journal of Gerontology, 40,* 208–210.

Makishima, K. (1978). Arteriosclerosis as a cause of presbycusis. *Otolaryngology, 86,* 322–326.

Marston, L. E., & Goetzinger, C. P. (1972). A comparison of sensitized words and sentences for distinguishing nonperipheral auditory changes as a function of aging. *Cortex, 8,* 213–223.

Martin, D. R., & Cranford, J. L. (1989). Evoked potential evidence of reduced binaural processing in elderly persons. *The Hearing Journal, 42,* 18–23.

Maurizi, M., Altissimi, G., Ottaviani, F., Paludetti, G., & Bambini, M. (1982). Auditory brainstem responses (ABR) in the aged. *Scandinavian Audiology, 11,* 213–221.

Mayer, C. (1975). *The perception of speech in noise as a function of age.* Unpublished doctoral dissertation. New York: City University of New York.

McCroskey, R. L., & Kasten, R. N. (1981). Assessment of central auditory processing. In R. R. Rupp & K. Stockdell (Eds.), *Speech audiometry,* (pp. 126–142). New York: Grune & Stratton.

Mehta, Z. (1999). *Speech perception in older adulthood.* Unpublished paper. Wichita, KS: Wichita State University.

Michalewski, H. J., Thompson, L. W., Patterson, J. V., Bowman, T. E., & Litzelman, D. (1980). Sex differences in the amplitudes and latencies of the human auditory brainstem potential. *Electroencephalography and Clinical Neurophysiology, 48,* 351–356.

Miller, M., & Ort, R. (1965). Hearing problems in a home for the aged. *Acta Otolaryngologica, 59,* 33–44.

Nabelek, A. K. (1988). Identification of vowels in quiet, noise, and reverberation: Relationships with age and hearing loss. *Journal of the Acoustical Society of America, 84,* 476–484.

Nabelek, A. K., & Robinson, P. K. (1982). Monaural and binaural speech perception in reverberation for listeners of various ages. *Journal of the Acoustical Society of America, 71,* 1242–1248.

Nabelek, A. K., & Mason, D. (1981). Effect of noise and reverberation on binaural and monaural word identification by subjects with various audiograms. *Journal of Speech and Hearing Research, 24,* 385–383.

National Advisory Neurological Diseases and Stroke Council. (1980). *Human communication and its disorders* (NIH Monograph No. 20). Bethesda, MD: National Institutes of Health, National Institute of Neurological, Communicative Disorders and Stroke.

National Center For Health Statistics. (1994a). *Current estimates from the National Health Interview Survey, 1990.* Vital Health Statistics, *10,* 1991, 181.

National Center For Health Statistics. (1994b). *Prevalence and characteristics of persons with hearing trouble* (Series 10. No. 188). Data From The National Health Survey. DHHS, PHS, 5–10.

National Center for Health Statistics. (1981). *Prevalence of selected impairments* (DHHS Pub. no [PHS] 82–1562). Washington, DC: Author.

National Center For Health Statistics. (1975). *Persons with Impaired hearing; United States.* Vital Health Statistics 10, 101.

Orchik, D. J., & Burgess, J. (1977). Synthetic sentence identification as a function of the age of the listener. *Journal of the American Audiological Society, 3,* 42–46.

Palva, A., & Jokinen, K. (1970). Presbycusis v. filtered speech test. *Acta Otolaryngologica, 70,* 232–241.

Patterson, J. V., Michalewski, H. J., Thompson, K. W., Bowman, T. E., & Litzelman, D. K. (1981). Age and sex differences in the human auditory brainstem responses. *Journal of Gerontology, 36,* 455–462.

Pestalozza, G., & Shore, I. (1955). Clinical evaluation of presbycusis on the basis of different tests of auditory function. *Laryngoscope, 65,* 136–163.

Pfefferbaum, A., Ford, J. M., Roth, W. T., Hopkins, W. F., & Kopell, B. S. (1979). Event-related potential changes in healthy aged females. *Electroencephalography and Clinical Neurophysiology, 46,* 81–86.

Pfefferbaum, A., Ford, J. M., Roth, W. T., & Kopell, B. S. (1980). Age-related changes in auditory event-related potentials. *Electroencephalography and Clinical Neurophysiology, 49,* 266–276.

Pfefferbaum, A., Wenegrat, B. G., Ford, J. M., Roth, W. T., & Kopell, B. S. (1984). Clinical application of the P3 component of event-related potentials: II. Dementia, depression and schizophrenia. *Electroencephalography and Clinical Neurophysiology, 59,* 104–124.

Poon, L. (1985). Differences in human memory with aging: Nature, causes, and clinical implications. In J. Birren & K. Schaie (Eds.), *Handbook of the psychology of aging* (pp. 427–462). New York: Van Nostrand Reinhold.

Poon, L., Walsh-Sweeney, L., & Fozard, J. (1980). Memory skill training for the elderly: Salient issues on the use of memory mnemonics. In Poon, et al., (Eds.), *Proceedings of the George A. Talland Memorial Conference* (pp. 123–145). Hillsdale, NJ: Lawrence Erlbaum.

Proctor, B. (1961). Chronic progressive deafness. *Archives Of Otolaryngology, 73,* 444–499, 565–615.

Psatta, D. & Matei, M. (1988). Age-dependent amplitude variation of brainstem auditory evoked potentials. *Electroencephalography and Clinical Neurophysiology, 71,* 27–32.

Puce, A., Donnan, G. A., & Bladin, P. F. (1989). Comparative effects of age on limbic and scalp P3. *Electroencephalography and Clinical Neurophysiology, 74,* 385–393.

Ramadan, H. H., & Schuknecht, H. F. (1989). Is there a conductive type of presbycusis? *Otolaryngology—Head, Neck Surgery, 100,* 30–34.

Rizzo, S. R., & Gutnick, H. N. (1991). Cochlear versus retrocochlear presbycusis: Clinical correlates. *Ear and Hearing, 12,* 61–63.

Rodriguez, G. P., DiSarno, N. J., & Hardiman, C. J. (1990). Central auditory processing in normal-hearing elderly adults. *Audiology, 29,* 85–92.

Rosen, S., Bergman, M., Plester, D., El-Mofty, A., & Satti, M. (1962). Presbycusis study of a relatively noise-free population of the Sudan. *Annals of Otology, Rhinology and Laryngology, 79,* 18–32.

Rosenhamer, H. J., Lindstrom, B., & Lundborg, T. (1980). On the use of click-evoked responses in audiological diagnosis: I. the variability of the normal response. *Scandinavian Audiology, 7,* 193–205.

Rosenwasser, H. (1964). Otitic problems in the aged. *Geriatrics, 19,* 11–17.

Rowe, M. J. (1978). Normal variability of the brainstem auditory evoked response in young and old adult subjects. *Electroencephalography and Clinical Neurophysiology, 44,* 459–470.

Salthouse, T. (1982). *Adult cognition.* New York: Springer.

Salthouse, T., & Kail, R. (1983). Memory development throughout the life span: The role of processing rate. In P. Bates & O. Brim (Eds.), *Life span development and behavior, 5,* (pp. 82–110). New York: Academic Press.

Schaie, K., Warner, P., & Strother, C. (1964). A study of auditory sensitivity in advanced age. *Journal of Gerontology, 19,* 453–457.

Schmitt, J. F. (1983). The effects of time compression and time expansion on passage comprehension by elderly listeners. *Journal of Speech and Hearing Research, 26,* 373–377.

Schmitt, J. F., & Carroll, M. R. (1985). Older listeners' ability to comprehend speaker-generated rate alteration of passages. *Journal of Speech and Hearing Research, 28,* 309–312.

Schmitt, J. F., & McCroskey, R. (1981). Sentence comprehension in elderly listeners: The factor of rate. *Journal of Gerontology, 36,* 441–445.

Schmitt, J. F., & Moore, J. R. (1989). Natural alteration of speaking rate: the effect on passage comprehension by listeners over 75 years of age. *Journal of Speech and Hearing Research, 32,* 445–450.

Schock, N. W., Greulich, R. C., Andres, R. Arenberg, D., Costa, P. T. Jr., Lakatta, E. G., & Tobin, J. D. (1984). *Normal human aging: The Baltimore Longitudinal Study of Aging* (pp. 89–112). NIH Publication No. 84–2450. Washington, DC: U.S. Government Printing Office.

Schow, R. L., & Nerbonne, M. A. (1980). Hearing levels among elderly nursing home residents. *Journal of Speech and Hearing Disorders, 45,* 124–132.

Schuknecht, H. (1974). The pathology of presbycusis. Paper presented at a *Workshop on Geriatric Aural Rehabilitation,* Denver, CO.

Schuknecht, H. (1964). Further observations on the pathology of presbycusis. *Archives of Otolaryngology, 80,* 369–82.

Schuknecht, H., & Woellner, R. (1955). An experimental and clinical study of deafness from lesions of the cochlear nerve. *Journal of Laryngology and Otology, 69,* 75–97.

Schuknecht, H. F., & Gacek, M. R. (1993). Cochlear pathology in presbycusis. *Annals of Otology, Rhinology, and Laryngology, 102,* 1–16.

Senturia, B. (1957). *Diseases of the external ear.* Springfield, IL: Charles C. Thomas.

Smith, R. A., & Prather, W. F. (1971). Phoneme discrimination in older persons with varying signal-to-noise conditions. *Journal of Speech and Hearing Research, 14,* 630–638.

Spoor, A. (1967) Presbycusis values in relation to noise induced hearing loss. *International Audiology, 6,* 48–57.

Stach, B. A. (1990). Central auditory processing disorders and amplification applications. *Research Sympo-*

sium: Communication Sciences and Disorders and Aging—ASHA Reports Series, 19, 150–156.

Stach, B. A., Spretnjak, M. L., & Jerger, J. (1990). The prevalence of central presbycusis in a clinical population. *Journal of the American Academy of Audiology, 1*, 109–115.

Stevens, K., & House, A. (1972). Speech perception. In Tobias, J. (Ed.), *Foundations of modern auditory theory*, Vol. 2. New York: Academic Press.

Suga, F., & Lindsay, J. R. (1976). Histopathological observations of presbycusis. *Annals of Otology, Rhinology, and Laryngology, 85*, 169–184.

Thomas, J., & Ruben, J. (1973). Age and mnemonic techniques in paired associate learning. Presented before *The Gerontological Society*, Miami, FL.

Thomsen, J., Terkeldsen, K., & Osterhammel, P. (1978). Auditory brainstem responses in patients with acoustic neuromas. *Scandinavian Audiology, 7*, 179–183.

Tobias, J. V. (1988). Working group on speech understanding and aging. *Journal of the Acoustical Society of America, 83*, 859–895.

Tobias, J. V., Bilger, R. C., Brody, H. K., Haskell, G., Howard, D., Marshall, L. A., Nerbonne, M. A., & Pickett, J. A. (1988). Speech understanding and aging. *Journal of the Acoustical Society of America, 83*, 859–894.

Townsend, T. J., & Bess, F. H. (1980). Effects of age and sensorineural hearing loss on word recognition. *Scandinavian Audiology, 9*, 245–248.

Traynor, R., & Hull, R. (1974). *Pure-tone thresholds among a confined elderly population*. Unpublished research. Greeley, CO: University of Northern Colorado.

Vaughan, N. E., & Letowski, T. (1997). Effects of age, speech rate, and type of test on temporal auditory processing. *Journal of Speech-Language and Hearing Research, 40*, 1192–1200.

Waugh, N., & Barr, R. (1982). Encoding deficits in aging. In F. Craik & S. Trehub (Eds.), *Aging and cognitive processes* (pp. 189–211). New York: Plenum.

Waugh, N., Thomas, J., & Fozard, J. (1978). Retrieval time from different memory stores. *Journal of Gerontology, 33*, 718–724.

Weg, R. (1975). Changing physiology of aging: Normal and pathological. In D. Woodruff & J. Birren (Eds.), *Aging: Scientific perspectives and social issues* (pp. 163–190). New York: D. Van Nostrand

Welsh, L. W., Welsh, J. J., and Healy, M. P. (1985). Central presbycusis. *Laryngoscope, 95*, 128–136.

Welsh, O. L., Luterman, D. M., & Bell, M. (1969). The effects of aging on response to filtered speech. *Journal of Gerontology, 24*, 189–192.

Willeford, J. (1971). The geriatric patient. In D. Rose (Ed.), *Audiological assessment* (pp. 107–121). Englewood Cliffs, NJ: Prentice Hall.

Wingfield, A., Poon, L.W., Lombardi, L., & Lowe, D. (1985). Speed of processing in normal aging: Effects of speech rate, linguistic structure and processing time. *Journal of Gerontology, 40*, 579–585.

Working Group on Speech Understanding and Aging. (1988). Speech understanding and aging. *Journal of the Acoustical Society of America, 83*, 859–894.

Zafar, H. (1994). *Implications of frequency selectivity and temporal resolution for amplification in the elderly*. Unpublished doctoral dissertation. Wichita, KS: Wichita State University.

Zwaardemaker, H. (1894). The presbycusic law. *Archives of Otology, 23*, 228–234.

Zwaardemaker, H. (1891). Der Verlust an hohen Tonen mitzundem Alter. Ein neues Gesetz. *Archives für Ohrenheilkunde, 32*, 53–56.

END OF CHAPTER EXAMINATION QUESTIONS

CHAPTER 17

1. What is presbycusis?

2. Describe the structural changes of the auditory system in aging (include the pinna, external auditory meatus, middle ear, cochlea, and brainstem).

3. Describe three tests of degraded speech used to assess central auditory processing difficulties found among older adults.

4. Name Schuknecht's four types of presbycusis.
   a.
   b.
   c.
   d.

5. The loss of hearing acuity in the_____ frequencies in aging is typically found as part of the process of aging.
   a. lower
   b. higher
   c. middle
   d. all of the above

6. At age 65 and above, the incidence of a hearing impairment is estimated at:
   a. 23%
   b. 29%
   c. 60%
   d. 5%

7. What are two characteristic auditory manifestations of presbycusis observed by the audiologist?
   a.
   b.

8. Presbycusis is typically characterized by both _____and_____ hearing loss.

END OF CHAPTER ANSWER SHEET

Name _____ Date _____

CHAPTER 17

1. _____

   _____

   _____

   _____

   _____

   _____

2. _____

   _____

   _____

   _____

   _____

   _____

   _____

   _____

3. a.

   b.

   c.

4. a.

   b.

   c.

   d.

5. Which one(s)?   a   b   c   d

6. Which one(s)?   a   b   c   d

7. a. _____

   b. _____

   _____

8. _____

   _____

9. _____

   _____

   _____

   _____

10. _____

9. A characteristic of hearing loss in older adult-hood has been coined "phoneme regression" which, defined, refers to _____
_____.

10. Adults more than age 65 years have been found to do (better, worse) than younger adults on listening tasks that involve degraded speech.

CHAPTER 18

The Impact of Hearing Loss on Older Persons

RAYMOND H. HULL, PH.D.

From the information presented in Chapter 17, it is clear that the effects of aging on individuals are as unique as their response to the process. When the effects of aging begin to impact negatively on sensory processes that previously permitted efficient personal and social functioning, then it may become even more difficult to cope with older age. The sensory deficit discussed here is presbycusis, or hearing impairment as a result of the process of aging.

THE IMPACT

Whatever the cause of the disorder called presbycusis, the effects on the some 20 million persons who possess it are, in many respects, the same. The disappointment of not having been able to understand what their children and grandchildren were saying at the last family reunion can be frustrating to say the least. It becomes easier to withdraw from situations where communication with others may take place rather than face embarrassment from frequent misunderstandings of statements and inappropriate responses. To respond to the question, "How did you sleep last night?" with "At home of course!" is embarrassing, particularly when other misinterpretations may have occurred within the same conversation and continue with increasing regularity. An older person, who may be an otherwise alert, intelligent adult, will understandably be concerned about such misunderstandings. Many elderly adults who experience such difficulties feel that perhaps they are "losing their senses," particularly when they may not know the cause for the speech understanding problems. Perhaps their greatest concern is that their family may feel that they are losing the ability to function independently and that the personal aspects of life for which they are responsible will be taken away.

Communication is such an integral part of financial dealings, for example, that elderly persons may also question their own ability to maintain a responsible position in the family, although in the end they may not wish to withdraw from those responsibilities. The self-questioning that may occur can be further aggravated by well-meaning comments by others. A comment by a concerned son or daughter such as, "Dad, why don't you think about selling the house and moving into an apartment? You know this house is too much for you to care for," can be defeating. Even though an elderly family member may be adequately caring for the house, cooking nutritious meals, and looking forward to each spring so that he or she can work in the garden, a seed of doubt about one's ability to maintain a house and other life requirements adequately because of age has been planted. A statement by his or her physician such as, "Of course you're having aches and pains, you're not a spring chicken any more," can bring about doubts of survival.

Compounding these self-doubts may be a growing inability to understand what others are saying because of presbycusis. It becomes easier, for lack of other alternatives, to withdraw from communicative situations in which embarrassment or fear of embarrassment may occur. If forced into such a difficult situation, the easiest avenue is to become noncommunicative rather than to attempt responses to questions and fail, thus instilling doubts in younger family members' minds about one's ability to maintain independent living. If forced into responding to questions that are not fully understood because an important word is missed or misunderstood, frustration by both the elderly person and the family can result.

HOW DO OLDER PERSONS REACT TO THEIR HEARING IMPAIRMENT?

Feelings of embarrassment, frustration, anger, and ultimate withdrawal from situations that require communication are very real among older persons who have hearing impairment and those who interact with them. When so much else is taken away from many older adults, including leadership in a family, a steady income, a spouse or friend who may have recently passed away, convenient transportation, and a regular social life, a gradual decrease in one's ability to hear and understand what others are saying can be debilitating. As one elderly person said, "I would like to participate socially, but I feel isolated when I cannot hear."

Many older adults feel so frustrated by their inability to understand what the minister is saying at church, what their friends are saying at the senior center, or what the speaker at an anticipated meeting is saying, that they withdraw from such situations. They may be described by their family or others with whom they associate as noncommunicating, uncooperative, withdrawn, and, most unkind of all, senile. An inability to use hearing aids as well as expected may further result in fear by the older adult or his or her family that, perhaps, the disorder is mental rather than auditory.

It has been observed by this writer that, in some instances, a portion of the depression experienced by older persons who have hearing impairment is brought about by feelings that breakdowns in communication being experienced, "are all my fault because it is my hearing impairment." It may not occur to them that the disorder of hearing may be magnified by family members who do not speak plainly or by being placed in communicative environments that are so noisy and otherwise distracting that only a person with normal auditory function would be able to hear and understand the speech of others. Those, for example, may include attempting to listen to a speaker in an auditorium with poor acoustics and the only seat left when he or she arrived was toward the rear of the room, watching a 20-year-old television set with distorted-sound speakers, or attempting to understand what his or her shy 3-year-old granddaughter is saying.

Some older persons who have hearing impairment become so defeated in their attempts at communication that it does not dawn on them that they might be better able to understand what others are saying if those with whom they are communicating would either improve their manner of speaking or improve the communicative environment. However, many elderly persons have resigned themselves to "not be a bother" rather than assert themselves by criticizing their family's manner of speaking or the environments in which they are asked to communicate. Rather, older adults may simply visit their families less frequently, even though they desire to be with their daughter or son and grandchildren. In the end, however, they may withdraw into isolation at home rather than attempt to maintain social or family contacts where they have previously felt frustration and embarrassment.

HOW DO OTHERS REACT TO OLDER PERSONS WHO POSSESS PRESBYCUSIS?

One elderly person with hearing impairment has quite eloquently stated to this author, "For every poor ear, there is at least one poor speaker!" He is probably quite accurate.

As stated earlier, many elderly persons have placed themselves in a position of "not being a bother," perhaps not realizing that at least a portion of their difficulties in communication with others may be the result of attempting to talk to persons who do not speak clearly or being asked to communicate in environments that may cause even a person with normal hearing to have difficulty. However, even though an elderly person's adult child may lack good speech skills, the blame for miscommunication or misunderstanding by the elderly parent with hearing impairment may be placed on them, and not the speaker, without attempting to analyze the problems of two-way communication.

Generally, the initial visible frustration with an elderly person's inability to understand what is being said is noticed by a listener. A lesser reaction may have resulted in a simple request for repetition or rephrasing of the statement for clarification. When an elderly listener with hearing impairment fails to understand a statement after several repetitions of a difficult word, it is usually he or she who first notices the apparent frustration on the face of the speaker, rather than the speaker her or himself. Increased self-imposed pressure to succeed in understanding a problem word within a speaker's sentence tends to increase anxiety and heighten the probability of failure to understand it. One of two reactions generally follows. The most frequent on the part of an elderly listener is to become frustrated, apologize, and withdraw from the situation. The second probable response is a feeling of anger coupled with frustration and embarrassment and either a covert or overt expression of, "Why don't you speak more clearly!"

Who initiated this trying situation? In all probability it was the speaker rather than the elderly listener. The speaker's initial unspoken display of frustration at the elderly listener's inability to understand the statement or question may have caused heightened anxiety on the elderly person's part. Anxiety, in that situation, breeds failure, failure breeds frustration, frustration breeds further failure, and on and on, until some resolution to cease the conversation, leave the situation, or continue to display anger and frustration is reached.

Did the initial attempt at the conversation prompt this less-than-tolerable situation? Probably not. The elderly person who has been frustrated in attempting to hold conversations on previous occasions usually develops a fairly immediate awareness of signs of anxiety, frustration, or concern that are reflected in a speaker when a nonunderstood word or phrase leads to a delay in the conversation. After failure in various communicative environments on many occasions and perhaps occurring with greater regularity, an elderly

person begins to anticipate a speaker's response, perhaps prematurely in some instances in anticipation of a *possible* negative response. In any event, a speaker at some time has planted the seed of suspicion that he or she was frustrated, concerned, and perhaps even angry at the elderly person's failure to understand or interpret what he or she was saying.

The second party's negative response to the older person's obvious difficulty in understanding what he or she is saying may be the result of an unanticipated interruption in the flow of a conversation. Otherwise, the reasons may be a lack of desire to really communicate with the elderly person, a lack of tolerance for a disorder that is not readily visible and therefore disconcerting to the nonimpaired person, or a lack of knowledge regarding ways in which the situation could be made more comfortable for both the listener who has hearing impairment and the speaker.

A nonimpaired person will typically assist a person who is physically disabled in crossing a busy street or guide a person who is visually handicapped through a maze of chairs. In those situations, however, the impairment and the manner in which assistance can be offered are both obvious to a person who may, in fact, know little about the handicapping effects of those disorders. But verbal communication, which is generally experienced as an ongoing set of events, when interrupted by a nonvisible disorder such as hearing impairment, may be disconcerting to the nonimpaired person. This is particularly true when a hearing aid is not worn or otherwise displayed.

Communication for a brief instant no longer exists. At that point the person with normal hearing may not know how to resolve the situation. The misunderstood word or phrase is repeated, but perhaps to no avail. The person who has hearing impairment still misinterprets the verbal message. A natural response is to repeat the word or phrase once again in a louder voice, perhaps with emphasis and facial expression that reveals at least some frustration, as the speaker may have not yet determined why the listener is having such great difficulty. The evident frustration may, in turn, concern the listener who has hearing impairment, and communication is at a stalemate.

If the impaired auditory system of a person with impaired hearing was as noticeable as the impaired limbs of person with paraplegia or the eyes of a person who is blind, perhaps the perplexing frustrations that occur could at least be reduced. Presbycusis is so complex, however, that simply raising the intensity of one's voice may do little to ease the difficulty. In fact, in some instances, the misinterpretations can actually increase from increased anxiety. In other words, the frustrations experienced by persons who communicate with a person of any age who has hearing impairment do exist and are shared among the persons who have hearing impairment themselves.

HEARING-IMPAIRED OLDER PERSONS VERSUS OTHERS WHO ARE HEARING-IMPAIRED

Why do family members, friends, or spouses of elderly persons with presbycusis appear to be more frustrated than persons who, for example, must communicate with children who have hearing impairment? Adults and children, perhaps, tend to be more compassionate toward children and young adults who have difficulty communicating as the result of hearing impairment. That is not to say that there are not instances in which attempts at getting a message across to a child who has hearing impairment fail in frustration for both the child and the speaker. Accommodations by nonimpaired children and adults, however, appear to be made willingly in most instances, because they know a child is likely to have difficulty understanding their verbal message, either because of the hearing impairment per se or as the result of language delay. On the other hand, the nonimpaired person who is frustrated at attempts to communicate with an elderly person who has hearing impairment may rationalize the reason as simply being because the person is "old."

Are the frustrations and resulting tension expressed because a listener is an older person? Perhaps in a few instances this may be true, but probably not as a general rule. Frustrations of persons who may have known an elderly person for some time before the onset of the auditory difficulties may be because this person "was always quite alert." For reasons unknown to them, however, frustrating and failed attempts at "communicating with Dad" are causing friction within their family. "Dad's mind seems to be failing. I told him yesterday to get the safety inspection sticker for his car renewed and he asked, 'Who was safe?' Maybe we should get him a hearing aid or take his car away from him." When a hearing aid is purchased for this elder by a well-meaning son or daughter, but he refuses to wear it because, as he says, "It doesn't help," he may be then described by his family as stubborn. Or they may feel that, "He refuses to do anything to improve himself," when in reality the hearing aid did not provide significant improvement. So, how do others who associate with the elderly person with presbycusis react to him or her? As one family member said to this writer:

We are concerned about Dad. We used to have a good time talking about the good old days and about what he wanted to do after he retired. Now that he can't seem to hear us or understand what we say, we all get angry. He can't understand what we are saying no matter how loud we talk, and all he does is get mad because no matter how many times we repeat what we say, he still can't get it. We bought him a hearing aid, but he won't wear it. He says it doesn't help. For $800, it *should* do something for him, but we all feel that he just can't get used to something new. Besides, he's just stubborn, we think. Our whole lives have changed since this hearing problem has gotten worse. We don't communicate anymore. We don't even like to have him over anymore and no one goes to visit him. He just sits. We are embarrassed to take him out to restaurants because he can't understand the waiters and then becomes angry when we try to interpret what they are saying. And, he talks so loud! So we just let him sit at his house. We told him to sell the house and move into an apartment complex where older persons live. He says that if we try to sell his house he'll lock the doors and windows and never come out until the hearse takes him away. His hearing problem has changed all of our lives for the worse. We really are at our wits' end.

Such statements are made many times by concerned and frustrated children, friends, and spouses of older persons who have hearing impairment. But many of these persons can be helped if those who serve them take the time to listen to their responses to their auditory disorder and their state in life and to carefully evaluate their hearing disorder. From this information viable service programs can be developed, not only for older persons who have hearing impairment, but also for those who most closely associate with them.

REACTIONS OF OLDER ADULTS TO THEIR HEARING LOSS: A DIALOGUE

How do older adults with hearing impairment react to the disorder and the difficulties they have in attempting to communicate with others? The following statements from clients reflect their feelings about their hearing loss. They are taken from initial pretreatment interviews with 10 older clients who have hearing impairment and were recorded on videotape by this author. This type of personalized information provides important insights into the feelings and desires of elderly clients that are not only important in the counseling process, but also in the development of treatment programs on their clients' behalf.

CASE STUDIES

The Interviewees

All of the interviewees are of an average socioeconomic level and are bright, articulate older adults.

All, however, possess a frustrating impairment of hearing.

OCCUPATIONAL HISTORY. Two women were teachers, one at the elementary and the other at high school level. One man managed a grain elevator in a rural community. He had no formal education past the sixth grade. One man is a retired agricultural agent for Weld County, CO. One man was a farmer, with no formal education past the third grade. Four women still consider themselves to be housewives and not retired. One man is a retired missionary. Four of these clients presently reside in a health care facility and the remainder are living in the community in their own homes.

STATE OF HEALTH AND MOBILITY. The six clients interviewed who reside in the community all describe themselves as being well. They feel that they are mobile, although only one of the women drives a car. All of the men who do not reside in a health care facility drive their own car. The women who do not drive a car said that transportation was occasionally a problem, but that city bus service was generally adequate, or friends or relatives take them where they want to go. All clients interviewed, except one man who was troubled with gout, stated that they sometimes walked where they needed to go, mostly for exercise.

No clients interviewed who resided in health care facilities drove a car. Transportation was stated as being generally adequate through local bus service or by the health care facility's "ambulo-bus" service. The clients who reside in health care facilities generally described the reason for placement there as health reasons, except for one who felt that she was simply deposited there. Health and physical problems among those confined persons include heart problems, kidney dysfunction, Parkinson disease, cataracts, and hearing loss. Walking was described by all as difficult. Two clients were confined to wheelchairs—one because of Parkinson disease and one because of arthritis.

AGE. Ages of the clients included here ranged from 66 to 95 years. The mean age was 76 years.

REASON FOR REFERRAL. All persons interviewed for this discussion had been referred for aural rehabilitation services or had sought out the service. All had consented to participate in aural rehabilitation treatment on an individual or group basis after an initial hearing evaluation and counseling.

THE DIALOGUE. The following are the interviewees' descriptions of themselves and the impact of their hearing impairment on them. The dialogue is taken from videotaped responses by each client to the question, "How do you feel about yourself at this time and your ability to communicate with others? Such videotaped interviews are held with each client seen by this author prior to aural rehabilitation services and again at the program's conclusion. The purpose for all pre- and postvideotaped interviews is to allow clients to confront themselves and their feelings about their ability to function in their communicating worlds. Changes in their opinions of themselves and their ability to function communicatively are thus more easily mapped. Clients are further allowed the opportunity to note changes in themselves and their opinions of their ability to communicate with others by watching and listening to their own statements.

The following are brief but descriptive excerpts of statements by clients.

Case 1

Age: 70 *Sex*: Female
Residence: Community (In own house)
Marital Status: Never married
Prior Occupation: Elementary educator
Health: Good
Mobility: Good
Dialogue:
I try to say, "What did you say?" but sometimes they begin to appear angry. I become frustrated—so—so frustrated that I then become angry at my-

self, because I have become angry at those with whom I am talking. Do other people have problems where they cannot understand what people are saying? Am I the only one?

I didn't realize why I had begun to dislike going to meetings until I realized I was not understanding what they were saying. I had been blaming my friends—and they had been secretly blaming me. I hope I can retain their friendship after I explain to them that the problems weren't all their fault.

Discussion: This woman's comments indicate concern over the difficulties she is experiencing in her attempts at interacting with others. She is, however, not resigned to continued failure. She is still striving to retain friendships with others. Further, she is still enrolled in aural rehabilitation treatment and making satisfactory progress in learning to make positive change in her communication environments.

Case 2

Age: 72 years *Sex*: Female
Resident: Health care facility
Marital status: Widow
Prior Occupation: Housewife
Health: Arthritis, renal disease
Mobility: Confined to wheelchair. Mobility severely limited.
Dialogue:
I feel handicapped. Anymore, I don't know what the demands are, or what capabilities I have. I try so hard to hear that I become so very tired. I may pass away any day. Is there hope for me? I want to talk to my children more than anything else, but they are so busy and can't come to see me very often. I want to hear what the minister here is saying at the chapel. Church means a great deal to me now.

I feel so alone when I can't participate in things I want to do. I can't weed out what I want to hear from the noises around me. The most important thing is communication. I desperately want it. My grandchildren—I pray that I can someday spend a pleasant afternoon with them.

Discussion: This woman feels despondent. She is, however, an alert person and desires that her situation will improve. She is enrolled in an aural rehabilitation treatment program, but her state of depression has not improved significantly. She says that if her family would visit her, it would help. Most importantly, she desires to have someone to communicate with.

Case 3

Age: 76 years *Sex*: Male
Residence: Community (In own house)
Marital Status: Widower
Prior Occupation: Grain elevator manager
Health: Generally good. Has known cardiovascular problems. Some dizziness noted on occasion.
Mobility: Good. Drives own car and is physically mobile. He is mentally alert and always seems to have a joke for the occasion. But, in most respects, he is a man of few words.
Dialogue:

It's embarrassing. When people find out that you have trouble hearing, they don't seem to want to talk to you anymore. If you ask them to speak up, sometimes they look angry.

I feel that time is lost when I go to a meeting I have looked forward to going to and I can't understand a word they are saying. Most people do not seem to have good speech habits. On the other hand, my poor hearing doesn't help a bit either.

My main goal in coming here is to learn to hear a woman's voice better, maybe a woman's companionship won't be so hard to come by. As they say, a woman's voice may not be as pretty as the song of a bird, but it's awful darn close!

Discussion: This man possesses a significant speech discrimination deficit, and strongly desires that aural rehabilitative services be of help to him. He feels that he has much to live for and is willing to work to improve his auditory problems. Assertiveness training and manipulation of

his communicative environments has supported those efforts.

Case 4

Age: 95 years *Sex*: Female
Residence: Health care facility
Marital Status: Widow
Prior Occupation: Housewife
Health: Parkinson disease
Mobility: Severely limited. Is confined to a wheelchair.
Dialogue:

I would like to be free, to drive, to go visit children and friends. I would like to get away from confinement. I would like to be able to hear again—to be able to be a part of the conversations that take place in this home. It would be pleasant to hear the minister again or to talk to my children. They live far away, though, and can't come often.

My main concern is death right now. I know that the infirmity I have will end in death. I don't know if I'm ready. If I could hear the minister, maybe I would know.

Discussion: These comments are typical of many elderly persons who are confined to a health care facility. They feel so many needs, but few can be fulfilled. This woman is alert, however, and can respond to aural rehabilitation treatment. If, for example, accommodations can be made in the chapel so that she can participate in those services, then one of her desires would be fulfilled. Further, if learning to manipulate her more difficult communicative environments can be achieved so that she can function better within the confines of the health care facility, then her years will become less isolating.

Case 5

Age: 72 years *Sex*: Male
Residence: Health care facility (Post-hospitalization)
Marital Status: Married

Prior Occupation: County extension agent
Health: Intestinal blockage. Arthritis. Otherwise in generally good health.
Mobility: Generally good. Drives own car on occasion. Walks to many places.
Dialogue:

I feel lost sometimes. If I look at people right straight in the eye, then sometimes I get what they say. I get angry sometimes, but I've finally figured out that for every poor ear, there's a poor speaker!

It's rough to have poor ears. I have trouble hearing women's voices. I wish I could hear them, since I'm around women more now than ever before.

Maybe it's me, maybe I don't have good attention.

I wish I could hear my preacher. I go to church every Sunday, but I don't get much out of it.

I wish I could understand what people are saying in a crowd, like when our children and our grandchildren come back home to visit. If I'm talking to only one person, sometimes I do okay.

Discussion: This man expresses a great many "wishes," but so far has not extended himself a great deal in aural rehabilitation treatment. In other words, he desires to improve, but seems to feel that either he does not possess the capability to regain greater communication function, or simply does not want to put forth the effort. He appears to have great communicative needs, but does not yet seem to be convinced of their importance. Counseling is important here.

Case 6

Age: 71 *Sex*: Male
Residence: Community (In own house)
Marital Status: Widower
Prior Occupation: Farmer
Health: Excellent, except for gout, which restricts his mobility.
Mobility: Not as mobile as desired, because of the gout. Drives his own car and is an avid fisherman.
Dialogue:

In a crowd—I have my worst trouble. Riding in a car drives me crazy!

People don't talk with their mouth open.

My ears hum, and that hurts too, in terms of my ability to understand what people are saying.

Some people talk with their hands in front of their mouth; that is very disturbing.

I don't think that my children understand that my problem is my hearing—not my mind.

It just seems like the voices don't come through. I went to the doctor and he says my hearing is ruined. My hearing is my only handicap. My minister has an English brogue and I can't understand a word of what he is saying.

Groups sound kind of like a beehive. I feel embarrassed. Someone speaks to you and you give them the wrong answer. I like to go to social gatherings, but I still get embarrassed. However, I certainly am not going to give up.

Discussion: This man represents the almost ideal older client for aural rehabilitation services. He is alert and active and desires to maintain himself as an active social person. He has also found a female companion who is also an avid fisherman. What an ideal motivational factor for success in aural rehabilitation!

Case 7

Age: 81 years *Sex*: Male
Residence: Community (In own house with spouse)
Marital Status: Married
Prior Occupation: Missionary. Still functions as part-time minister for a local church. He receives many requests to serve on community and church committees.
Health: Excellent
Mobility: Excellent. Walks a great deal and drives own car.
Dialogue:

My greatest concern is my inability to participate in council meetings at church. In some cases, I am in charge of the meeting, but if I cannot understand what the members are saying, then my participation is made almost impossible. It distresses me tremendously that in some instances I cannot perform my duties. Maybe it's me? Maybe my concentration wanders. Maybe my mind is not working as well now, although I feel that it is. I have 20 to 30 members in the Sunday School class that I teach. I find that I have terrible problems determining what their questions are. If I do not know what their questions are, how can I respond to their needs?

Discussion: These statements are made by an obviously frustrated man. "How can I respond to their needs?" This man has a great deal to offer his community and church, but is beginning to feel defeated. The audiologist must consider this type of older client as a high priority and intervene as a strategist to aid the person in functioning more efficiently in his prioritized communicative environments.

Case 8

Age: 72 years *Sex*: Female
Residence: Community (In own house with spouse)
Marital Status: Married
Prior Occupation: Nonretired housewife
Health: Excellent
Mobility: Excellent, but has never learned to drive a car. Depends on husband or bus for transportation. Walks a great deal.
Dialogue:

My hearing loss has been a handicap to me. I ask people to speak up, and they sigh and sometimes I feel terribly embarrassed.

Sometimes they shout at me, which hurts in more ways than one.

I do wish people would speak more distinctly. Even with my family, they sometimes forget to speak up "for Mom."

On the telephone I tell people that I'm wearing a hearing aid whether I am or not. They usually speak up more after that.

My husband says I am a different person in this later age. I used to be full of fun, but now I don't even want to go to church. I don't like to go because I don't understand what others are saying.

It isn't all peaches and cream to be this way. It hurts more than anything when people laugh at you when you give the wrong answer to something they say. I just go home and cry.

People mumble when they talk.

I just sometimes want to get out of people's way. I don't want to be a bother to anyone—be a nuisance. I've lost my self-confidence and I don't know if I'll ever get it back.

Discussion: This otherwise vital woman was on the verge of giving up. Further, her husband was talking about placing her in a nursing home. After 30 weeks of individual aural rehabilitation treatment, she leaned to manipulate the majority of those communicative environments that were most difficult for her. Further, she has rejoined a women's social group from which she had previously resigned membership. The gradual progression from a depressed woman to one with renewed hope has been rewarding to observe.

Case 9

Age: 66 years *Sex*: Female
Residence: Community (In own house)
Marital Status: Single
Prior Occupation: Elementary educator
Health: Excellent
Mobility: Excellent
Dialogue:

I was feeling concern in as much as when people would ask me a question, I would know they were speaking, but I couldn't make sense out of it. I was afraid that my mind was going. I felt closed in, not comfortable—like I could hear, but little of it made sense—like I was losing my mind!

I think sometimes that people want me to go away. When I found out that my problem was with my hearing and not my mind, the relief was wonderful. Now I feel that I have something I can try to handle, where before I didn't think I had a chance.

If people will bear with me, I'll be able to talk with them. I'm going to stay in there just as long as I can.

Discussion: This woman benefitted greatly from an initial counseling session regarding her auditory problem and learning some reasons for the difficulties she was encountering. After she found that the communicative problems she was experiencing were "not the result of her mind," but rather her hearing, she was a ready candidate for a formal aural rehabilitation treatment program.

Case 10

Age: 79 years *Sex*: Female
Residence: Health care facility. Stated that she thought her daughter was looking for an apartment for her, but found herself in the health care facility instead.
Marital Status: Widow
Prior Occupation: Housewife (nonretired)
Health: Generally excellent except for broken hip two years ago
Mobility: Somewhat restricted because of fear of falling. Otherwise excellent. She takes the bus to those places she desires to go.
Dialogue:

I used to blame others for my inability to hear, but someone the other day told me it was my fault, me and my inability to hear.

A speaker at a meeting the other evening spoke for 45 minutes and I did not understand what she was saying. The disturbing thing was that she refused to use the microphone!

I was in a car with two friends the other day, I rode in the back seat. They were talking in the front seat. They were talking about a person I had not seen for quite a while. I heard them say something about a ball game, something about Omaha, and something about someone becoming very ill. I finally felt that I had to say something, so I asked, "She is well, isn't she?" Well, what they had said was that my friend had died! She became very ill during a ball game in Omaha and died while being taken by ambulance to the hospital. It was terribly embarrassing, but they don't become angry with me.

It is frustrating to try to do well, but continually fail. I try not to be irritable. I think I can overcome it.

Discussion: This is an example of an alert, intelligent woman who, because of factors beyond her control, fell and found herself unable to provide for her physical needs. She was thus placed in a health care facility—hopefully for a relatively short time. She has accepted such placement because of the evident short stay. She is responding well to aural rehabilitation treatment services, particularly in learning to cope within her most difficult environments. She has analyzed the reasons for many of her communicative difficulties, and is aware of her limitations.

SUMMARY

Auditory deficits as the result of presbycusis are as real as the people who possess the disorder. The disorder, however, affects each person in unique ways. One common denominator is evident, however, and that is that the resulting communication problems can be terribly frustrating and, in many instances, debilitating. The most common strain among the confessions of these elderly persons, however, is the isolation and loneliness that they experience.

END OF CHAPTER EXAMINATION QUESTIONS

CHAPTER 18

1. The greatest fear described by many hearing impaired older adults is that they are afraid that their family and friends will mistake their hearing loss for

2. What are three emotional reactions an older adult might have to the difficulties experienced as a result of her or his hearing impairment?

3. As hearing-impaired older adults communicate their feelings regarding their hearing loss to the author, the most common thread centers on _____ and _____.

4. The most common goal expressed by older hearing impaired adults to the author involved their desire to better communicate with

5. The inability of some hearing impaired older adults to utilize hearing aids well gives rise to even greater

6. When repeated attempts at communication fail, some hearing impaired older adults simply

7. (True/False). Presbycusis affects only older adults. Why?

8. (True/False). One concern of persons with presbycusis is that family members will feel that they are no longer able to function on an independent basis.

9. (True/False). According to the author, presbycusis affects all older persons in essentially the same way. Is this true or false? Briefly explain your choice.

END OF CHAPTER ANSWER SHEET

Name   Date

CHAPTER 18

1. _____

2. _____

3. _____

4. _____

5. _____

6. _____

_____

7. Circle one: True   False

_____

_____

_____

_____

8. Circle one: True   False

9. Circle one: True   False

_____

_____

_____

_____

Counseling the Older Adult Who is Hearing-Impaired

JAMES F. MAURER, Ph.D.
DOUGLAS R. MARTIN, Ph.D.

PSYCHOSOCIAL RESPONSES TO HEARING LOSS IN
OLDER AGE: TYPES AND CASE STUDIES
  Defending Against the Hearing Impairment
  Escaping from the Impairment

AN OPEN LETTER TO AN OLDER PERSON WHO HAS
HEARING IMPAIRMENT

SUMMARY

A hearing impairment experienced during the later years of life represents more than a communicative imposition. For many, it represents the superimposition of degraded auditory reception on a small galaxy of other problems, ranging from other sensory deficits to necessary changes in lifestyle. Presbycusis compounds the consequences of coexisting physical and social limitations. Butler and Lewis (Butler & Lewis, 1973) described it as "potentially the most problematic of the perceptual impairments" (p. 73).

THE IMPACT OF ENVIRONMENT ON THE OLDER CLIENT

No communication environment is a positive one for persons with a hearing impairment. Some are simply better than others. The some 2.5 million institutionalized aged, who constitute about 8% of the population, reside in environments that generally are not conducive to communication. Many senior adult centers also fall into this category. Nearly 30 years ago, Moriarity (1974) surveyed 25 group living environments for the elderly, including nursing homes, high-rise apartments, extended-care facilities, and senior adult centers. His conclusions were:

1. Most were located in high traffic areas, where average outside noise levels exceeded that of normal conversational speech.
2. Most were poorly insulated against the intrusion of outside noise.
3. Only 4 of the 25 facilities were adequately equipped with acoustic tile, drapes, and carpeting to dampen inside noise.
4. Nearly half of the buildings contained noise producing sources, such as vibrating fans and kitchen and laundry appliances, which were in close proximity to both recreation and meeting areas.

Even though the survey was conducted more than 26 years ago, few, if any, positive changes are currently observed in health care facility (nursing home) environments. In fact, most of today's facilities were built at the time of the Moriarity (1974) survey and most have not changed.

PLACES OF WORSHIP

Too few places of worship have been architecturally designed to accommodate individuals with hearing difficulties. Older persons generally are faced with vaulted ceilings, hard, flat resonating walls, and an unfavorable distance from the speaker to the listener. Sanctuaries that provide the all-too-familiar wall-mounted speakers and a pulpit microphone may offer some assistance, provided that listeners who have hearing impairment are near the speakers and not in the acoustically "dead" spaces throughout the sanctuary. Assistive listening devices, including FM and infrared systems that transmit directly to listeners, generally offer greater noise-free intelligibility of a message. However, "fortunately for most elderly worshipers, the familiarity of the message content may be the greatest blessing" (Maurer, 1976, p. 12).

Comprehending spoken messages, particularly in situations in which there is background noise, is one of the most common communication problems arising during older age. This and another enigma, difficulty interpreting rapidly spoken speech, are in near epidemic proportions by the eighth decade of life. Both problems can occur in advanced age, and both merit precounseling assessment of the everyday life situations in which they occur, as well as the development of realistic coping strategies.

In many situations where complaints about hearing in background noise are common, assistive listening devices (ALD) can significantly improve life satisfaction. Guidance in the selection of an appropriate ALD for a given situation calls for expertise by a counselor. The counselor, having assessed the nature of the difficulty, including the situation(s) in which it occurs, can deal with the problem realistically by selecting from an array of products designed to compensate for unfavorable listening situations. Problems that may be confounding and frustrating for older adults can often be rectified by such simple solutions by an informed counselor. Examples of problem solving that can occur through counseling by an audiologist are presented next.

Mrs. E. was invariably relegated the back seat of the family vehicle during weekend drives in the country. Her son and daughter-in-law sat in front conversing, occasionally raising their voices to include her in some of their conversation. She admitted not paying continuous attention, because most of what they said was lost in the rumble of the vehicle. The solution was an inexpensive battery-operated miniature public address system with a microphone in the front seat and a small speaker which was attached to the back of the headrest in front of Mrs. E.

Mr. B., who was in his early 70s and semiconfined to his apartment with prostate cancer and neuropathy involving his fingers, was regularly the focus of complaints from neighbors that he turned his television set up too loud. However, one of the most satisfying rewards in his life was watching baseball games on television. Because he was unable to regulate his hearing aid, his audiologist dispensed a wireless infrared system which transmitted the audio portion of the TV program directly into lightweight earphones, allowing him to hear as well as see the ball games with the television volume turned down.

Although knowledge about the effective use of assistive listening devices can now solve many communication breakdowns for aging individuals, there is no immediate remedy for comprehending the speech of people who simply talk too fast for the aging brain to comprehend the message. The simplest remedy is to coach the older person to say, "I'm sorry, could you speak a little slower for me?" The audiologist might also, for example, screen the various broadcast stations in the area and determine new reporters who tend to speak at a reasonable word per minute rate and direct the older adult to those television or radio stations.

PSYCHOSOCIAL ADJUSTMENT

The nucleus of individuals associated with the older person in his or her living environment is a key ingredient in psychosocial adjustment and counseling. What Comfort (1978) described as "childrenization" of the elderly all too frequently occurs within family constellations and among staff members in collective living environments. That is, there is a tendency to regard an older person from the standpoint of being "elderly," rather than attending to his or her needs. This attitude, when associated with ignorance about the problems of hearing impairment, may lead to dangerous misconceptions about an individual and his or her social communicative potential. As Hull (1997) has observed:

Hearing impairment as seen by the "lay person" is often mislabeled as senility because the elderly person will often times respond to questions or statements with wrong or inappropriate answers. Senility is without question seen among the geriatric patients, but non-senile hearing impaired patients often seem to demonstrate similar symptoms with inappropriate responses to questions, depression, anxiety, suspiciousness and withdrawal. (p. 298)

In some environments, there is virtually a collusion of anonymity operating against a person who has hearing impairment. Although collectively sharing in the person's general welfare, often no member of a nursing staff or family personally accepts responsibility for an older individual's auditory difficulties.

Such a situation has a powerful detrimental effect on an individual's success in social interaction. People communicate less because the older person does not understand them. The older person communicates less often to them, because of their lessening interest. They reciprocate by ignoring the older person's social presence. The older adult adjusts to this deprivation of interaction by interacting inwardly through thoughts and imageries that are intrinsically more reinforcing than the extrinsic social environment. Although the person is not regarded by family as "deaf," he or she often appears "preoccupied, unsociable, absentminded, or paranoid" (Joensen & Saunders, 1984). In the presence of other possible functional limitations, the person who is hearing impaired may suffer from depression, often closely followed by self-isolation

(LaFerle & LaFerle, 1988). Observers may remark how he or she has changed and how "he or she lives in a world all his or her own."

THE INFLUENCE OF FINANCES AND MOBILITY

Aging persons who are more self-sufficient financially, albeit equal in other respects, seem to adjust more readily to their hearing handicaps than those who have fewer means (Maurer, 1974). Of course, more alternatives for psychosocial adjustment are available to people who are more affluent. The cost of clinical and medical services, hearing aids, and other special listening systems such as telephone amplifiers are within their financial means. Although an auditory impairment may dampen elder's enthusiasm for some activities, a sound economy creates more options for compensating for a hearing loss.

The case is reversed among low-income persons, who have fewer alternatives available to them. In a comparative study made between the hearing levels of lower- versus higher-income elderly seeking intervention for hearing deficits, aging persons with low income had poorer hearing sensitivity by the time they obtained hearing aids (Project ARM, 1983).

Persons both from minority and low-income groups fare even worse. Data reflecting a hearing survey in low-income neighborhoods (Table 19-1) reveal that among those with communicatively significant hearing impairments, more African-Americans failed to seek professional intervention than Whites. African-Americans with low incomes also more frequently reported stress associated with hearing loss than did Whites with low incomes.

Older individuals who are economically more self-sufficient also tend to be more mobile. They can travel to community clinics for weekly aural rehabilitation sessions. They can seek more immediate adjustments for a hearing aid in need of repair. They can avail themselves of others, includ-

TABLE 19–1. Reactions to Hearing Impairment: A Comparison Between Black and Caucasian Elderly, 60–65 Years.

	Black	Caucasian
Failed to seek professional help	61%	18%
Hearing problem produced stress	70%	53%
Average hearing loss of group (PTA)	36 dB	32 dB
of those seeking professional help	42 dB	34 dB

Source: Project ARM. Data from Multi-Service Center, Action Center, Albina, Dahlke, Campbell Hotel, Portland, OR: Portland State University.
Note: N = 262 low-income persons, 81 black, 181 Caucasian.

ing friends and family members in distant places, who can provide emotional support.

Financial restrictions and lack of mobility can exacerbate negative influence of a hearing impairment. The person may isolate him- or herself to avoid the stress of communication that becomes increasingly difficult. When given an opportunity to extricate themselves from difficult situations, some older persons would rather not re-enter the world of sound because, apart from their hearing problem, they feel rejected by their environment.

THE INFLUENCE OF ATTITUDES AND FEELINGS

ADMITTING THE EXISTENCE OF A HEARING LOSS

Unlike blindness, deafness fails to make a visible appeal to human compassion. In fact, responses of family and friends to a hearing loss may be antagonistic. The communication breakdowns associated with the difficulty frequently become frustrating for the family as well, often accounting for the impetus to seek intervention.

Admission of hearing problems is also difficult, because the present generation of elderly is not far removed from the stigmatic association of "deafness" and "dumbness" that prevailed only a century ago. They are in an age bracket in which a number of friends and relatives may have tried hearing aids, often with marginal reported success. Even having educational information pertaining to hearing loss provided prior to rehabilitation does not guarantee a commitment to wearing a hearing aid (Warren & Daily, 1984). It seems that the desire to pass in social groups as "normal" or younger than one's years negates acceptance of hearing aid devices, which, in turn, diminishes public awareness of the disability, until difficulties in communication become apparent. Many hearing aid manufacturers continue to emphasize the concealability of the devices, a strategy that both pays homage to and abets potential negative self-concepts among potential wearers.

Some older persons, on the other hand, appear to be more accepting of the problem and less resistant toward intervention. One reason for this is that therapeutic gains are significantly greater for biologically younger individuals than for very old persons. Another reason is that amplification is gaining in popular acceptance, and younger old persons are more likely to move with the tide of public sentiment than individuals who are psychosocially older.

THE USE OF PROJECTION IN ADJUSTMENT TO STRESS

A common method of adjustment to stresses associated with presbycusis is "disprojection" (Maurer & Rupp, 1979). Older persons commonly attribute their own problems with the failure of others to speak clearly. This seems to be particularly true in cases of mild hearing loss, where hearing sensitivity is most depressed in the high frequencies. Thus, perhaps it is the low frequency information that sustains an individual's belief that his or her hearing is normal and that distortion is a result of the poor speaking habits of others.

Stress associated with hearing impairment does reveal itself clinically through counseling of older adults. It surfaces as a technique through which persons who have hearing impairment relieve anxiety. Methods of adjustment are developed early in life as mechanisms for defending against or escaping from stressful situations (Cameron, 1947).

THE INFLUENCE OF THE AUDIOLOGIST AS COUNSELOR

Surveys of practicing audiologists (Metcalf, 1993); Schow, Balsara, Smedley, & Whitcomb, 1993) have suggested that audiologists have expanded their role as counselor in recent years. This is most likely a result of the increased emphasis on the fitting of hearing aids and the counseling that must take place in the process. Although this is certainly encouraging, there remains some concern that the field of audiology has yet to firmly come to terms with both preparation and competence in this important aspect of audiological services (Clark, 1994).

It is important that audiologists be prepared to counsel their clients. By the very nature of their role in providing direct service on behalf of those with hearing impairment, counseling takes place each day of the audiologist's professional life.

INNOVATIONS IN COUNSELING

In recent years, professionals have investigated alternative means of delivering counseling services that have merit for use by all audiologists. Many of these investigations have involved the use of evolving technologies that may be appropriate in the clinical arena. For instance, Tye-Murray (1992) has reported on the use of computer-controlled videodisc technologies to provide counseling in the area of communication breakdowns and repair strategies for both the individual who has hearing impairment and his or her family. Palmer (1992) described an initial im-

plementation of a computerized administration of the Hearing Handicap Inventory for the Elderly. A study is currently underway at Portland State University investigating the effectiveness of a computer-controlled multimedia presentation in describing and demonstrating realistic expectations of hearing aids for new users (Martin & Sayre, 1994).

The degree to which these emerging technologies will influence the delivery of counseling services to older persons who have hearing impairment is yet to be seen. One of the obvious benefits of such counseling approaches is the ability to structure counseling sessions into self-directed exercises, with only limited demands placed on an audiologist's time. Some might argue that counseling is a process that, by its very nature, demands direct human interaction and, therefore, computer technology has no role to play. Certainly, there are aspects of counseling in an audiology setting that, without question, require direct person-to-person interactions. However, there remain components of the counseling process such as description of the normal hearing process, benefits and limitations of various amplification options, and role-playing scenarios in communication management that may lend themselves to interactive multimedia applications. Considerable research, within both laboratory and clinical domains, remains to be undertaken to fully explore these exciting possibilities.

PSYCHOSOCIAL RESPONSES TO HEARING LOSS IN OLDER AGE: TYPES AND CASE STUDIES

DEFENDING AGAINST THE HEARING IMPAIRMENT

Case Study. Mr. J. arrived at the clinic accompanied by his wife and dressed for a dinner party. The audiologist was prompted by his appearance to compliment Mr. J. on his attire. Mr. J. beamed, exhibiting head and torso movements while pro-claiming, "Well, this should go smoothly. What do you want me to do?"

Mrs. J. stared at her husband in disbelief. Later, she acknowledged, "I don't know what got into him this morning. He hasn't worn that suit since we took an ocean voyage four years ago."

Comment. Since Mr. J.'s impeccable dress and youthful behaviors were inconsistent with his usual attire and demeanor, one might justifiably raise the question whether these efforts were de-signed to reduce stress by drawing attention away from the real problem. Later, when the test results became known, Mr. J. appeared deflated and the youthful mannerisms were gone.

Case Study. Mrs. R. listened patiently while the audiologist gave instructions about pure-tone test-ing. Then she announced, "I didn't sleep well last night, so I doubt if you would get very good re-sults on me today." After the examination, she re-flected, "I'm not sure I pushed the button every time I heard the sound. Those earphones pressing on my head really bothered me."

Comment. Mrs. R. presented very good reasons for not performing well in the test suite. However, the validity of her excuses is highly questionable. The real message of her rationalizing might be summed up as, "My hearing is quite normal. I'm just having a bad day."

Attention-getting and rationalization are de-fense techniques that avoid the stress or anxiety of a perceived problem. In these two cases, they rep-resented mechanisms for drawing attention away from or denying a possible hearing impairment. They are avoidance behaviors in the sense that they are aimed at preventing the occurrence of a potentially aversive consequence. Defense tech-niques that act in similar ways are identification, compensation, and projection.

Identification relieves stress in an individual who temporarily assumes new roles or attributes. As examples, a 74-year-old woman about to undergo a hearing test announced that she had "the ears of a cat." A 61-year-old man about to start a hearing

evaluation irrelevantly indicated that he had just completed a thorough physical examination and the diagnostician had told him he, "had the arter-ies of a 40-year-old."

Compensation avoids stressful encounters by substituting less aversive activities in their place. A 74-year-old retiree rejected the need for amplifi-cation because, "I don't go out much anymore. I mostly just watch television."

Projection defends an individual against a prob-lem by referring it to others. Clinically, it seems al-most commonplace to hear variations on the state-ment, "I can hear others fine, but my wife doesn't speak clearly."

ESCAPING FROM THE IMPAIRMENT

Insulation

Case Study. Mrs. O. was asked, during the coun-seling session that followed the hearing test, "What changes in your life have been necessary because of your reduced hearing?"

"Quite honestly," she began, "the only change I deeply regret is church attendance. Our pastor has a soft voice and the services always contain a lot of music. And there's something about that build-ing—that sanctuary—that makes it difficult to hear. I reached the point where I would spend most of my time sitting there, thinking about oth-er things." She shook her head. "Finally, I just gave up on it."

Comment. Mrs. O. seems to recognize that in the church situation she has insulated herself from her problem by avoiding certain stimuli that pro-duce it. Insulation represents a retreat from situa-tions in which an impairment causes problems. A very positive aspect of her conversation is that she has not insulated herself from her clinician. She is willing to discuss her actions. Moreover her pos-sessive description of "our pastor" and her use of present tense verbs suggest that she really has not "given up on it."

Another example of insulation was observed in the behavior of a woman who had hearing impairment who was seated at a group dining table in a nursing home. In the midst of conversations around her, she maintained a stereotyped expression on her face, avoiding any eye contact with others at the table. Her expression seemed to convey the message, "I am thinking about something terribly important and do not wish to be disturbed."

Negativism

Negativism, on the other hand, reduces stress by opposition. Older persons may argue that they "can't learn to lipread" or they "can't stand any object" in their ears.

Some potentially stressful situations or events are simply eliminated from the elderly person's repertoire. At least momentarily, repression reduces anxiety by excluding the problem. The individual may selectively forget to wear a hearing aid, although the eye glasses are never forgotten. In addition, auditory experiences that have not been perceived for a number of years may be inhibited. One older man was asked, "How long has it been since you heard a whisper?" The question provoked a smile and then, shaking his head incredulously, he replied, "A whisper! I've never even thought of it until you mentioned it. Why, it's been years!"

Regression

Regression is a mechanism that permits a client to retreat from a problem by assuming a dependent role, one that contraindicates participation in a conflict. As another method of adjustment to stress, fantasy is often equated with daydreaming. Although this behavior reportedly is not more frequent in the aging population than in younger age groups, its frequency has not been studied among the elderly who have hearing impairment (Giambra, personal communication,

1989). Clinically, fantasy is manifested in the older person who, frustrated by not being able to keep up with or comprehend a group conversation, simply tunes it out and permits thoughts to wander to other topics.

In brief, the "geriapathy syndrome" begins when an individual feels disengaged from group interaction. Apathy ensues, the product of the fatigue that sets in from the relentless effort of straining to hear. Frustration, kindled by begging too many pardons, gives way to subterfuges that disguise misunderstandings. The head nods in agreement with conversation only vaguely interpreted. The voice registers approval of words often void of meaning. The ear strives for some redundancy that will make the message clearer. Finally, acquiescing to fatigue and frustration, thoughts may stray from the conversation to mental imageries that are unburdened by the defective hearing mechanism (Maurer, 1976, p. 60)

AN OPEN LETTER TO AN OLDER PERSON WHO HAS HEARING IMPAIRMENT

The changes during senescence that accompany hearing impairment may range from subtle to profound. Similarly, adjustive behaviors may range from minor irritation to self-imposed isolation. If there is one thread of professional continuity between such extremes, it must be the discipline of audiology.

It was in this spirit that the following "Open letter to the older person who has hearing difficulties" was written.

"You don't listen to me"
An Open Letter to an Older Person
Who Has Hearing Difficulties

Dear Grandperson:

Your problems are very real. They are witnessed a thousand times in countless places where people are talking to you. Their mouths move and sounds reach your ears, but somehow they don't say what they are talking about. Or their message arrives on a slow train, and you respond too late to avoid the flashing signals of concern. Sometimes they frown, their voices kindling a spark of exasperation that illuminates everyone's attention on your dilemma. Too often they take the path of lesser effort and, oblivious to the strain of your forward head movements and raised eyebrow, they continue to mouth their sounds to others. The space you occupy is disregarded.

Is it any wonder that you sneak an occasional rendezvous with yourself? At least your inner thoughts are not burdened by speakers who mumble and patchwork conversations that have no meaning.

Your complaints are altogether familiar. The television newscaster seems bent on cramming as many words into a minute as is humanly possible. The musical background gets in the way of the actor's voice. Everyone talks at once on that show. Who decided that woman should appear on national TV? And when did they take the tick out of watches?

Places are annoying, too. The city transit service is a foreign country, where people seem to speak in tongues against the drones and hisses of spasmodic motion. Restaurants—couldn't we find a quiet place where the dishes don't clatter, the music doesn't overwhelm, and the waitress was once a state elocution champion? Churches—the architect who designed them must have borrowed the plans from the Tower of Babel. The open banking system—whatever happened to the dignity of discussing one's fixed income in the quiet confines of a private office?

People—those teenage children who converse in short, accelerated bursts of unintelligible enthusiasm. Conversation stoppers, such as "Don't you remember?" Heart stoppers, such as the voice that appears suddenly at your elbow or the bicycle that materializes on soundless tires. Whispers—Their secrets are well guarded, as you don't have the remotest idea what they are talking about.

Your complaints are very reasonable, and the communication problems that you are experiencing extend well beyond your diminishing hearing ability. But how do you tell others to speak slowly and clearly without shouting, to call your name before addressing you so that your attention can surface, to turn the background noise down so you can understand? How do you tell them without exposing "the old person" in you? How do you project your difficulties on a society that is one or two generations away from sharing your experience? If only for a moment they could listen to the future through your ears!

Unfortunately, they cannot. However, there are a number of things they can do. They can learn to speak to you more slowly and clearly. They can select quiet places to communicate with you. They can turn off distracting noises before addressing you. They can touch you to gain your attention and look at you when they talk. And they can pause in their conversation long enough for your train of thought to catch up with their meaning. These things they can do for you, if you will muster the courage to step outside of your older person and assert yourself. Your problem must be shared with your listener.

You must not give up. You must not relinquish one listening experience that contains a shred of satisfaction. You must not withdraw from one conversation that invites your participation. Communication must be regarded as your personal invitation against mental aging.

Finally, you will need to adopt the attitude that the emotional cost of trying to hear again is minuscule compared to the depersonalizing experience of disengagement. Once you have resolutely determined to master your handicap, you will find that you are no longer a helpless spectator in the traffic of language, but a willing participant in the wonderful world of word transaction. This is human communication.

And the next time someone says, "You aren't listening to me," try responding with a smile and a gentle reminder, "Perhaps you are not talking to me."

REFERENCES

Butler, R., & Lewis, M. I. (1973). *Aging and mental health*. St. Louis, MO: C. V. Mosby.

Cain, L. D., Fine, M. A., & Maurer, J.F. (1974, November). *Responses of elderly to socialization demands in the move to public high rise housing*. Paper presented at the 27th annual Meeting of the Gerontology Society, Portland, OR.

Cameron, N. (1947). Basic adjustive techniques. In N. Cameron (Ed.), *The psychology of behavior disorders* (pp. 141–186). Boston: Houghton-Mifflin.

Clark, J. G. (1994). Audiologists' counseling purview. In J. G. Clark & F. N. Martin (Eds.), *Effective counseling in audiology: Perspectives and practice*. Englewood Cliffs, NJ: Prentice-Hall.

Comfort, A. (1978, April). *Perceptions of aging*. Keynote address at the 24th annual meeting of the Gerontology Society, Tucson, AZ.

Hull, R. H. (1997). Hearing loss in older adulthood. In R. H. Hull (Ed.), *Aural rehabilitation* (pp. 291–321). San Diego: Singular Publishing Group.

Joensen, J.P., & Saunders, D.J. (1984). Psychological correlates of geriatric hearing loss. *The Hearing Journal*, *38*(5), 24–27.

LaFerle, K. R., & LaFerle, K. (1988). Senility and its impact on the hearing instrument delivery. *Hearing Instruments*, *39*(2), 32–35.

Martin, D. R., & Sayre, C. (1994). *Prefitting hearing aid counseling delivered via an interactive multimedia application*. Unpublished paper, Portland State University, Speech and Hearing Sciences Program, Portland, OR.

Maurer, J. F. (1974). Auditory impairment and aging. In B. Jacobs (Ed.), *Working with the impaired elderly* (pp. 59–84). Washington, DC: The National Council on Aging.

Maurer, J. F., & Rupp, R. R. (1979). *Hearing and aging: Tactics for intervention*. New York: Grune & Stratton.

Metcalf, A. (1993). *Aural rehabilitation services provided to hearing impaired clients in the private sector*. Unpublished masters thesis. Portland, OR: Portland State University.

Miller, M.H. (1967). Audiological rehabilitation of the geriatric patient. *Maico Audiological Library Series*, *2*, 3.

Moriarity, M. (1974). *A survey of noise levels in senior adult environments*. Unpublished paper, Portland State University, Speech and Hearing Sciences Program, Portland, OR.

Palmer, C. (1992). Computer administration of hearing performance inventories. *American Journal of Audiology*, *1*(4), 13–14.

Project ARM. (1983). [Reaction to hearing impairment: A comparison between black and Caucasian elderly]. Unpublished raw data.

Schow, R. L., Balsara, N. R., Smedley, T. C., & Whitcomb, C. J. (1993). Aural rehabilitation by ASHA audiologists: 1980–1990. *American Journal of Audiology*, *2*(3), 28–37.

Tye-Murray, N. (1992). Laser videodisc technology in the aural rehabilitation setting: Good news for people with severe and profound hearing impairments. *American Journal of Audiology*, *1*(2), 33–36.

Warren, V. G., & Daily, L. B. (1984). Efficacy of aural rehabilitation with geriatic hearing impaired. *The Hearing Journal*, *37*(3), 15–19.

END OF CHAPTER EXAMINATION QUESTIONS

CHAPTER 19

1. In this chapter, a survey by Moriarity was described that concluded that group-living environments adversely affect hearing-impaired older adults. Describe those environments.

2. According to the author, one ingredient in listening environments appears to cause more problems in speech understanding for hearing-impaired older adults than any other. What is that ingredient? Why?

3. In many situations in which complaints about hearing in background noise are common, a specific strategy will, according to the authors, in many instances provide relief. What is it?

4. According to the authors, what is the key ingredient in psychological adjustment and counseling for hearing impaired older adults? Briefly explain this.

5. A statement by Hull is presented in this chapter that illustrates misinterpretations by lay persons as it relates to hearing loss in older adults. How might the "lay person" interpret hearing loss and the misunderstandings that are common to hearing impaired older adults?

6. What appears to most negatively affect an older hearing-impaired person's successes in social interaction?

7. What role do finances play in reference to hearing handicap among older adults?

8. Why have audiologists expanded their role into the realm of counseling? Are they prepared to do so at the present time?

END OF CHAPTER ANSWER SHEET

Name   Date

CHAPTER 19

1. _____

   _____

   _____

   _____

2. _____

   _____

   _____

   _____

3. _____

   _____

   _____

   _____

4. _____

   _____

   _____

   _____

5. _____

_____

_____

_____

6. _____

_____

_____

_____

7. _____

_____

8. _____

_____

_____

■ CHAPTER 20 ■

Considerations for the Use and Orientation to Hearing Aids for Older Adults

■ RAYMOND H. HULL, Ph.D. ■

FACTORS INFLUENCING SUCCESSFUL HEARING AID
USE BY OLDER ADULTS

ASSESSING THE POTENTIAL SUCCESS OF HEARING
AID USE

MODIFICATIONS OF HEARING AID EVALUATION AND
FITTING PROCEDURES FOR OLDER ADULTS

MODIFICATIONS ACCORDING TO DIFFERENT
POPULATIONS OF OLDER ADULTS
  The Independent Older Adult
  The Semi-Independent Older Adult
  The Dependent Older Adult
  The Extremely Dependent Older Adult

(continued)

NON-HEARING AID ASSISTIVE LISTENING DEVICES
FOR OLDER ADULTS

HEARING AID ORIENTATION

SUMMARY

The process and tests for evaluating and prescribing hearing aids, as well as the various styles, parts of hearing aids, and circuits are covered partially in Chapter 4 of this text and in several other texts. Therefore, the focus of this chapter is on how amplification must be considered as part of the aural rehabilitation program for older adults.

The fitting and dispensing of hearing aids and other amplification systems and devices is a very important aspect of the process of aural rehabilitation. When an older adult's level of auditory acuity is brought to a more efficient level through the appropriate fitting of a hearing aid, then other components of the auditory habilitation or rehabilitation program are facilitated. For many older individuals, a properly fitted and properly used hearing aid will enhance their ability to interact more competently and more enjoyably in their social and personal worlds.

FACTORS INFLUENCING SUCCESSFUL HEARING AID USE BY OLDER ADULTS

As discussed in Chapter 17, hearing loss and accompanying auditory impairment found among many older adults is quite complex. In individuals with both a sensorineural hearing loss and a compounding central auditory impairment, a hearing aid per se may not resolve all of the hearing problems being experienced by the person (Stach, 1990). Hull (1988, 1992, 1995) discussed the additive factors that an older person experiences when attempting to understand speech through a peripheral and central auditory system that is no longer programmed for the speed required for comprehending rapid speech and less than beneficial extrinsic/environmental influences with which the auditory system must contend.

Stach (1990) found that persons with a combined central auditory processing disorder and a peripheral hearing loss do not benefit from hearing aids as one would expect from studying the person's audiogram. In other words, it is important to consider the possibility that a hearing aid candidate's audiogram may not reveal all that is important when recommending the individual for a hearing aid fitting.

According to Kasten (1992), there are nine important factors that must be considered when determining the appropriateness of amplification for hearing-impaired older adults: (1) motivation, (2) adaptability, (3) personal appraisal, (4) money, (5) social context, (6) personal influences, (7) mobility, (8) vanity, and (9) dexterity.

Motivation

In their early writings, Rupp, Higgins, and Maurer (1977) consider motivation as being the most important factor in their feasibility scale for predicting successful hearing aid use. They point out that those who show less personal motivation and depend more on the urging of others to procure a hearing aid are less likely to be successful in the use of amplification. Likewise, the individual who has a great desire to continue to lead a mentally, physically, and emotionally active life and to participate in the affairs of society is more likely to be a successful user of hearing aids. On the other hand, those who have lost interest in their surroundings and are willing to withdraw from society may have little motivation or desire to be successful in the use of amplification. Thus, the probability of these persons being successfully rehabilitated through hearing aid use becomes correspondingly less.

Adaptability

One of the more important factors concerning the use of amplification are the expectations of each individual. Until a person becomes hearing impaired and finds that he or she may need some type of amplification or until he or she interacts with a spouse or friend who has hearing impairment, it is unlikely that the person will have a clear-cut expectation about the use of a hearing aid.

New hearing aid users are sometimes quite surprised when they first hear with amplification. It is likely that some people expect a hearing aid to restore their hearing to the efficiency that it had many years previously, and others may expect an aid to be nothing but a nuisance. It is almost certain that neither of these levels of expectation is realistic or correct. If an individual expects essentially complete correction of the hearing deficiency, he or she almost certainly will be disappointed. Conversely, if an individual has so little optimism as to think that the hearing aid will be of no help, then he or she is likely to be unwilling to put forth the effort necessary to become oriented to and consequently wear the instrument(s). In other words, the person may simply be unwilling to give amplification a chance. If a person is unwilling to try something that is new or unusual, then major changes in attitude are necessary before successful hearing aid use will be noted.

Personal Appraisal

An individual's personal assessment and emotional feelings about his or her communication problems are extremely important factors in the degree of success in the use of amplification. Rupp et al. (1977) approached this matter with the attitude that audiological assessment data are appropriate in determining the degree of hearing loss, but that self-assessment is also important and should be carried out with one of the available scales for determining the degree of communication disability. Suggested communication scales include those by Demorest and Erdman (1987), Hull (1992), Kaplan, Bally, and Brandt (1990), Noble and Atherley (1970), or Ventry and Weinstein (1982). Another possibility would be to use one of the abbreviated scales designed by Allen and Rupp (1975) or Shotola and Maurer (1974). There is generally good agreement on the degree of disability as determined by audiological data and by a self-inventory using one of the self-assessment scales.

Successful use of amplification is most likely when there is strong correlation between the two sets of information (i.e., audiometric data and self-assessment). One who is able to appraise his or her personal disability objectively and with accuracy is generally in a position to at least accept the resulting communication problems and assist in developing a realistic approach to the possibilities, as well as to the specific procedures, needed in rehabilitation.

Money

The financial status of a person can certainly have a profound effect on his or her interest or lack of interest in hearing aids. For the majority of potential users, however, the purchase of hearing aids is not impossible. On the other hand, hearing aids still may be in the category of a luxury and would probably be purchased only if the person who has hearing impairment is convinced that they will meet his or her needs. Many people are aware that their friends and, perhaps they themselves, have spent hundreds of dollars for one or more hearing aids that proved to be unsatisfactory and were relegated to a dresser drawer or closet shelf. Thus, some people are unwilling to spend the money necessary to obtain hearing aids. When an individual is living on a fixed income from a pension plan and is only meeting living expenses, then the matter of hearing aid purchase may become financially difficult.

Those who are eligible for Medicaid assistance can sometimes obtain help from that source in buying a hearing aid (if their state Medicaid laws provide for hearing aids). However, some states (e.g., California, Kansas, and others only provide one hearing aid every 3 years unless the patient has special circumstances, such as blindness). Hearing aid banks can be an important resource and there may be other possibilities for financial assistance by civic organizations. However, these sources also may have restrictions that present problems in carrying out a purchase.

Social Context

The older client who has hearing impairment, as any other person, may fit anywhere along a continuum from one who is socially active to one who is socially withdrawn. Those who are active in various aspects of social life are ones who are likely to desire to maintain contact with other people and to communicate actively. Those who are withdrawn, on the other hand, may have lost interest in such contact. Thus, it becomes the task of the audiologist to determine if a withdrawal is due to hearing loss and, if so, how to rehabilitate the person.

It seems reasonable to assume that those who are engaged in social activities would be the ones most likely to be successful in rehabilitation utilizing hearing aids. At least they would have the desire and motivation for this type of achievement. Conversely, those who are withdrawn or who lack social awareness might be the ones least likely to be successful in rehabilitation utilizing hearing aids.

The large remaining group includes those who are neither extremely active socially nor completely withdrawn. They are, in fact, the ones who are in the process of losing their interest in social contact, because there is too great an effort needed to maintain communication with their friends. Although their lagging interest in social affairs would make them less than ideal candidates for the use of amplification, it is also highly possible that satisfactory selection of amplification and the use of appropriate rehabilitation procedures can improve the probability of reentry into social activities.

Personal/Functional Influences

The attitudes, interests, and activities of the friends of the older client who has hearing impairment can have a great deal of influence on his or her attitudes and desires. If the person is still employed or active in volunteer or avocational activities that involve him or her with communication and, if the people who are associated with the person who has hearing impairment are sympathetic, understanding, and stimulating in their conversations, then the elderly person's desire to utilize amplification will be enhanced. Conversely, if the living situation and the people involved in the life process of the older person lack stimulating ingredients, then the individual who has hearing impairment is likely to have little reason for wanting to try to obtain or adjust to the use of amplification.

Mobility

The ability of persons who have hearing impairment to be physically mobile and be involved in daily activities has a great effect on their desire to use hearing aids. For example, if an individual is able to be involved in various activities including church, theater, musical concerts, and favorite social clubs, then he or she is likely to be a good candidate for the use of amplification and improved communication. On the other hand, those who are limited in mobility and who rarely leave their living area for social or business contacts may have less desire or apparent need for communication and, therefore, less need and/or desire for amplification. There are those who essentially live alone and seem to have little desire for communication with others. They may feel a great deal of loneliness, yet they are unable or unwilling to make the effort to maintain contact with other people.

These persons may have a need for the communicative assistance that can be obtained through amplification, yet they often are physically and emotionally limited in their ability and/or desire to become involved in social activities, and, thus, their ability or desire to utilize amplification. They might have arthritis, a cardiac condition, or some other type of debilitating problem in addition to the hearing impairment, yet they could participate in social activities, for example, if transportation were available. However, the hearing problem presents an additional barrier and the combination results in greater physical isolation, which means they are less likely to be successful from the standpoint of a desire or need for improvement in their ability to communicate.

Vanity

Vanity is an aspect of human nature that can have a great impact on a person's interest in trying to adjust to hearing aids. Corrective lenses for the eyes illustrate how a prosthetic appliance can be accepted or rejected. Many people would prefer not to wear eyeglasses, but, nevertheless, a large majority of our society eventually needs to wear some type of visual correction. In fact, most people accept the use of corrective lenses at some time in their lives and may even consider it stylish to wear them. Once an individual has accepted the necessity of eyeglasses, he or she may go to extremes by purchasing large and gaudy eyewear, which definitely calls attention to the prostheses. On the other hand, based on their own opinions of appearance of self or the opinions of others, persons may try to use contact lenses to conceal a sight problem as completely as possible. Sunglasses are thought of as glamorous and most people, young and old, wear them for utility *and* style.

Hearing aids have not received the same level of acceptance as eyeglasses. And, it is unlikely that anyone would buy an overly large or conspicuous hearing aid in the same way that some people buy large or unusual pairs of glasses. On the contrary, people are interested in being fit with hearing aids that are as small and inconspicuous as possible. This seems to be true for most people, regardless of their age or lifestyle. A behind-the-ear instrument is frequently rejected in favor of a smaller all-in-the-ear model, simply because the person feels that this would be less conspicuous. Some older persons state strongly that they might accept an in-the-ear instrument, but would not even consider a postauricle aid, even though it might provide them better hearing.

On the other hand, some people are unwilling to wear an instrument of any kind, because they do not wish to advertise that they have a hearing problem. They would prefer to try to "get by" and conceal their problem. This type of attitude has historically presented a barrier in acceptance of amplification. However, this view appears to be diminishing, as people of this generation take charge of their own destiny by doing whatever is necessary to reduce barriers to their lives.

Dexterity

Hearing aids and their controls continue to become smaller. This reduction in size has made hearing aids far more acceptable to a larger number of people than ever before. For the vast majority of the population, the smaller size has not presented a great problem. However, with advancing age, the reduction in the dimensions of instruments and the resulting decrease in the size of the controls can present difficulties.

With age, acuity of touch may diminish, and people find it difficult to know precisely if they are correctly seating a hearing aid or ear mold into the concha. Many an elderly person may be seen with a hearing aid hanging precariously from his or her ear or with an ear mold that is far from being seated properly. In most cases the individual is unaware about the situation even though he or she has just put on the hearing aid. Such individuals often com-plain that the hearing aid does not work properly or that it hurts the ear; both complaints are easily resolved by ensuring that the aid is properly seated in the ear. Likewise, an older person may have such a poor sense of touch that he or she is unable to find the volume control or the off–on switch. When the person tries to move a control to a de-sired location, the person may not be certain whether the movement was successful. In addition, older persons may have reduced finger mobility because of poor muscle control or arthritis. They find it difficult to manipulate the controls even if they know what they need to do.

Thus, good manual dexterity and a good sense of touch can help a great deal in the successful use of amplification. On the other hand, reduced dexterity and sense of touch can be strong deterrents to success, and almost certainly require the assistance of some relative or other person to overcome this difficulty. A mandatory portion of every hearing aid fitting with an older individual should include a dexterity check to determine if the person can use the controls, fit the aids to the ears, and actually handle and change batteries. The fitter should note any problems and consider the need for larger or stacked volume controls.

ASSESSING THE POTENTIAL SUCCESS OF HEARING AID USE

The previously discussed factors are by no means unique. It was mentioned previously that as early as 1977, Rupp et al. proposed "A Feasibility Scale for Predicting Hearing Aid Use with Older Individuals." Their scale incorporates 11 prognostic areas or factors that should be considered when dealing with aged persons. The scoring sheet used with this scale is shown in Figure 20–1, and a guide for use in scoring the Feasibility Scale is presented in Figure 20–2.

The prognostic areas are not only listed and explained, but they are also weighted according to relative importance. One should also note similarities between the prognostic areas associated with the feasibility scale and the factors listed earlier in this chapter. The important consideration for all individuals who deal with fitting hearing aids with older persons is the realization that complex and interactive issues must be dealt with to ensure successful hearing aid use.

To a large extent, those of us who work with older hearing aid users must be able to examine their probable success within the framework of various factors or prognostic areas. We must also learn to accept certain guidelines as they relate to successful hearing aid use. Many older individuals view themselves as having completed the most active phases of their lives and they are now living out the remainder of their life according to their own prescribed rules. Many view themselves as having made it through the rigors and difficulties of adult life and they, therefore, feel that they have insight into life that is far more complete and comprehensive than younger persons. They have established their own game plan for the coming years, and they feel strongly that the game plan should not be modified. They look back on their previous years as authority figures, either in occupations or in families and realize that oftentimes their present state of authority is only an honorary award. More specifically, they acknowledge that

PROGNOSTIC FACTORS/DESCRIPTIONS (continuum, high to low)	ASSESSMENT 5-High: 0-Low	WEIGHT	WEIGHTED SCORE (Possible) Actual	
1. Motivation and referral (self . . . family)	5 4 3 2 1 0	× 4	(20)_____	1.
2. Self-assessment of listening difficulties (realistic . . . denial)	5 4 3 2 1 0	× 2	(10)_____	2.
3. Verbalization as to "fault" of communication difficulties (self caused . . . projection)	5 4 3 2 1 0	× 1	(5)_____	3.
4. Magnitude of loss: amplification results				4.
A. Shift in spondaic threshold: _____	5 4 3 2 1 0	× 1	(5)_____	
B. Discrimination in quiet: _____at _____BB HTL	5 4 3 2 1 0	× 1	(5)_____	
C. Discrimination in noise: _____at _____dB HTL	5 4 3 2 1 0	× 1	(5)_____	
5. Informal verbalizations during Hearing Aid Evaluation Re: quality of sound, mold, size (acceptable . . . awful)	5 4 3 2 1 0	× 1	(5)_____	5.
6. Flexibility and adaptability versus senility (relates outwardly . . . self)	5 4 3 2 1 0	× 2	(10)_____	6.
7. Age: 95 90 85 80 75 70 65 < (0 0 1 2 3 4 5)	5 4 3 2 1 0	× 1.5	(7.5)_____	7.
8. Manual hand, finger dexterity, and general mobility (good . . . limited)	5 4 3 2 1 0	× 1.5	(7.5)_____	8.
9. Visual ability (adequate with glasses . . . limited)	5 4 3 2 1 0	× 1	(5)_____	9.
10. Financial resources (adequate . . . very limited)	5 4 3 2 1 0	× 1.5	(7.5)_____	10.
11. Significant other person to assist individual (available . . . none)	5 4 3 2 1 0	× 1.5	(7.5)_____	11.
12. Other factors, please cite				12.

Client _____

Age _____

Date _____

Audiologist _____

FSPHAU:
Very limited	0 to 40%
Limited	41 to 60%
Equivocal	61 to 75%
Positive	76 to 100%

_____% Total Score

Figure 20–1. A feasibility scale for predicting hearing aid use. An analytic approach to predicting the probable success of a provisional hearing aid user. (Reprinted from Rupp, R. R., Higgins, J., & Maurer, J. F. [1977]. A feasibility scale for predicting hearing aid use with older individuals. *Journal of the Academy of Rehabilitative Audiology, 10*, 95–96, with permission).

1. Motivation/Referral	5.	Completely on own behalf
	4.	Mostly on own behalf
	3.	Generally on own behalf
	2.	Half self; half others
	1.	Little self; mostly others
	0.	Totally at urging of others

2. Self Assessment	5.	Complete agreement
	4.	Strong agreement
	3.	General agreement
	2.	Some agreement
	1.	Little agreement
	0.	No agreement

3. Verbalization as to "fault" of communicative difficulties	5.	Clearly created by hearing loss
	4.	Usually by loss
	3.	Loss and others
	2.	Environments and others
	1.	Mostly of others
	0.	Others totally at fault

4. Magnitude of loss; and results of amplification*		ST shift	in quiet at —dB HTL	in noise at —dB HTL
	5.	30 + dB	90%	70%
	4.	25	80–88	60–68
	3.	20	70–78	50–58
	2.	15	60–68	40–48
	1.	10	50–58	30–38
	0.	5	48	28

5. Informal verbalizations during hearing aid evaluation re: quality of sound, mold, size, weight, look	5.	Completely positive
	4.	Generally positive
	3.	Somewhat positive
	2.	Guarded
	1.	Generally negative
	0.	Completely negative

6. Flexibility and Adaptability A. Questionnaire and observation B. Raven's Progressive Matrices C. Face/Hand Sensory Test	5.	90th percentile
	4.	70
	3.	50
	2.	25
	1.	10
	0.	5

7. Age	5.	65 years
	4.	70
	3.	75
	2.	80
	1.	85
	0.	90 +

Figure 20–2. Scoring the Feasibility Scale items. Reprinted from Rupp, R. R., Higgins, J., & Maurer, J. F. (1977). A feasibility scale for predicting hearing aid use with older individuals. *Journal of the Academy of Rehabilitative Audiology, 10*, 97. (With permission).

(continued)

Figure 20–2. *(continued)*

8.	Manual/Hand Dexterity via Purdue Peg Board and Symbol Digit Modalities Test	5.	Superior
		4.	Adequate
		3.	Slow but steady
		2.	Slow and shaky
		1.	Slow and awkward
		0.	"Arthritic"
9.	Visual Ability (with glasses)	5.	Very good—no problems
		4.	Corrected, adequate
		3.	Adequate but safeguarded
		2.	Limited visibility
		1.	Very limited
		0.	Blind
10.	Financial Resources	5.	Unlimited resources
		4.	Generally unrestricted
		3.	Adequate
		2.	Adequate but close
		1.	Dipping into savings
		0.	Poverty level, on assistance
11.	Significant other person	5.	Always available
		4.	Often
		3.	Sometimes
		2.	Occasionally
		1.	Seldom
		0.	Never

*Alternate scoring scheme for factor 4 in cases where the ST shift was minimal due to loss in high frequencies only.

(Average threshold shift at 2000 and 3000 Hz)	5.	25 + dB
	4.	21–25 dB
	3.	16–20 dB
	2.	11–15 dB
	1.	6–10 dB
	0.	0–5 dB

many of their aged counterparts exhibit difficulties with hearing and this particular deficit is one that simply should be accepted and tolerated. Most importantly, however, they frequently know or have heard of any number of individuals who have invested sizable amounts of money from their generally limited resources in their unsuccessful search for improved hearing through amplification.

One can recognize the effects that these circumstances can have on the outlook of an older individual toward the successful use of amplification. Further, the person may simply doubt that a pros-

thetic device will change their lifestyle and social function, and, further, may not be fully certain that a change will really be beneficial to them. They may feel that a device so small can only be of limited benefit, but at the same time also appear firmly convinced that this small device will call undue attention to the fact that yet another physical affliction has taken its toll. In short, the aged individual often has a sizeable number of apparently logical arguments against the use of amplification. Before successful hearing aid use can be instituted, those arguments must be defused.

MODIFICATIONS OF HEARING AID EVALUATION AND FITTING PROCEDURES FOR OLDER CLIENTS

Since the development of the wearable hearing aid, procedures have been developed to compare the performance of different hearing instruments. Early procedures by Alpiner (1975); Carhart (1946, 1950); Hayes and Jerger (1978); Jeffers (1960); McConnell, Silber, and McDonald (1960); Reddell and Calvert (1966); Ross (1972); Zerlin (1962), and others have been developed for determining hearing aid candidacy and hearing aid fittings. This has been done to provide as much assurance as possible that a potential wearer would obtain hearing aids that would be of substantial benefit for that individual.

Today, 2cc coupler and real-ear probe microphone measurements provide more objective measures of hearing aid function and in the latter case, hearing aid function in relation to a client's ear canal resonance. No matter what method is used to evaluate hearing aid function, however, it is not possible to state unequivocally that every recommended instrument is the most efficient for each individual. Procedures have, of course, been developed that take into account many different acoustic and personal factors in an effort to fit each individual appropriately. The degree of success in obtaining this goal undoubtedly varies, but it is believed that these procedures avoid selection of an instrument that would be unsuitable for the individual concerned.

McCarthy (1987) emphasized the need for modifications in hearing aid evaluation procedures that take advantage of the abilities that an older client may possess. For example, she encouraged the audiologist to consider the modification of traditional comparative hearing evaluation procedures using speech stimuli by both presentation and response modes. The testing procedures to determine the potential usefulness of hearing aids should not be so difficult and task-oriented that the hearing aids will be rejected because the older client does not feel that he or she can pass the audiologist's tests.

With the aging population, it is increasingly necessary to mold the evaluation procedures to fit the individual. One cannot talk about a single evaluation procedure anymore than one can talk about a single population of aging individuals. In short, it is necessary for the evaluator and fitter of hearing aids to employ a broad array of procedures and tailor these procedures to the specific requirements of each potential hearing aid user.

It has been stressed throughout this section of this book that aging individuals have hearing impairments that present unique problems as a result of their age and their psychosocial and economic status. These factors are particularly important when one considers procedures to be used in the selection and fitting of hearing aids for these persons. There is no question that the same purposes and philosophies apply to the selection of hearing aids for this group as for any other group. But, their unique needs, abilities, and limitations demand that the selection and fitting procedures be modified to some extent. The selection procedures used in choosing amplification for older clients must take those special characteristics of aging persons into account.

MODIFICATIONS ACCORDING TO DIFFERENT POPULATIONS OF OLDER ADULTS

There are several populations of older adults that must be considered, and the differences among these populations influence the potential use of hearing aids. According to Kasten (1992), the differences among these populations influence the procedures that can be used for selecting a suitable hearing aid.

THE INDEPENDENT OLDER ADULT

Older individuals in the independent-living group are frequently the easiest to work with and the most successful in terms of hearing aid use. They continue to be in control of their lifestyles and they enter into the process of hearing aid use with their eyes open, albeit sometimes reluctantly. It is with this particular group that a high score on the feasibility scale of Rupp et al. (1977) is most encouraging. For the factors or prognostic areas that predict hearing aid use, individuals in this population are most frequently amenable to change. These individuals often continue to see a great many varied opportunities available to themselves and frequently are willing to modify behavior and attitudes for their own betterment and for the benefit of their spouse or friends.

According to Kasten (1992), with the independent-living population, *motivation* is the critical factor. When motivation exists, even to a limited degree, appropriate counseling can bring about positive change in a client. Sympathetic support on the part of a spouse or friend can clearly help to strengthen the degree of communicative success.

To a large degree, potential success with hearing aids is directly tied to the extent that a potential hearing aid user can see and experience success in significant and meaningful communication situations. Success in communication can cause a heightened social awareness and can lead to a genuine desire to expand social horizons and to modify an individual's personal everyday life.

Fitting the Hearing Aid

Great care must be taken to see that all clients are able to handle and adjust their own hearing aids. They must be given opportunities during the evaluation and orientation to work with specific hearing aid models and to demonstrate their ability to both use and adjust them. If they are unable to accomplish these tasks on their own, they must understand that successful hearing aid use will require either a larger instrument or the assistance of other persons. These facts must be emphasized to prevent the individual from later rejecting the instrument or finding that it simply cannot be used. Some individuals will be willing to rely on a significant other person and, in this case, clinicians can do their best to satisfy their desires by including the other person in the process. Those who are strongly independent in terms of their personal care, however, must be made aware that hearing aids should be of a size and construction that will allow them to make necessary manipulations.

It is extremely important to convince the potential hearing aid user that he or she is not being pushed into purchasing an instrument that is not desired or that will not be personally satisfactory. Because the elderly client has a lifetime of knowledge and experience behind him or her, it is important for the person to have the opportunity to experience aided hearing and to make a decision without undue pressure from the evaluator or dispenser.

During the trial period, it is imperative that a potential hearing aid purchaser be provided with counseling to ensure that he or she and everyone concerned with the aged person who has hearing impairment knows how to use the hearing aid. This period also provides the maximum opportunity to make any necessary adjustments of the instrument or of the client's own attitudes, to become a truly successful hearing aid user.

THE SEMI-INDEPENDENT OLDER ADULT

When clinicians work with the semi-independent population, according to Kasten (1992), they are faced with a different set of circumstances. These individuals frequently have large portions of their lifestyles dictated by those who control the environment in which they live. Very often, this direction is provided by well-meaning but communicatively naive sons or daughters in whose homes the older person may reside. All too often, this group of older individuals find themselves living in a relatively comfortable, albeit controlled, environment, and they may think that their only other option is nursing home placement. As a result, their psychological set and their attitude toward the factors relating to successful hearing aid use are consciously or subconsciously dictated to them by the individual or individuals governing their living accommodations.

With this population, it is frequently necessary to spend as much time with the persons who control the living environment as with the older individuals, themselves. If the well-meaning son or daughter is not sold on the value of hearing aids, then the older individual may not be convinced that they will help. If the son or daughter feels that hearing aids are too expensive to warrant purchase, the likelihood is high that the older individual will find no way to afford the purchase. If the son or daughter strongly states that the older person does not seem to have enough of a problem to warrant hearing aid use, then chances are that the older person will at least verbalize a similar statement. If the son or daughter feels that the older person does not have a wide enough range of activities or experiences to benefit from a hearing aid, then the likelihood is quite high that the older person will reflect the same belief and, even worse, may demonstrate it.

In spite of the apparent needs of an older individual, decisions about amplification and attitudes toward amplification may be shaped by others who are not directly experiencing the problem. On the other hand, family members can also be a catalyst in the successful use of hearing aids.

The former situation creates an awkward position for the older individual who has hearing impairment. He or she may readily recognize the need for the kind of assistance that can be obtained from amplification, but genuinely fear the consequences of a decision that goes contrary to the power structure in his or her environment. Although often not intentional, the older individual in the semi-independent population may become the *recipient* of attitudes and decisions rather than the *originator* of the attitudes and decisions.

THE DEPENDENT OLDER ADULT

The dependent-living population frequently requires a different approach and demands serious moral judgments on the part of the audiologist or the hearing aid dispenser. According to Kasten (1992), individuals in this population may be almost totally controlled and cared for as the result of their physical, emotional, or mental condition. If this population is viewed objectively in terms of hearing aid use, clinicians are faced with the fact that they may have poor motivation, little adaptability, limited insight in terms of personal appraisement, little available money, poor social awareness, and a restricted social environment, as well as limited mobility and finger dexterity.

In addition to these factors, we must realize that these people oftentimes are cared for by well-meaning and hard-working staff members who know almost nothing about hearing aid use and who are primarily concerned with physical factors relating to the maintenance of life. Taken as a group, the prospects for successful hearing aid use are limited. This has been substantiated in early reports of Alpiner (1963), Gaitz and Warshaw (1964), and Grossman (1955). In particular, Alpiner in his early writings (1963) discussed three general attitudes that appear among dependent older individuals who chose not to become involved in hearing aid use. They presented a definite denial that a problem was present, displayed a general attitude of hopelessness, and expressed a recognition of the hearing loss, but indicated no desire for any type of rehabilitation.

Successful Hearing Aid Use
For Dependent Older Persons

For dependent older persons, the key to any successful hearing aid use will be the staff members who care for the individual or the volunteers who help in activities of daily living. These people must be trained in proper hearing aid use and maintenance and must be schooled on the importance of hearing aids for communication. By explaining in detail the methods and procedures they can use to convey information to the older individual who has hearing impairment, they receive extensive knowledge about hearing aid use and care.

Clinicians must realize, however, that there generally is a relatively high turnover of staff in many health care facilities. As a rule, the work is hard, the hours are long, and the pay is often not commensurate with the work involved. As a result, many individuals stay with a particular job only until they are able to find something else that will provide them with more satisfaction or more money. With this in mind, clinicians must realize that in-service training that deals with hearing aid use and care must be performed on a recurring basis and must include a great deal of demonstration and some rather thorough follow-up evaluations.

With the dependent group, clinicians must remember that well-fitted hearing aids are not an end unto themselves. Hearing aid use will be successful only if there is a need for communication, a desire for personal interaction, and support that includes family and staff encouragement and understanding. Hearing aid use will be successful only when older individuals can demonstrate to themselves a real benefit from the process. Services on behalf of the confined older adult are discussed in Chapter 22.

THE EXTREMELY DEPENDENT OLDER ADULT

These are individuals who are truly physically, mentally, or emotionally dependent. In many cases, they have only limited ability to communicate, but improved hearing may make it possible to make their care easier and provide them with some additional contact with the outside world. With individuals of this group, formal testing procedures are often not useable and decisions concern-

ing the value of amplification may necessarily be made only by observation.

Before actually attempting the use of hearing aids, it is necessary to make some type of estimate concerning the degree of hearing impairment. It may be necessary for these tests to be conducted with the presentation of various sounds combined with subjective observation of types or levels of response. Predictive acoustic reflex testing should also be accomplished. Also, otoacoustic emission (OAE) testing is providing yet another objective means of evaluating patients' hearing, especially those who will not or cannot respond to traditional tests. Although these procedures may provide only an approximation of the hearing capacity, the audiologist will garner information regarding the status of the client's hearing and some indication as to whether the use of amplification is or is not indicated. Obviously, any type of information concerning the degree of hearing impairment is most helpful, including the person's ability to hear and understand speech.

As soon as the degree of hearing impairment has been determined, it would be appropriate to evaluate performance with a series of listening devices while the audiologist carefully observes responses to sound. One might notice whether the individual responds to voice or environmental noises or if the use of both visual and auditory clues are used in making contact with those around him or her. The observer also should watch for any behavioral changes, tolerance reactions, vestibular effects, or aggression toward amplification.

This procedure may appear to lack the strict objectivity that audiologists strive for in evaluating performance with hearing aids. But, if one can observe and document behavioral changes that result from amplification, it is reasonable to recommend use of an instrument based on these results. However, if one can observe no changes between the unaided and aided behaviors and there is no evidence of improvement, then the recommendation for hearing aids may not be justified.

A Final Consideration as It Relates To The Extremely Dependent

One final factor is essential to consider when dealing with the extremely dependent aged population. By definition, individuals in this group are incapable of caring for themselves and require the constant attendance of others who care for them. For the hearing aid user within this group, a significant other person must be knowledgeable and proficient in terms of hearing aid use. He or she must be able to ensure that the hearing aids are working properly, the batteries are appropriate and working, the earmolds or hearing aids are inserted properly, and the hearing aids are set as they should be for the individual. Although these do not seem to be overwhelming tasks, they can be major hurdles for an overworked health care facility staff member who has had no experience with hearing aid use.

Because there is a relatively high turnover in nursing home staff, this means that an ongoing program of hearing aid familiarization is necessary to ensure proper hearing aid use for both dependent and extremely dependent individuals. The audiologist must maintain close contact with the health care facility administrators and nursing staff so that he or she can be available when staff turnover requires a new staff training program. In this way, continuous care for hearing aid users is assured.

NON-HEARING AID ASSISTIVE LISTENING DEVICES FOR OLDER LISTENERS

Assistive listening devices for adults who possess impaired hearing are providing them with alternatives to hearing aids for specific listening environments. Most involve: (1) infrared, (2) FM amplification, (3) AM amplification, (4) hardwire amplification systems, and (5) various telephone amplifying systems. A review of hearing health care business publications revealed there are presently more than 85 U.S. companies, along with more than 50 overseas companies, that are marketing and distributing the most common types of assistive listening devices (International Directory of Hearing Health Care Products, 1999).

In 1990, Hull studied the most common forms of assistive listening devices. They were systematically evaluated by older adult listeners, ages 70–80 years, who possessed sufficient hearing impairment to interfere with their desired level of social activity. The types of assistive listening devices evaluated included (1) infrared, (2) FM, (3) AM, and (4) hardwire systems. The older adults used each type of assistive listening device for 6 weeks in various preselected listening environments including church, meeting rooms, restaurants, gathering places such as senior centers, their home, the theater, and viewing television.

The results revealed that infrared systems were ranked by the older listeners as the most satisfactory in most environments, including church, community gathering places, television viewing, and at the theater. FM systems were also found to be satisfactory, but in fewer environments. Hardwire systems were found to be useable only in restaurants and for home television viewing. They were ranked as the least satisfactory. The results of this study are shown in Figure 20–3. These older listeners enjoyed the experience of being able to hear well with the assistive listening devices and affirmed the need for the availability of nonhearing aid assistive listening devices for special environments in which hearing aids may be less than effective.

HEARING AID ORIENTATION

The importance of adequate orientation to one's hearing aid(s) has been stressed throughout this chapter, but a separate discussion of the essential elements of that important aspect of hearing aid fitting and use is important. Orientation to the use

Environment	Listening Device			
	Best ◄————————► Worse			
1. Church sanctuary/meeting rooms	Infrared	FM	AM	Hardwire
2. Restaurants	None	Hardwire	Fm	Infrared
3. Senior center/community gathering places	Infrared	FM	AM	Hardwire
4. At home—living rooms/dining rooms	None	Hardwire	Infrared	FM
5. Home-television viewing	Infrared	Hardwire	AM	FM
6. The theatre	Infrared	FM	Hardwire	AM

Figure 20–3. Rankings of various non-hearing aid assistive listening devices by older hearing impaired listeners.

of hearing aids is an essential part of the ongoing aural rehabilitation program. The fitting and dispensing of hearing aids is just the beginning of the process. If a client is not comfortable with a hearing aid, its uses, benefits, and limitations, it will probably not be successfully employed by the client.

According to McLauchlin (1992), there are seven important components of a hearing orientation program:

1. An understanding of the function of the component parts and adjustments of hearing aids;
2. Practice in fitting, adjusting, and maintaining the hearing aid;
3. An understanding of the limitations of amplification;
4. Knowledge of why the particular hearing aid was selected for him or her;
5. How to begin using a newly selected hearing aid;
6. How to troubleshoot hearing aid problems; and
7. How to exercise a hearing aid user's legal rights.

Depending on the state of health, alertness, and physical ability of the client, those key elements should guide the hearing aid orientation program. The hearing aid orientation program, according to McLauchlin (1992), need not be restricted to a spe-

cified time frame. If the client is part of an ongoing aural rehabilitation program, hearing aid orientation is integral. The client asks questions, receives answers from the audiologist, requests adjustments regarding the fit of the amplification, and in this regard, receives comprehensive orientation and adjustment service over time.

If the client is among the dependent population, it becomes critical that his or her family, significant other, or health care facility staff become integral members of the hearing aid orientation program, as they may be the ones who fit the client with the hearing aid each day. Chapter 22 describes the ongoing service that family and health care facility staff can provide on behalf of the dependent older client.

Clients and their significant other(s) should be provided practical information about the care and maintenance of the hearing aid(s), and their uses. For example:

1. The client should receive general information about hearing aids, what they are, what they do, what they do not do, and the component parts. There is so much misinformation presented in advertisements about hearing aids, that it behooves the audiologist to provide accurate and informative details.

2. Information on adjusting to one's hearing aid is critical to the orientation process. This involves practicing placing the hearing aid in one's ear and removing it; what to expect from the hearing aid in noisy or otherwise distracting environments; and how to adjust the aid.

3. The care of one's hearing aid, including the potential harm from water, hair spray, excessive heat, perspiration, and other factors are important parts of the orientation process. Receiving information on cleaning and caring for one's hearing aid is as important as learning how to use it.

4. Telephone use with a hearing aid with or without a telecoil should be a part of the orientation process.

5. Information on what causes "whistles and squeals" is also important for clients to receive. This can be a part of the information presented on "When do hearing aids need repair?"

6. Battery sizes, materials, life expectancy, increasing battery life, and other information about batteries is also critical to the orientation process. There is almost as much misinformation available to hearing aid users about batteries as there is about hearing aids, themselves.

An effective and efficient hearing aid orientation process is a critically important part of the fitting of hearing aids. The effectiveness of this part of the aural rehabilitation process can enhance or doom the willingness of clients to use their hearing aid(s) in constructive ways.

SUMMARY

The older individual who has hearing impairment may belong to one of several different populations who demonstrate a wide range of skills and abilities. Therefore, it is frequently necessary to modify the procedures for selecting and fitting hearing aids to succssfully meet each client's amplification needs.

It matters little which dependency category an aged person may fit into. Each individual presents a unique set of capabilities and/or limitations and audiologists must be aware of all as they pertain to each individual to deal effectively with these clients.

The growing population of aged individuals poses a unique challenge to all persons involved in the hearing health care team. The audiologist must be particularly aware that he or she is not dealing with one large homogeneous group of individuals, but rather with several subgroups who have advanced age as a common factor and their individual level of ability as a distinctive feature.

REFERENCES

Alpiner, J. G. (1963). Audiologic problems of the aged. *Geriatrics, 18*, 19–26.

Alpiner, J. G. (1975). Hearing aid selection for adults. In M. Pollack (Ed.), *Amplification for the hearing impaired* (pp. 247–263). New York: Grune & Stratton.

Allen, C., & Rupp, R. R. (1975). *Comparative evaluation of a self-assessment hearing handicap scale given to elderly women from low and high socio-economic groups.* Paper presented at the annual convention of the American Speech and Hearing Association, Washington, DC.

Carhart, R. (1946). Selection of hearing aids. *Archives of Otolaryngology, 44*, 1–18.

Carhart, R. (1950). Hearing aid selection by university clinics. *Journal of Speech and Hearing Disorders, 15*, 106–113.

Demorest, M. E., & Erdman, S. A. (1987). Development of the communication profile for the hearing impaired. *Journal of Speech and Hearing Disorders, 52*, 129–143.

Gaitz, C., & Warshaw, M. S. (1964). Obstacles encountered in correcting hearing loss in the elderly. *Geriatrics, 19*, 83–86.

Grossman, B. (1955) Hard of hearing persons in a home for the aged. *Hearing News, 23*, 11–12, 17–18, 20.

Hayes, D., & Jerger, J. (1978). A new method of hearing aid evaluation. *Journal of the Academy of Rehabilitative Audiology, 11*, 57–65.

Hull, R. H. (1988). Evaluation of ALDs by older adult listeners. *Hearing Instruments, 39*, 10–12.

Hull, R. H. (1990). Evaluation of ALDs by older adult listeners. *Hearing Instruments, 39,* 10–12.

Hull, R. H. (1992). UNC Communication Appraisal and Priorities Profile. In R. H. Hull (Ed.), *Aural rehabilitation* (pp. 223–225). San Diego, CA: Singular Publishing Group.

Hull, R. H. (1995). *Hearing in aging.* San Diego, CA: Singular Publishing Group.

International Directory of Hearing Health Care Products (1993). *Hearing Instruments, 51,* 14–133.

Jeffers, J. (1960). Quality judgment in hearing aid selection. *Journal of Speech and Hearing Disorders, 25,* 259–266.

Kaplan, H., Bally, S. J., & Brandt, F. D. (1990). *Communication Skill Scale.* Washington, DC: Gallaudet University.

Kasten, R.N. (1992). Considerations for the use and orientation to hearing aids for older adults. In R. H. Hull (Ed.), *Aural rehabilitation* (2nd ed., pp. 265–277). San Diego, CA: Singular Publishing Group.

McCarthy, P. A. (1987). Rehabilitation of the hearing impaired geriatric client. In J. G. Alpiner & P. A. McCarthy (Eds.), *Rehabilitative audiology: Children and adults.* Baltimore: Williams and Wilkins.

McConnell, F., Silber, E. F., & McDonald, D. (1960). Test-retest consistency of clinical hearing aid tests. *Journal of Speech and Hearing Disorders, 25,* 273–280.

McLauchlin, R. M. (1992). Hearing aid orientation for adult clients. In R. H. Hull (Ed.), *Aural rehabilitation* (2nd ed., pp. 327–342). San Diego, CA: Singular Publishing Group.

Noble, W., & Atherley, G. (1970). The hearing measure scale: A questionnaire for the assessment of auditory disability. *Journal of Auditory Research, 10,* 229–250.

Reddell, R. C., & Calvert, D. R. (1966). Selecting a hearing aid by interpreting audiological data. *Journal of Auditory Research, 6,* 445–452

Ross, M. (1972). Hearing aid evaluation. In J. Katz (Ed.), *Handbook of clinical audiology* (pp. 482–513). Baltimore: Williams and Wilkins.

Rupp, R. R., Higgins, J., & Maurer, J. F. (1977). A feasibility scale for predicting hearing aid use (FSPHAU) with other individuals. *Journal of the Academy of Rehabilitative Audiology, 10,* 81–104.

Shotola, R., & Maurer, J. (1974). *The development and use of a short screening form for detection of hearing loss in older adults.* Paper presented at the annual meeting of the Western Gerontological Society, Tucson, AZ.

Stach, B. A. (1990). Central auditory processing disorders and amplification applications. Research Symposium: Communication sciences and disorders aging. *ASHA Reports Series, 19,* 150–156.

Ventry, I. M. & Weinstein, B. E. (1982). The hearing-handicap inventory for the elderly: A new tool. *Ear and Hearing, 3,* 128–134

END OF CHAPTER EXAMINATION QUESTIONS

CHAPTER 20

1. The author presents nine factors that should be considered when determining the appropriateness of amplification for hearing-impaired older adults. Name and describe all nine of those factors.

   a.

   b.

   c.

   d.

   e.

   f.

   g.

   h.

   i.

2. The author presents a number of elements that must be taken into consideration when recommending and fitting hearing aids for older adults who have hearing impairment.

   Compare and contrast those for the following groups; (1) the independent older adult,(2) the semi-independent older adult, (3) the dependent older adult, and (4) the extremely dependent older adult.

3. What are 5 non-hearing aid assistive listening devices that may provide benefit on behalf of hearing impaired older adults. What are they? What are their benefits?

   a.

   b.

   c.

   d.

   e.

END OF CHAPTER ANSWER SHEET

Name   Date

CHAPTER 20

1. a.

   b.

   c.

   d.

   e.

   f.

   g.

   h.

   i.

2. _____

   _____

   _____

   _____

   _____

   _____.

3. a.

   b.

   c.

   d.

   e.

Techniques for Aural Rehabilitation for Aging Adults Who are Hearing Impaired

■ RAYMOND H. HULL, Ph.D. ■

THE PROCESS OF AURAL REHABILITATION
The Ongoing Aural Rehabilitation Program
Use of Residual Hearing With Supplemental Visual Clues
Linguistic, Content, and Environmental Redundancies
Reducing Auditory or Visual Confusions
Communicating Under Adverse Conditions
Other Approaches to Aural Rehabilitation Treatment
Summary

The process of aural rehabilitation[1] with older clients is exciting. To be involved in the recovery of communication skills that may have previously caused an adult to withdraw from a communicating world is rewarding. Both the client and the audiologist can rejoice in the recovery of those skills. Some elderly clients recover skills that allow them to participate on a social basis once again, at least with a greater degree of efficiency. Others may simply regain the ability to communicate with their family with greater ease. In light of those gains and, perhaps, a step toward a reinstatement of communicative independence, a client and his or her audiologist have reason to rejoice.

Clinicians cannot, under any circumstances, hope to benefit every older hearing-impaired person. But, in attempting to do so, if some are helped who had previously submitted to a self-imposed withdrawal from family and friends because of the embarrassment resulting from responding inappropriately to misunderstood questions, then professionals can be satisfied that our work is worthwhile.

Because most older adults who have hearing impairment have experienced normal to near-normal auditory function during their younger years, and because they are generally fully aware of the communicative difficulties they face, it is important that our services address their specific communicative needs. And, as it is being confirmed that auditory disorders found in older adults is quite complex (e.g., that is not only peripheral in nature but also involves the central auditory system according to Bergman, 1980; Hull, 1988; Jerger & Chmiel, 1997; Kasten, 1981; McCroskey & Kasten, 1980; Stach, 1990; Welsh, Welsh, & Healy, 1985; and others), approaches to aural rehabilitation must accommodate the communication difficulties experienced as a result of those compounding problems (see Chapter 17). The audiologist is, indeed, serving complex people who possess a complex auditory disorder.

---

[1] It is emphasized that the procedures presented in this chapter are ones that can be successfully used with any age of adult client.

INDIVIDUAL VERSUS GROUP TREATMENT

INDIVIDUAL TREATMENT

Some individuals will require such concentrated aural rehabilitation treatment efforts that individual sessions will be necessary. In instances in which clients are experiencing communicative difficulties that are not conducive to a group therapy environment, individual sessions are warranted.

For example, a semiretired physician came to this author with a desire for more efficient communication within his office and examination room. The sessions centered on the specific difficulties he was experiencing in that environment, and he did not desire that they be opened up into group aural rehabilitation sessions.

Another client's concern was that her granddaughter's wedding was forthcoming, and she felt that she was not going to be able to hear and understand what people were saying while she stood in the reception line. Her request was to receive some hints on how to "not embarrass herself and her family" by responding inappropriately to what people were saying to her in the reverberant environment of their local Moose Lodge. The aural rehabilitation program was based on three sessions of problem solving and supportive/informational counseling. After successfully working through the potential pitfalls of the communicative demands of her granddaughter's wedding, the woman returned to enter group therapy.

The sessions held for this woman were rather personal in regard to the difficulties she was anticipating and, in that instance, were not conducive to a group therapy environment, at least at that time. So, her desire for individual sessions was fulfilled.

Other circumstances in which individual treatment sessions would be appropriate include:

1. The client's hearing impairment and concomitant communicative difficulties are so severe that the client requires concentrated effort to resolve them to the greatest degree possible before entering a group environment;
2. The client's emotional response to the auditory impairment and the resulting communicative difficulties is such that group involvement, at a particular time, is contraindicated.

GROUP TREATMENT

Group aural rehabilitative treatment, as discussed later in this chapter, can be extremely motivating for most older adults who have hearing impairment. Once the problems and difficulties that are specific to individual clients have been resolved to the degree possible through work on an individual basis, clients should move into group therapy.

Individuals in group treatment find strength in hearing of others' successes and failures in their own communicative environments. They gain insights through group discussions and problem-solving into how to best cope in spite of their hearing impairment. The camaraderie that develops can be rewarding to group members as their confidence grows in their ability to take charge of the difficulties that they have been having in their own communicative worlds

COMPONENTS OF AURAL REHABILITATION SERVICES FOR OLDER CLIENTS

The following are important elements in aural rehabilitation service programs for older adults that are applicable for either the well adult in the community or those who are confined to a health care facility. They include:

1. Counseling
2. Hearing aid orientation
3. Adjusting the listening environment

4. Development of positive assertiveness
5. Developing compensatory skills in the use of residual hearing and supplemental visual cues
6. Involvement of family and significant others.

COUNSELING

As this author talks with his students about aural rehabilitation services for older adults, it is emphasized that counseling, for lack of a better term, is one of the most important aspects and is intertwined throughout the process of aural rehabilitation. It is not something that occurs alone and out of context. It is an integral part of everything an audiologist does when working with his or her clients. It is called **talking**. It is called **instilling confidence** in a client who became discouraged when he or she did not do as well as expected on a given communicative task. It is called **listening** to the innermost feelings a client reveals about him- or herself and that person's relationship with an intolerant family or roommate. And, it is called **trust** that must develop between audiologist and client. Counseling is the **discussion** that develops when a client desires to talk about an incident in which he or she had particular difficulty understanding what another person was saying and also includes the **problem solving** to unravel the possible reasons for the difficulty.

This aspect of the process of aural rehabilitation is, again, for lack of a better term, called **counseling**. But, whatever it is called, it involves **listening, talking, problem solving, facilitating adjustment** to a sometimes infuriating disability, and the **development of trust** between client and audiologist.

When an audiologist encounters an older client who has hearing impairment who says, "I do not desire to be helped. I am old and I do not know how much longer I will live," the attitude of the person certainly will influence how much potential progress that he or she will make. This is particularly true if the person has isolated him- or herself from the outside world and is resigned to not seek help because of advanced age.

The Audiologist as Counselor

If there are no other significant contraindicating factors that would hinder responsiveness to aural rehabilitation services, the audiologist is in a position to intervene in a counseling role. It is possible that this person has said what was said because he or she has been told by others that "you are too old." A well-meaning physician may have said, "You know you're no spring chicken any more." Or, a child may have said unthinkingly, "Mom, you know you can't care for yourself as well as you used to, so we should start thinking about moving you to a care facility," not realizing that the older adult is convinced that placement in a "care facility" will be terminal. Such statements, even said in a well-meaning way, are understandably unsettling and sometimes demeaning to an older adult.

One of this author's clients, a woman of 89 years, told me that her 50-year-old daughter told her they should sell her house and she should then move into an efficiency apartment. She was so hurt and angry that she could not think of anything to say. She felt convinced that if her mature daughter felt that she could not care for her house, then she must be doing a worse job than she thought. I asked her what she would have said if her daughter would have suggested that to her when she was 45 years old and her daughter was 15. She said she would have asked her why she would say such a thing, but, she said, "When you are 89 years old, perhaps it is not worth it."

If the medical records of an individual indicate satisfactory health, and there appears to be nothing that would contraindicate the provision of aural rehabilitative services, then the self-defeating attitude of the potential client may be the only thing that stands between the provision of services and reasonable progress in aural rehabilitation. Although an older person's realistic view of becoming older may be a healthy one, long-term mourning because of age and the possibility of death is not. The audiologist can be a positive catalyst in encouraging adjustment to aging, particularly for those who are barred from social interaction as a result of their auditory deficit.

Feelings to Which the Audiologist Must Respond

Phrases exemplifying attitudes typical of many older adults who have hearing impairment have been recorded by this author during initial aural rehabilitation interviews with hundreds of older clients. The feelings that prompted these revealing statements are those that can and do stifle the desire for aural rehabilitative services or the progress they may be capable of. They are, further, those to which the audiologist must respond. The following are a few of those statements, out of context, recorded by this author:

- "I feel that I'm on trial, incompetent."
- "My son is right behind me. He comes down to see me as often as he can, but he has a lot of business to handle there. I don't see him very often anymore."
- "I can't hear and my eyes bother me. Surgery won't help my ears or my eyes. I'm told that I'm too old."
- "My arthritis bothers me all over, especially with the weather. I used to walk a lot. I can't hear now. I'm too old."
- "I fear being alone—being melancholy—with no future to look forward to. I need to find some way to be useful. I can stand a lot. I'm still sturdy."
- "I would like, more than anything, to be able to get out, to socialize, but I can't hear very well. I would like to go to church, but the children don't come on Sundays and there is no one to take me."

One statement stands out from all of the rest. It is a statement by a physically strong and mentally alert 82-year-old man who has hearing impairment and who is torn between giving up or submitting to the opportunity to improve his ability to function communicatively through aural rehabilitation treatment. The statement is, "I'd like to put a younger person on my shoulders to ride intellectually and hear for me and to go on from there. I suppose I need to learn to rely on myself . . . relationships with people are important, but do I have the potential?"

The statements are representative of those heard by audiologists who accept the opportunity to provide a significant rehabilitative service to adults who have hearing impairment. These people are, in many ways, wishing to be recognized not simply as older persons, but as adults who have grown older, who have something to offer, and who do not want to be left alone. Their resolution to "not be a bother" and their resignation to "being old" is, in some cases, the most logical choice in their minds for lack of alternatives. The audiologist can be a catalyst in developing a desire for self-improvement.

The audiologist must not be afraid to work with these clients in a close, but professional manner. He or she must not be hesitant to intervene in a counseling role, but must be cognizant of those instances when a client's emotional problems are beyond the scope of the audiologist's knowledge. For those persons, it is the responsibility of the audiologist to refer the individual to other appropriate professionals. Above all, a client must be confident in the audiologist who is providing the aural rehabilitation service. The client must realize that the audiologist understands the communicative impact of presbycusis through his or her experience in working with other elderly clients. The client must know that the audiologist feels that he or she can, indeed, be helped to communicate more efficiently through aural rehabilitative services, and that feeling has justification on the basis of evaluation, not sympathy. A feeling of justified trust is the true key to motivational counseling.

Listen-talk-empathize-listen—encourage where appropriate—remember the status and age of the client—provide support—counsel—listen—ask questions—expect answers—listen—provide guidance. Add an appropriate amount of inspiration for what may be the key to successful motivational counseling.

Counseling as a part of the aural rehabilitation process is presented later in this chapter under "The Process of Aural Rehabilitation."

HEARING AID ORIENTATION

Information in Chapter 20 deals with considerations of hearing aids for older adults. As stated in that chapter, the process of adjustment to the use of hearing aids and orientation to their efficient use can be facilitated with greater ease for some elderly clients than others; this depends on prior exposure to and knowledge of the use of hearing aids and factors of memory, manual dexterity, and others. The process of adjustment to hearing aids and orientation to their use can be logically carried into daily or weekly aural rehabilitation treatment sessions, as can the trial use of various assisting listening devices.

Through carryover of hearing aid orientation into the aural rehabilitation treatment program, slight adjustments to the hearing aids can, for example, be made to alleviate communicative problems encountered during the previous week. Questions can be answered regarding their use, and discussions regarding certain difficult listen-

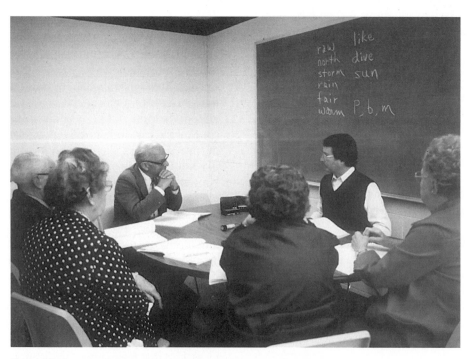

Figure 21–1. Older adults who are hearing impaired deserve our best services.

ing environments can be entertained that may benefit not only that individual client, but others in a group session. More experienced hearing aid users can be an important catalyst in a new user's successful adjustment to amplification. Further, experimental adjustments in hearing aid gain and frequency response can be made in accordance with the activities in various treatment sessions.

Carryover of the hearing aid orientation process into aural rehabilitation treatment sessions can be as important as the orientation process, itself, and is a logical extension. The consistency of client contact is a valuable asset in facilitating adjustment to amplification. In group treatment sessions, the catharsis and camaraderie that arise as various clients describe their own difficulties experienced during the initial adjustment period is a healthy environment for efficient adjustment to hearing aid use. Procedures for hearing aid orientation applicable for older adults are well outlined by Downs (1970), modified by Traynor and Peterson (1972), in McLauchlin (1992), and in Chapters 13 and 20 in this text. An excellent hearing aid orientation program for the confined elderly has been prepared by Smith and Fay (1977).

ADJUSTING/MANIPULATING THE LISTENING ENVIRONMENT

As is observed in "The Process" section of this chapter, elderly clients are initially asked to set priorities for communication situations in which they desire to function more efficiently. After this is completed, they are asked to choose one or two in which they *most* desire to learn to function more efficiently. They are, of course, requested to be reasonable in their selections. In this way, the aural rehabilitation treatment program can be designed to meet their specific communication needs. In instances in which a client's auditory difficulties are so severe that group sessions are not practical or cannot be tolerated by the client, individual treatment is scheduled. The goal, however, is to integrate the client into a group situation as soon

as possible, if at all possible. Another situation in which it is desirable that individual treatment be instituted is in the case of a client whose priority communication environment is so unique as to warrant individual work.

A situation in point is a client who was provided services individually by this author. His most difficult communication environment as a teacher in a middle school in Colorado was his classroom. His treatment sessions, therefore, centered on physical/environmental adjustments in that specific room. His priority communication environment did not warrant exposure in group sessions. He, further, did not desire that his difficulty be exposed to the group at that time. He had little difficulty in other more social environments.

Group Discussions of Problem Environments

Group sessions center on discussions of the clients' chosen and priority communication environments. Priority environments most frequently center on church (understanding the minister or Sunday school teacher, or participating in church committee meetings), other social environments in which groups of people meet, understanding what women or children are saying, and understanding what people are saying in environmentally distracting environments, such as on the street corner, in a restaurant, or at the theater. The inevitable commonality of their choices allows for group sessions that are beneficial for everyone, as the majority of clients can enter into each discussion as it relates to him or her.

A problem specific to a certain environment is brought before the group by one of the therapy group members. The client who presented the communication problem is asked to describe it in detail by giving examples of instances when it has occurred and the physical environment of each. As the physical environment is described, the audiologist or the client diagrams it on the chalkboard as accurately as possible. The room or other physical environment is drawn on the chalkboard (including windows, doors, partitions, furniture, and so on). The remainder of the group is then asked to give suggestions, as they see it, about how this client may have adjusted to that communication environment by manipulating it, making physical adjustments, or manipulating the speaker to, in their opinion, resolve the client's difficulty in that environment.

As those suggestions are made, the audiologist lists suggestions and makes the suggested adjustments on the chalkboard diagram, for example, (1) moving the client's chair into a better situation for listening, (2) changing position away from a window, (3) moving closer to a public address system speaker, (4) asking the person being conversed with to move closer, (5) walking out into a hallway where it is quieter, and so on.

The group participation in this treatment activity can be extremely motivating. As the client joins the group discussion by explaining the difficult environment more fully and as questions or assumptions are made, ways in which he or she may have been able to manipulate the listening environment or those within it to his or her benefit become more clear. Others in the group also benefit because most may have or may find themselves in a similar environment.

CREATING POSITIVE ASSERTIVENESS

A trait that appears to become more typical as some people grow older is to be less assertive or more passive. This is particularly true of older adults who have been placed in a health care facility, or who have moved from their home to a retirement complex, not of their own will, or who are trying to maintain their independence by remaining at home. Some may seem "stubborn," but those responses are generally out of self-defense, perhaps because they may not have heard or understood what was expected of them, or they suspect that they are being put-upon rather than being allowed to make indepndent decisions about their life. Then, in all too many instances, older persons

in health care facilities simply are not told what is going to be done to them. Rather than continuing to react against the health care facility personnel and, thus, being listed as "uncooperative," such patients generally become more passive.

Whether an older person is residing in a health care facility or in the community, it regrettably becomes more usual for dramatic and sometimes unpleasant things to occur in that person's life. In light of the unexpected occurrences that are prompted by people doing things *to* elderly persons rather than *for* them, it becomes easier to remain passive and wait rather than to become assertive and say "no," as force may be used to make one do it, anyway. "Dad is getting stubborn in his old age," may be the label placed on the older person. Many elderly persons feel powerless, because of a lack of independence. It is difficult to respond to a rapidly changing world when one does not possess the finances, transportation, physical mobility, quickness of analytical thought, or strength to manipulate one's environment.

Examples of Passive Behavior

One of this author's clients, a 78-year-old man, was asked to chair a committee in his church because of his knowledge of religion. He was flattered to be asked to accept that position, but then shortly resigned because he could not understand what his committee members were saying. When I asked him why he did not ask the members to speak up, he said that he did once. He further stated that it worked for a short time, but then they returned to their old speaking habits. When I asked him why he did not change the room arrangements so he could place himself in a more advantageous position for communication, he said that the room had been in that same arrangement for years, and he did not want to disrupt it. Those attitudes can defeat an otherwise potentially productive person.

Another example that illustrates the feelings of many older adults who have hearing impairment is one that involved a 72-year-old female client who had just returned from a lecture on Southeast Asia that she had been looking forward to attending for some time. She explained that the lecturer, a woman who had a rather soft voice, began talking and then walked away from the public address system microphone and sat down in front of the podium with the statement, "I'm sure that you can all hear me without the microphone."

The client said that she hardly understood a word the speaker said throughout the next hour, but she was too embarrassed to leave the auditorium. When I asked her why she did not say, "Please use the microphone," when the speaker moved away from it, her reply was that she just could not bring herself to do it. She wanted to, but was too embarrassed, "Besides," she said, "maybe I was the only person there who couldn't hear her." When I asked her if she was important enough to warrant that speaker's consideration, this client's response was simply, "I hope so." I said, "Don't you think that the microphone was put there for a purpose? A public address system generally helps everyone to hear more comfortably. If you would have said something, I am sure that others in the audience would have been pleased that she had returned to the podium and used the microphone." Her reply was that she had not thought of that. "But still," she said, "I didn't want to make a nuisance of myself. I'm just an old woman who can't hear very well."

Learning to Help Themselves

The attitude just described is one that must be altered, if possible, if persons are to learn to cope and function more efficiently in their communicative worlds. In light of the fact that some people are simply not willing to accommodate older persons who have hearing impairment or, perhaps, are not aware of what accommodations can be made to facilitate communication, older persons must be taught ways to become assertive enough to manipulate their communication environment and those with whom they desire to communicate.

Altering Passive Behaviors

As stated earlier, one way to alter passivity is by asking individual clients to describe difficult communication situations in which they have found themselves during the past week or month. The situation in which the 72-year-old woman found herself, as described previously, is a prime example of the problems that are brought to the treatment sessions. Suggestions by group members are brought forth after individual questions by the group members and the audiologist have been satisfied. When group members courageously state what **they** would have done in that situation (e.g., to have told the woman speaker that, "I would appreciate it if you would use the microphone") in front of the audience, they are asked if they really would have done it. If they hold fast to their commitment, they are asked to do it at the next lecture they attend when the speaker hesitates to use the microphone. Occasionally, a group member returns after such an experience and triumphantly proclaims, "I did it!" On occasion, another member of the aural rehabilitation treatment group may have been in attendance at that meeting and confirms that the individual did a very nice job in changing a poor listening situation to a more pleasant one. Also, others at the meeting may have thanked our client for asking the speaker to use the microphone by saying, "We just did not have the courage to speak up like that!" The triumph is great and does much toward encouraging the other clients to also become more assertive.

Other difficult situations brought before the groups may include family dinners, going to a noisy restaurant, talking to timid grandchildren, talking to one's attorney with other members of the family in attendance, following more than one request in a sequence, and many others. The bywords in these treatment sessions are, "If those with whom we desire to or must communicate do not seem to be accommodating, then we must **assert** ourselves by showing them how they can best communicate with us!" Suggestions or adjustments must be made without hesitation. To do otherwise is to "place ourselves back where we started." These are powerful treatment sessions that instill confidence in clients in whom it may not have existed for some time.

INVOLVEMENT OF FAMILY AND SIGNIFICANT OTHERS

The client's family and significant others in the client's life are critical elements for a successful aural rehabilitation treatment program. This is particularly true if a client's significant other is willing to become involved in the aural rehabilitation process. This includes attending individual or group treatment sessions and participating in follow-up assignments.

A significant other's involvement in the aural rehabilitation treatment process provides a person with a better understanding of the difficulties and frustrations with which the friend, spouse, or family member undergoing treatment is faced, particularly if he or she can attend the first sessions when discussions of hearing loss and difficult communication situations are emphasized. It further aids the client's significant other to understand the commonality of communication difficulties when other clients discuss similar problems. The involvement prompts a realization that the communication difficulties that have arisen because of the auditory deficit are not limited only to their spouse, family member, or friend, but are found in others as well. That enhanced understanding hopefully will be passed on to others who are close to the client.

This author frequently requests that those who attend the treatment sessions with individual clients be fit with noise suppressing ear plugs and participate in various activities during the sessions. Some of the same frustrations revealed by the clients are often felt by the significant others during that brief period of time. It is explained to them, however, that ear plugs do not replicate the speech recognition problems being encountered by the person with whom they are attending the sessions, but simply demonstrate a moderate loss of auditory acuity. Still, their use enhances a feeling of empathy for the frustrations the hearing-impaired person must feel.

One important byproduct of encouraging the involvement of a significant other in the aural rehabilitation treatment program is that carryover of the treatment process into the everyday life of a client can be greatly enhanced. If, for example, an elderly client asserts him- or herself before the remainder of the family by suggesting certain adjustments regarding seating arrangements for Thanksgiving dinner so that he or she can become involved in the conversation with greater efficiency, the significant other can reinforce and strengthen that positive step.

It is, further, not as much fun to go to a restaurant or the movie by oneself. The significant other can not only strengthen and encourage carryover, but also make some potentially apprehensive situations more enjoyable. It helps to have someone there to back you up when the going gets rough.

One of the most discouraging aspects of the provision of any rehabilitative service to elderly clients is the lack of family involvement. In many instances, if a spouse has passed away, the remainder of the family may live quite a distance from the client. Children may visit only once a year if the distance is great, and that may be for only a few days around a principal holiday. Even if grown children live in the same community, their desire for involvement with their parent on a social basis may be lacking, let alone a desire to become an important part of their mother's or father's rehabilitation program. The excuse is generally, "We just don't have time." In this remarkably advanced society, it is sad that we lose sight of the needs of

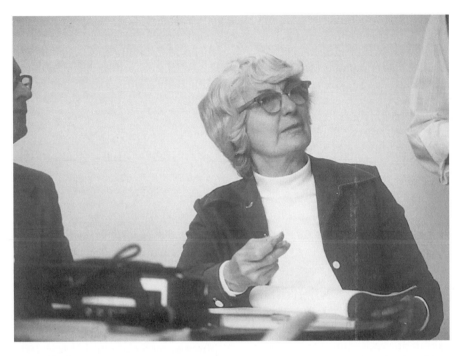

Figure 21–2. Assertiveness training sometimes brings out strengths in our adult clients that they did not know they possessed.

our family. But, it seems to be the case, and alternative means for carryover support for elderly clients must, in many cases, be sought.

As stated earlier, a client's spouse can be the most effective significant other, if the spouse is emotionally supportive of his or her husband or wife. If the spouse is not willing or capable of aiding in the support or carryover process, then a friend is appropriate and can be a most effective partner in the aural rehabilitation process. In fact, at times it is common for people to discuss feelings with supportive friends prior to bringing them before a spouse or other family members. In any event, a close friend can be a very significant other.

A case in point is that of a 70-year-old male client who was provided aural rehabilitation services by this author. He had been a widower for 4 years. On the first day of his group aural rehabili-

tation program, he brought a female companion. Both loved to fish and were almost inseparable. They both enjoyed attending social gatherings together, but my client was experiencing great difficulty hearing and, in particular, understanding what was being said in such environments. His female companion was willing to explain what was being said, but was becoming discouraged at the consistency with which she had to function in the capacity of interpreter.

In this instance, she attended all treatment sessions with the client, she wearing her ear plugs and he his hearing aid. A great deal of warmth and understanding developed between them and, as his ability to function communicatively increased, so did her willingness to aid in the treatment process through carryover. The assignments, which included experimentation at social gatherings, were carried out in an excellent manner. Problem situations that were to be discussed during treatment sessions lessened and, likewise, his dependence on his female companion for communicative support became less frequent.

The support and carryover by this significant other was instrumental in this client's achievements in learning to use his residual hearing, to use supplemental visual clues, and to manipulate his most difficult listening environments. Without such support and assistance, an audiologist may have great difficulty facilitating such improvements. In the end, he or she may never be able to aid the client in making such significant and positive strides as will the significant other.

THE PROCESS OF AURAL REHABILITATION

The aural rehabilitation program for an older adult client should include:

1. Knowledge of the client's desires and needs for communication through setting priorities;
2. Ongoing motivational counseling as an integral part of the process;
3. Carryover of hearing aid orientation, at least for those who are felt to benefit from amplification;
4. Learning how to manipulate one's environment to enhance communication;
5. Learning to become positively assertive;
6. Throughout everything listed, learning to use one's residual hearing and supplemental visual cues to enhance comprehension of verbal messages

To put all of this together into a meaningful aural rehabilitation treatment program for an older adult is not really difficult. As a matter of fact, the process becomes quite logical, once a number of older clients have critiqued your approach in relation to its meaningfulness and benefit to them.

The following is an example of an approach to aural rehabilitation treatment for elderly adult clients, employing and intermingling the six listed areas. This process has been found effective for use with both confined and community-based older adults.

THE ONGOING AURAL REHABILITATION PROGRAM

Reasons for Successful and Unsuccessful Treatment Programs

Some structure in the treatment process is desired by the majority of older clients. But, on the other hand, overly structured sessions can be counterproductive. For example, it is not uncommon for audiologists who utilize traditional speechreading (lipreading) approaches that emphasize a progression from phoneme analysis to syllables, words, phrases, sentences, and stories (which, for example, stress several like phonemes), to begin to realize in a fairly short time that the clients who seemed motivated initially are attending speechreading sessions with less regularity. Soon they may cease attending altogether. Excuses generally range from, "My family is coming to visit and I will be spending time with them," to "We have several church suppers coming up, and I have to help with them." It is embarrassing to see such persons downtown later with apparently nothing to do. They may, further, call to tell your secretary that they really do not feel the need to come to "class" anymore, even though the audiologist knows that they have made little or no progress in treatment.

Those clients are telling us something we *should* receive loudly and clearly. That is, if they felt that aural rehabilitation services were benefitting them they probably still would be attending, as they evidently were motivated when they began.

If the aural rehabilitation treatment program had been geared to their specific needs, they would probably be taking advantage of the audiologist's expert services. But, for those reasons, and because the audiologist perhaps began the first session from a book of strict unalterable approaches to speechreading, the clients were not interested in receiving those services anymore. A few faithful clients might continue to attend, but they probably will leave the final session as able or unable to communicate with others as he or she was in the beginning.

The audiologist may wonder why these otherwise apparently alert older persons have not improved, even though they may say, "I enjoyed your class," and pat him or her on the shoulder. Further, why does this audiologist have to coerce clients in health care facilities to attend aural rehabilitation treatment sessions or have to depend on a gracious activity director to bring them from their rooms to attend sessions that should be helping them cope in the everyday world more efficiently? Again, it may be because the audiologist has lost sight of the fact that the treatment must be designed with the needs of the clients in mind. Other treatment procedures used by speech-language pathologists, occupational therapists, physical therapists, and others are based on a *treatment plan* designed around the *assessed needs* of each client. Why, then, are some audiologists still opening their "lipreading" lesson book and beginning at page 1 to provide services to clients who have varied and individual communication deficits and needs? Those speechreading books too often are used as hymnals, and the session begins with the audiologist saying, "And for the next session we will turn to page 15." That is not treatment.

Individualizing the Approach

How does one develop a meaningful approach to aural rehabilitation treatment for the elder client? More than 20 years ago Hardick (1977) described basic characteristics of a successful aural rehabilitation program for older adults. They are well defined and provide comprehensive guidance for those who intend to provide services for older clients. Those characteristics are:

1. The program must be client-centered.
2. The program must revolve around amplification and/or modifying a client's communication environment.
3. All programs consist of group therapy, with some individualized help when necessary.
4. The group must contain normally hearing friends or relatives of the person who has hearing impairment.
5. Aural rehabilitation programs are short-term.
6. The program is consumer-oriented.
7. Promotion of a better realization by colleagues and other professionals of the existence of aural rehabilitation programs and their potential benefits.
8. Make use of "successful graduates" as resource people in group activities whenever possible. (pp. 60–62)

These characteristics are extremely important for consideration prior to the initiation of aural rehabilitation programs for an older adult. They go far beyond the more traditional "lipreading" procedures that continue to be employed by some. Even though Hardick (1977) and others recommended group treatment for the elderly, some will require individual sessions. As has been noted by this author, there is a tendency among some to hesitate or refuse to participate in individual treatment unless they, themselves, have requested it.

Other client-centered approaches to aural rehabilitation are discussed by Alpiner, (1963); Alpiner and McCarthy (1987), Colton (1977), Colton and O'Neill (1976), Giolas (1994), Hull (1982, 1992, 1997), McCarthy and Alpiner (1978), M. Miller and Ort (1965), O'Neill and Oyer (1981), Sanders (1982), Sanders (1993), and others. The aspect stressed by these authors is that older adult clients possess needs that are specific to them and each client's aural rehabilitation program must be centered on his or her needs and priorities.

If the ingredients presented on the previous pages are combined properly, a possible sequence of services emerges. An example of such a sequence is provided below.

Awareness of Reasons for Auditory Dysfunction

UNDERSTANDING HEARING LOSS. Facilitating an awareness of the reason for auditory communication difficulties through an understanding of the process of aging and its effect on the auditory mechanism is an important part of the aural rehabilitation process. Included is a discussion of the central processing of auditory/linguistic information and the effect of aging on the speed and precision of that important component in communication, particularly in noisy or otherwise distracting environments. The level of terminology is determined by the individual or group in question. The audiologist is cautioned *never* to speak down to clients. It is important to use the correct technical terminology, but immediately explain it at the level of the persons involved. Clinicians must always remember that the audience is adult, no matter what their educational level or age. They deserve to be treated as such.

Charts need to be used in such discussions, perhaps along with a 35-mm slide presentation on the ear. If individuals in the group are severely hard of hearing, projected slides should be used only if enough light can remain in the room to facilitate the use of visual clues. Charts, diagrams, slides, and chalkboard drawings are used for these discussions, including presentations on (1) the aging ear, (2) uses, benefits, and limitations of hearing aids, (3) environmental factors that affect communication, (4) poor speakers versus good speakers and their makeup; and (5) a general discussion of the aging process.

The basis for the first session (or sessions) is to facilitate a basis of understanding for the remainder of the treatment program, to develop a better understanding among the clients of what has occurred to them, and to assure them that in all probability they can improve, at least to some degree. Most persons leave such session or sessions with a better understanding and greater acceptance of what is occurring to them and a desire to participate in the aural rehabilitation treatment program.

It cannot be emphasized enough that a significant other in each client's life should attend these sessions. Whether it be a spouse or a family member such as a child or a friend, he or she will gain much greater insight into the auditory/communication problems with which the person is attempting to cope.

PRIORITIZED COMMUNICATIVE NEEDS. The second step in the aural rehabilitation treatment programs is, as stated earlier, to ask each client to list those difficulties in communication which most affect him or her. The Wichita State University Communication Appraisal and Priorities Profile (CAPP), as presented in Figure 21–3, can be used in this process. They may include specific communication environments, such as a meeting room, church, certain restaurant, table arrangement at their child's home, and so on. They also may list certain individuals who they have difficulty understanding.

The next step is for clients to set priorities for these situations or persons, from most important to least important, and, if they had their choice, in which of those would they most like to improve. They are asked, of course, to be realistic in their final choices. For some, the choice is a simple one. For others, it is more difficult. It is important to note, however, that if gains are made in one category, there is the probability that clients will observe improvement in others.

They are asked to discuss their choices, present a situation in which they had difficulty, and explain what prompted them to make those choices. Particularly in a group situation, it is interesting to note the general consistency of priority areas that emerge. The clients generally appreciate the camaraderie that develops out of this discussion. For the first time, many of them realize that they are

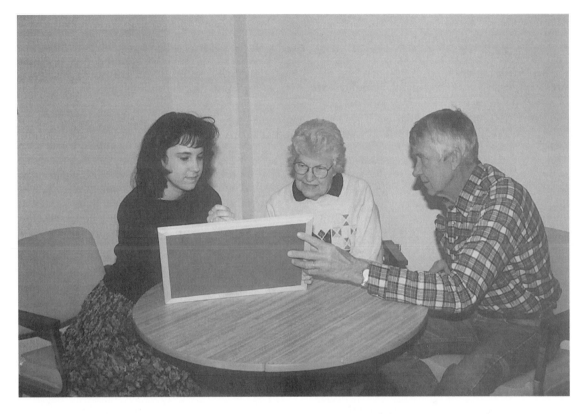

Figure 21–3. A spouse or other family members can add to the strength of aural rehabilitation services.

not the only ones who have difficulty in certain environments.

In many instances, clients put part of the blame for their auditory/communicative difficulties on others who display poor speech habits. That is acknowledged and discussed. The discussion centers on the fact that there are, indeed, many poor speakers in this world. A demonstration of some of the habits that interfere with efficient communication is appropriate. Clients generally immediately recognize poor speaking habits. Even though there are many poor speakers, persons with impaired hearing must develop ways to cope in those communication environments. The encouraging

acknowledgment that they can, in many instances, manipulate such difficult situations to function more efficiently in them, and that they will be working on those situations, ends the discussion on a positive note.

These items generally do not consume more than 1 or 2 full-hour sessions. The discussions of priority difficulties and circumstances that interfere with efficient communication should not be curtailed, however, because the airing of frustrations and concerns will greatly facilitate future progress. For many, this may be the first time those concerns have been discussed. To prematurely conclude such a discussion simply on the basis of a rigid schedule can stifle the airing of emotions and adjustment that may have otherwise not be made.

ON BECOMING ASSERTIVE. Weekly assignments for each client are made and include noting a communication situation in which they had particular difficulty that, in the end, interfered with communication. As discussed earlier, they write about situations and diagram the physical environment if necessary (or simply recall it as accurately as possible). In any event, clients are to bring the specifics of the situation to the next treatment session for presentation and discussion. Each client (or in the case of individual treatment, the client) presents his or her difficult situation, if one has been noted. It is imperative that the client who was involved in the situation be the one who presents it and not the significant other who may accompany the client.

After a thorough presentation, with diagrams if possible, the situation is discussed by the group (or in the event of individual treatment, by the client, the audiologist, and the accompanying significant other, if he or she was involved). Suggestions regarding possible ways the client might have manipulated the communication environment to his or her best advantage, including the physical environment or the speaker, are made by the group under the guidance of the audiologist and are accepted as viable or discarded.

As stated by this author previously (Hull, 1980), insights into ways of manipulating the communication environment to their best advantage, along with methods of coping with and adjusting to frustrating situations are, in turn, developed among clients under the guidance of the audiologist. This form of self- and group analysis is an extremely important part of the aural rehabilitation program. Clients, then, are helped to develop their own insights into methods of adjusting to situations where communication is difficult. If, for some reason, they find that it is impossible for them to make the necessary adjustments, perhaps they

can, in a positive-supportive-assertive manner, ease their difficulty by requesting that others make certain adjustments. Perhaps they could request that the physical environment be adjusted so that they can function more efficiently in it or they can make adjustments on their own.

It becomes difficult for some older clients to develop even mildly assertive behaviors. They do not want to be noticed as a "demanding" older person. Many do feel rather vulnerable, perhaps feeling that the people who invited them to a party did so more out of obligation than desire. They may feel that if they request those seeking conversation change positions by moving to a quieter place to talk, or request that someone change the position of his or her chair to be in a better position to talk then, perhaps, the hosts will feel that it is more trouble than it is worth to invite them again. In light of such fears, it becomes quite logical to avoid that possibility by simply remaining quiet and being fearful that if asked a question, he or she might be embarrassed by answering inappropriately. Those fears are occasionally brought forth by clients and should be discussed as they arise.

Examples of those discussions include one that was initiated by one of this author's clients who was being seen on a group basis. The woman in question was discussing a situation involving another woman with whom she had morning coffee on almost a daily basis for a number of years. The client's complaint was that her friend was an incessant gum chewer and as chewing continued as she talked, it interfered with precise articulation and two-way conversation. Her friend interpreted the client's inability to understand what she was saying to be the result of the hearing impairment, not her imprecise manner of speaking from her enthusiastic gum chewing, compounded by the client's hearing loss. This apparent interpretation of the situation infuriated my client. But, she continued the morning coffee time, because there were few other women her age in that geographic area and, besides, they had been friends since childhood.

This woman's major concern was how to tell her friend that her manner of speaking and gum chewing had, for several years, interfered with her ability to understand what she was saying and, in the end, made what might have been a pleasant conversation, a difficult one. She was particularly afraid to say anything because of the embarrassment her friend might feel because the situation had been going on for so long and nothing had previously been said. "Almost like," as the client said, "being associated with a person for a long time and never knowing her name. As the days pass, you become increasingly embarrassed about asking her name, particularly when she knows yours." The suggestions that came from the group varied from an enthusiastic, "Tell her that if she wants to talk to you, to take her gum out of her mouth!" to a timid, "If you value your friendship, maybe it is best to say nothing and simply tolerate the situation." The latter suggestion was discarded. The ultimate conclusion was to simply tell the truth.

It was the consensus of the group that they would respect their own friend more if he or she would say something like, "You know, we've been friends for a long time. You realize, as I do, that I have some difficulty hearing what people say to me. I have particular difficulty with men who wear mustaches or beards, people who do not move their lips enough, or people who talk with their hand near their mouth, as I depend upon seeing the face of persons with whom I am talking. You know, I have difficulty understanding what you say sometimes and I think that I may have discovered why. I know that you like to chew gum a great deal and, like me, it helps my mouth not to become so dry. I do think, however, that because you—probably not realizing it—chew your gum while we are talking, it doesn't allow me to see your lips move properly and, besides, you aren't able to talk as plainly when you chew it so hard. I just bet that if you don't chew gum while we are having our coffee, I will be able to understand you better and we'll have a nicer time talking. Do you want to give it a try?" *Positive assertiveness* are

the key words in this instance. For that client, the strategy she and the remainder of the group determined as most effective did prove to be successful. She maintained the friendship.

OTHER TOPICS TO FACILITATE COMMUNICATION. Other topics for discussion and for the development of communicative strategies may include (1) weekly socials at private homes where the furniture arrangements interfere with efficient communication. Some, as experienced through this author's work with older clients, involve (2) the table arrangement at one client's son's home where they usually had Thanksgiving dinner, (3) the television set at a male client's friend's home, (4) the seating arrangement and acoustics at a church meeting room, and others. Even though the discussions and thought-provoking suggestions generally aid the individual whose situation is being discussed, they also provide insights for the remainder of the group on how they, too, may be able to manipulate similar communicative environments.

These assertiveness discussions can be extremely stimulating for the involved clients and for their significant other in attendance. Clients have told this author that those sessions are probably the most valuable for them, particularly because we are working and sharing on behalf of their problems in communication. As clients identify with other clients' difficult communication situations and relate to solutions as they see them, insights into solutions for their own difficult situations emerge and are strengthened.

Self-confidence reawakens when clients return to state that the solution contrived during the last session did not work as planned, but with a few adjustments developed by him- or herself, it did. Most older clients, no matter the level of hearing impairment or how distraught they may be as a result of their inability to communicate, can benefit from these assertiveness sessions. The topics of **self-worth** and, **"I'm important too"** that become a part of the discussions are an extremely important part of the total aural rehabilitation program.

The WSU Communication
Appraisal and Priorities Profile

Date_____

Name_____ Age_____ Sex____

Address_____ Phone_____

Please indicate below those situations in which you are able to communicate best, those that are difficult for you in some instances, and those that are a definite problem. Under "explain," please tell us more if you desire, such as certain instances when you experience more difficulty than others, certain types of speakers, certain places, and so on.

	No problems	Only in specific instances	Definite problem	Priority
1. At parties or other social events	____	____	____	____

Explain_____

_____

2. At the dinner table	____	____	____	____

Explain_____

_____

3. On the telephone	____	____	____	____

Explain_____

_____

4. At home	____	____	____	____

Explain_____

_____

5. With males	____	____	____	____

Explain_____

_____

6. With females	____	____	____	____

Explain_____

_____

7. With children	____	____	____	____

Explain_____

_____

8. In groups	____	____	____	____

Explain_____

_____

(continued)

Figure 21–4. The Wichita State University Communication Appraisal and Priorities Profile (CAPP). (See Appendix J for the profile in its entirety.)

Figure 21–4. *(continued)*

	No problems	Only in specific instances	Definite problem	Priority
9. With certain important individuals	____	____	____	____
Explain_____				
_____				
10. At Church	____	____	____	____
Explain_____				
_____				
11. At meetings	____	____	____	____
Explain_____				
_____				
12. Watching TV	____	____	____	____
Explain_____				
_____				
13. At the theater	____	____	____	____
Explain_____				
_____				
14. At work	____	____	____	____
Explain_____				
_____				
15. Other (please specify)	____	____	____	____
Explain_____				
_____				

Do you have specific preferences in regard to things you would like to improve as they relate to your abiity to communicate with others?_____
_____

USE OF RESIDUAL HEARING WITH SUPPLEMENTAL VISUAL CLUES

Even though the use of visual clues and every possible bit of residual hearing individual clients can muster is discussed and practiced throughout all aspects of the aural rehabilitation program, sessions should also emphasize those aspects of communication. Again, it is suggested that strict approaches to speechreading/auditory training not be emphasized. Rather, the fact that the majority of older clients possess normal to near-normal language function should be capitalized on to encourage the use of in-novative and useful approaches toward increased efficiency in the use of a very natural complement to communication, that is, the complement of vision to audition.

The premise on which these sessions are based is that speech (including the phonemic patterns of words in the English language, the use of gestures, inflectional clues, and the English language, itself) is generally quite predictable, although, understandably, there are differences among individual's speech patterns, use of gestures, words, and so on. A further premise is that the average listener has been taking advantage of the redundancies inherent in American English speech and language patterns to aid in verbal comprehension for the majority of his or her life. When hearing declines with age, along with the precision and speed of the processing of phonemic verbal/linguistic elements of speech, it becomes more difficult to comprehend (understand) what others are saying. This is particularly true in environmentally distracting or otherwise difficult listening situations.

The purpose of these sessions, therefore, is to remind clients of what they have been doing for years at an almost subliminal level—that is, using important parts of auditory/verbal messages, when heard, and supplementing what was not heard with visual clues. By visual clues, this author means the face of the speaker, including lip, tongue, and mandibular movements, gestures, facial expression, shoulder movements, and so on used to "fill in the gaps" between what was heard, what was not heard, and what was observed visually.

A further purpose of these sessions is to discuss the redundancies of the phonemic and linguistic aspects of spoken American English and to encourage clients to take advantage of them when they are communicating with others. This aspect of the aural rehabilitation treatment program is called, for lack of a better descriptive title, "A Linguistic Approach to the Teaching of Speechreading" described by this author (Hull, 1976). It essentially depends on clients possessing normal language function. Further, a great deal of time is spent using the chalkboard. If, however, a client has visual impairment, these sessions help to enhance auditory closure. The term "closure" is the byword during these sessions, as the reader soon will realize.

Linguistic Closure

As the reader will observe in this section, clients are asked to determine the correct information within sentences from the least number of words provided. Clients are asked to imagine that the word or words written on the chalkboard are those that were heard. Blanks are placed between words, representing those not heard or not heard well. Clients are, first of all, asked to tell the audiologist what the sentence is about (out of context), when, perhaps, only 1 word is provided out of a total of 7, with 6 blanks indicating that those words were not heard.

Clients are encouraged to venture guesses as to what the sentence might be. Let us say, for example, that the word presented is "street," located as the last word in the sentence. The clients are asked to let their minds wander. "Take a guess." As clients accept that encouragement and begin to guess, the fear of being wrong appears to decrease. Many are genuinely surprised, in fact, to find that their "educated" guesses are often extremely close, if not correct. Guesses in this instance may, for example, range from "the man was walking down the street," to "a horse was seen running up the street." They are, however, encouraged to be rational in their decisions. The question may appropriately be asked, "How many times have you heard someone say, 'A giraffe was running up the street'?" The clinician continues, "Think more realistically about the possibilities. The word, 'street' as the last word in a sentence tells you what? It tells you, generally, that *something* is happening. If the word came as the second word in a sentence, maybe after the word 'the,' I may have been describing the street, such as, 'the street was very bumpy.' But, as it is located at the end of the sentence, we know that something is probably happening either on or to the street.

"Now, let's set the stage. Let us say that your neighbor's child, Billy, has run away. You and other people from around the neighborhood are searching for him. Suddenly, someone runs to you and says something about, "____ ____ ____ ____ ____ street!" You observed that the speaker had obviously been running, and was pointing up the street as he was talking. Now, what do you imagine the speaker was telling you?" As the audiologist has now set the stage for the clients, their guesses will probably be quite close to what he or she had intended.

The audiologist's next step is to say, **"Now I am going to allow you to fill in the gaps by observing my face and gestures as I take the place of the excited neighbor who is talking to you."** The audiologist then presents the sentence in a slightly audible manner and with full visible face and gestures. If clients are not able to "make closure," then another word is added to the chalkboard, and the clients are allowed to try again. An example of the sequence of presentation, if additional words are required, is presented below.

1. ____ ____ ____ ____ ____ ____ street!
2. ____ ____ is ____ ____ ____street!
3. ____ ____ is ____ down ____ street!
4. ____ ____ is running down ____ street!
5. ____ is running down ____ street!
6. ____ is running down the street!
7. A horse is running down the street!

As clients become aware of what the message is, the audiologist continues by discussing **(1)** the importance of the position of each word within the sentence that was required before they were able to determine its content, **(2)** their linguistic value in terms of the probability of situations in the meaning of the sentence, **(3)** the importance of the environmental clues that were available to them, and **(4)** the supplemental use of visual clues.

An important element involved in any of these sessions is the audiologist's enthusiasm for the fact that, perhaps, the clients needed only to "hear" one or two words out of a sentence to make closure and grasp the meaning of the sentence. It is encouraging for older clients to understand that, with their knowledge of the English language and their successful use of visual and auditory clues, they were able to determine what a message was.

On more difficult sentences and more complex contrived situations, clients may require more "heard" words to be provided via the chalkboard. Nevertheless, they are being reminded that with a relatively small amount of visual, auditory, and environmental information, they are generally able to determine, at least, the thought of what is being said.

LINGUISTIC, CONTENT, AND ENVIRONMENTAL REDUNDANCIES

Linguistic Redundancies

The American English language is redundant in its formal usage in relation to the position of various parts of speech. In other words, the positions of principal words, such as nouns, pronouns, and direct objects, are generally constant, as are function words, descripters such as adjectives and adverbs, and action words such as verbs. Some dialects within the United States do, however, deviate from those standard rules. During these sessions, although the technical names of the parts of speech are not stressed, the importance of those words that fall within various positions in verbal messages are discussed as they relate to deriving the meaning of those messages.

This aspect of treatment capitalizes on the fact that most older clients who have hearing impairment will possess at least near-normal language function. It stresses that as people listen to others, they zero in on words within conversations that permit them to at least derive the thought of what is being said, so that the conversation can be followed. In some distracting environments, less of the message may actually be heard, but most persons can still maintain the content or intent of what is being said. It is normal in those circumstances to ask a speaker to repeat a word, if one was missed, because it appeared to be an important one regarding the content of the statement.

The point that is stressed to the clients is that the reason a listener was able to determine that the word was an important one in following the conversation is that most listeners have an almost innate knowledge of the structure of the American English language that has progressively expanded since early childhood. This provides the listener with a distinct advantage even in light of a loss of hearing.

The treatment sessions that stress this important aspect of efficient listening revolve around bringing that functional language capability to a more conscious level. Occasionally, clients have become so despondent over an inability to communicate with others that such otherwise natural compensatory skills have become repressed.

Content and Environmental Redundancies

These discussions stress that, as we observe human behavior, it is discovered that not only do the same

people generally say similar things on similar occasions, but they also say them in similar places. In other words, in a given environment, depending on who the person is with whom one will be speaking, what the listener knows about him or her and if the listener is aware of those influences, the general content of some conversations can be predicted with reasonable accuracy.

Clients are asked to describe the environments they frequent. In all probability they will be those that were set as priorities earlier. They are also asked to describe those persons who are generally there, including their speaking habits, their facial characteristics, and their known interests. During these treatment sessions, the clients also are asked to write down the most frequent topics of conversations that are observed among those whom they have described. These not only include frequent topics, but also words and phrases that those people may use habitually. They are asked to keep those lists and add to them as they remember additional items or as they find out more about the person after speaking with him or her. Clients also are asked to begin new lists as they meet new people. The more one knows and remembers about a person, the more communication is enhanced.

An awareness of the predictability, or redundancy, of people and what they will say within known environments is sometimes surprising to older adults who have hearing impairment. If it is surprising, it is generally because they had not really thought about it prior to that time. If nurtured, however, this awareness can facilitate increased efficiency in communication.

REDUCING AUDITORY OR VISUAL CONFUSIONS

Other activities that, by necessity, are important for adults may include information on why certain confusions of words occur in conversations. This particularly concerns older adults, because word confusions may be occurring with some frequency. These discussions not only include information that the nature of the majority of auditory disorders that older adults face enhances the probability of auditory confusions, but also that the nature of certain sound and visual elements within many words enhances the probability of confusions because they either sound like or look like other words. When words are confused with others, the meaning of a sentence or conversation may appear to be different than what was intended. Words used as examples to illustrate words that are homophenous (visually similar) and potentially confusing include, for example:

1. found-vowed
2. purred-bird
3. head-hen
4. vine-fried
5. geese-keys
6. neck-deck

An example of an activity that can bring about an awareness of how these confusions can occur is based on typed lists of sentences or sentences written on the chalkboard. It is generally best to use those sentences that contain visually and/or auditorily confusing words within mock conversations to exemplify most accurately the clients' real-world difficulties. In this instance, the first sentence on the clients' list may be presented by the audiologist within a short "conversation." The conversation is presented with voice, but as close to the clients' auditory thresholds as possible. Full-face observations and gestures are used.

When the sentence within the "conversation" is presented, the clients are asked to determine if the sentence the audiologist said was "the same as" or "different" from the one on their list. If they determine that there was a word or words that were different than observed in the sentence on their list, then they are asked to explain why they felt that there were differences. On the other hand, if they felt that the sentence presented by the audiol-

ogist was the same as the one on their sheet or on the chalkboard, they also are asked to explain why.

If, in the context of the short conversation the clients determine what word or words in that sentence "threw them off course," they not only are asked to analyze those confusing words, but attempt to determine why they were confusing. They also are asked, in light of what they derived from the remainder of the conversation, to determine the words (or the thought) that the sentence should have contained so that it makes sense. When that analysis is completed, the clients again are asked to listen to and observe the conversation and the possibly confusing sentence to determine if it then appears to be what they thought it should have been within the context of the intended message. If the word or words within the sentence still do not appear to be what they should have been to complete the thought of the conversation, then they again are asked to attempt to determine what the confusion was.

An example of the type of brief conversation and stimulus sentence used in this exercise is:

1. **Stimulus sentence:** *She bought a new coat.*
2. **Stimulus conversation:** "Alice came over yesterday to see me, and had some news to share. She said that she now has a new friend who is soft, black and white, and weighs about 1 pound. Well, she bought a new coat. She named him Mike."

In this stimulus conversation, the possible visual confusion occurs with the word coat, which was given to the clients within the stimulus sentence they were expecting as per their list of sentences. Again, if clients, in this instance, determine that the word in the sentence they were expecting did not make sense within the context of the conversation, they are asked to explain why that word seemed to be misplaced, and what the word should have been. Further, the visual and auditory similarities and differences between the word they were expecting and the one they saw and heard are discussed.

These exercises should progress toward truly homophenous (visually similar) and homophonous (acoustically similar) words within sentences. The "mental gymnastics" required during these sessions allows for practice in making on-the-spot decisions regarding misunderstood messages by determining why a sentence within a conversation was visually and/or auditorily confusing, or otherwise did not make sense. The process generally involves:

1. Analyzing the information derived from the previous portions of a conversation;
2. Determining that a confusing word has been received that may change the content of what is being said;
3. Sifting mentally through other words that look and/or sound like one that would make more sense in light of the previous portions of the conversations;
4. Simultaneously projecting what that word "should have been" from the ongoing conversation.

COMMUNICATING UNDER ADVERSE CONDITIONS

One of the most frequent communication problems that older adult clients view as their most difficult is communication in noisy environments including social events and meetings. Many clients' primary complaint, after finding themselves in an adverse listening environment, is that the noise and the resulting difficulties they experience in attempting to sort out the primary message from the chatter of other voices makes them tense and nervous. They describe the nervousness as, perhaps, the greatest detriment to their ability to manage a conversation successfully in those environments. They tell this author that as they begin

to experience difficulty within a noisy communicative environment, they begin to feel nervous. The nervousness, as they describe it, results in a further deterioration of their ability to cope in that environment and, thus, their ability to sort the primary message from the noise.

For many, the only alternative that appears to be available is to excuse themselves from the situation by ceasing the conversation. By submitting to that less-than-satisfactory option, however, they generally feel some embarrassment. Unless they are quite resilient, many will simply avoid those situations in which they consistently fail. Because situations include social events, meetings, the theater, church, and other desirable environments, the decision to avoid them can be self-defeating. The torment of those with hearing impairment may continue, as they still want to function communicatively in those environments and are torn between making another attempt at coping or giving up altogether.

In an attempt to ease such communication problems, treatment sessions need not only be designed to aid clients in the development of skills for communicating in those distracting environments, but also to develop coping strategies. The terms "desensitization," "reciprocal inhibition," and others may be appropriate to use here, but "coping behaviors" stand as the most meaningful for this discussion.

Within this framework, clients again choose as priorities those environments in which they have most difficulty and/or those within which they most desire to function with greater efficiently. Those situations are recreated within the treatment room as accurately as possible, based on individual clients' description of their chosen difficult environments. It is stressed that in the treatment environment, no one can fail but can feel free to discuss his or her concerns or frustrations as they arise. Use of the language-based speechreading instruction previously discussed is further emphasized during these sessions. The areas stressed in the dis-

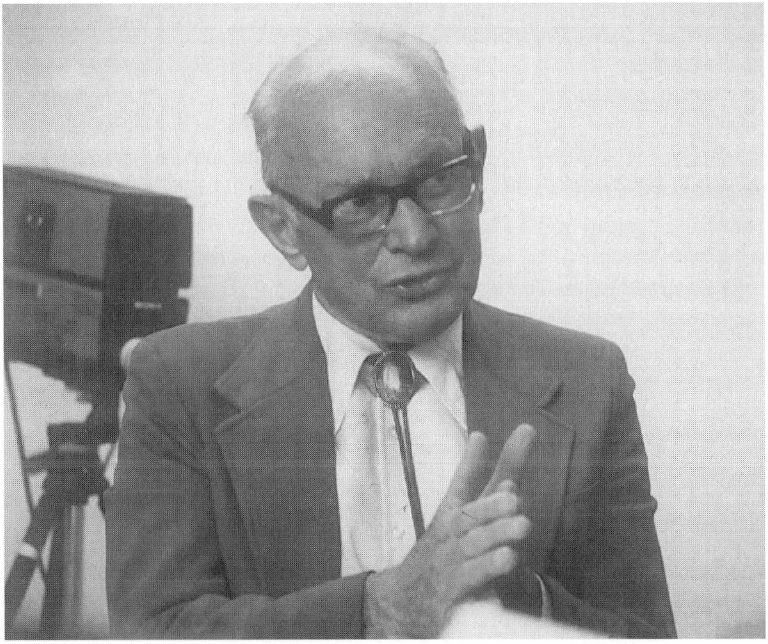

Figure 21–5. Problem-solving of difficult listening situations provides tangible rewards.

cussions during these noise exercises, but not in order of importance, are outlined in Table 21–1.

These sessions are used as the culminating treatment experience. Clients are asked to take everything that they have gained from the previous sessions and put them to use here. Some may never learn to cope in environmentally distracting situations. Others develop such self-confidence that they feel more comfortable in the most adverse environments.

One aspect of coping is stressed. That is that few persons, whether they possess normally functioning auditory mechanisms or have hearing impairment, can tolerate every noise environment. They must learn to recognize their limits in attempting to develop coping behaviors.

Introducing Noise Into the Treatment Environment

As each client's difficult communication environment is recreated by the audiologist and other members of the treatment group, taped noise that is the same as or similar to the environment the client(s) described is introduced into the room. It is best to use a stereophonic tape system to recreate the noise environment most accurately. The noise is introduced gradually at the beginning of these sessions and increased as tolerance and coping behavior likewise increase, until the noise is presented at such a level as to become difficult to tolerate. If clients wear hearing aids, they also are asked to experiment with them as they participate in the mock noisy communication environments.

TABLE 21–1. Responses Stressed During Auditory Treatment Sessions.

- Relaxation under stressful conditions.

- Confidence that clients can, indeed, piece together the thought of the verbal message, even though not all of it was heard.

- Remembering that, because of their normal language function and their knowledge of the predictability of American English, they can determine what is being said, if supplemental visual cues are used, along with as much auditory information as is possible under the environmental circumstance.

- Knowledge that other people in the same environment may also be having difficulty understanding what others are saying and that they also may or may not be coping successfully with the stress.

- Freedom to manipulate the communication environment as much as possible by, for example, asking the person with whom they are speaking to move with them to a slightly quieter corner where they can talk with greater ease or move his or her chair to a more advantageous position so the speaker can be seen and/or heard more clearly, or other positive steps to enhance communication.

- Remembering that, if difficulty in a communication environment seems to be increasing, and feelings of concern or nervousness begin to become evident, they should feel free to interrupt the conversation and talk about the noise or the activity around them that seems to be causing the difficulties. The other person will probably agree with that observation and, in talking about it, feelings of stress may be reduced and communication may be enhanced.

- Remembering that the amount of example noise used in treatment sessions is probably greater than will be experienced in most other environments. If success was noted in their treatment sessions, then similar success may be carried over into other stressful environments.

The clients are told that the situation during treatment is going to be made more difficult in regard to noise levels and/or visual distractions than they will probably experience in the "real world." Clients inevitably desire such an approach, as they would rather practice in such difficult situations in the friendly environment of the treatment room than among less tolerant people.

Discussions of Adverse Listening Environments

Discussions of noise per se and its natural effect on speech perception are introduced before the actual re-creations begin. An awareness of different types of noise, the general acoustical characteristics, emotional impact, and other factors give clients a better understanding of the "situation" as they see it. When one begins to gain an understanding of feared elements, the fear generally subsides.

Almost without fail, some persons begin to become nervous and frustrated during the noise sessions. The susceptibility of certain clients to an intolerance for noise can be observed by an alert audiologist, even when low levels of noise are introduced.

If the group (or individuals) begin to become obviously frustrated, the audiologist, rather than ceasing the activity immediately, terminates it momentarily at a logical point and begins to discuss general feelings about the noise rather than attempting to pinpoint individual personal feelings about it. The audiologist might appropriately say, "Noise makes me feel nervous. How about you? Sometimes during these sessions I want to turn it off. When I'm in a situation where I can't turn it off, it even makes me angry sometimes. Is that a little like the feelings you have when you find yourself in a situation like that?" Generally the response will be affirmative and clients will agree that those feelings are real for them, also.

The time-out periods are used to talk about feelings about noise. When feelings of frustration and even anger are expressed freely among clients, the reality that those feelings are not uncommon among others occasionally brings relief to those who, perhaps, thought that they were among only a few older adults who had such difficult time. These persons are, thus, learning to cope with their feelings and realizing that they are normal reactions to adverse and frustrating communication environments.

Discussing those feelings freely, without fear of negative responses from others, is an important part of the aural rehabilitation process. As frustrations and anger are expressed regarding their difficulties tolerating and communicating in a noisy world—and occasionally at the whole process of growing older—the way opens for the aural rehabilitation program to move forward toward the development of coping behaviors and techniques for manipulating their communication environments as positive, assertive attributes. As one of this author's clients has so aptly stated, "In a noisy world of generally poor speakers, we usually have to fend for ourselves. But, we are looking to you to teach us how, and to give inspiration to use what we learn."

OTHER APPROACHES TO AURAL REHABILITATION TREATMENT

Other components of effective aural rehabilitation sessions, as utilized by this author (Hull, 1980, 1989, 1992, 1997) involve the following elements.

The Use of Time-Compressed Speech

In light of the probability of a slowing of the speed of central nervous system processing of auditory-linguistic information with advancing age (Madden, 1985; Marshall, 1981; Schmitt & McCroskey, 1981; Stach 1990; Welsh et al., 1985; and others), the use of time compression of speech has been found by this author to be a method through which clients can learn to compensate to

some degree for that decline. Some older clients can increase their ability to comprehend speech with speed and precision that is greater than they had before the training.

Clients practice by listening to progressively time-compressed sentences and paragraphs, attempting over an 8- to 10-week sequence of sessions to increase the speed with which they are able to synthesize and make auditory/linguistic closure. Some clients have increased their accuracy of speech comprehension for sentences and paragraphs up to 40% at time-compression levels of 35% (65% of the message received over time). These same older clients have been found to correspondingly increase their accuracy of auditory-only speech recognition by as much as 24% (Hull, 1988).

This is a very exciting and tangible method for enhancing the speed and accuracy of speech comprehension among individual clients who can tolerate the demands of the process. Usable aided or unaided hearing is a prerequisite, however, because this is an auditory-only task.

Interactive Laser-Video Training in Speed and Accuracy of Visual Synthesis and Closure

Interactive laser video technology recently has evolved for use in training Olympic athletes, Air Force fighter pilots, and radar observers to increase their speed and accuracy in visual closure, tracking, and synthesis. This technology also has been found by this author to be an effective and motivational way of training adults who have hearing impairment to increase their visual compensatory skills, particularly as it relates to speed, accuracy, and visual vigilance (Hull, 1989).

Environmental Design

Hull (1989) described avenues for the training of older clients who have hearing impairment in techniques and strategies of environmental design. This involves modifying the acoustical/environmental design of their homes, offices and other communicative environments to their listening/communicative advantage. Training also involves how to make modifications in those and other situations in which they find themselves, including social environments, meetings, and business environments that otherwise may have placed them at a communicative disadvantage. These can be very powerful aural rehabilitation sessions that provide clients with tangible methods for modifying their most difficult communication situations.

SUMMARY

It is important for older clients to be given the opportunity to make decisions regarding areas of communication in which they desire to improve. Even though many may feel discouraged because of the embarrassing difficulties they experience in their attempts at understanding what others are saying, they have communicative priorities that must be addressed through their aural rehabilitation programs.

As adults who probably possessed normal hearing during the majority of their life and whose case histories may reveal nothing more than that they have become older, they deserve to participate in the decisions regarding their treatment program. However, guidance must be provided by the audiologist.

REFERENCES

Alpiner, J. G. (1963). Audiological problems of the aged. *Geriatrics, 18*, 19–26.

Alpiner, J., & McCarthy, P. (Eds.). (1987). *Rehabilitative audiology: Children and adults* (Vol. 3.) Baltimore: Williams & Wilkins.

Bergman, M. (1980). *Aging and the perception of speech.* Baltimore: University Park Press.

Colton, J. (1977). Student participation in aural rehabilitation programs. *Journal of the Academy of Rehabilitative Audiology, 10*, 31–35.

Colton, J., & O'Neill, J. (1976). A cooperative outreach program for the elderly. *Journal of the Academy of Rehabilitative Audiology, 9*, 38–41.

Downs, M. (1970). *You and your hearing aid.* Unpublished manual. Denver: University of Colorado Medical Center, Department of Otolaryngology, Division of Audiology.

Giolas, T. G. (1994). Aural rehabilitation of adults with hearing impairment. In J. Katz (Ed.), *Handbook of clinical audiology* (pp. 776–792). Baltimore: Williams and Wilkins.

Hardick, E. J. (1977). Aural rehabilitation programs for the aged can be successful. *Journal of the Academy of Rehabilitative Audiology, 10*, 51–66.

Hull, R. H. (1976). A linguistic approach to the teaching of speechreading: theoretical and practical concepts. *Journal of the Academy of Rehabilitative Audiology, 9*, 14–19.

Hull, R. H. (1980). Aural rehabilitation for the elderly. In R. L. Schow & M. A. Nerbonne (Eds.), *Introduction to aural rehabilitation* (pp. 311–348). Baltimore: University Park Press.

Hull, R. H. (1982). *Rehabilitative audiology.* New York: Grune & Stratton.

Hull, R. H. (1988). *Hearing in aging.* Presentation before the national invitational conference on Geriatric Rehabilitation. Department of Health and Human Services, PHS, Washington, DC.

Hull, R. H. (1989, November). *The use of interactive laser/video technology for training in visual synthesis and closure with hearing impaired elderly clients.* Presentation before the annual convention of the American Speech-Language-Hearing Association, St. Louis, MO.

Hull, R. H. (1992). Techniques for aural rehabilitation with elderly clients. In R. H. Hull (Ed.), *Aural rehabilitation* (pp. 278–292). San Diego: Singular Publishing Group.

Hull, R. H. (1997). Techniques for aural rehabilitation treatment for older adults who are hearing impaired. *Aural rehabilitation: Serving children and adults* (pp. 367–393). San Diego: Singular Publishing Group.

Jerger, J., & Chmiel, R. (1997). Factor analytic structure of auditory impairment in elderly persons. *Journal of the American Academy of Audiology, 7*, 269–276.

Kasten, R. N. (1981). The impact of aging on auditory perception. In R. H. Hull (Ed.), *The communicatively disordered elderly* (pp. 33–51). New York: Thieme-Stratton.

Madden, D. (1985). Age-related slowing in the retrieval of information from long-term memory. *Journal of Gerontology, 40,* 208–210.

Marshall, L. (1981). Auditory processing in aging listeners. *Journal of Speech and Hearing Disorders, 46,* 226–240.

McCarthy, P. A., & Alpiner, J. G. (1978). The remediation process. In J. G. Alpiner (Ed.), *Handbook of adult rehabilitative audiology* (pp. 88–111). Baltimore: Williams and Wilkins.

McCroskey, R. L., & Kasten, R. N. (1981). Assessment of central auditory processing. In R. Rupp & K. Stockdell (Eds.), *Speech protocols in audiology* (pp. 121–132). New York: Grune & Stratton.

McLauchlin, R. (1992). Hearing aid orientation for hearing impaired adults. In R. H. Hull (Ed.), *Aural rehabilitation* (pp. 178–201). San Diego: Singular Publishing Group.

Miller, W. E. (1976, November). *An investigation of the effectiveness of aural rehabilitation for nursing home residents.* Paper presented at the annual Convention of the American Speech and Hearing Association, Houston, TX.

Miller, M., & Ort, R. (1965). Hearing problems in a home for the aged. *Acta Oto-Laryngologica, 59,* 33–44.

O'Neill, J. J., & Oyer, H. J. (1981). *Visual communication for the hard of hearing.* Englewood Cliffs, NJ: Prentice-Hall.

Sanders, D. A. (1982). *Aural rehabilitation.* Englewood Cliffs, NJ: Prentice-Hall.

Sanders, D. A. (1993). *Management of hearing handicap.* Englewood Cliffs, NJ: Prentice-Hall.

Schmitt, J. F., & McCroskey, R. L. (1981). Sentence comprehension in elderly listeners: The factor rate. *Journal of Gerontology, 36,* 441–445.

Smith, C. R., & Fay, T. H. (1977). A program of auditory rehabilitation for aged persons in a chronic disease hospital. *Journal of the American Speech and Hearing Association, 19,* 417–420.

Stach, B. A. (1990). Central auditory processing disorders and amplification applications. *Research symposium: Communication sciences and disorders and aging—ASHA Reports Series, 19,* 150–156.

Traynor, R., & Peterson, K. (1972). *Adjusting to your new hearing aid.* Unpublished manual, Greeley, CO.

Welsh, J., Welsh, L., & Healy, M. (1985). Central presbycusis. *Laryngoscope, 95,* 128–136.

END OF CHAPTER EXAMINATION QUESTIONS

CHAPTER 21

1. The author describes two circumstances in which individual treatment sessions would be appropriate for adult clients. What are they?

    a.

    b.

2. Some older adults begin to exhibit passive behaviors in communication situations in which one would expect them to "take charge" of the environment or person causing the problem. Why may passivity begin to take the place of positive assertiveness among older persons who are hearing-impaired?

3. Describe the role of a "significant other" in the aural rehabilitation process.

4. List and describe the six components of aural rehabilitation services for adult clients as described in this chapter.

    a.

    b.

    c.

    d.

    e.

    f.

5. Briefly explain the process that seeks to help a client be less passive and more assertive in making positive change in difficult listening environments.

6. The author describes reasons why some approaches to aural rehabilitation work and why others do not. Briefly describe those reasons.

END OF CHAPTER ANSWER SHEET

Name _____ Date _____

CHAPTER 21

1. a. _____

    b. _____

2. _____

    _____

    _____

    _____ .

3. _____

    _____

    _____

    _____ .

4. a. _____

    b. _____

    c. _____

    d. _____

    e. _____

    f. _____

5. _____

_____

_____

_____

_____ .

6. _____

_____

_____

_____

_____

_____ .

7. Which one(s)?   a   b   c   d

8. Which one(s)?   a   b   c   d

9. Which one(s)?   a   b   c   d   e

10. _____

_____ .

7. To improve a client's communicative environ-
    ment, the audiologist might suggest:
    a. that the client move closer to the speaker;
    b. that the client move away from a window
       that may be casting shadows on the speak-
       er's face;
    c. that the client move to a quieter place,
       where communication can take place;
    d. all of the above.

8. Individualizing an aural rehabilitation treat-
    ment program for a client involves
    a. focusing on the family's concerns
    b. group therapy
    c. a long-term AR program
    d. focusing, first, on the client's communica-
       tion concerns and priorities.

9. "Counseling" involves:
    a. listening;
    b. building the client's confidence in him/
       herself;
    c. all members of the family;
    d. giving the client current information about
       hearing loss and hearing aids;
    e. all of the above.

10. What is the complement of vision to audition?

Special Considerations in Aural Rehabilitation for Older Adults in Health Care Facilities

■ RAYMOND H. HULL, Ph.D. ■

ESTABLISHING AURAL REHABILITATION PROGRAMS IN HEALTH CARE FACILITIES
    Addressing the Need of Health Care Facility Residents
    Developing Realistic Expectations
    Determining the Need for Services

THE ONGOING AURAL REHABILITATION PROGRAM
    In-Service Training for Health Care Facility Personnel and
        Families of the Residents
    Provisions of Aural Rehabilitation Treatment Services in
        the Health Care Facility

SUMMARY

THE POPULATION OF CONFINED OLDER ADULTS IN THE U.S.

Approximately 6% of all persons beyond age 65 years reside in various levels of health care facilities (Ignatavicius & Bayne, 1995). Of the some 34 million persons over age 65 years, that percentage represents more than 2 million persons (Health Care Financing Administration, 1998). According to Bayles and Kaszniak (1987), placement rates for the young-old persons aged 65–74 have fallen, especially for older men. But, among persons aged 75–84, these rates have increased, particularly for women. Older women who are most likely to be placed in a health care facility are poor, widowed, living alone, and very old. In 1972, Atchley reported that over 14% of persons age 85 or over were institutionalized. Of those, most were placed in nursing homes or other personal care facilities. On the other hand, in 1987, Stone, Cafferata, and Sangl reported that 21% of

persons age 85 years and beyond were recipients of specialized care either in nursing homes, by home health care agencies, or by family. In 1996, the Administration on Aging placed the number of persons over age 70 years who were residing in nursing homes at more than 2 million. As persons continue to live to greater ages, the number who will require special care environments will continue to grow.

In 1996, more than 20% of older persons were limited in their activity because of chronic health conditions, that is, 14% for persons age 65–74 years, 26% for persons 75–84 years, and 48% for those beyond age 85 years (Administration on Aging, 1996). Further, about 92% of older persons wear glasses and approximately 50%–60% have hearing impairment to a sufficient degree to interfere with their activities of daily living (Administration on Aging, 1996; Hull, 1997). According to Hull (1993), approximately 92% of persons residing in health care facilities possess hearing impairment of sufficient degree to interfere with communication. Twenty years ago, Schow and Nerbonne (1980) found an incidence of hearing loss among health care facility residents to be 80%.

Although many of these persons will, for all practical purposes, remain confined for the remainder of their lives because of chronic illness and other physical or mental problems, many can benefit from aural rehabilitation services from an audiologist. They deserve the opportunity for enhanced communicative skills in spite of impaired hearing and to experience the heightened social and personal communication that may result.

Further, with effective inservice education for health care facility personnel on the topics of hearing impairment, the use of hearing aids, and communication with older adults who have hearing impairment, the daily lives of elderly persons (and the staff) within a health care facility can be enhanced. However, these services must be coordinated with educational programming for elderly persons and their families.

HEALTH CARE FACILITIES

Before this discussion of services for confined older persons proceeds, a description of what is meant by "health care facility" is appropriate.

Health care facility is a currently accepted term denoting any facility that provides long- or short-term residential care for older adults who require medical or other health services other than that provided by hospitals. The facilities may provide intensive care services, including 24-hour-a-day nursing care for posthospitalized stroke patients or simply a place to live near nursing or other health care.

OUTPATIENT RESIDENTIAL FACILITIES

These facilities may include apartment or condominium living for ambulatory older persons. The apartments, or condominiums, in this instance,

are a part of a health care facility, perhaps in a separate wing or simply on the same grounds. Health care is usually a button push away. Older persons who reside in an outpatient or residential facility may have been ill enough at some recent time to desire the proximity of those services. These facilities most nearly resemble retirement communities. The only difference is they may be a part of a health care facility complex.

SHORT-TERM CARE FACILITIES

Many health care facilities have an intensive care or a skilled nursing wing or may be an intensive-care or skilled nursing facility. These are generally considered short-term care facilities. A stroke patient, for example, when known to be recovering, but still too ill to return to his or her own home because of the need for rather constant monitoring and nursing care, may be released from the hospital and taken to the short-term care facility. The stay may be only a few days or may last for several weeks. These facilities play an important role, not only for recuperative purposes, but also as an alterative to higher-cost extended hospital stays. For stroke patients and others who may require other services, rehabilitation personnel such as occupational therapists, audiologists, speech-language pathologists, and others are generally available, at least on a contractual basis.

When placed in a short-term facility, it is expected that the patient will be released within a fairly short time. The most desirable destination is the patient's home. Unfortunately, however, for some older adults, the destination is to an intermediate or long-term care facility, for lack of other alternatives.

INTERMEDIATE AND LONG-TERM CARE FACILITIES

The most frequently observed facilities for older adults are most often called "nursing homes."

They are facilities where older adults reside who may require nursing or other health care. Although the primary reason for placement is generally a health or psychologically related problem, recent studies have shown that some persons who reside in intermediate or long-term care facilities do not have health or mental problems. Intermediate care facilities all too frequently become long-term in nature. For example, placement in these health care facilities may be because (1) no place else to live, (2) a spouse has passed away and the elderly survivor fears living alone, or (3) the most frustrating to older persons: the elderly person's family "feels that it is best." As one older woman told this author, "I thought my daughter was out looking for an apartment for me and I ended up here!"

These facilities offer a room (usually with a roommate), balanced meals, some social and recreational activities, and a nursing staff. Larger health care facilities may have a social services director, an activity director, and rehabilitative services such as occupational therapy, speech-language therapy, and physical therapy. Some facilities are Medicare- and/or Medicaid-approved, but for those programs to provide payment for services and residence, a medically related problem must be the reason for placement in the facility. Further, some health care facilities do not want to be approved by either program because of the relatively low rate of reimbursement for care of the residents.

THE RESIDENTS OF HEALTH CARE FACILITIES

The older adults who are placed in skilled or intensive-care wings of health care facilities or in skilled nursing care facilities are there because of specific health or mental reasons. They may have been transferred from a hospital to the skilled nursing facility because they are still too weak or unable to care for themselves at home, but well enough to be released from the hospital. It is anticipated that the facility and the 24 hour-per-day nursing care that is available will, in that respect, be the "halfway house" for the patient between hospitalization and home. In some instances, however, because of lack of sufficient recovery, some older patients must be transferred to an extended-care facility because they are not able to care for themselves sufficiently to live at home and, further, there may not be others at home to help the person. Therefore, the adult is placed in a longer-term health care facility so that the necessary services for daily needs are available.

In all too many instances, an elderly person views such placement as terminal. It is a fear that can interfere with the elderly person's desire for rehabilitative or health services. The audiologist and other health care professionals must be aware of this, as well as other responses and feelings that can interfere with client desire for supportive services.

REASONS FOR PLACEMENT

What are the reasons for placement in extended care facilities? Because placement for any reason can result in a lessening of desire for self-maintenance and/or improvement, the audiologist should be aware of them. According to Atchley (1972), and Gatz, Bengston, and Blum (1990), the major factor in placement of persons in health care facilities (nursing homes or other residences) appears to be their state of mental or physical health, their previous residential setting, or the family system. Older people in nursing and other health care facilities tend not to have a spouse or children who live nearby, although many have living children. Indications are that many older people would be able to avoid institutionalization, if they had relatives to help care for them (Gatz et al., 1990) and if they had adequate finances. A breakdown in the support system appears to be the primary cause for placement in nursing homes or other forms of residential facilities. Others include loss of residence because of urban renewal projects, a child who has urged them to sell a house (that according to the child is just too much for the elderly family member to care for), or other reasons.

The placement of an elderly person in a health care facility does not generally occur rapidly. A series of events usually take place prior to placement. Those events may include serious illness. They may include attempts at residence with relatives who, in the end, find the older person to be too much of an emotional or financial burden. For whatever reason, placement in a health care facility (nursing home) was felt to be a necessity and the factors leading to that decision frequently may effect the morale of the older person and his or her family.

THE IMPACT OF PLACEMENT

As the majority of older adults view residence in a nursing home as a last resort—in all probability terminal placement—its impact on an older person can have a number of negative implications, which the audiologist or other health professionals who may attempt to provide diagnostic and rehabilitative services must recognize. The negative effects include:

1. Depression.
2. Loneliness.
3. A growing lack of desire to receive rehabilitative services when they may be indicated.
4. The shock and stress associated with the move from a residence where the person may have lived for many years to the nursing home.
5. A lessening of self-image due to the routine of the nursing home.
6. Gradual dependency on persons who, for all practical purposes, are strangers.

7. A lessening of awareness of occurrences in the outside world due to the isolating effect of the nursing home.
8. Personality changes resulting from isolation and/or certain medications.
9. A loss of independence.
10. A loss of personal control including who his or her roommate will be, time for sleeping and eating, and other aspects of life.
11. The depressing influence of illness.
12. The dehumanization of people which can occur in more institutionalized nursing homes.
13. A lack of personal stimulation, which occurs from a loss of close interpersonal communication.
14. A reduction of sensory capabilities that comes with age, including sense of smell, touch, sight, and hearing.

These effects and many others not mentioned are difficult to overcome. Therefore, the elderly resident of a nursing home may not readily accept an audiologist's services.

THE IMPACT OF PLACEMENT ON A DESIRE FOR REHABILITATION SERVICES

When depressed communicative function due to presbycusis is only one of many distressing aspects of an elderly person's life state, should he or she be forced to make a choice as to which is most important? No, a choice should not be forced. However, when an inability to communicate with other people, watch television, or participate in other enjoyable activities may be one of the reasons for increasing depression and decreased feelings of self-worth, then it is reasonable that the service offered by the audiologist should be presented to residents as being very important. When so much else is taken away, an enhanced ability to communicate with other people can encourage increased personal, emotional, and physical function, plus a desire for survival.

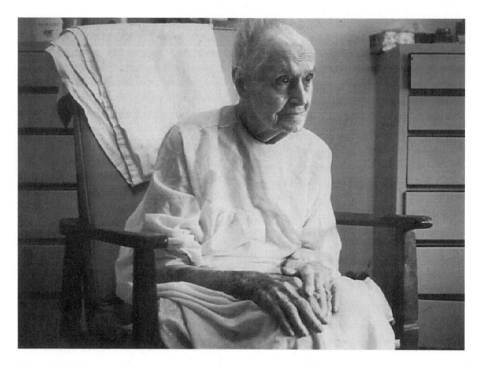

Figure 22-1. Placement in a health care facility for any reason is difficult for all concerned.

ESTABLISHING AURAL REHABILITATION PROGRAMS IN HEALTH CARE FACILITIES

The large population of persons who have hearing impairment who reside in various levels of health care facilities were, for many years, either ignored or avoided because it was felt they possessed little rehabilitative potential. Others believed they were experiencing so many other problems that it was probably best to leave them alone. Further, many audiology services on behalf of elderly nursing home clients have been provided as parts of practicum experiences by graduate students in audiology training programs. In the greatest majority of instances, however, those students did not possess the insights into aging and aging persons to provide effective aural rehabilitation services. Rather, they may have begun with "lesson num-

ber one" in a book of speechreading lessons and proceeded to provide "speechreading instruction" that had little or no meaning for the clients involved. The majority of clients, then, had to be "rounded-up" before each weekly session, and the gradually disillusioned graduate student clinician wondered why so many would not leave their room to come to "class."

This experience is discouraging to a clinician, to say the least. The clinician may have felt that the book of speechreading lessons must contain **something** that would benefit the older clients or else it would not have been written. More importantly, the clients were told that the aural rehabilitation program may help them learn to communicate more efficiently with others in spite of impaired hearing, only to realize later that it did not.

It is no wonder, then, that so few audiologists graduating from training programs have had a desire to initiate audiology service programs in health care facilities. The fact is that many of those graduate students may not have had a positive practicum experience in that setting. They also may not have had a positive instructor mentor who provided concrete information and personal examples on how to provide meaningful services to elderly clients. Further, many professionals who could have effectively served older adults who have hearing impairment may not have taken the time to **listen** to their potential clients, to find out what their functional needs and desires were. That information is probably the most critical for developing a viable rehabilitation program for elderly clients.

ADDRESSING THE NEEDS OF HEALTH CARE FACILITY RESIDENTS

It is important to remember that residents of health care facilities are individuals who have specific goals and needs. Among the 92% of health care facility residents who possess some degree of hearing impairment, the sense of need and urgency for interpersonal communication is as great as for other persons. After all, verbal communication is one of the traits that identifies us as humans. The isolation that occurs as the result of impaired hearing can be even more devastating to persons who are already isolated because of their confinement in a nursing home. Their sense of urgency to break through the barriers to communication caused by an inability to hear and understand what others are saying or, at least, to watch television and understand what is being said may be much greater than evidenced by their statements or emotions. They, further, may have suppressed a desire to accept those services, as they may feel that perhaps nothing will help at their late stage of life.

In Chapter 21, suggested procedures for aural rehabilitation services for older adult clients were presented. If geared toward the specific needs and priorities of the client, those procedures will also benefit residents of health care facilities who have hearing impairment. Before beginning rehabilitation, however, the clients must be encouraged to develop a desire to at least "give it a try." If the desire is awakened or reawakened, it is then the responsibility of the audiologist to demonstrate to the client that his or her communication needs and priorities are of prime importance in the treatment program. Additionally, within reason, improvements can be made if they also accept responsibility as adults to participate.

Above and beyond the service aspect is the important fact that the audiologist is working with adults, no matter what the age or temperament. They are adults who, beyond their desire or control have become older. And with age, an increasing inability to efficiently hear and understand what others are saying has added to the isolation and depression they may be experiencing. If the audiologist offers the time, energy, and commitment to learn about the process of aging and listen to what his or her clients are saying about their needs, desires, and concerns, then viable aural rehabilitation treatment programs can be developed.

DEVELOPING REALISTIC EXPECTATIONS

Another important aspect of this fascinating work must be acknowledged. That is, the audiologist must be realistic in her or his efforts and expectations when serving this population. There are some, no matter how much we would like to effectively serve all persons, who, because of physical or mental problems, do not have the potential to benefit from aural rehabilitation services and others may benefit only marginally. On the other hand, the audiologist must refrain from providing services only on behalf of those who will benefit most to the exclusion of those who may benefit slightly. Even a terminally ill, bedridden person's last weeks or months may be brightened by a health care facility nursing staff who have learned from the audiologists' inser-

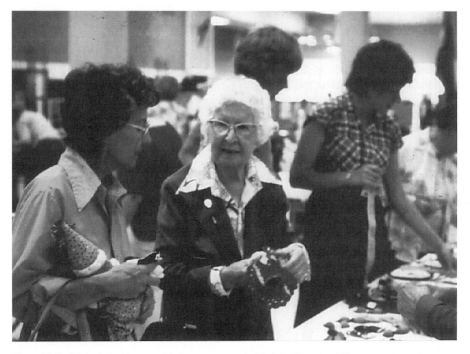

Figure 22-2. It is important to remember that, no matter what their health and mobility status, older adults have specific goals and needs.

vices how to communicate more efficiently with persons who have hearing impairment. This, in itself, can be a significant service. *These are quality (not quantity) of life issues.*

DETERMINING THE NEED FOR SERVICES

Establishing the Benefits

In most health care facilities, it can be assumed there are at least a number of persons who reside there who are hearing impaired and can benefit from some aspect of an assessment and aural rehabilitation program. The benefits of initiating an aural rehabilitation program should be presented to the director and his or her staff. The benefits stressed in that meeting include:

1. The fact that effective in-service education can enhance communication between health care facility personnel and residents who have hearing impairment and, thus, ease one reason for frayed nerves on both parts.
2. Recommendations for alterations in the furniture arrangement in a lounge area or other central gathering place that can enhance communication will be of great service to a health care facility. Otherwise, residents may avoid an important area where the greatest amount of activity and communication could take place.
3. Effective hearing aid orientation programs can provide the impetus for previously inefficient users of hearing aids to benefit from them in their daily activities.
4. An effective assessment program can identify persons who have hearing impairment who

may have been thought to be noncommunicating or confused for other reasons.

5. Further, a well-designed aural rehabilitation treatment program can provide enhanced communicative skill for those who can benefit from that service. For others, the aural rehabilitation program may consist of discussions of their most difficult communication environments and suggestions for manipulation of the physical environment or those persons with whom they have difficulty communicating.

These programs, if geared toward clients' specific communication needs, can be extremely beneficial for confined elderly residents. It is also generally found that most persons in the health care facility environment can benefit from at least some aspect of these services.

Surveying for Hearing Impairment

The determination of the need for any of the services discussed previously must begin with a survey of the residents of the health care facility and, in specific terms, a presentation of the results of the survey to the health care facility administration. Those include the director, the head of nursing, the activity director, and the social services director. It is suggested that all residents who can respond to a hearing evaluation should be included in the survey.

A typical hearing screening at a fixed intensity level has generally not been found to be a satisfactory method for use in a health care facility, because such large numbers fail. An efficient procedure was described 25 years ago by Traynor (1975) and includes establishment of pure-tone thresholds and the use of immittance audiometry to confirm the type of loss. Even if a quiet environment for assessment can be found, the use of impedance audiometry is important, because of the probability of even low noise levels interfering with bone-conduction testing.

For those who are found to have hearing impairment, assessment of speech recognition ability with and without visual clues provides relevant information for initial discussions with the health care facility staff about each individual client's disability and the need for aural rehabilitation services. Speech recognition, in the absence of a sound-treated room and audiometer with speech capabilities, can be assessed with relative accuracy by live voice, with the audiologist seated approximately 4 to 6 feet from the client. Monosyllabic words, CID Everyday Sentences, and brief conversation with and without visual clues and with and/or without the use of amplification administered at a comfortable listening level for the client, is a reasonable mode of test administration. However, this should only be conducted by a skilled audiologist.

Presentation of Survey Results

Results of the survey are presented to the administration of the health care facility and, if that facility is a part of a corporate body, a representative of the corporation. If the administration is convinced that an aural rehabilitation program is desired, the program format is outlined. It is stressed that the initial screening/threshold survey be conducted only after the administration has contracted for the assessment program and the avenue for reimbursement of that service has been established.

The survey, alone, will provide important information for the health care facility staff. Residents who may have previously been described as confused and/or disoriented may be found to possess a severe enough auditory impairment to account for at least a portion of that behavior. Modifications in patterns of communication by health care facility staff alone may result in positive behavior change on the part of such residents. Those modifications in communication strategies by the staff, for example, can result from an effective staff in-service program. An elderly man, previously described as stubborn, inattentive, withdrawn, and antisocial, may begin to interact more with his environment when communication with staff is likewise improved. Others may demonstrate positive personality change as the result of properly fitted hearing aids, combined with modifications of speaking habits by health care facility staff as the result of an effective in-service program.

With information on the incidence, severity, and communicative impact of hearing loss within a health care facility that will be available for discussion with the administration, a full assessment and aural rehabilitation program can be outlined and initiated. This includes a discussion of the possible positive impact of a viable aural rehabilitation program on the residents, on the health care facility staff, and on the other programs within the facility.

Client Records

Records of progress for each client must be maintained on an ongoing basis, along with records of physician, staff, family contact, and referrals. Records of social progress, continuing service, medical records, staff notification of audiometric test results, physician and family notification, and progress in the aural rehabilitation program are integral parts of the audiologist's record-keeping procedures. Such reports should be kept both in the client's master file in the health care facility and as a part of the audiologist's file on each client.

Patient Care Plan

A patient care plan is developed in cooperation with the audiologist, the speech-language pathologist, social services personnel, and other staff that have daily contact with the person, including the activities director. The plan contains the goals and objectives for each aural rehabilitation client, along with methods and approaches and the problem or concern. An example of a patient care plan is in Figure 22–3.

Continuing Service Records

Continuing service records must be maintained on an ongoing basis. Each note, dated and signed, relates, for example, to progress in specific aural rehabilitation efforts, a contact made by the audiologist with that client for hearing aid maintenance, statements regarding communicative progress, or a contact by a family member or the client's physician.

Communication Progress Forms

Communication progress forms are also integral to the record-keeping efforts on behalf of the health care facility program. The client's baseline of communicative behavior is noted on each form. Each form for each member of the evaluation team is placed in a client's file. As each person notes specific changes in communicative behavior, they are noted on his or her own form for each client. At weekly or monthly staff meetings, the ratings for each client are compared, and a consensus as to progress or lack of it is noted in the client's continuing service record.

Reimbursement for Services

In discussing the auditory assessment program, the aural rehabilitation program, and reimbursement issues with the health care facility administration, it should be emphasized that Medicare and, in many states, Medicaid covers auditory diagnostic evaluations, including special assessment procedures, in accordance with charges which are reasonable and typical in that geographic area. The testing must be justified on an individual basis. Routine testing will not be reimbursed. Audiologists who are certified, or are eligible for certification as audiologists by the American Speech-Language-Hearing Association, or licensed by states having licensure laws, are eligible to become Medicare approved providers of audiology services by award of a Medicare provider number (Hull, 1988). If the audiologist has been awarded a provider number, he or she

```
┌─────────────────────────────────────────────────────────────────┐
│                        KENTON MANOR                             │
│                     AUDIOLOGY CARE PLAN                          │
│                                                                 │
│   RESIDENT:                          ROOM LOCATION:             │
│                                                                 │
│   A.  PROBLEM OR CONCERN:                                       │
│      _____           │
│      _____           │
│      _____           │
│                                                                 │
│   B.  GOALS OF CARE TEAM:                                      │
│      _____           │
│      _____           │
│      _____           │
│                                                                 │
│   C.  METHODS AND APPROACHES:                                  │
│      _____           │
│      _____           │
│      _____           │
│                                                                 │
│   D.  COMMENTS:                                                 │
│      _____           │
│      _____           │
│      _____           │
│                                                                 │
│   NAME:                                                         │
│   TITLE:                                                        │
│   DATE:                                                         │
└─────────────────────────────────────────────────────────────────┘
```

Figure 22–3. Audiology Services Care Plan utilized in a program for the hearing impaired older client (Courtesy of Wichita State University Audiology Clinic).

can bill for services directly. If the health care facility is Medicare-approved, its own accounting office can bill for the service. In whatever manner, an agreement for the avenue for reimbursement for services should, in all instances, be arranged before the initial survey.

THE ONGOING AURAL REHABILITATION PROGRAM

The remaining components of an aural rehabilitation program are next described.

IN-SERVICE TRAINING OF HEALTH CARE FACILITY PERSONNEL AND FAMILIES OF THE RESIDENTS

In-service training for health care facility administration, staff, and the residents' families not only supports an assessment and aural rehabilitation treatment program, but also provides carryover of the treatment aspects into the daily life of the clients. In-service provides administration, staff, and families with insights into (1) the cause and effects of presbycusis on residents' ability for communication, (2) the resulting psychosocial impact, (3) the structure of the aural rehabilitation program, (4) what hearing aids can and cannot do, (5) troubleshooting procedures for hearing aid malfunction, and (6) methods for more efficient communication with residents who have hearing impairment.

Included during in-services are discussions of individual residents who are involved as clients in the program. Discussions include the hearing impairment those clients possess, the impact of the hearing impairment on their communicative function, their progress (or lack of it) as a result of the aural rehabilitation treatment program, and the development of plans for follow-through and carryover of those clients' programs into their daily lives in the health care facility. The health care facility staff, including the director of nurses, activity director, physical therapist, occupational therapist, and other personnel, including the cooks and custodians, can all be vital forces in the carryover process. This, importantly, includes the families of the residents.

Techniques offered through in-service for more efficient communication with older persons who have hearing impairment can enhance the lives of the staff, the residents' families, and the residents. It is generally found, to everyone's relief, that some of the emotional encounters resulting from futile attempts at communication between residents who have hearing impairment and staff members are sometimes soothed after utilization of the techniques for communication that the staff learned during in-service and that the elderly clients are learning during their treatment sessions.

Topics for in-service training should include:

1. **The structure of the auditory mechanism** and theories as to the cause of presbycusis.
2. **The manifestations of presbycusis** and its impact on an elderly person's ability to function communicatively. This discussion includes presentations of audiometric configurations and examples of what the client who possesses presbycusis might hear, compared with a normally hearing person.
3. **Hearing aids, their uses and misuses**, are discussed relative to what hearing aids are, what they sound like, what they can do, and what they cannot do. The reasons why some persons cannot benefit from hearing aids are also discussed, along with the necessity for a thorough hearing aid evaluation by a hearing professional.
4. **Instruction on the use of hearing aids**, placing the earmold properly in the ear, the switches (including the use of the gain control), the battery, the care of ear molds, and others are presented, in turn, to alleviate some of the difficulties some elderly residents have because of manual dexterity or memory problems. The staff of health care facilities can, further, aid the carryover of hearing aid orientation for recently fitted residents, if they are familiar with the component parts and their use.
5. **Hearing aid trouble-shooting procedures** also are stressed and include:
   a. Knowledge of the causes of acoustic feedback
   b. Battery longevity and placement

c. Checking for cerumen in earmolds or receiver tubing

d. Procedures for cleaning ear molds

e. Correct use of the telephone switch and other controls

Instructions to the staff of the health care facility on the care of hearing aids can be invaluable. The staff should be instructed to check to see that hearing aids do not go into the shower, the laundry, or denture cups, and that the hearing aid does not accidently get tossed out with soiled tissue paper.

The nurse aide, for example, can reduce a patient's stresses involved in adjusting to hearing aids by having the knowledge required to conduct a quick check on hearing aids that a frustrated elderly resident feels are not working. A simple adjustment of battery placement or reminding the resident that the earmolds need cleaning can eliminate non-use of otherwise beneficial hearing aids. Because these adjustments and reminders may be necessary when the audiologist is not in the health care facility, this aspect of in-service is extremely important. Hearing aid loss and malfunction are two of the most frequently observed problems for health care facility residents who have hearing impairment.

6. The components of an aural rehabilitation program are discussed so that administration and staff are aware of the intricacies involved not only in the assessment of auditory function, but also in treatment sessions. These insights and a resulting staff knowledgeable of the role of the audiologist, permits an enhanced working relationship between audiologist and staff. A program that flows more smoothly generally results.

The role of the staff in carryover is also discussed. This includes the fact that the staff can be the vital catalyst in providing an enhanced climate for communication in the health care facility.

7. Discussing methods for effective communication with hearing-impaired elderly persons is a critical part of in-service training. The stresses that grow out of frustrated attempts at communication, both on the part of residents and staff, can stifle an otherwise pleasant living environment. The suggestions provided the staff include the Thirteen Commandments for Communicating with Hearing Impaired Older Adults (Hull, 1980) presented in Table 22–1.

PROVISION OF AURAL REHABILITATION TREATMENT SERVICES IN THE HEALTH CARE FACILITY

The specific strategies for providing aural rehabilitation treatment services on behalf of older adult clients in the health care facility remain essentially the same as those outlined in Chapter 21. They are procedures that lend themselves to any level of client impairment. There are, however, some considerations that will benefit both a client and the audiologist when providing aural rehabilitation services for confined elderly clients, including:

1. Motivation of clients,
2. The environment of the health care facility,
3. The health state of individual clients,
4. Family involvement, and
5. Compounding visual problems.

Motivation

Some audiologists prefer not to attempt to provide aural rehabilitation services on behalf of older persons who reside in health care facilities. They reason that many potential clients lack motivation to receive services. As clinicians observe these clients, many of them have good reason for their lack of motivation. Clinicians can, however, blame themselves in some instances for not being able to

TABLE 22-1. THE THIRTEEN COMMANDMENTS FOR COMMUNICATING WITH HEARING IMPAIRED OLDER ADULTS

- Speak at a slightly greater than normal intensity.

- Speak at your normal rate, but not too rapidly.

- Do not speak to the elderly person at a greater distance than 6 feet but no less than 3 feet.

- Concentrate light on the speaker's face for greater visibility of lip movements, facial expression, and gestures.

- Do not speak to the elderly person unless you are visible to him or her (e.g., not from another room while he or she is reading the newspaper or watching TV).

- Do not force the elderly person to listen to you when there is a great deal of environmental noise. That type of environment can be difficult for a younger, normally hearing person. It can, on the other hand, be defeating for the hearing impaired elderly.

- Never, under any circumstances, speak directly into the person's ear. Not only can the person not make use of visual clues, but the speaker may be causing an already distorting auditory system to distort the speech signal further. In other words, clarity may be depressed as loudness is increased.

- If the elderly person does not appear to understand what is being said, rephrase the statement rather than simply repeating the misunderstood words. An otherwise frustrating situation can be avoided in that way.

- Do not over-articulate. Over-articulation not only distorts the sounds of speech, but also the speaker's face, thus making the use of visual clues more difficult.

- Arrange the room (living room or meeting room) where communication will take place so that no speaker or listener is more than 6 feet apart, and all are completely visible. Using this direct approach, communication for all parties involved will be enhanced.

- Include the elderly person in all discussions about him or her. Hearing-impaired persons sometimes feel quite vulnerable. This approach will help alleviate some of those feelings.

- In meetings or any group activity where there is a speaker presenting information (church meetings, civic organizations, etc.) make it mandatory that the speaker(s) use the public address system. One of the most frequent complaints among elderly persons is that they may enjoy attending meetings of various kinds, but all too often the speaker, for whatever reason, tries to avoid using a microphone. Many elderly persons do not desire to assert themselves by asking a speaker who has just said, "I am sure that you can all hear me if I do not use the microphone," to **please** use it. Most persons begin to avoid public or organizational meetings if they cannot hear what the speaker is saying. This point cannot be stressed enough.

- Above all, treat elderly persons as adults. They, of anyone, deserve that respect.

Reproduced with permission from Hull, R. H. (1980). The thirteen commandments for talking to the hearing impaired older person. *Journal of the American Speech and Hearing Association, 22,* 427.

provide motivation. Cohen (1990) has described a number of reasons for lack of motivation among many elderly persons. Lack of available finances, the death of a spouse or friends, lack of efficient modes of transportation, children living a great distance away, and physical problems that may restrict mobility are among problems of older adults.

REASONS FOR LACK OF MOTIVATION. As clinicians view elderly residents of health care facilities, they observe other more dramatic effects that impact on this population's motivation to receive rehabilitation services. According to Atchley (1972) and Smyer, Zarit, and Qualls (1990), the most depressing aspect of placement in a health care facility (nursing home) is the move from a home where the person may have lived for many years to a strange and, to that person, a probable final residence. The events leading to placement in the health care facility were, in all probability, equally depressing, including, perhaps, the loss of a spouse, the loss of a home due to rezoning laws or lack of finances, severe enough illness to require constant nursing care, or slowly declining health simply because of advancing age. If the elderly resident has read the statistics on the longevity of residents of nursing homes, he or she will know that the probability of survival after the first month of placement is only about 73%. Further, only about 20% ever leave health care facilities except for burial (Moss & Halamandaris, 1997).

The well elderly in the community may not experience the reasons for depression, nor are they experiencing that single dramatic change in their lives. The fear of the necessity for a move to a health care facility can, however, result in motivation to work toward preventing it.

For those who can benefit from aural rehabilitation services, efforts toward motivation should be made. If for no other reason than to enhance communication abilities with family and friends in the confined environment of the health care facility, to be able to enjoy watching television once again, or to participate more efficiently in social activities within the health care facility, motivation for receiving aural rehabilitation services should be given a high priority. It must be kept in mind, however, as was discussed in Chapter 21, that the aural rehabilitation treatment program must be developed around the clients' priority communication needs and no others.

Once an older client is motivated to receive aural rehabilitation services, working lesson by lesson through an activity manual on speechreading can be self-defeating, and initial motivation can be quickly lost. The audiologist has, then, lost the trust of the clients. "She said that aural rehabilitation treatment would help, and that learning to communicate in spite of hearing impairment would be a priority, and all we did was try to figure out what the sounds, words, and sentences were from a book she was giving our lessons from. Is that aural rehabilitation?" That is a common complaint by previously motivated clients who desire to be helped.

Treatment Environment

Discovering an area within the health care facility where aural rehabilitation services can be provided in a pleasant and least restrictive environment can be challenging. Most health care facilities do, however, have an area that is, at least, a pleasant place to be. That area may be an activity room, a lounge that is not the main lounge or lobby area, a staff dining room, or other sections of the health care facility that are not considered by the residents as ones where, for example, people go when they are "not well." Places to avoid include the infirmary and the chapel. The chapel has special meaning for many persons and it is not a place where therapy is held. Further, the infirmary is usually thought of as a place to avoid and it is not a place where one voluntarily goes once or twice a week for self-improvement.

The only available space where frequent disturbances may not occur may be an esthetically undesirable space, such as the laundry room or the rear portion of the cafeteria. In that instance, modifications will be necessary. This is not always greeted with enthusiasm by health care facility administrators, particularly with the tight budgets faced by many. Such modifications for improvement of the therapy environment, however, may be necessary for the aural rehabilitation program to be effective to any degree.

Some remodeling of an otherwise drab room can be done inexpensively. Some wallpaper, a moveable partition, some paint, and carpeting can do wonders for the environment. There are few health care facilities that do not have at least a small amount of money for such improvements. If an audiologist has some talent for painting and minor carpentry, then labor costs may be reduced. Even some of the health care facility residents may enjoy chipping in on the labor. A retired carpenter or painter may find it a joy to lend an experienced hand. Women who can make curtains may enjoy reawakening that skill for the good of the "Audiology Room." If the health care facility agrees to hire professionals to do the remodeling work, then such innovations may not be necessary.

At the University of Northern Colorado Aural Rehabilitation Program for the Aging (Hull & Traynor, 1975), renovations for the installation of sound-treated rooms and audiometers, including carpentry, electrical work, painting, and others were funded by the health care facilities involved. When one health care facility was being constructed, the corporate owner's plans included a sound-treated room as part of the initial construction in support of their aural rehabilitation program. The room was, further, to double as a staff lounge. That aspect, for obvious reasons, was not a satisfactory arrangement and the staff later found other quarters for coffee and conversation.

Another health care facility remodeled a large linen closet, one provided a large vacant resident room, another provided remodeled space in what originally was an alcove area off a hallway, and yet another built new walls for a new room for the audiology services. Interest level in the program varies from facility to facility, but the general commitment remains the same. Figure 22–4 illustrates a desirable room arrangement for the provision of aural rehabilitation services, including counseling, hearing aid orientation, and speechreading/auditory training.

The Health Status of Clients

As stated earlier, an audiologist must be realistic regarding an elderly client's potential to respond to aural rehabilitation services. A terminally ill resident of a skilled nursing wing of a health care facility may possess impaired hearing, but not be able to respond to a diagnostic evaluation. It is not reasonable to ask that person to participate in a complex aural rehabilitation program. A knowledgeable staff, however, as the result of effective in-service, may ease some of the frustrations the resident may be having because of an inability to understand what they are saying. If the state of health of some individuals was the catalyst for placement in the health care facility, but those persons can, indeed, benefit from audiology services, additional considerations will be necessary. For example, accommodations for persons who are confined to a wheelchair are mandatory. Ramps into sound-treated testing booths, tables used in therapy that conform to the height of wheelchairs, and doors that permit maneuvering in and out of the rooms are necessary.

Attention Span

Many elderly persons cannot tolerate long periods of concentrated effort on any task. Audiometric evaluations in which attention to an almost inaudible pure tone is required, or aural rehabilitation sessions that instruct on more efficient means for communication, can become intolerable for some elderly persons, even when the program is specifically designed around their needs. This is equally frustrating to some audiologists who have difficulty understanding the reason for the low attention/tolerance span. The problem does exist, however and it must be accounted for.

It may be necessary to break audiological evaluations into two or even three short periods, particularly if a hearing aid evaluation is included. Speechreading/auditory training sessions should not extend for more than 45 minutes. If clients appear to be less tolerant on a specific day, short breaks during which time something else is talked about will be necessary. An alert audiologist will realize when the "stretch breaks" are required.

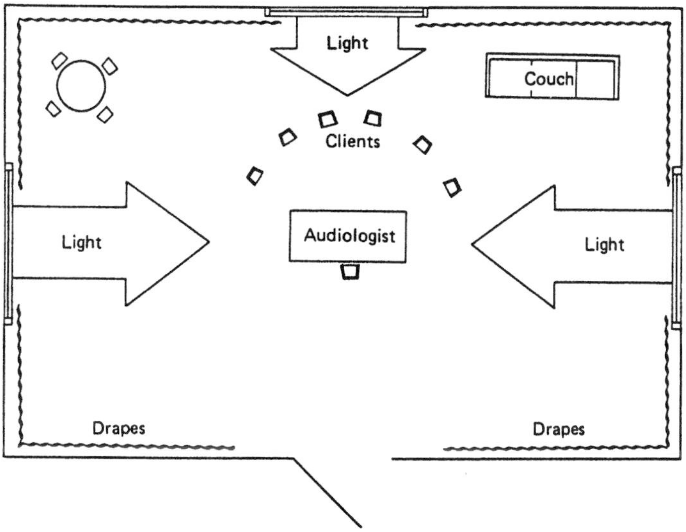

Figure 22–4. Desirable room arrangement for aural rehabilitation services for older adults.

Number of Clients

The number of clients for optimal group interaction ranges from six to eight. Aural rehabilitation groups should not exceed this number. If at all possible, it is important to control admittance to specific groups to assure that hearing levels and levels of mental functioning among participants are as equal as possible. It can become frustrating for the group members, the audiologist, and the client, if one client has extreme difficulty communicating and, thus, great difficulty participating in the group. The audiologist, out of necessity, will tend to spend most of the group time attempting to facilitate that person's participation. The latter does not enhance positive and facilitatory group interaction. As the clients make progress in their communicative skill, the development of advanced classes may be warranted, depending on the needs of the clients.

Individual Versus Group Treatment

The more severely impaired individuals will require individual aural rehabilitation treatment. If a person progresses to the point that group involvement is possible, then he or she should be referred to that treatment setting. Some audiologists prefer to begin all clients' treatment on an individual basis so as to attend to any immediate needs they may have.

Acoustics and Lighting

Consideration of the acoustic and visual environment of an aural rehabilitation treatment facility is critical. At least initially, the environment should be a quiet one, free of undue reverberation, and with adequate lighting. Noting that older eyes will generally require at least twice as much light as younger eyes, lighting is an important consideration.

Visual Aspects

Fluorescent lighting is not suggested for use with elderly clients. Both the hue of the light and the "flicker" can cause visual difficulties, inattentiveness, and even seizures. Indirect and incandescent lighting is suggested, but glare from hard tables, floors, walls, and ceilings is to be avoided at all costs. Aging results in a thickening of the lens of the eye and a narrowing of the pupil aperture. Further, the muscles of the eye do not function as well, so that accommodation of light changes is not as efficient.

Fozard (1990) and Woodruff (1975) have advised that it takes almost twice the light energy to have the same effect on the older eye as the younger eye. In other words, the older eye is less responsive to light and cannot compensate for changes in light as quickly as it could when it was younger. It behooves the audiologist, therefore, to avoid moving from light to shadows as he or she is involved in aural rehabilitation treatment sessions.

Acoustic Needs

The suggested acoustic environment is one that consists of non-plush carpeted floors, textured walls or walls that are carpeted one-third up from the floors, spackled acoustic tile ceilings or spackled dry wall, and chairs that at least have a padded seat and back. From this initial design, the audiologist can modify it to suit his or her own acoustic desires relative to aural rehabilitative tasks engaged in.

The room should not become so padded that it becomes anechoic, nor should it become too reverberant. A little reverberation gives sound "life." But, too much causes distortion of the acoustic aspects of speech. Bergman et al. (1976) determined that unfavorable acoustics (reverberated speech) contributed most to difficulties in speech discrimination among older persons who have hearing impairment.

Time of Day for Treatment

The process involved in aural rehabilitation treatment is fatiguing for both the client and the audiologist. In providing services, particularly on behalf of the older adult clients, the factors of fatigue and alertness must be kept in mind. That includes remembering that most people function better at certain times of the day and that attention span and periods of maximum alertness are different as one becomes older.

In working with older adults, the period immediately following lunch and anytime in the evening provides the least benefit for clients. The inefficiency of those times is seen most dramatically among the confined or less active older person.

The time periods most advantageous for older clients and an audiologist are those toward the middle of the morning and perhaps 1 to 2 hours after lunch. The audiologist should be alert to the behaviors of his or her clients and change times as needed. It is generally best to ask a client to suggest the time of day when he or she feels best.

The length of aural rehabilitation sessions must also be considered. This author has found that most alert, active older adults can work for at least 1 hour, as long as periodic breaks are taken that include brief chats about things other than the treatment session. Many older clients will not be able to tolerate strenuous sessions for longer than 30 minutes. The alert audiologist will be able to judge the tolerance levels of his or her clients.

Family

Although the role of the family or other significant others in the aural rehabilitation process is discussed throughout this text, it is a critically important aspect to be presented as per the elderly resident who is confined to the health care facility. The discouraging component of this discussion, however, is that many family members of these persons either do not wish to become involved or live such a great distance away that they cannot be involved in any consistent manner. It is disheartening, not only on the part of the audiologist, but more so on the part of the elderly client, to observe a family member who agreed to come to the health care facility to become involved in the aural rehabilitation process, who eventually dissolves the commitment. If such a possibility exists, it is generally better to not ask the family member to participate at all. A genuine commitment is necessary before such participation is initiated, mostly for the mental health of the elderly resident. The anguish felt by elderly persons, who eventually realize that their child or other family member apparently did not genuinely desire to become involved, is heartbreaking.

If family involvement is possible, however, the enhanced awareness about the potential for communication by and with their elderly family member can enhance family bonds. The importance of this involvement cannot be stressed enough.

Compounding Problems of Vision

The multiple handicaps of vision and hearing impairment are very real among elderly persons. Many of those with significant visual problems can be found within health care facilities, particularly if they have not been able to remain mobile and self-sufficient in their own homes.

For persons who have rehabilitative potential, the aural rehabilitation process revolves around working toward enhancement of auditory function, as visual clues may be of little advantage. The audiologist's efforts must be combined with those of a vision specialist who can work to assist a person in becoming more mobile, including correcting furniture arrangements in his or her room, safe use of cosmetics, and self-help skills. That team effort, along with the help of a facility activity director can supplant the isolation that may otherwise face the elderly resident. The audiologist can play a vital role in providing input to the person's rehabilitation programs.

SUMMARY

This chapter has presented considerations for the provision of services on behalf of persons who reside in health care facilities. It is stressed that, as with other clients, these persons' communication needs must be addressed as priorities. Even though they are residing within the confines of the health care facility, they are still individuals and, most importantly, they are individual adults with unique goals and concerns. The audiologist and other professionals who serve these people must be constantly aware of that fact. On the other hand, clients must be fully aware that they are involved in treatment, not simply another activity within the health care facility. They must be aware of the reasons for the communication problems they are experiencing, the steps that will be taken to help them, and the strategies involved. Only then will the services and the audiologist be accepted.

REFERENCES

Administration on Aging and the American Association of Retired Persons. *Profile Of Older Americans: 1996* (Pub. No. PF3049, 1090). Washington, DC.

Atchley, R. C. (1972). *The social forces in later life*. Belmont, CA: Wadsworth.

Bayles, K. A., & Kaszniak, A. W. (1987). *Communication and cognition in normal aging and dementia*. Boston: Little Brown.

Bergman, M., Blumenfeld, V., Cascardo, D., Dash, B., Levitt, H., & Margulies, M. (1976). Age-related decrement in hearing for speech. *Journal of Gerontology, 31,* 533–538.

Cohen, G. D. (1990). Psychopathology and mental health in the mature and elderly adult. In J. E. Birren & K. W. Schaie (Eds.), *Handbook of the psychology of aging* (pp. 642–667). New York: Academic Press.

Fozard, J. (1990). Vision and hearing in aging. In J. E. Birren & K. W. Schaie (Eds.), *Handbook of the psychology of aging* (pp. 329–342). New York: Academic Press

Gatz, M., Bengtson, V. L., & Blum, M. J. (1990). Caregiving families. In J. Birren & K. W. Schaie (Eds.), *Hand-*

book of the psychology of aging (pp. 886–914). New York: Academic Press.

Health Care Financing Administration (1998). *Incidence of health care facility placement in the U.S. Personal communication*. Washington, DC: Public Health Service.

Hull, R. H. (1977). *Hearing impairment among aging persons*. Lincoln, NE: Cliff Notes.

Hull, R. H. (1980). The thirteen commandments for talking to the hearing impaired older person. *Journal of the American Speech and Hearing Association, 22*, 427.

Hull, R. H. (1988). *Hearing in aging*. Presentation before the National Invitational Conference on Geriatric Rehabilitation. Washington, DC: PHS, DHHS.

Hull, R. H. (1993). Incidence of hearing loss in a nursing home population. Unpublished study. Wichita State University, Wichita, KS.

Hull, R. H. (1997). *Hearing in aging*. San Diego: Singular Publishing Group.

Hull, R. H., & Traynor, R. (1976). A community-wide program in geriatric aural rehabilitation. *Journal of the American Speech-Language-Hearing Association, 14*, 33–34, 47–48.

Ignatavicius, D. D., & Bayne, M. V. (1995). *Medical-surgical nursing*. Philadelphia: W. B. Saunders.

Moss, F. E., & Halamandaris, F. E. (1997). *Too old, too sick, too bad: Nursing homes in America*. Germantown, MD: Aspen Systems.

Schow, R. L., & Nerbonne, M. A. (1980). Hearing levels in elderly nursing home residents. *Journal of Speech and Hearing Disorders, 45*, 124–132.

Smyer, M. A., Zarit, S. H., & Qualls, S. H. (1990). Psychological intervention with the aging individual. In J. E. Birren & K. W. Schaie (Eds.), *Handbook of the psychology of aging* (pp. 375–394). New York: Academic Press.

Stone, R., Cafferata, G.L., & Sangl, J. (1987). Caregivers of the frail elderly: A national profile. *The Gerontologist, 36*, 616–626.

Traynor, R. L. (1975). *A method of audiological assessment for the non-ambulatory geriatric patient*. Unpublished doctoral dissertation. Greeley, CO: University of Northern Colorado.

Woodruff, D. S. (1975). A physiological perspective of the psychology of aging. In D. S. Woodruff & J. E. Birren (Eds.), *Aging: Scientific perspectives and social issues* (pp. 179–198). New York: Van Nostrand.

END OF CHAPTER EXAMINATION QUESTIONS

CHAPTER 22

1. Among persons residing in health care facilities, approximately _____ possess hearing impairment of sufficient degree to interfere with communication.
   a. 15%
   b. 38%
   c. 56%
   d. 92%

2. Describe the possible benefits a resident of a health care facility may realize from aural rehabilitation treatment.

3. Define the term: "health care facility" and briefly compare and contrast the three levels of care that they may provide.

4. Briefly discuss how the attitude of a person toward residing in a health care facility may affect his or her desire for rehabilitative services.

5. Which of the following is **not** felt to be a major factor in placement of persons in health care facilities?
   a. Their previous residential setting
   b. Their children regarding them as "inconvenient"
   c. Their state of mental or physical health
   d. Their family setting

6. The scope of the audiologist's services in health care facilities should include
   a. The resident's family
   b. The medical/support staff
   c. The resident
   d. All of the above

END OF CHAPTER ANSWER SHEET

Name   Date

CHAPTER 22

1. Which one?   a   b   c   d

2. _____

   _____

   _____

   _____

   _____

   _____

3. _____

   _____

   _____

   _____

   _____

   _____

4. _____

   _____

   _____

5. Which one(s)? a b c d

6. Which one(s)? a b c d

7. Which one(s)? a b c d

8. a. _____

   b. _____

   c. _____

   d. _____

   e. _____

9. a. _____

   b. _____

10. a. _____

   b. _____

   c. _____

   d. _____

   e. _____

7. The most efficient screening process recommended for the identification of residents with hearing impairment includes:
   a. Fixed intensity level screening
   b. A conversational voice test
   c. Pure-tone thresholds and impedance audiometry
   d. Interviewing family members and/or caregivers

8. List five (5) possible in-service training topics which the audiologist could share with facility staff members and administrators.
   a.
   b.
   c.
   d.
   e.

9. The author suggests two optimal time periods for scheduling aural rehabilitation. What are those times and why might they prove advantageous?
   a.
   b.

10. The author describes five considerations that should guide the establishment of aural rehabilitation services on behalf of the residents. What are they? Briefly describe each.
   a.
   b.
   c.
   d.
   e.

PART V

Evaluation in the Aural Rehabilitation Process

Evaluation in Aural Rehabilitation Treatment for Adults who are Hearing Impaired

■ RAYMOND H. HULL, Ph.D. ■

IMPORTANT ASSESSMENT FACTORS

ASSESSMENT
   Elements to be Assessed
   Historical Perspectives
   Assessment Through Bisensory Modalities
   Scales of Communicative Function
   Assessment Based on Communicative Priorities
   Profiles
   Scales for Older Adults who are Hearing Impaired

(continued)

> Evaluating Communicative Function
> Communication Scales and Profiles
>
> A COMPREHENSIVE APPROACH TO ASSESSMENT OF
> COMMUNICATIVE FUNCTION

One of the many historically challenging aspects of aural rehabilitation services on behalf of adult clients has been the attempts at assessing the impact of those services on their communicative behaviors. Perhaps the most discouraging have been those instances in which persons from other professions, or within our own have asked us to show them *how much* improvement a given client has made when, in fact, the instruments to measure those gains were not available. It is simpler to note the speech and language progress of a child who has congenital hearing impairment, or to plot the increase in speech reception thresholds after a hearing aid fitting, than to pinpoint the social gains as a result of aural rehabilitation services on behalf of an adult who has adventitious hearing impairment. It is equally challenging to assess the psychosocial and personal handicap of hearing loss on an otherwise active adult client when the assessment tools available to us may not be sensitive to the elements of life and communication faced daily by that person.

IMPORTANT ASSESSMENT FACTORS

Several factors that must be considered when assessing communication skills or the impact of hearing loss on adult clients include the following:

1. **The person's emotional response to his or her auditorily based communication difficulties.** Occasionally positive change in a client's emotional response to his or her auditory difficulties will reflect itself in increased attempts at communication and/or enhanced communication with others.

2. **A clients' most frequented communication environments.** Audiologists must realize that not all persons require an active social life, but rather they may be content to remain at home with family or a friend. Their requirements regarding aural rehabilitation services are, thus, based on such environments, and the tools for assessing communication abilities and subsequent determination of improvements or lack of them resulting from aural rehabilitation services must be sensitive to such differences among adult clients.

3. **The communication priorities of a client.** Linked to the previous factor, but important to discuss further, is the establishment of priorities by the client about his or her communication needs. In Chapters 11 and 21, this author discuss prioritization as an important part of the provision of aural rehabilitation services for older clients. If the communicative priorities of each client are the basis on which treatment services are developed and provided, then any evaluation of progress must also be based on

them. Only then can progress or lack of it be determined.

4. **Determining realistic goals for the client.** Besides establishing client needs or desires for communication as a basis for services and subsequent evaluation, the *importance of determining those that are realistic for individual clients is critical.* If, for example, a client who has profound hearing impairment has established as a priority the ability to communicate with absolute precision at social gatherings, that goal may not be realistic for that person. If the goal is held at that level, treatment may be doomed to failure and the evaluation will reflect little or no improvement. However, a realistic goal of increased skill in social communication within optimal environments may be reached, and pre- and postrehabilitation evaluation may reveal those gains. This is not to say, however, that goals should be set so low that improvement in communication skills is inevitable.

The point stressed here is that goals for individual clients should not be set so high that failure is probable. A perceptive audiologist will be aware of the communicative heights to be attempted. The most important criteria for goals, however, are the communication needs of individual clients. The author finds that most adults are realistic in their expectations and in their knowledge of their limitations. It is sad to observe audiologists who have established the same aural rehabilitation goals for all clients or, perhaps, had established no real individual goals at all at the initiation of aural rehabilitation services for a group of adult clients.

ASSESSMENT

ELEMENTS TO BE ASSESSED

Research designed to investigate factors that influence the ability of persons who have hearing impairment to communicate has historically included such areas as the visibility of phonemes of speech, intelligence versus lipreading ability, factors of memory, synthetic abilities among good and poor lipreaders, and others. Those and other studies have led to the conclusion that a person's language level is one of the most important factors that influence compensation for a hearing loss (Lowell, 1969). This not only includes vocabulary level, but also a client's ability to use the level of language efficiently that he or she possesses. This involves the rules of language and the ability to make closure when not all of the linguistic information is available within a given moment of communication. This also inevitably involves factors in the processing of linguistic information from moment to moment.

Impressive mental gymnastics are involved when a person who has hearing impairment is required to take the threads of phonemic and linguistic information obtained through an impaired receptive auditory system and combine them with what is received visually (if the speaker is visible) and derive information from what is being said. To measure that ability appears to be equally difficult, especially when we are dealing with complex older clients who differ greatly in relation to:

1. Their response to their hearing impairment,
2. Their communication environments,
3. Their response to noise and other distractions,
4. Those with whom they communicate, and
5. The multiple interrelated parameters of peripheral and central auditory function.

These important aspects are, in one way or another, addressed in most scales of communicative function. In terms of evaluating changes in social/communication behavior, the use of such scales may also be leading us in the right direction.

In view of the complex nature of the requirements for efficient communication that may be complicated by a hearing impairment and/or advanced age, the remainder of this chapter concentrates on sorting through the factors involved in assessment of progress in communicative function for adult clients who are involved in aural rehabilitation treatment. Even though there is evident diversity among philosophies related to assessment of speechreading, general communication abilities, and other factors involved in communication by those with hearing impairment, common denominators appear to be emerging.

HISTORICAL PERSPECTIVES

Filmed Tests

Studies of filmed tests of lipreading ability have generally demonstrated that persons who have hearing impairment perform at least similar to persons who have normal hearing. Further, they have generally shown that adult clients perform as well or as poorly on such tests after completion of a speechreading treatment program as when they began. Most important, it has been demonstrated that it is difficult to separate the quality or efficiency of aural rehabilitation treatment procedures from persons' performance on these tests.

MORKOVIN LIFE SITUATION FILMS. Early filmed tests include those that were introduced in the 1940s as an attempt to both evaluate and teach lipreading. Mason (1943) developed a series of 30 silent films for lipreading instruction. Morkovin (1948) introduced the "Morkovin Life Situations Films." These films depicted various "real-life" situations for lipreading therapy that advocated a theme approach. They were also utilized as an approach to assessing lipreading skills. The films were made with sound and, for example, depicted a girl and her mother buying shoes at the shoe store, youngsters receiving dancing lessons, and Monty Montana, the cowboy movie star, demonstrating cowboy rope tricks for children. The films were generally interesting, but difficult to use either for instruction or for assessment. They, further,

became quickly dated because of the actors' clothing and mannerisms. In the majority of instances, they were certainly not suitable for work with adults.

UTLEY TEST. The first actual filmed test of lipreading was developed by Utley (1946). It has also received the majority of attention by researchers. This silent film was developed from the most frequently used words in Thorndike's *First Word Dictionary*. It is not known whether the use of those words hindered the validity of her test or not, as the words contained in that dictionary were the most frequently written words, not the most frequently spoken.

The test contained three parts. *Part 1* utilized words and *Part 2* contained sentences. Both Parts 1 and 2 were filmed in black and white. *Part 3* was a five-part story test filmed in color. Utley investigated the reliability of the forms of the tests and found that in Parts 1 and 2, the internal reliability of each portion was high enough to be significant. For standardization, those parts were presented to 761 subjects who were deaf or hard of hearing, for purposes of standardization.

The validity of the Utley test has been investigated on numerous occasions. DiCarlo and Kataja (1951), for example, found that the test was probably, although not necessarily, reliable. Even though they found a 0.77 correlation level between the Utley test and the Morkovin "Family Dinner" film, they questioned the validity of both tests. They felt, because of the method of filming and its length and speed of presentation, that the test primarily assessed persistence and the frustration tolerance of the viewers.

O'Neill and Stephens (1959) studied the Mason, the Utley, and the Morkovin films. They did not find a significant correlation between the responses for viewers of the Utley and Morkovin films, but did find a correlation between the Mason films and Parts 1 and 2 of the Utley film test and the Morkovin films. They concluded that the lack of correlation between the Utley Tests and the Morkovin films was probably because the Morkovin films were originally constructed as a series of lessons and not as an assessment tool.

Simmons (1959) concluded that the Utley and Mason films seem to measure something related to lipreading ability. But, the "something" was thought to be only a vague part of the general ability of persons who have hearing impairment to communicate in face-to-face situations.

Pestone (1962) determined that no filmed tests met all the criteria that are needed in a test. She felt that a filmed test should utilize presentation of material by two speakers—one male and one female. Further, she advocated that the films should be in color to make them more realistic, two equivalent forms should be developed to facilitate measurements, and the test should have a wide range of difficulty and be easy to score. Pestone used this philosophy to develop a filmed test that utilized sentences evenly divided between statements and questions. She found the test to be reliable, but it has not been heard to any extent since the early 1960s.

JOHN TRACY TEST OF LIPREADING. Donnelly and Marshall (1967) developed a filmed multiple-choice test of lipreading using the John Tracy Clinic Test of Lipreading. The test was filmed in color and with sound. College-age students who had hearing impairment were utilized as subjects in a study to assess its reliability. The subjects individually controlled the intensity of the sound.

Multiple choice answers were based on (1) the correct answer, (2) the most frequently incorrect response of persons tested previously, and (3) the second most frequently missed. Donnelly and Marshall found the test to be reliable.

SUMMARY OF THIS SECTION. Even though filmed tests of lipreading have consistently shown at least some level of reliability on test-retest and between tests, their validity has continually been questioned. Perhaps Lashley (1961) stated it best by saying, "It is possible that validity of lipreading tests will not be established until an understanding of what factors involved in lipreading are agreed upon" (p. 182). Alpiner (1978a) has listed criticisms of filmed or videotaped tests (see Table 23-1).

Other Earlier Attempts at Assessment

Other attempts at measuring speechreading or lipreading abilities included interview procedures to determine the communicative function of persons who have hearing impairment. These have included clients' lipreading ability and the notation of progress or lack of it. For example, the basis on which Simmons (1959) attempted the use of interviews rather than previous standard tests of lipreading was the lack of quantitative measures of lipreading ability. She felt this was the major problem in attempting to establish a relationship

TABLE 23–1. Criticisms of Filmed or Videotaped Tests of Lipreading.

- The distractions caused by the tester on the film holding up a card with the number of the test item.
- The stolid appearance of the presenter.
- The usual presentation mode of showing the speaker from the shoulders upward.
- The erratic rate of presentation of stimulus materials.
- The dated clothing and hair styles which may prove distracting to the client.

Reprinted with permission from Alpiner, J. G. (1978). *Handbook of adult rehabilitative audiology* (p. 36). Baltimore: Williams and Wilkins.

between lipreading ability and other physical or psychological factors.

INTERVIEW METHODS. Simmons (1959) used five judges who were qualified therapists of adults who were hard of hearing to attempt to determine the reliability of an interview method for assessing lipreading abilities. Subjects included 12 men and 12 women. All possessed hearing loss with a mean pure-tone average of 33.8 dB and mean speech recognition scores of 58.7%. The rating scale devised was based on three simple categories of "good, average, and poor" lipreading abilities. Each classification had its own set of criteria for determining the level of skill. The judges engaged in "everyday" conversation with the subjects, keeping their voices at an intensity level that was below the speech reception threshold of each subject. Comparison of the judges' decision as to lipreading ability of individual clients yielded a relationship of 0.92, indicating a high positive correlation.

If such correlations can be maintained, perhaps such interview techniques could be used with success. Close monitoring of the intensity level of the judge's voice below, at, or above clients' thresholds could yield important pre- and posttreatment information about their ability to utilize visual and supplemental auditory clues in everyday speech. The most difficult aspect when dealing with such methods, however, is the scoring procedure. It is suggested that further investigation of such approaches be made relative to their possible routine use with older adults.

MULTIPLE-CHOICE TESTS. Other procedures, such as that developed by Hutton (1959), included the use of multiple-choice tests. Hutton's procedure, for example, utilized two simultaneous word presentations in visual-only, auditory-only, and auditory-visual modes. The subjects were asked to choose the correct word from a multiple-choice answer sheet of eight words.

Furthermore, Black, O'Reilly, and Peck (1963) developed a self-administered multiple-choice procedure that was presented on silent film. The filmed stimulus items were used for training in lipreading. The projector speed could be slowed or speeded. Subjects were first tested using the normal speed of projection. The film was then slowed to 15% and subjects were tested again. The subjects, after reviewing their scores, were permitted to adjust the speed of the projector until they could achieve a score of 100%. Results revealed that even with that brief period of practice, subjects improved their ability to lipread even when viewing a different speaker. Although this procedure was basically self-administered training in lipreading, the assessment aspect was unique.

ASSESSMENT THROUGH BISENSORY MODALITIES

The current consensus is that assessment of the ability of persons who have hearing impairment to understand speech should combine use of vision and audition. Innumerable studies confirm the reciprocal complement of vision and audition (Binnie, 1973; Binnie, Montgomery, & Jackson, 1974; Duffy, 1967; Erber, 1971, 1975, 1979; Ewertsen, Nielsen, & Nielsen, 1970; Hutton, Curry, & Armstrong, 1959; Miller & Nicely, 1955; O'Neill, 1954; Sumby & Pollack, 1954; Van Uden, 1960). Their results, as do the results of numbers of other studies, continually confirm the benefits of bisensory modalities for speech reception. No matter how restricted the auditory component, the complement continues to exist. If an individual client's ability to recognize the visimes of speech or to discriminate auditorily is to be assessed, then those sensory modalities must be isolated. If assessment of the ability to communicate is held as a priority, however, then both vision and audition should be combined.

Use of Live-Voice Tests

The criticisms of filmed or videotaped tests of lipreading cited earlier by Alpiner (1978a) are valid. Further, people do not communicate with others via film or videotape in the course of everyday conversations. Therefore, the use of live voice for the presentation of assessment materials to determine skill in the reception of speech by clients who have hearing impairment is generally preferred, although the problem remains of maintaining a constant stimulus level when live voice is used.

For live-voice testing, the use of sentences is preferred over single words. Sentences as stimulus items most closely approximate the types of stimuli found in the everyday lives of clients who have hearing impairment. Sentences also lend themselves to greater ease of scoring. Even though paragraphs most closely resemble the conversations that people listen to in the everyday world, they are more difficult to score and other compounding factors such as auditory and visual memory may influence the results. For a more accurate determination of skill in auditory-visual reception of speech, sentences continue to be beneficial.

Sentence materials that lend themselves well to assessment of speechreading skills include the Central Institute for the Deaf (CID) Everyday Speech Sentences (Davis & Silverman, 1970), the Denver Scale Quick Test (Alpiner, 1978b), and WSU Sentence Test of Speechreading Ability (Hull, 1992). All are in the Appendixes of this book.

The CID Everyday Speech Sentences include 10 lists of 10 sentences each. The sentences vary in length and are common to most adults. (See the Appendixes of this book for the CID lists of sentences, Lists A through J.)

The Denver Scale Quick Test is made up of 20 simple sentences, 8 questions, and 12 declarative statements. Although no information is available regarding consistency of sentence ease or difficulty or consistency of phonemic visibility, the list lends itself well to assessing client abilities in the identification of sentence material. It is suggested by Alpiner (1978b) that the test be administered under the visual-only condition, although it can be used with an auditory-visual mode. Each stimulus item has a value of 5%, and scoring is based only on identifying the thought of the sentence rather than on verbatim repetition. (See the Denver Scale Quick Test in the Appendixes of this book.)

The WSU Sentence Test of Speechreading (1992) is based on a study by Hull and Alpiner (1976) in which they investigated linguistic factors in speechreading. Three lists of 12 sentences each were developed based on a sentence length of 8 words, which was found by Taaffe and Wong (1957) to be as visually intelligible as shorter sentences. Because shorter sentences are limited in content and complexity, it was felt that longer sentences would provide a greater opportunity for comparisons between conditions and allow for greater experimental manipulation. Further, the sentences were developed according to specific requirements (see Table 23-2).

Scoring is based on the thought, or idea, of the sentence. Each sentence is valued at 3 points for a total possible score of 60 points and it is suggested that the lists be presented live voice at a just-audible level for the client (see the Appendixes for the WSU Sentences). If a verbatim scoring is desired, then each word of each sentence is valued at 1 point each.

Presentation of Sentence Material

Recorded videotaped assessment materials can be presented in the same room as the client at a distance of approximately 5 feet, with the voice of the tester adjusted so that it is just audible to the client. The speaker must be videotaped with head and shoulders in full view, with plain background, and no shadows. The determination of audibility can be made by asking the client to close his or her eyes while the tester presents sample words or sentences that were recorded on the same videotape.

TABLE 23–2. Guidelines to Development of Sentences for WSU Sentence Test of Speechreading.

- An equal number of interrogative and declarative sentences (45 each).
- All sentences contained an equal number of words (8).
- All words within each sentence were taken from the Jones and Wepman (1966) list of 1,000 most commonly spoken words.
- Parts of speech within each sentence were varied as much as possible in terms of position, so identifying cues could not be obtained from word position.
- Percentage of words among parts of speech was based on norms established by Templin (1957) regarding the structure of the English language.
- No common phrases such as "good morning," "in the U.S.," or "how are you" were used in the sentences developed.
- No contractions that might be confusing in terms of completing written answers were included.
- No bisyllabic proper nouns that might be confusing were included.
- No highly visible words that could influence the visual intelligibility of sentences were included (Fisher, 1968).

The client is to judge when the tester's voice is audible, but the stimulus items are not understood.

Another method of live-voice presentation that has been found to be useful is the use of a sound-treated audiometric suite where a window separates the tester from the client. If lighting can be adjusted so that the face and shoulders of the tester are clearly observable, the free-field speech system of the audiometer can be used for presentation of the auditory portion. Further, the just-audible level, or other intensity levels, of voice presentation can be more easily established and the intensity levels varied when needed. The most difficult aspect of the use of an audiometric sound-treated suite is the visibility of the tester, particularly through the two to four panels of glass between prefabricated enclosures.

SCALES OF COMMUNICATIVE FUNCTION

A viable approach to assessing the handicap of hearing loss in adult clients, as well as changes that

occur as the result of aural rehabilitation treatment, are rating scales of communicative function. Selected scales that have been tested and published over the past 30 years are discussed next.

Hearing Handicap Scale

One forerunner of the current scales is the Hearing Handicap Scale (HHS) developed by High, Fairbanks, and Glorig (1964). Both forms of this scale are presented in the Appendixes of this book. As can be seen, the scale concentrates on questions related to communication—that is, the impact of hearing impairment on communication in various environments. It does not delve into other aspects related to hearing, such as the social or psychological impact of hearing impairment, which appears to be one of its weaknesses (Giolas, 1970; Sanders, 1975). Responses for this scale include the options of (1) almost always, (2) usually, (3) sometimes, (4) rarely, and (5) almost never.

Even though the scale is somewhat limited by probing only into various communication settings (including the impact of distance on communication) those questions do lend themselves well for interviewing adult clients who have hearing impairment. Clients' subjective judgments about their ability to function communicatively within typical environments provide important treatment data. Because there are two forms for the scale that are similar in terms of the area of communication queried, the scale can be used pre- and postassessment to determine if clients' opinions of their ability to communicate in various similar environments have changed for the positive or the negative. Further, the pretreatment administration can, as with other scales, be used to guide the emphasis of treatment and procedures. Lack of the psychosocial impact of hearing impairment in the scale is, as stated before, a drawback to its possible usefulness. It does, however, provide some specific information on clients' attitudes regarding their ability to function in common everyday communication environments.

The Denver Scale of Communication Function

The Denver Scale of Communication Function (Alpiner, Chevrette, Glascoe, Metz, & Olsen, 1978) is an attitude scale that provides adults who have hearing impairment the opportunity to make subjective judgments relative to the impact of their hearing impairment on relationships with family, their ability to communicate with others, image of self, and the impact of the hearing impairment on the social and/or vocational aspects of life and other areas. (This scale is presented in the Appendixes of this book.)

It is suggested by Alpiner et al. (1978) that the scale be administered prior to initiating aural rehabilitation treatment so that a client's responses will not be influenced by discussions that take place in the process. Clients respond to 25 statements on a 7-level semantic differential continuum from 1 (agree) to 7 (disagree). The scale contains four categories: family, self, social-vocational, and general communication experience. Alpiner (1978b) recommended a time limit of 15 minutes for administration of the scale.

Client responses are recorded on the Denver Scale Profile form (Alpiner et al., 1978). The abscissa numbers represent the statements on the scale, and the ordinate points represent the client's responses to each statement, ranging from agree to disagree. The responses are plotted along the abscissa and lines are drawn from response to response. The profile is studied by the client and audiologist in relation to the communication problems that need attention. That information is then used to design individual client's aural rehabilitation treatment programs.

One aspect of the scale has been confusing to some clients and their ratings are, therefore, probably affected. That aspect is that the middle point on the semantic differential, exactly between 1 (agree) and 7 (disagree), is meant to be marked if the statement on the scale is, to an individual client, "irrelevant or unassociated" with his or her communication situation. Some clients, perhaps not understanding the instructions, have placed marks in that position believing that their response would then mean that it is somewhere between agree and disagree, perhaps as a "maybe."

Even though this scale is not designed specifically with the older adult in mind, it is applicable and useful for pinpointing areas of communication that concern individual clients. These are important in planning the treatment program. The majority of the Denver Scale is also applicable for noninstitutionalized older adults. Zarnoch and Alpiner (1977) have developed a modified version of the Denver Scale designed for the older adult who is confined to a health care facility (nursing home). This scale is discussed later.

Test of Actual Performance

A brief scale to assess the communication habits of persons who have hearing impairment has been developed by Koniditsiotis (1971). (The test is shown in the Appendixes of this book.) The purpose of the design of the test was to study the extent of a relationship between the amount of hearing loss as determined by pure-tone and speech audiometry and the actual disability experienced by a person with hearing loss. The test contains 7 items that are scored as 1 (poor), 2 (adequate), 3 (good), or 4 (excellent). Little correlation between the test judgments and actual hearing impairment has been found. The lowest correlation was found when comparing the test judgments and client scores for speech discrimination.

The strongest limitation to the test is that the test judgments are made by the clinicians who work with the clients and not by the clients, themselves.

The Hearing Measurement Scale

Noble and Atherley (1970) devised the Hearing Measurement Scale (HMS), which was designed to probe the disability of hearing impairment. Even though the purpose of their scale is to assess disability of hearing loss acquired as the result of industrial noise, all of the questions lend themselves well for use with other persons, including the elderly. (This scale is shown in the Appendixes of this book.)

The scale is divided into seven sections.

Section 1: Speech Hearing

Section 2: Acuity for Nonspeech Sounds

Section 3: Localization

Section 4: Reaction to Handicap

Section 5: Speech Distortion

Section 6: Tinnitus

Section 7: Personal Opinion of Hearing Loss

The HMS contains a valuable assortment of questions that not only aid in the determination of a client's opinions of the extent of his or her hearing impairment, but also those aspects that interfere most, and his or her reactions to the disability. A set of instructions accompany the assessment forms. Noble and Atherley (1970) stressed that the scale cannot be administered without reading the instruction manual.

Profile Questionnaire for Rating Communicative Performance

A Profile Questionnaire for Communicative Performance was developed by Sanders (1975). Two aspects of the profile—"Communicative Performance in a Home Environment" and "Communicative Performance in a Social Environment"— are quite applicable for older adults. A third profile is the questionnaire entitled "Performance in an Occupational Environment." The former two profiles are suitable for the noninstitutionalized older client. For older adult clients in a health care facility environment, responses to the profile relating to the home environment would need to be interpreted as being their typical environment (The profiles on social and home environments are presented in the Appendixes of this book.)

These profiles and the Hearing Handicap Scale (High et al., 1964) discussed earlier differ from the Denver Scale because they probe into specific communication environments, rather than a client's attitudes regarding his or her ability to communicate. All, however, provide valuable pre- and posttreatment information for assessment of progress or lack of it.

The scales or profiles discussed previously by Alpiner et al. (1978), High et al. (1964), Noble and Atherley (1970), and Sanders (1975) can be used appropriately with noninstitutionalized adult clients. They can also be used with older clients who are confined at home or in a health care facility, but in those instances, the questions must be interpreted in relation to their frequented environment(s).

ASSESSMENT BASED ON COMMUNICATIVE PRIORITIES

Priority-based assessment, developed, among others, by Hull (1982), can be used with both community-based adults and elderly clients and confined older adults. Its premise is that a client's highest priority communication environments should be stressed in planning aural rehabilitation treatment and assessment of successes or lack of them should also be based on those environments. A scale that addresses the priorities of the client is the WSU Communication Appraisal and Priorities Profile (CAPP) (Hull, 1992), found in the Appendixes of this book.

Prior to the initiation of treatment, clients are asked to rank the difficulty they experience in a variety of communication environments. The ratings of difficulty range from 1 (no problem) through 2 (only in specific instances) to 3 (definite problem). A section for "Other" is included on the form in anticipation that an environment not included in the list may be felt to be important to an individual client. After they have rated those 13 communication environments, they are asked to choose those that are most important to them. When that task is completed, they are requested to rank environment in terms of their priority, from highest to lowest. The priorities, if realistic for individual clients, are used as the basis for the design of their treatment program and evaluation of successes or lack of progress.

At the conclusion of a specified number of treatment sessions, clients are again asked to complete an identical form and rank the communication environments in terms of the difficulty they experience in them. The client and the audiologist then review both the pre- and posttest ratings, particularly noting communication environments considered high priority by the client. Success or lack of it is based only on changes in client attitudes relative to their priority environments. It is interesting to note, however, that on occasion, if positive progress is noted on one priority item, there appears to be a progression of attitude change regarding other "near" environments, as they are ranked according to their difficulty. For example, if participation in church group meetings was rated as the highest priority communication environment by an individual client, but other "near" environments such as other formal meetings, at the

dinner table, and at parties or other social events were also ranked as being a definite problem, but not as high of a priority, the client's rating in those other environments also may begin to change.

In any event, evaluation of progress or lack of it based on clients' priority communication environments appears to have merit. Further, clients feel a sense of confidence in audiologists who hold their priorities as preeminent in aural rehabilitation treatment and evaluation.

PROFILES

Hearing Performance Inventory

The assessment tool entitled the Hearing Performance Inventory, was developed by Giolas, Owens, Lamb, and Schubert (1979). It probes six areas that can either influence or involve communication. Those areas are:

1. Understanding the speech of various talkers;
2. Intensity, or the person's awareness of social and nonsocial sounds in his or her environment;
3. Response to auditory failure;
4. Social, or the person's ability to converse in groups of two or more persons in social environments;
5. Personal, or the person's feelings about his or her hearing impairment in relation to its personal impact; and
6. Occupational.

This inventory can be used effectively with all ages of adults. Because of its length, partial use of only some categories may be needed to establish priorities for aural rehabilitation treatment and for assessment.

The Communication Profile for the Hearing Impaired

The Communication Profile for the Hearing Impaired (CPHI) (Demorest & Erdman, 1987), was, according to the authors, designed to provide a systematic and comprehensive assessment of a broad range of communication problems. It was developed at Walter Reed Army Medical Center for use with patients in their Aural Rehabilitation Program. The profile was developed for use with all ages of adults who have hearing impairment. Although it was developed for use with a military population, the authors chose not to use materials that are specific to military life.

The final version of the CPHI contains 145 items and 25 scores. The scales of the profile are organized into four areas: (1) Communication Performance, (2) Communication Environment, (3) Communication Strategies, and (4) Personal Adjustment. The scoring process for the scales was chosen to have low scores always indicating potential problem areas regardless of the name of the scale and identifying areas in need of rehabilitative intervention. When the scores are plotted graphically, it permits a rapid visual scan of the profile. Thus, according to Demorest and Erdman (1987), a low score on Self-Acceptance, for example, indicates a low level of self-acceptance, but a low score on Communication Need indicates a high level of need for communication. The Communication Profile for the Hearing Impaired is presented in the Appendixes of this book.

SCALES FOR OLDER ADULTS WHO ARE HEARING IMPAIRED

It is evident that all scales discussed in this chapter can be used in assessing or discussing the impact of hearing loss on various aspects of older adults' lives. Aside from the sections that are specific to one's occupational life, most others are applicable. In the long run, because the majority of adults who audiologists serve are beyond age 60 years, all of the adult scales must necessarily be designed to serve them to some degree.

Two scales have been designed specifically for the confined elderly client. One is the Denver Scale of Communication Function for Senior Citizens Living in Retirement Centers (Zarnoch & Alpiner, 1977) and the other is the Hearing Handicap Inventory for the Elderly (HHIE) (Ventry &

Weinstein, 1982). Both are in the Appendixes of this book.

The Denver Scale of Communication Function for Senior Citizens

The Denver Scale of Communication Function for Senior Citizens Living in Retirement Centers is the result of a modification of the Denver Scale of Communication Function and was developed by Zarnoch and Alpiner (1977). The content of the questions has been designed to be suitable for confined elderly clients. Further, rather than being self-administered as in the original Denver Scale (Alpiner, 1978b; Alpiner et al., 1978), the questions are presented to the clients, who respond verbally. This provides control for variables, such as a client's inability to respond to written tests, or fatigue. The Scale for Senior Citizens is based on seven major questions regarding their feelings about themselves and their communication abilities. Each question is followed by probe effect questions that delve more extensively into the principal questions. The number of probe effect questions range from two to five, depending on the principal question. To determine the relevance of the principal question and the probe effect questions, exploration effect questions are also asked.

Each of the seven major questions, including the probe effect and exploration effect questions, is categorized according to family, emotional, other persons, general communication, self-concept, group situations, or rehabilitation theme. Responses are based on yes or no answers, and scores are indicated by a plus or a minus. Scoring is identical in relation to the principal questions, the probe effects, and exploration effects.

As stated earlier, the Denver Scale for Senior Citizens appears very useful for interviewing a confined elderly person on a pre- and posttreatment basis. The only drawback observed by this author is the scoring procedure. A semantic differential format that allows for degrees of yes-to-no responses is generally more desirable for any age of client. Otherwise, the scale provides valuable information for the development of aural rehabilitation treatment programs and evaluation of progress based on the attitudes a client has about him- or herself.

The Hearing Handicap Inventory for the Elderly

The Hearing Handicap Inventory for the Elderly (HHIE) (Ventry & Weinstein, 1982), according to the authors, represents a disability assessment technique designed to quantify the emotional and social/situational effects of hearing impairment on noninstitutionalized elderly persons. They state that this inventory differs from other instruments in that the focus is on the psychosocial effects of hearing impairment specific to the elderly. The inventory consists of 25 questions that address the client's social and personal life, identified as **E** (emotional), and **S** (social) on the questionnaire.

The HHIE was studied to compare self-assessed hearing disability utilizing that inventory with pure-tone sensitivity and word recognition utility among 100 elderly individuals (Weinstein & Ventry, 1983). The authors found a high correlation between the HHIE responses and subjects' pure-tone sensitivity loss. They found significantly less correlation between the HHIE and word recognition scores. The HHIE (Ventry & Weinstein, 1982) is in the Appendixes of this book.

EVALUATING COMMUNICATIVE FUNCTION

Whatever method is used to determine if a person who has hearing impairment can perceive speech, communicative function in some form is being evaluated. The methods may include (1) determining if phonemes, words, or sentences can be recognized visually; (2) determining if residual hearing can be utilized to recognize units of speech; (3) determining if both vision and hearing can be used to recognize speech; or (4) determining if various factors of language can be utilized to determine the meaning of statements. *What matters is the emphasis placed on the interpretation of the results of the evaluation.*

Phoneme Identification

If lipreading ability for phonemes is intended to be measured, then a visible mouth, mandible, and neck may be all that is necessary to determine if a person can identify the various vowels, consonants, and diphthongs as they are viewed on film, on slides, or in ink-drawn pictures. If the score that is derived is presented as that person's score for the recognition of phonemes of American English in isolation, then it would be described accurately.

If the score was described as a measure of communicative ability, however, then it would be misrepresented, as would that client's probable ability to communicate. The emphasis would have been inappropriately placed, although a high score may indicate that the person has less difficulty recognizing phonemes of speech, which is, indeed, a part of communication. The score does not, however, tell us how well that person may be able to recognize those same phonemes within continuous discourse. The score also does not tell us how well the person can communicate in his or her frequented communicative environments.

Word Identification

Tests of lipreading ability that include filmed, videotaped, or live visual-only presentations of single words out of context as test items do not provide information about the ability of a person who has hearing impairment to recognize words within continuous discourse or his or her ability to communicate in various social or business environments. However, the scores are still used by some to predict abilities in social communication, even though they may only provide information regarding a person's visual recognition of those words. On the other hand, this procedure can provide important bits of diagnostic information regarding auditory and visual recognition of speech. If the mode of presentation includes both the auditory and visual portions of the stimulus items, then information may be obtained regarding a person's ability to utilize the additive complement of vision to audition and vice versa.

Although the components discussed previously can provide important information regarding the ability of an individual who has hearing impairment to utilize audition and vision in the recognition of phoneme and word elements, they do not provide information as to that person's ability to communicate in his or her most frequented environments. This has been a historic drawback to these test procedures.

Sentences and Paragraphs

The use of sentences and paragraphs as stimulus items for assessment of a person's ability to communicate in spite of hearing impairment have been recommended. (Hirsh, 1952) but, again, the use of sentences still leaves the audiologist without important information regarding a client's ability to function in his or her communication environments. Assessment of a person's ability to receive and interpret at least the thought of sentences does, however, provide information on that person's ability to receive and synthesize content while using the visual and auditory modalities.

The use of paragraphs in examining a person's ability to use visual and auditory clues is generally compounded by such factors as memory and attentiveness. Difficulties in administration of test batteries that utilize paragraphs, standardization of the tests, client variables such as a person's emotional response to his or her hearing impairment, and the testing environment, make the use of paragraphs relatively inefficient as measures of communicative efficiency or of improvements in

communicative ability. This is further compounded by problems of scoring.

Vision Versus Audition

The visual-only mode of presentation of test batteries generally is not satisfactory for determining efficiency of communication. Few adults lack all usable hearing, no matter how severe their speech recognition problem. **Any formal assessment and treatment procedure should include the use of both audition (including amplification) and vision**. Because clients will seldom find themselves in situations where they will not be using both hearing and vision, any assessment of the ability to receive and interpret verbal information should emphasize the advantage of the bisensory mode of speech reception. Among persons with severe visual disorders, assessment and treatment will obviously involve the use of residual hearing as the primary sensory modality.

COMMUNICATION SCALES AND PROFILES

Scales of communicative function, including those that stress attitudes of people who have hearing impairment and those concentrating on situations or communication environments, seem to be going in the right direction. This is particularly true when attempting to assess the communicative behaviors and needs of an older client. The majority of the scales and profiles appear to be based on the important fact that the audiologist is dealing with adult clients who have communication needs and priorities unique to them. Even though many persons may benefit from work on enhancing visual and/or auditory awareness and skill, they also desire that the efforts involved have meaning for them and that the treatments have relevance to their specific communication needs.

Assessment and treatment based on the feelings, attitudes, and priority communication environments of elderly clients will surely add an element of maturity and relevance to aural rehabilitation services. These procedures have brought clinicians a long way from the days of the filmed tests of lipreading.

Validity

The scales of communication function face similar questions of validity as have tests of lipreading and other procedures. Test-retest reliability among the various scales and profiles has been generally found to be acceptable. A major question that is inevitably asked, however, is: Do audiologists know that clients are answering the questions or responding to the statements honestly? In that regard, the reliability of a client is in question. Hopefully, a wise audiologist will be able to, in the majority of cases, "see through" the client who appears to be attempting to fool the audiologist or, perhaps more regrettably, fool him- or herself.

Occasionally, there are clients who provide answers they feel the provider of services *wants* to hear. Clients do not like to see audiologists fail, either. It is up to the audiologist to assure clients that their answers or responses are to be honest ones. How else can real progress, or lack of it, be noted? How can adjustments in the treatment program be made, if they are needed?

The question of validity is, indeed, for lack of a better phrase, a valid one. However, Alpiner (1978b) responded to that question well when he stated that, "Their [the scales or profiles] successful use depends on the audiologists' judgment, not on tests of validity" (p. 32).

A COMPREHENSIVE APPROACH TO ASSESSMENT OF COMMUNICATIVE FUNCTION

It is difficult to recommend an approach to assessment that can determine the degree of disability that adult clients are experiencing as a result of an auditory disorder, that also assesses the results of

aural rehabilitation treatment. In the end, however, the audiologist is responsible for determining the aspects of communicative function to be assessed and treated, as well as the assessment of the value of the treatment procedures utilized.

In this regard, a comprehensive approach to assessment is recommended. This includes:

1. Observing the results of the case history relative to the possible causes of the auditory deficit, its duration, and the current social and environmental status of the elderly client.
2. Utilizing audiometric results, particularly the type, degree, and configuration of the hearing loss, and very importantly the results of assessment of speech recognition.
3. Assessing the results of a hearing aid evaluation and the possible benefits of amplification as determined both by the audiologist and the client.
4. Assessing a clients' ability to utilize visual clues with minimal auditory information. This assessment may include (1) monosyllabic words, (2) sentences, and (3) everyday conversation. Sentence lists recommended are the Denver Quick Test of Lipreading, the CID Everyday Sentences, or the WSU Sentence Test of Speechreading.
5. Assessing the impact of the hearing impairment by the use of one of the scales of communication function. Those recommended are (1) the Denver Scale of Communication Function, (2) the Denver Scale of Communication Function for Senior Citizens, (3) the Profile Questionnaires (Home and Social), (4) the Communicative Priorities Assessment, or (5) the WSU Communication Appraisal and Priorities Profile (CAPP), all of which are in the Appendixes of this text.
6. Plans for aural rehabilitation treatment and posttreatment assessment should solely be based on a clients' communicative needs and priorities. Only then will the audiologist be adding validity to his or her treatment goals.

"Cookbook" approaches usually do nothing more than consume valuable time.

7. Most importantly, clinicians must listen to what clients are telling them as it relates to the difficulties they are experiencing and the services that are being provided on their behalf. If they are benefitting from those services, they will let us know.

REFERENCES

Alpiner, J. G. (1978a). Evaluation of communication function. In J. G. Alpiner (Ed.), *Handbook of adult rehabilitative audiology* (pp. 236–252). Baltimore: Williams and Wilkins.

Alpiner, J. G. (1978b). *Handbook of adult rehabilitative audiology* (p. 36). Baltimore: Williams and Wilkins.

Alpiner, J. G., Chevrette, W., Glascoe, G., Metz, M., & Olsen, B. (1978). The Denver Scale of Communication Function. In J. G. Alpiner (Ed.), *Adult rehabilitative audiology* (pp. 36, 53–56). Baltimore: Williams and Wilkins.

Binnie, C. A. (1973). Bi-sensory articulation functions for normal hearing and sensorineural hearing loss patients. *Journal of the Academy of Rehabilitative Audiology, 6*, 43–53.

Binnie, C. A., Montgomery, A. A., & Jackson, P. L. (1974). Auditory and visual contributions to the perception of consonants. *Journal of Speech and Hearing Research, 17*, 619–630.

Black, J. W., O'Reilly, P. P., & Peck, L. (1963). Self-administered training in lipreading. *Journal of Speech and Hearing Disorders, 28*, 183–186.

Davis, H., & Silverman, S. R. (1970). *Hearing and deafness.* New York: Holt, Rinehart and Winston.

Demorest, M. E., & Erdman, S. A. (1987). Development of the communication profile for the hearing impaired. *Journal of Speech and Hearing Disorders, 52*, 129–143.

DiCarlo, L. M., & Kataja, R. (1951). An analysis of the Utley Lipreading Test. *Journal of Speech and Hearing Disorders, 16*, 226–240.

Donnelly, K. G., & Marshall, W. J. (1967). Development of a multiple-choice test of lipreading. *Journal of Speech and Hearing Research, 10*, 565–569.

Duffy, J. K. (1967). Audio-visual speech audiometry and a new audio and audio-visual speech perception index. *Maico Audiological Series, 5*, 9.

Erber, N. P. (1971). Auditory and audiovisual reception of words in low-frequency noise by children with normal hearing and by children with impaired hearing. *Journal of Speech and Hearing Research, 14*, 496–512.

Erber, N. P. (1975). Auditory-visual perception of speech. *Journal of Speech and Hearing Disorders, 40*, 481–492.

Erber, N. P. (1979). Auditory-visual perception of speech with reduced opitical clarity. *Journal of Speech and Hearing Research, 22*, 212–223.

Ewertsen, H. W., Nielsen, H. B., & Neilsen, S. S. (1970). Audio-visual speech perception. *Acta Otolaryngologica 263* (Suppl.), 229–230

Giolas, T. G. (1970). The measurement of hearing handicap: A point of view. *Maico Audiological Library Series, 8*, 6.

Giolas, T. G., Owens, E., Lamb, S. H., & Schubert, E. E. (1979). Hearing performance inventory. *Journal of Speech and Hearing Disorders, 44*, 169–195.

High, W. S., Fairbanks, G., & Glorig, A. (1964). Scale for self-assessment of hearing handicap. *Journal of Speech and Hearing Disorders, 29*, 215–230.

Hirsh, I. J. (1952). *The measurement of hearing.* New York: McGraw-Hill.

Hull, R. H. (1971, November). *Sentence test of speechreading.* Paper presented at the annual convention of the American Speech and Hearing Association, Houston.

Hull, R. H. (1982). *Rehabilitative audiology.* New York: Grune & Stratton.

Hull, R. H. (1992). In R. H. Hull (Ed.), *Aural rehabilitation* (pp. 305–319). San Diego: Singular Publishing Group.

Hull, R. H., & Alpiner, J. G. (1976). The effect of syntactic word variations on the predictability of sentence content in speechreading. *Journal of the Academy of Rehabilitative Audiology, 9*, 42–56.

Hutton, C. (1959). Combining auditory and visual stimuli in aural rehabilitation. *Volta Review, 6*, 316–319.

Hutton, C., Curry, E. T., & Armstrong, M. B. (1959). Semidiagnostic test materials for aural rehabilitation. *Journal of Speech and Hearing Disorders, 24*, 318–329.

Koniditsiotis, C. Y. (1971). The use of hearing tests to provide information about the extent to which an individual's hearing loss handicaps him. *Maico Audiological Series, 9*, 10.

Lashley, K. S. (1961). The problem of serial order in behavior. In S. Saporta (Ed.), *Psycholinguistics* (pp. 180–198). New York: Holt, Rinehart and Winston.

Lowell, E. L. (1969). Rehabilitation of auditory disorders. *Human communication and its disorders—An overview* (Monograph No. 10). Bethesda, MD: National Advisory Neurological Diseases and Stroke Council, National Institutes of Health.

Mason, M. K. (1943). A Cinematic technique for testing visual speech comprehension. *Journal of Speech Disorders, 8*, 271–278.

Miller, G. A., & Nicely, P. E. (1955). An analysis of perceptual confusions among some English consonants. *Journal of the Acoustical Society of America, 27*, 338–352.

Morkovin, B. S. (1948). *Life-situation speechreading through the cooperation of senses* (film). University of Southern California, Los Angeles.

Noble, W. G. (1978). *Assessment of impaired hearing: A critique and a new method.* New York: Academic Press.

Noble, W. G. & Atherley, G. R. C. (1970). The hearing measurement scale: A questionnaire for the assessment of auditory disability. *Journal of Audiology Research, 10*, 229–250.

O'Neill, J. J. (1954). Contributions of the visual components of oral symbols to speech communication. *Journal of Speech and Hearing Disorders, 19*, 429–439.

O'Neill, J. J., & Stephens, M. C. (1959). Relationships among three filmed lipreading tests. *Journal of Speech and Hearing Research, 2*, 61–65.

Pestone, M. J. (1962). Selection of items for a speechreading test by means of scalogram analysis. *Journal of Speech and Hearing Disorders, 27*, 71–75.

Sanders, D. (1975). Hearing aid orientation and counseling. In M. C. Pollack (Ed.), *Amplification for the hearing impaired* (pp. 132–145). New York: Grune & Stratton.

Simmons, A. A. (1959). Factors related to lipreading. *Journal of Speech and Hearing Research, 2*, 340–352.

Sumby, W. H., & Pollack, I. (1954). Visual contributions to speech intelligibility in noise. *Journal of the Acoustical Society of America, 26*, 212–215.

Taaffe, G., & Wong, W. (1957). Study of variables in lipreading stimulus material. *John Tracy Clinic Research Papers III.* Los Angeles: The John Tracy Clinic.

Utley, J. (1946). Factors involved in the teaching and testing of lipreading ability through the use of motion pictures. *Volta Review, 38*, 657–659.

Van Uden, A. A. (1960). A Sound-perceptive method. In A. W. G. Ewing (Ed.), *The modern educational treatment of deafness* (pp. 3–19). Washington, DC: Volta Bureau.

Ventry, I. M., & Weinstein, B. E. (1982). The Hearing Handicap Inventory for the Elderly: a new tool. *Ear and Hearing, 3*, 128.

Weinstein, B. E., & Ventry, I. M. (1983). Audiometric correlates of the Hearing Handicap Inventory for the Elderly. *Journal of Speech and Hearing Disorders, 48*, 379–384.

Zarnoch, J. M., & Alpiner, J. G. (1977). *The Denver Scale of Communication Function for Senior Citizens Living in Retirement Centers.* Unpublished study, University of Denver.

END OF CHAPTER EXAMINATION QUESTIONS

CHAPTER 23

1. The author of this chapter presents factors that must be considered when assessing communication skills and/or the impact of hearing loss on adult clients. What are they? List and describe them.

2. When setting aural rehabilitation goals for a specific client, it is important that the goals
   a. be set very high so that the client must always reach a little higher than he or she can actually accomplish;
   b. be set at an achievable level so that failure is not probable;
   c. be established in accordance with the client's family's desires as they will know what is best for him or her.

3. Studies of film tests of lipreading have shown that people who are hearing impaired perform _____ as compared to people with normal hearing.
   a. better
   b. worse
   c. equally

4. Who developed the first film test of lipreading? Was it found to be valid in its ability to measure skill in lipreading?

5. In regard to the early methods for assessment of speechreading (lipreading) abilities, various procedures were utilized including (a) interview methods, (b) multiple choice tests, (c) bisensory modalities, (d) live-voice tests, and (e) use of sentence and paragraph materials. Were any of these methods found to be reliable in regard to assessing one's communication abilities? If so, which one(s)?

END OF CHAPTER ANSWER SHEET

Name   Date

CHAPTER 23

1 _____

_____

_____

_____

_____

_____

_____

2. Which one(s)?   a   b   c

3. Which one(s)?   a   b   c

4. _____

_____

_____

5. _____

_____

_____

_____

_____

_____

6. _____

_____

_____

_____

_____

7. _____

_____

_____

_____

_____

_____

_____

_____

_____

_____

_____

6. Among the various scales of communication described in this chapter, has one or more of them been found to reliably assess the ability of hearing impaired individuals to communicate? If so, which one or which ones?

7. At the conclusion of this chapter, the author presents his concept of a comprehensive approach to the assessment of hearing impaired adults. It includes seven components. What are they? List and explain them.

■ APPENDIXES ■

Materials and Scales for Assessment of Communication for the Hearing Impaired

The following appendixes present an array of assessment tools and scales of handicap that are appropriate for use with adults and elderly clients who are hearing impaired. All are designed for use with either adult or elderly clients, except for "The Communication Scale" by Kaplan, Bally, and Brandt (1990), which is designed also for younger adults, including high school and college-age students. However, it is also designed to be utilized with adults beyond college age.

The tools and scales in the appendixes include the following:

A. CID Everyday Sentences;
B. The Denver Scale Quick Test (Alpiner, 1978);
C. The WSU Sentence Test of Speechreading Ability (Hull, 1992a);
D. Hearing-Handicap Scale (High, Fairbanks, & Glorig, 1964);
E. The Denver Scale of Communication Function (Alpiner, Glascoe, Metz, & Olsen, 1971);
F. Test of Actual Performance (Konditsiotis, 1971);
G. The Hearing Measurement Scale (Noble & Atherley, 1970);
H. Profile Questionnaire for Rating Communicative Performance in a Home and Social Environment (Sanders, 1975);
I. The Denver Scale of Communication Function for Senior Citizens Living in Retirement Centers (Zarnoch & Alpiner, 1978);
J. Wichita State University (WSU) Communication Appraisal and Priorities Profile (CAPP) (Hull, 1992a);
K. The Hearing Handicap Inventory for the Elderly (Ventry & Weinstein, 1982);
L. The Communication Profile for the Hearing Impaired (Demorest & Erdman, 1987); and
M. Communication Skill Scale (Kaplan, Bally, & Brandt, 1990).

CID Everyday Sentences

LIST A

1. Walking's my favorite exercise.
2. Here's a nice quiet place to rest.
3. Our janitor sweeps the floors every night.
4. It would be much easier if everyone would help.
5. Good morning.
6. Open your window before you go to bed!
7. Do you think that she should stay out so late?
8. How do you feel about changing the time when we begin work?
9. Here we go.
10. Move out of the way!

LIST B

1. The water's too cold for swimming.
2. Why should I get up so early in the morning?
3. Here are your shoes.
4. It's raining.
5. Where are you going?
6. Come here when I call you!
7. Don't try to get out of it this time!
8. Should we let little children go to the movies by themselves?
9. There isn't enough paint to finish the room.
10. Do you want an egg for breakfast?

LIST C

1. Everybody should brush his teeth after meals.
2. Everything's all right.
3. Don't use up all the paper when you write your letter.
4. That's right.
5. People ought to see a doctor once a year.
6. Those windows are so dirty I can't see anything outside.
7. Pass the bread and butter please.
8. Don't forget to pay your bill before the first of the month.
9. Don't let the dog out of the house.
10. There's a good ball game this afternoon.

LIST D

1. It's time to go.
2. If you don't want these old magazines, throw them out.
3. Do you want to wash up?
4. It's a real dark night so watch your driving.
5. I'll carry the package for you.
6. Did you forget to shut off the water?
7. Fishing in a mountain stream is my idea of a good time.
8. Fathers spend more time with their children than they used to.
9. Be careful not to break your glasses.
10. I'm sorry.

LIST E

1. You can catch the bus across the street.
2. Call her on the phone and tell her the news.
3. I'll catch up with you later.
4. I'll think it over.
5. I don't want to go to the movies tonight.
6. If your tooth hurts that much you ought to see a dentist.
7. Put the cookie back in the box!
8. Stop fooling around!
9. Time's up.
10. How do you spell your name?

LIST F

1. Music always cheers me up.
2. My brother's in town for a short while on business.
3. We live a few miles from the main road.
4. This suit needs to go to the cleaners.
5. They ate enough green apples to make them sick for a week.
6. Where have you been all this time?
7. Have you been working hard lately?
8. There's not enough room in the kitchen for a new table.
9. Where is he?
10. Look out!

LIST G

1. I'll see you right after lunch.
2. See you later.
3. White shoes are awful to keep clean.
4. Stand there and don't move until I tell you.
5. There's a big piece of cake left over from dinner.
6. Wait for me at the corner in front of the drugstore.
7. It's no trouble at all.
8. Hurry up!
9. The morning paper didn't say anything about rain this afternoon or tonight.
10. The phone call's for you.

LIST H

1. Believe me!
2. Let's get a cup of coffee.
3. Let's get out of here before it's too late.
4. I hate driving at night.
5. There was water in the cellar after that heavy rain yesterday.
6. She'll only be a few minutes.
7. How do you know?
8. Children like candy.
9. If we don't get rain soon, we'll have no grass.
10. They're not listed in the new phone book.

LIST I

1. Where can I find a place to work?
2. I like those big red apples we always get in the fall.
3. You'll get fat eating candy.
4. The show's over.
5. Why don't they paint their walls some other color?
6. What's new?
7. What are you hiding under your coat?
8. How come I should always be the one to go first?
9. I'll take sugar and cream in my coffee.
10. Wait just a minute!

LIST J

1. Breakfast is ready.
2. I don't know what's wrong with the car, but it won't start.
3. It sure takes a sharp knife to cut this meat.
4. I haven't read a newspaper since we bought a television set.
5. Weeds are spoiling the yard.
6. Call me a little later!
7. Do you have change for a $5 bill?
8. How are you?
9. I'd like some ice cream with my pie.
10. I don't think I'll have any dessert.

■ APPENDIX B ■

The Denver Scale Quick Test

REHABILITATIVE AUDIOLOGY (ADULTS)

1. Good morning.
2. How old are you?
3. I live in (state of residence).
4. I only have one dollar.
5. There is somebody at the door.
6. Is that all?
7. Where are you going?
8. Let's have a coffee break.
9. Park your car in the lot.
10. What is your address?
11. May I help you?
12. I feel fine.
13. It is time for dinner.
14. Turn right at the corner.
15. Are you ready to order?
16. Is this charge or cash?
17. What time is it?
18. I have a headache.
19. How about going out tonight?
20. Please lend me 50 cents.

Reproduced with permission by Alpiner, J. G. Evaluation of communication function. In J. G. Alpiner (Ed.), *Handbook of adult rehabilitative audiology.* Baltimore, MD: Williams and Wilkins, l978, p. 36.

The WSU Sentence Test of Speechreading Ability

LIST 1

1. It was such a great day for hiking.
2. Have you read the sports page this morning?
3. The cost of living will make you poor.
4. He serves excellent food in all his restaurants.
5. What kind of a car do you drive?
6. The weather for the game was almost perfect.
7. Why was the picnic called off this time?
8. I like white houses with large covered porches.
9. Did the white-and-black cat have kittens?
10. Slow music always makes me feel like sleeping.
11. Why did you go there for your vacation?
12. How much snow did we have last night?

LIST 2

1. Will you come with me to see him?
2. Snow always looks pretty on the mountain side.
3. Is your whole family getting together for Thanksgiving?
4. Do you have an umbrella with you today?
5. Fathers should spend more time with their children.
6. Are you going grocery shopping while in town?
7. The wind is blowing from the northeast again.
8. It is time to go back home now.
9. Did you forget to shut off the water?
10. (Name) has been considered this state's favorite sport.
11. Where do you usually work during the winter?
12. It is a good day for playing golf.

Hull, R. H. Unpublished materials. Wichita, KS: Wichita State University, 1992a.

LIST 3

1. What time was it when you arrived?
2. Have you any brothers or sisters at home?
3. It has rained for the past 3 days.
4. Do you have a dog or a cat?
5. What does the judge say about him now?
6. A soft rain makes grass grow in spring.
7. Did you buy a new car this year?
8. You should brush your teeth three times daily.
9. Children go to school at around age 6.
10. He let the dog out of the house.
11. Hockey is often a rough and tumble sport.
12. Would you like to go to the show?

■ APPENDIX D ■

Hearing-Handicap Scale

FORM A

1. If you are 6 to 12 feet from the loudspeaker of a radio do you understand speech well?
2. Can you carry on a telephone conversation without difficulty?
3. If you are 6 to 12 feet from a television set, do you understand most of what is said?
4. Can you carry on a conversation with one other person when you are on a noisy street corner?
5. Do you hear all right when you are in a street car, airplane, bus, or train?
6. If there are noises from other voices, typewriters, traffic, music, etc., can you understand when someone speaks to you?
7. Can you understand a person when you are seated beside him and cannot see his face?
8. Can you understand if someone speaks to you while you are chewing crisp foods, such as potato chips or celery?
9. Can you carry on a conversation with one other person when you are in a noisy place, such as a restaurant or at a party?
10. Can you understand if someone speaks to you in a whisper and you can't see his or her face?
11. When you talk with a bus driver, waiter, ticket salesman, etc., can you understand all right?
12. Can you carry on a conversation if you are seated across the room from someone who speaks in a normal tone of voice?
13. Can you understand women when they talk?
14. Can you carry on a conversation with one other person when you are out of doors and it is reasonably quiet?
15. When you are in a meeting or at a large dinner table, would you know the speaker was talking if you could not see his lips moving?
16. Can you follow the conversation when you are at a large dinner table or in a meeting with a small group?
17. If you are seated under the balcony of a theater or auditorium, can you hear well enough to follow what is going on?
18. When you are in a large formal gathering (a church, lodge, lecture hall, etc.) can you hear what is said when the speaker *does not* use a microphone?
19. Can you hear the telephone ring when you are in the room where it is located?
20. Can you hear warning signals, such as automobile horns, railway crossing bells, or emergency vehicle sirens?

Reproduced with permission from High, E. S., Fairbanks, G., & Glorig, A. (1964). Scale for Self-Assessment of Hearing Handicap. *Journal of Speech and Hearing Disorders, 29*, 215–230.

FORM B

1. When you are listening to the radio or watching television, can you hear adequately when the volume is comfortable for most other people?
2. Can you carry on a conversation with one other person when you are riding in an automobile with the windows *closed*?
3. Can you carry on a conversation with one other person when you are riding in an automobile with the window *open*?
4. Can you carry on a conversation with one other person if there is a radio or television in the same room playing at normal loudness?
5. Can you hear when someone calls to you from another room?
6. Can you understand when someone speaks to you from another room?
7. When you buy something in a store, do you easily understand the clerk?
8. Can you carry on a conversation with someone who does not speak as loudly as most people?
9. Can you tell if a person is talking when you are seated beside him and cannot see his face?
10. When you ask someone for directions, do you understand what he or she says?
11. If you are within 3 or 4 feet of a person who speaks in a normal tone of voice (assume you are facing one another), can you hear everything he or she says?
12. Do you recognize the voices of speakers when you don't see them?
13. When you are introduced to someone, can you understand the name the first time it is spoken?
14. Can you hear adequately when you are conversing with more than one person?
15. If you are in an audience, such as in a church or theater and you are seated near the *front*, can you understand most of what is said?
16. Can you carry on everyday conversations with members of your family without difficulty?
17. If you are in an audience, such as in a church or theater and you are seated near the *rear*, can you understand most of what is said?
18. When you are in a large formal gathering (a church, lodge, lecture hall, etc.) can you hear what is said when the speaker *does* use a microphone?
19. Can you hear the telephone ring when you are in the next room?
20. Can you hear night sounds, such as distant trains, bells, dogs barking, trucks passing, and so forth?

■ APPENDIX E ■

The Denver Scale of Communication Function

Preservice _____ Postservice _____

Date _____ Case No. _____

Name _____ Age _____ Sex _____

Address _____

_____
(City)   (State)   (Zip)

Lives Alone _____ In Apartment _____ Retired _____
                                     (if no, specify)

Occupation _____

Audiogram (Examination Date _____ Agency _____)

Pure Tone:

	250	500	1000	2000	4000	8000	Hz
RE	____	____	____	____	____	____	
LE	____	____	____	____	____	____	dB (re:ANSI)

Speech:

	SRT		*Discrimination Score (%)* Quiet Noise (S/N=_____)
RE	_____	dB	RE _____
LE	_____	dB	LE _____

Hearing Aid Information:

Aided _____ For How Long _____ Aid Type _____

Satisfaction _____

EXAMINER _____

The following questionnaire was designed to evaluate your communication ability as you view it. You are asked to judge or scale each statement in the following manner.

If you judge the statement to be very closely related to either extreme, please place your check mark as follows:

Agree _____ _____ _____ _____ _____ _____ _____ Disagree

or

Agree _____ _____ _____ _____ _____ _____ _____ Disagree

If you judge the statement to be *closely related* to either end of the scale, please mark as follows:

Agree _____ _____ _____ _____ _____ _____ _____ Disagree

or

Agree _____ _____ _____ _____ _____ _____ _____ Disagree

If you judge the statement to be only *slightly related* to either end of the scale, please mark as follows:

Agree _____ _____ _____ _____ _____ _____ _____ Disagree

or

Agree _____ _____ _____ _____ _____ _____ _____ Disagree

If you consider the statement to be *irrelevant* or *unassociated* to your communication situation, please mark as follows:

Agree _____ _____ _____ _____ _____ _____ _____ Disagree

PLEASE NOTE: Check a scale for every statement. Put only one checkmark on each scale. Make a separate judgment for each statement.

ALSO: You may comment on each statement in the space provided.

1. The members of my family are annoyed with my loss of hearing.
   Agree _____ _____ _____ _____ _____ _____ _____ Disagree
   Comments: _____

2. The members of my family sometimes leave me out of conversations or discussions.
   Agree _____ _____ _____ _____ _____ _____ _____ Disagree
   Comments: _____

3. Sometimes my family makes decisions for me because I have a hard time following discussions.
   Agree _____ _____ _____ _____ _____ _____ _____ Disagree
   Comments: _____

4. My family becomes annoyed when I ask them to repeat what was said because I did not hear them.
   Agree _____ _____ _____ _____ _____ _____ _____ Disagree
   Comments: _____

5. I am not an "outgoing" person because I have a hearing loss.

Agree _____ _____ _____ _____ _____ _____ _____ Disagree

Comments: _____

6. I now take less of an interest in many things as compared to when I did not have a hearing problem.

Agree _____ _____ _____ _____ _____ _____ _____ Disagree

Comments: _____

7. Other people do not realize how frustrated I get when I cannot hear or understand.

Agree _____ _____ _____ _____ _____ _____ _____ Disagree

Comments: _____

8. People sometimes avoid me because of my hearing loss.

Agree _____ _____ _____ _____ _____ _____ _____ Disagree

Comments: _____

9. I am not a calm person because of my hearing loss

Agree _____ _____ _____ _____ _____ _____ _____ Disagree

Comments: _____

10. I tend to be negative about life in general because of my hearing loss.

Agree _____ _____ _____ _____ _____ _____ _____ Disagree

Comments: _____

11. I do not socialize as much as I did before I began to lose my hearing.

Agree _____ _____ _____ _____ _____ _____ _____ Disagree

Comments: _____

12. Since I have trouble hearing, I do not like to go places with friends.

Agree _____ _____ _____ _____ _____ _____ _____ Disagree

Comments: _____

13. Since I have trouble hearing, I hesitate to meet new people.

Agree _____ _____ _____ _____ _____ _____ _____ Disagree

Comments: _____

14. I do not enjoy my job as much as I did before I began to lose my hearing.

Agree _____ _____ _____ _____ _____ _____ _____ Disagree

Comments: _____

15. Other people do not understand what it is like to have a hearing loss.

Agree _____ _____ _____ _____ _____ _____ _____ Disagree

Comments: _____

16. Because I have difficulty understanding what is said to me, I sometimes answer questions wrong.

Agree _____ _____ _____ _____ _____ _____ _____ Disagree

Comments: _____

17. I do not feel relaxed in a communicative situation.

Agree _____ _____ _____ _____ _____ _____ _____ Disagree

Comments: _____

18. I do not feel comfortable in most communication situations.

Agree _____ _____ _____ _____ _____ _____ _____ Disagree

Comments: _____

19. Conversations in a noisy room prevent me from attempting to communicate with others.

Agree _____ _____ _____ _____ _____ _____ _____ Disagree

Comments: _____

20. I am not comfortable having to speak in a group situation.

Agree _____ _____ _____ _____ _____ _____ _____ Disagree

Comments: _____

21. In general I do not find listening relaxing.

Agree _____ _____ _____ _____ _____ _____ _____ Disagree

Comments: _____

22. I feel threatened by many communication situations due to difficulty hearing.

Agree _____ _____ _____ _____ _____ _____ _____ Disagree

Comments: _____

23. I seldom watch other people's facial expressions when talking to them.

Agree _____ _____ _____ _____ _____ _____ _____ Disagree

Comments: _____

24. I hesitate to ask people to repeat if I do not understand them the first time they speak.

Agree _____ _____ _____ _____ _____ _____ _____ Disagree

Comments: _____

25. Because I have difficulty understanding what is said to me, I sometimes make comments that do not fit into the conversation.

Agree _____ _____ _____ _____ _____ _____ _____ Disagree

Comments: _____

Test of Actual Performance

How well does he or she:

	Poor	Adequate	Good	Excellent
1. Pay attention in the group? (daydreams, restlessness, changes the subject)	_____	_____	_____	_____
2. Communicate ideas verbally?	_____	_____	_____	_____
3. Use speech intelligibly?	_____	_____	_____	_____
4. Respond to others? (shares similar experiences, agrees, disagrees)	_____	_____	_____	_____
5. Hear speech when noise was going on around him/her? (like at parties) him/her? (like at parties)	_____	_____	_____	_____
6. Understand speech when not able to see the speaker?	_____	_____	_____	_____
7. Monitor the loudness of his or her own speech?	_____	_____	_____	_____

Reproduced with permission by Konditsiotis, C. Y. The use of hearing test to provide information about the extent to which an individual's hearing loss handicaps him. *Maico Audiological Library Series*, 1971, *9*, 10.

APPENDIX G

The Hearing Measurement Scale

SECTION 1

SPEECH HEARING

1. Do you ever have difficulty hearing in the conversation when you're with one other person at home?
2. Do you ever have difficulty hearing in the conversation when you're with one other person outside?
3. Do you ever have difficulty in group conversation at home?
4. Do you ever have difficulty in group conversation outside?
5. Do you ever have difficulty hearing conversation at work?
5a. Is this due to your hearing, due to the noise, or a bit of both?
6. Do you ever have difficulty hearing the speaker at a public gathering?
7. Can you always hear what's being said in a TV program?
8. Can you always hear what's being said in TV news?
9. Can you always hear what's being said in a radio program?
10. Can you always hear what's being said in radio news?
11. Do you ever have difficulty hearing what's said in a film at the cinema?

Revised with permission. Noble, W. G., & Atherley, G. R. C. The hearing measurement scale: A questionnaire for assessment of auditory disability. *Journal of Audiological Research*, 1970, *10*, 229–250.

SECTION 2

ACUITY FOR NONSPEECH SOUND

1. Do you have any pets at home? (Type_____) Can you hear it when it barks, mews, etc.?
2. Can you hear it when someone rings the doorbell or knocks on the door?
3. Can you hear a motor horn in the street when you're outside?
4. Can you hear the sound of footsteps outside when you're inside?
5. Can you hear the sound of the door opening when you're inside that room?
6. Can you hear the clock ticking in the room?
7. Can you hear the tap running when you turn it on?
8. Can you hear water boiling in a pan when you're in the kitchen?

SECTION 3

LOCALIZATION

1. When you hear the sound of people talking and they're in another room would you be able to tell from where this sound was coming?
2. If you're with a group of people and someone you can't see starts to speak would you be able to tell where that person was sitting?
3. If you hear a motor horn or a bell can you always tell in which direction it's sounding?
4. Do you ever turn your head the wrong way when someone calls to you?
5. Can you usually tell from the sound, how far away a person is when he calls to you?
6. Have you ever noticed outside that a car you thought, by its sound, was far away turned out to be much closer in fact?
7. Outside, do you always move out of the way of something coming up from behind, for instance a car, a trolley, or someone walking faster?

SECTION 4

REACTION TO HANDICAP

1. Do you think that you are more irritable than other people or less so?
2. Do you ever give the wrong answer to someone because you've misheard them?
3. When you do this, do you treat it lightly or do you get upset?
4. How does the other person react? Does he get irritated or make little of it?
5. Do you think people are tolerant in this way or do they make fun of you?
6. Do you ever get bothered or upset if you are unable to follow a conversation?
7. Do you ever get the feeling of being cut off from things because of difficulty in hearing?
7a. Does this feeling upset you at all?

SECTION 5

SPEECH DISTORTION

1. Do you find that people fail to speak clearly?
2. What about speakers on TV or radio? Do they fail to speak clearly?
3. Do you ever have difficulty, in everyday conversation, understanding what someone is saying even though you can hear what's being said?

SECTION 6

TINNITUS

1. Do you ever get a noise in your ears or in your head?
2a. to 2e. A series of items on the nature and incidence of tinnitus.
3. Does it ever stop you from sleeping?
4. Does it upset you?

SECTION 7

PERSONAL OPINION OF HEARING L0SS

1. Do you think your hearing is normal?
2. Do you think any difficulty with your hearing is particularly serious?
3. Does any difficulty with your hearing restrict your social or personal life?
4a. to 4f. A series of items on Temporary Threshold Shift, specifically for those with chronic acoustic trauma, on the relative importance of eyesight over hearing and on other difficult hearing situations not mentioned in the interview.

Profile Questionnaire for Rating Communicative Performance in a Home and Social Environment

HOME ENVIRONMENT

1. (a) In my living room, when I can see the speaker's face, I have

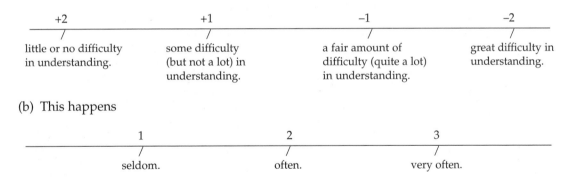

+2	+1	−1	−2
little or no difficulty in understanding.	some difficulty (but not a lot) in understanding.	a fair amount of difficulty (quite a lot) in understanding.	great difficulty in understanding.

(b) This happens

1	2	3
seldom.	often.	very often.

Reproduced with permission by Sanders, D. A. Hearing aid orientation and counseling, in M. C. Pollack (Ed.), *Amplification for the hearing impaired*. New York: Grune and Stratton, 1975, pp. 363–372.

2. (a) If I am talking with a person in my living room or family room while the television, radio, or record player is on, I have

+2	+1	−1	−2
little or no difficulty in understanding.	some difficulty (but not a lot) in understanding.	a fair amount of difficulty (quite a lot) in understanding.	great difficulty in understanding.

(b) This happens

1	2	3
seldom.	often.	very often.

3. (a) In a quiet room in my house, if I cannot see the speaker's face I have

+2	+1	−1	−2
little or no difficulty in understanding.	some difficulty (but not a lot) in understanding.	a fair amount of difficulty (quite a lot) in understanding.	great difficulty in understanding.

(b) This happens

1	2	3
seldom.	often.	very often.

4. (a) If someone in my home speaks to me from another room on the same floor, I experience

+2	+1	−1	−2
little or no difficulty in understanding.	some difficulty (but not a lot) in understanding.	a fair amount of difficulty (quite a lot) in understanding.	great difficulty in understanding.

(b) This happens

1	2	3
seldom.	often.	very often.

5. (a) If someone calls me from upstairs when I am downstairs, or from the window when I am in the garden, I will experience

+2	+1	−1	−2
little or no difficulty in understanding.	some difficulty (but not a lot) in understanding.	a fair amount of difficulty (quite a lot) in understanding.	great difficulty in understanding.

(b) This happens

1	2	3
seldom.	often.	very often.

6. (a) Understanding people at the dinner table gives me

+2	+1	−1	−2
little or no difficulty in understanding.	some difficulty (but not a lot) in understanding.	a fair amount of difficulty (quite a lot) in understanding.	great difficulty in understanding.

(b) This happens

1	2	3
seldom.	often.	very often.

7. (a) When I sit talking with friends in a quiet room I have

+2	+1	−1	−2
little or no difficulty in understanding.	some difficulty (but not a lot) in understanding.	a fair amount of difficulty (quite a lot) in understanding.	great difficulty in understanding.

(b) This happens

1	2	3
seldom.	often.	very often.

8. (a) Listening to the radio. record player, or watching TV gives me

+2	+1	−1	−2
little or no difficulty in understanding.	some difficulty (but not a lot) in understanding.	a fair amount of difficulty (quite a lot) in understanding.	great difficulty in understanding.

(b) This happens

1	2	3
seldom.	often.	very often.

9. (a) When I use the phone at home, I have

+2	+1	−1	−2
little or no difficulty in understanding.	some difficulty (but not a lot) in understanding.	a fair amount of difficulty (quite a lot) in understanding.	great difficulty in understanding.

(b) This happens

1	2	3
seldom.	often.	very often.

SOCIAL ENVIRONMENT

1. (a) If we are entertaining a group of friends, understanding someone against the background of other talking gives me

+2	+1	−1	−2
little or no difficulty in understanding.	some difficulty (but not a lot) in understanding.	a fair amount of difficulty (quite a lot) in understanding.	great difficulty in understanding.

(b) This happens

1	2	3
seldom.	often.	very often.

2. (a) If we are playing cards, understanding my partner gives me

+2	+1	−1	−2
little or no difficulty in understanding.	some difficulty (but not a lot) in understanding.	a fair amount of difficulty (quite a lot) in understanding.	great difficulty in understanding.

(b) This happens

1	2	3
seldom.	often.	very often.

3. (a) When I am at the theater or the movies, I have

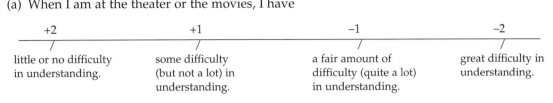

+2	+1	−1	−2
little or no difficulty in understanding.	some difficulty (but not a lot) in understanding.	a fair amount of difficulty (quite a lot) in understanding.	great difficulty in understanding.

(b) This happens

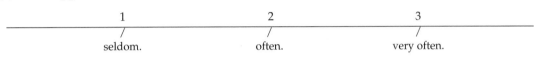

1	2	3
seldom.	often.	very often.

4. (a) In church, when the minister gives the sermon, I have

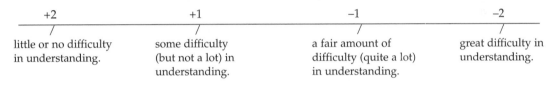

+2	+1	−1	−2
little or no difficulty in understanding.	some difficulty (but not a lot) in understanding.	a fair amount of difficulty (quite a lot) in understanding.	great difficulty in understanding.

(b) This happens

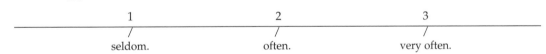

1	2	3
seldom.	often.	very often.

5. (a) When you eat out, following the conversation I have

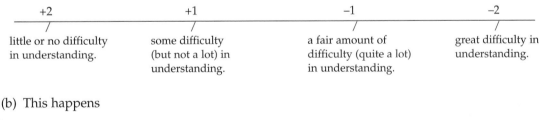

+2	+1	−1	−2
little or no difficulty in understanding.	some difficulty (but not a lot) in understanding.	a fair amount of difficulty (quite a lot) in understanding.	great difficulty in understanding.

(b) This happens

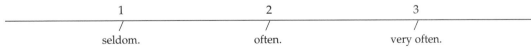

1	2	3
seldom.	often.	very often.

6. (a) In the car, I find that understanding what people are saying gives me

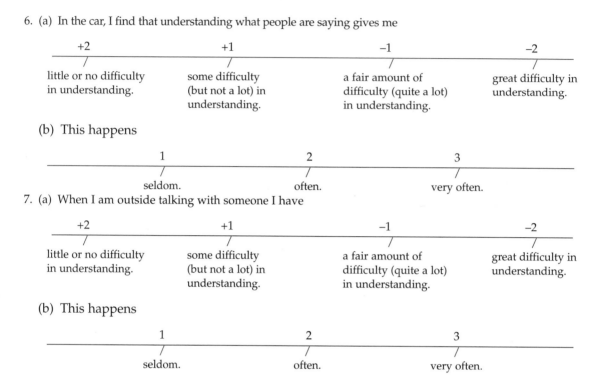

+2	+1	−1	−2
little or no difficulty in understanding.	some difficulty (but not a lot) in understanding.	a fair amount of difficulty (quite a lot) in understanding.	great difficulty in understanding.

(b) This happens

1	2	3
seldom.	often.	very often.

7. (a) When I am outside talking with someone I have

+2	+1	−1	−2
little or no difficulty in understanding.	some difficulty (but not a lot) in understanding.	a fair amount of difficulty (quite a lot) in understanding.	great difficulty in understanding.

(b) This happens

1	2	3
seldom.	often.	very often.

■ APPENDIX I ■

The Denver Scale of Communication Function for Senior Citizens Living in Retirement Centers

Name _____   Date of Pretest_____

Address _____   Date of Post-test _____

Age _____   Examiner _____

Sex _____

1. Do you have trouble communicating with your family because of your hearing problem?

   Yes_____ No_____

   Probe Effect I

   a. Does your family make decisions for you because of your hearing problem?

   Yes_____ No_____

   b. Does your family leave you out of discussions because of your hearing problem?

   Yes_____ No_____

   c. Does your family get angry or annoyed with you because of your hearing problem?

   Yes_____ No_____

Reproduced with permission by Zarnoch, J. M., & Alpiner, J. G. The Denver scale of communication function for senior citizens living in retirement centers, in J. G. Alpiner (Ed.), *Handbook of adult rehabilitative audiology*. Baltimore: Williams and Wilkins, 1978, pp. 166–168.

Exploration Effect
a. Do you have a family?   Yes_____   No_____
b. How often does your family visit you? _____
c. How far away does your family live?_____ In a city _____ Other_____
d. How often do you visit your family?_____

2. Do you get upset when you cannot hear or understand what is being said?
   Yes_____   No_____
   Probe Effect I (to be used only if person responds yes)
   a. Do your friends know you get upset?   Yes_____   No_____
   b. Does your family know you get upset?   Yes_____   No_____
   c. Does the staff know you get upset?   Yes_____   No_____
   Probe Effect II (to be used only if person responds no)
   a. Do your friends realize you are not upset?   Yes_____   No_____
   b. Does your family realize you are not upset?   Yes_____   No_____
   c. Does the staff realize you are not upset?   Yes_____   No_____
   Exploration Effect (to be used only if person responds yes)
   a. How does your behavior change when you become upset? _____

3. Do you think your family, your friends, and the staff understand what it is like to have a hearing
   problem?   Yes_____   No_____
   Probe Effect
   a. Do they avoid you because of your hearing problem? Yes_____ No_____
   b. Do they leave you out of discussions?   Yes_____   No_____
   c. Do they hesitate to ask you to socialize with them? Yes_____ No_____
   Exploration Effect
   a. Family   Yes_____   No_____
   b. Friends   Yes_____   No_____
   c. Staff   Yes_____   No_____

4. Do you avoid communicating with other people because of your hearing problem?   Yes_____
   No_____
   Probe Effect
   a. Do you communicate with people during meal times? Yes_____ No_____
   b. Do you communicate with your roommate(s)?   Yes_____ No_____
   c. Do you communicate during the social activities in the home?
      Yes_____   No_____

d. Do you communicate with visiting family or friends? Yes _____ No_____

e. Do you communicate with the staff?   Yes_____ No_____

Exploration Effect

a. Is your roommate capable of communication? Yes_____ No_____

b. What are the social activities of the home?_____

c. Which ones do you attend? _____

5. Do you feel that you are a relaxed person?   Yes_____ No_____

Probe Effect

a. Do you think you are an irritable person because of your hearing problem?   Yes_____ No_____

b. Do you think you are an irritable person because of your age?
   Yes_____ No_____

c. Do you think you are an irritable person because you live in this home?
   Yes_____ No_____

Exploration Effect

a. Do you have to live in this home?   Yes_____ No_____

6. Do you feel relaxed in group communication situations? Yes_____ No_____

Probe Effect

a. Do you get nervous when you have to ask people to repeat what they have said if you have not understood them? Yes_____ No_____

b. Do you feel nervous if you have to tell a person that you have a hearing problem?   Yes_____ No_____

Exploration Effect

a. Do you watch facial expressions?   Yes_____ No_____

b. Do you watch gestures?   Yes_____ No_____

c. Do you think you are a good listener?   Yes_____ No_____

d. Do you have a hearing aid?   Yes_____ No_____

e. Do you wear your aid?   Yes_____ No_____

7. Do you think you need help in overcoming your hearing problem?
   Yes_____ No_____

Probe Effect

a. If lipreading training was available, would you attend?
   Yes_____ No_____

b. Do you think this home provides adequate activities to make you want to communicate?
   Yes_____ No_____

Exploration Effect I

a. Can a person improve communication ability by using lipreading (or speechreading), which means watching the speaker's lips, facial expressions, and gestures when he or she is speaking?

Yes_____ No_____

b. Do you agree with the above as a definition of lipreading?

Yes_____ No_____

Exploration Effect II

a. Is your vision adequate? Yes_____ No_____

b. Are you able to get around unassisted? Yes_____ No_____

Wichita State University (WSU) Communication Appraisal and Priorities Profile (CAPP)

Date_____

Name_____ Age_____ Sex _____

Address_____ Phone_____

Please indicate below those situations in which you are able to communicate best, those that are difficult for you in some instances, and those that are a definite problem. Under "explain," please tell us more if you desire, such as certain instances when you experience more difficulty than others, certain types of speakers, certain places, and so on.

	No problems	Only in specific instances	Definite problem	Priority
1. At parties or other social events	_____	_____	_____	_____
	Explain _____			
	_____			
2. At the dinner table	_____	_____	_____	_____
	Explain _____			
	_____			

Hull, R. H. Unpublished scale. Wichita: Wichita State University, 1992a.

	No problems	Only in specific instances	Definite problem	Priority
3. On the telephone	_____	_____	_____	_____

Explain _____

_____

| 4. At home | _____ | _____ | _____ | _____ |

Explain _____

_____

| 5. With males | _____ | _____ | _____ | _____ |

Explain _____

_____

| 6. With females | _____ | _____ | _____ | _____ |

Explain _____

_____

| 7. With children | _____ | _____ | _____ | _____ |

Explain _____

_____

| 8. In groups | _____ | _____ | _____ | _____ |

Explain _____

_____

| 9. With certain important individuals | _____ | _____ | _____ | _____ |

Explain _____

_____

	No problems	Only in specific instances	Definite problem	Priority
10. At church	_____	_____	_____	_____

Explain _____

_____

11. At meetings	_____	_____	_____	_____

Explain _____

_____

12. Watching TV	_____	_____	_____	_____

Explain _____

_____

13. At the theater	_____	_____	_____	_____

Explain _____

_____

14. At work	_____	_____	_____	_____

Explain _____

_____

15. Other (please specify)	_____	_____	_____	_____

Explain _____

_____

Do you have specific preferences in regard to things you would like to improve as they relate to your ability to communicate with others? _____

_____

_____

The Hearing Handicap Inventory for the Elderly

The purpose of this scale is to identify the problems your hearing loss may be causing. Answer YES, SOMETIMES, or NO for each question. Do not skip a question if you avoid a situation because of your hearing problem. If you use a hearing aid, please answer the way you hear without the aid.

		YES (4)	SOMETIMES (2)	NO (0)
S-1.	Does a hearing problem cause you to use the phone less often than you would like?	_____	_____	_____
E-2.	Does a hearing problem cause you to feel embarrassed when meeting new people?	_____	_____	_____
S-3.	Does a hearing problem cause you to avoid groups of people?	_____	_____	_____
E-4.	Does a hearing problem make you irritable?	_____	_____	_____
E-5.	Does a hearing problem cause you to feel frustrated when talking to members of your family?	_____	_____	_____
S-6.	Does a hearing problem cause you difficulty when attending a party?	_____	_____	_____
E-7.	Does a hearing problem cause you to feel "stupid" or "dumb?"	_____	_____	_____

Reproduced with permission by Ventry, I. J., and Weinstein, B. (1982). The hearing handicap inventory for the elderly: A new tool. *Ear and Hearing*, 3, 128–134.

	YES (4)	SOMETIMES (2)	NO (0)
S-8. Do you have difficulty hearing when someone speaks in a whisper?	_____	_____	_____
E-9. Do you feel handicapped by a hearing problem?	_____	_____	_____
S-10. Does a hearing problem cause you difficulty when visiting friends, relatives, or neighbors?	_____	_____	_____
S-11. Does a hearing problem cause you to attend religious services less often than you would like?	_____	_____	_____
E-12. Does a hearing problem cause you to be nervous?	_____	_____	_____
S-13. Does a hearing problem cause you to visit friends, relatives, or neighbors less often than you would like?	_____	_____	_____
E-14. Does a hearing problem cause you to have arguments with your family members?	_____	_____	_____
S-15. Does a hearing problem cause you difficulty when listening to TV or radio?	_____	_____	_____
S-16. Does a hearing problem cause you to go shopping less often than you would like?	_____	_____	_____
S-17. Does any problem or difficulty with your hearing upset you at all?	_____	_____	_____
S-18. Does a hearing problem cause you to want to be by yourself?	_____	_____	_____
S-19. Does a hearing problem cause you to talk to family members less often than you would like?	_____	_____	_____
E-20. Do you feel that any difficulty with your hearing limits or hampers your personal or social life?	_____	_____	_____

	YES (4)	SOMETIMES (2)	NO (0)
S-21. Does a hearing problem cause you difficulty when in a restaurant with relatives or friends?	_____	_____	_____
S-22. Does a hearing problem cause you to feel depressed?	_____	_____	_____
S-23. Does a hearing problem cause you to listen to TV or radio less often than you would like?	_____	_____	_____
E-24. Does a hearing problem cause you to feel uncomfortable when talking to friends?	_____	_____	_____
E-25. Does a hearing problem cause you to feel left out when you are with a group of people?	_____	_____	_____

FOR CLINICIANS USE ONLY: Total Score: _____

Subtotal E: _____

Subtotal S: _____

APPENDIX L

The Communication Profile for the Hearing Impaired

The purpose of this questionnaire is to find out how your hearing loss affects your daily life and what problems, if any, you may be having as a result. Most of the items deal in some way with communication and your interactions with other people, but there are also items that describe your feelings and your reactions in a variety of situations.

PART I

This section of the questionnaire asks you to describe how often you feel you are able to communicate effectively with others. Mark "1" if you *Rarely* or *Almost Never* communicate effectively in that situation. Use "2" for *Occasionally* or *Sometimes*; use "3" for *About Half the Time*; use "4" for *Frequently* or *Often*; and use "5 " if you *Usually* or *Almost Always* communicate effectively.

We would also like to know how important these situations are to you. That is, we would like to know which types of situations really matter to you and which ones don't. If a particular situation occurs quite often, or if it's essential for you to communicate effectively in that situation, indicate this by marking "5" for *Essential* on the response sheet. On the other hand, if the situation occurs rarely, or if it does not really matter if you communicate in that situation, then mark "1" for *Not Important* on the response sheet. Use "2" for *Somewhat Important*, use "3" for *Important*; and use "4" for *Very Important*.

Reproduced with permission by Demorest, M. E., and Erdman, S. A. (1987). Development of the communication profile for the hearing impaired. *Journal of Speech and Hearing Disorders, 52,* 129–143.

The CPHI is *not* reproduced in its entirety here, but rather as an example of the profile. Those who intend to use the CPHI clinically should become thoroughly familiar with the items, scales, and interpretation of the instrument. This information is available in: Erdman, S. A., and Demorest, M. E. (1990). *CPHI manual: A guide to clinical use.* Simpsonville, MD.

_____ 1. Someone in your family is talking to you while you're driving or riding in a car.

_____ 2. You're at a social gathering with music or other noise in the background.

_____ 3. You're at the dinner table with your family.

_____ 4. You're at work and someone is talking to you from another room.

_____ 5. You're at a restaurant ordering food or drink.

_____ 6. You're talking on the telephone when you're at work.

_____ 7. You're at an outdoor picnic.

_____ 8. Someone's talking to you while you're watching TV or listening to the stereo.

_____ 9. You're listening for information at a lecture, briefing, or class.

_____ 10. You're talking with someone in an office.

_____ 11. You're at home talking on the telephone.

_____ 12. You're at a dinner party with several other people.

_____ 13. You're listening to someone speak at religious services.

_____ 14. You're at a meeting with several other people.

_____ 15. You're at home and someone is talking to you from another room.

_____ 16. You're having a conversation at a social gathering while others are talking nearby.

_____ 17. You're talking with a friend or family member in a quiet room.

_____ 18. You're giving or following work instructions outdoors.

PART II

In this section of the questionnaire you're asked to describe the kinds of experiences you have when you're communicating with others. What kinds of things happen when you're trying to carry on a conversation? What do you do when you have trouble understanding what someone has said? What kinds of things do other people do that make it harder or easier for you to communicate with them?

Mark "1" if the item describes something that *Rarely* happens or that is *Almost Never* true for you. Mark "2" for *Occasionally* or *Sometimes*; mark "3" for *About Half the Time*; mark "4" for *Frequently* or *Often*; and mark "5" for *Almost Always*.

_____ 19. One way I get people to repeat what they said is by ignoring them.

_____ 20. If someone repeats what they've said and I still don't understand, I ask them to repeat again.

_____ 21. I have to talk with others when there's a lot of background noise.

_____ 22. If I hear part of what someone has said, I only ask them to repeat what I didn't hear.

_____ 23. My family gets annoyed when I don't hear things.

_____ 24. I try to give the impression of normal hearing.

_____ 25. Others think I'm ignoring them if I don't answer when they speak to me.

_____	26. In difficult listening situations, I try to position myself so that I can hear as well as possible.
_____	27. I have conversations with others when I'm home.
_____	28. People think I'm not paying attention if I don't answer them when they speak to me.
_____	29. I have to communicate with others in a group situation.
_____	30. I interrupt others when listening to them is difficult.
_____	31. I've asked my family to get my attention before speaking to me.
_____	32. I tend to dominate conversations so I don't have to listen to others.
_____	33. Members of my family speak to me when they're not facing me.
_____	34. When I don't understand what someone has said, I ask them to repeat it.
_____	35. People who know I have a hearing loss accuse me of hearing only what I want to hear.
_____	36. When I have trouble understanding someone, I pay close attention to his or her face.
_____	37. If someone seems irritated at having to repeat, I stop asking them to do so and pretend to understand.
_____	38. I tend to avoid situations where I think I'll have problems hearing.
_____	39. I get bothered or upset when I'm unable to follow a conversation.
_____	40. I have to talk to others in noisy areas.
_____	41. I avoid conversing with others because of my hearing loss.
_____	42. If I'm sitting where I can't hear, I'll move to another seat.
_____	43. My job required me to use the telephone.
_____	44. When I don't understand what someone has said, I pretend that I understood it.
_____	45. At parties or other social gatherings I try to stay in a well-lighted area so I can see the speaker's face.
_____	46. People treat me as if I'm stupid because I can't understand what they say.
_____	47. When I'm having trouble understanding friends or family members, I remind them that I have a hearing problem.
_____	48. I avoid talking to strangers because of my hearing loss.
_____	49. People get annoyed when I ask them to repeat what they've said.
_____	50. During the day I have to communicate with others.
_____	51. My job involves talking to people who speak quietly.
_____	52. Members of my family leave me out of conversations or discussions.
_____	53. When I must listen in a group, I try to sit where I'll be able to hear better.
_____	54. Others become impatient because I don't always understand.
_____	55. Members of my family refuse to repeat what they've said more than once or twice.
_____	56. Members of my family talk to me from another room.
_____	57. I feel stupid when I have to ask someone to repeat what they've said.

_____ 58. When I don't understand what someone has said, I ignore them.

_____ 59. People act frustrated when I don't understand what they say.

_____ 60. People who know I have a hearing loss don't speak clearly enough when they're speaking to me.

_____ 61. People don't remember to get my attention before speaking.

_____ 62. My job involves communicating with others.

_____ 63. I try to hide my hearing problem.

_____ 64. When there's background noise I position myself so that it's less distracting.

_____ 65. I've asked friends and people I work with to get my attention before speaking to me.

_____ 66. People who know I have a hearing loss don't speak up when they're talking to me.

_____ 67. When I don't understand what someone has said, I explain that I have a hearing loss.

_____ 68. People say, "Never mind" or "Forget it" if I ask them to repeat more than once.

_____ 69. When I'm having trouble following a conversation, I listen carefully and try to catch the main points.

_____ 70. I feel foolish when I misunderstand what someone has said.

_____ 71. When I think a person is speaking too softly, I ask them to speak up.

_____ 72. If possible, I try to watch a person's face when he or she is speaking.

_____ 73. People mumble when they're talking to me.

_____ 74. I get mad at myself when I can't understand what people are saying.

_____ 75. Others think I'm not interested in what they're saying.

_____ 76. I feel embarrassed when I have to ask someone to repeat what they've said.

PART III

The items in this section describe a variety of feelings, attitudes, and beliefs about hearing loss and communication. If the statement accurately describes your beliefs, feelings, attitudes, or experiences, mark "4" on the response sheet for *Agree* or "5" for *Strongly Agree*. If the statement doesn't accurately describe your feelings or reactions, mark "2" for *Disagree* or "1" for *Strongly Disagree*. Mark "3" if you're *Uncertain* or if you partly agree and partly disagree.

_____ 77. Sometimes I have trouble understanding what's being said when someone speaks to me from another room.

_____ 78. I feel threatened by many communication situations due to difficulty hearing.

_____ 79. My hearing loss is my problem and I hate to bother others with it.

_____ 80. I feel left out of conversations because I have trouble understanding.

_____ 81. People should be more patient when they're talking to me.

_____ 82. My hearing loss makes me mad.

_____ 83. Sometimes I'm ashamed of my hearing problems.

_____ 84. I withdraw from social talk because of my hearing loss.

_____ 85. I'm not very relaxed when conversing with others.

_____ 86. Others feel I use my hearing loss as an excuse for not paying attention.

_____ 87. Communicating with others is an important part of my daily activity.

_____ 88. I sometimes have trouble understanding others when there's background noise.

_____ 89. I feel guilty about asking people to repeat for me.

_____ 90. Sometimes I feel left out when I can't follow the conversation of those I'm with.

_____ 91. I sometimes get annoyed when I have trouble hearing.

_____ 92. I hate to ask others for special consideration just because I have a hearing problem.

_____ 93. There's a lot of background noise where I work.

_____ 94. When I have trouble hearing, I feel frustrated.

_____ 95. Because of my hearing loss, I sometimes have trouble communicating with others.

_____ 96. I'm not very comfortable in most communication situations.

_____ 97. Sometimes it's hard for me to understand what's being said in meetings, conferences, or other large groups.

_____ 98. At social gatherings I sometimes find it hard to follow conversations.

_____ 99. At times my hearing loss makes me feel incompetent.

_____ 100. It's frustrating when people refuse to repeat what they've said.

_____ 101. I get very tense because of my hearing loss.

_____ 102. Sometimes when I misunderstand what someone has said I feel foolish.

_____ 103. I get aggravated when others don't speak up.

_____ 104. Because of my hearing loss I keep to myself.

_____ 105. I'm sensitive about my hearing loss.

_____ 106. When I have trouble hearing, I become nervous.

_____ 107. I feel depressed as a result of my hearing loss.

_____ 108. I find it difficult to admit to others that I have a hearing problem.

_____ 109. Since I have trouble hearing, I don't enjoy going places with friends as much.

_____ 110. If people speak where I can't see them, they shouldn't expect me to answer them.

_____ 111. My family doesn't understand the strain and stress I feel from trying to understand what they say.

_____ 112. I get discouraged because of my hearing loss.

_____ 113. I worry about looking stupid when I can't understand what someone has said.

_____ 114. Straining to hear upsets me.

_____ 115. Communicating with others is an important part of my job.

_____ 116. I feel bad about the inconvenience I cause others because of my hearing loss.

_____ 117. I get impatient with people who aren't willing to repeat for me.

_____ 118. Because of my hearing loss I have feelings of inadequacy.

_____ 119. Questions about my hearing loss really irritate me.

_____ 120. It bothers me to admit that I have a hearing loss.

_____ 121. The problems I have communicating with others really get me down.

_____ 122. I sometimes get angry with myself when I can't hear what people are saying.

_____ 123. When I can't understand people, sometimes I just don't care anymore.

_____ 124. Sometimes it's difficult for me to follow a conversation when others are talking nearby.

_____ 125. I can't talk to people about my hearing loss.

_____ 126. If people want me to understand them, it's up to them to speak more clearly.

_____ 127. Sometimes I feel tense when I can't understand what someone is saying.

_____ 128. If someone talks to me while I'm watching TV, I sometimes have trouble understanding them.

_____ 129. Others should be more understanding about my hearing problems.

_____ 130. I sometimes feel embarrassed when I misunderstand what someone has said.

_____ 131. Sometimes I miss so much of what's being said that I feel left out.

_____ 132. I let my hearing problems get me down.

_____ 133. I have a hard time accepting the fact that I have a hearing loss.

_____ 134. I really get annoyed when people shout at me as if I'm deaf.

_____ 135. I try not to bother anyone else when I'm having trouble hearing.

_____ 136. I feel self-conscious because of my hearing loss.

_____ 137. When people mumble, they shouldn't expect me to understand them.

_____ 138. Feeling isolated is part of having a hearing impairment.

_____ 139. When I can't understand what's being said, I feel tense and anxious.

_____ 140. I'd rather miss part of a conversation than admit that I have a hearing loss.

_____ 141. I sometimes have trouble understanding what's being said when I can't see the speaker's face.

_____ 142. Not being able to understand is very discouraging.

_____ 143. I get angry when I can't understand what someone is saying.

_____ 144. I don't like to ask other people to help me with my hearing problems.

_____ 145. The difficulties I have with my hearing restrict my social and personal life.

Communication Skill Scale

IDENTIFYING INFORMATION

Name _____
      Last   First   Middle Initial

Social Security # _____
                  (Gallaudet Student use ID Number)

Age _____   Sex   ( ) Male   ( ) Female

When did you become deaf:

    ( ) 1) Birth - 2 years of age
    ( ) 2) Age 3 - 6 years of age
    ( ) 3) Age 6 - 12 years of age
    ( ) 4) Age 12 - 18 years of age
    ( ) 5) After age 18

Education:

    ( ) 1) Less than High School
    ( ) 2) High School Graduate
    ( ) 3) Some College
    ( ) 4) College Undergraduate Degree
    ( ) 5) Postgraduate
    ( ) 6) Ph.D.

The CSS is not reproduced here in its entirety, but rather as an example of the scale.

The Scale, Scoring Form, and Norms can be obtained from Dr. Harriet Kaplan, Department of Audiology, Gallaudet University, Washington, DC 20002.

How long did you attend each of the following:
(Enter 0 if you did not attend and .5 if you attended less than a full year.)

Residential School for the Deaf	_____ year(s)	_____ months
Private School for the Deaf	_____ year(s)	_____ months
Public School—Mainstreamed	_____ year(s)	_____ months
Public School—Special Class	_____ year(s)	_____ months
Private School—Mainstreamed	_____ year(s)	_____ months
Private School—Special Class	_____ year(s)	_____ months

How long did you attend each of the following:
(Enter 0 if you did not attend and .5 if you attended less than a full year.)

Gallaudet University	_____ year(s)	_____ months
National Technical Institute for the Deaf	_____ year(s)	_____ months
Other program for hearing impaired	_____ year(s)	_____ months
Hearing Jr. College, College or University	_____ year(s)	_____ months
Program not specifically for hearing impaired	_____ year(s)	_____ months

How do you communicate most of the time:

At Home:	( ) ASL	( ) PSE	( ) Speech
At School:	( ) ASL	( ) PSE	( ) Speech
At Work:	( ) ASL	( ) PSE	( ) Speech
In the Community:	( ) ASL	( ) PSE	( ) Speech

How often do you use a hearing aid now:

( ) 1) Do Not Own a Hearing Aid
( ) 2) Not At All
( ) 3) Occasionally
( ) 4) All the Time

Do you wear an aid in:

( )   One ear
( )   Both ears

Type of aid currently in use:

( ) 1) Behind-the-ear aid
( ) 2) In-the-ear aid
( ) 3) Body-worn or eyeglass aid
( ) 4) Vibrotactile aid
( ) 5) Cochlear implant

Indicate the degree of your hearing loss:

( ) 1) Mild
( ) 2) Moderate
( ) 3) Severe
( ) 4) Profound

INSTRUCTIONS

We want to find out how your hearing loss affects your daily life. The following questions are about different communication situations, ways of managing situations, and attitudes about different situations. If you have never experienced the situation do not answer the question. Go on to the next question.

Some of the items ask you whether you understand conversation. The word "understand" means knowing enough of what is said or signed to be able to answer appropriately. Always assume you are interested in what is being said.

We know that some people are easier to understand than others. Please answer the questions according to the way most people talk to you or understand you. We know that sounds and speakers vary. Please answer the questions as best you can.

If you wear a hearing aid, answer the questions as though you were wearing your aid.

SECTION I

Difficult Communication Situations

Please read each situation. Decide if the situation is true:

1. Almost always,
2. Sometimes, or
3. Almost never.

Then indicate if the situation is:

1. Very important to you,
2. Important to you,
3. Not important to you.

If you have not experienced this situation **DO NOT** answer the question. Go on to the next question.

Question #1.
    You are in class. The teacher is easy to lipread but is not signing. You understand _____ (frequency) _____ (importance)

Question #2.
    You meet a stranger on the street and ask for directions. He does not sign. You understand him _____ (frequency) _____ (importance)

Question #3.
    You are at work. It is quiet. Your supervisor gives you an order. She is not signing but her face is clearly visible. You understand her _____ (frequency) _____ (importance)

Question #4.
    You are at work. It is noisy. A hearing co-worker asks you to eat lunch with her. She does not sign but you can see her face. You understand her _____ (frequency) _____ (importance)

Question #5.
    You are visiting a friend. His hard-of-hearing child speaks to you about his school. The child does not sign. You understand _____ (frequency) _____ (importance)

Question #6.

    You are at a meeting. A hearing person speaks but does not sign. You know the subject. You understand _____ (frequency) _____ (importance)

Question #7.

    You are in class. A hearing person speaks but does not sign. You know the subject. You understand _____ (frequency) _____ (importance)

Question #8.

    You are at the dinner table at home. All your relatives are hearing. Your grandmother is talking. She does not sign. You do not know the topic. You understand her _____ (frequency) _____ (importance)

Question #9.

    You are introduced to a hearing person. You sign and speak at the same time. He understands you _____ (frequency) _____ (importance)

Question #10.

    You are at a meeting with five hearing people. No one signs but everyone's face can be seen. One person talks at a time. You understand the conversation _____ (frequency) _____ (importance)

Question #11.

    You are watching a movie on television. There is no captioning. It is quiet in the room. You understand _____ (frequency) _____ (importance)

Question #12.

    You are talking to the doctor. It is quiet. She does not sign. You can see her face clearly. You understand her _____ (frequency) _____ (importance)

Question #13.

    You are ordering lunch at McDonald's. You speak to the person behind the counter. She understands you _____ (frequency) _____ (importance)

Question #14.

    You are talking to one person at a noisy party. The person does not sign. You understand _____ (frequency) _____ (importance)

Question #15.

    You are talking to a family member on the telephone. It is quiet in the room. You understand _____ (frequency) _____ (importance)

Question #16.

    You are reading in a quiet room. Someone calls you from the next room. You hear the person's voice _____ (frequency) _____ (importance)

Question #17.

    You are sitting in a car next to the driver. The driver is talking. He is not signing. You understand him _____ (frequency) _____ (importance)

Question #18.

    You must give directions to hearing people at work. They understand your speech _____ (frequency) _____ (importance)

Question #19.
   I have trouble hearing fire alarms in buildings when other people can hear them _____ (frequency) _____ (importance)

Question #20.
   I have trouble hearing fire engines and ambulances when other people can hear them. _____ (frequency) _____ (importance)

Question #21.
   I have trouble hearing cars or buses when other people can hear them _____ (frequency) _____ (importance)

Question #22.
   I have trouble hearing the telephone when I am in the same room _____ (frequency) _____ (importance)

Question #23.
   I have trouble hearing the telephone when I am in the next room _____ (frequency) _____ (importance)

Question #24.
   I have trouble hearing the doorbell when other people can hear it _____ (frequency) _____ (importance)

Question #25.
   I have trouble hearing a knock on the door when other people can hear it _____ (frequency) _____ (importance)

Question #26.
   I have trouble hearing music when it is loud enough for other people _____ (frequency) _____ (importance)

Question #27.
   I have trouble hearing a person's voice when he is talking in the same room _____ (frequency) _____ (importance)

SECTION II

Communication Strategies

Please read each situation. Decide if the situation is true:
1. Almost always,
2. Sometimes, or
3. Almost never.

If you have not experienced this situation **DO NOT** answer the question. Go on to the next question.
Question #28.
   You are talking with someone you do not know well. You do not understand. You ask her to repeat. _____ (frequency)

Question #29.
   You are talking with two people. You are not understanding. You change the topic so that you can control the conversation. _____ (frequency)

Question #30.
   You ask a stranger for directions. You understand part of what he says. You tell him the part you understand and ask him to repeat the rest. _____ (frequency)

Question #31.
   You answer a question but the other person doesn't understand. You repeat the answer. _____ (frequency)

Question #32.
   You are at work. Your boss gives you instructions. You do not understand. You ask him to say the instructions in a different way. _____ (frequency)

Question #33.
   A friend introduces you to a new person. You do not understand the person's name. You ask the person to spell her name. _____ (frequency)

Question #34.
   A person asks you for your name. He does not understand your speech. You spell your name. _____ (frequency)

Question #35.
   A stranger spells his name for you. You miss the first two letters. You ask him to say each letter and a word starting with each letter (A as in Apple, B as in Boy). _____ (frequency)

Question #36.
   A person tells you his address. You do not understand. You ask him to repeat the street number, one number at a time _____ (frequency)

Question #37.
   You are talking with one person but are not understanding. You interrupt the person before he finishes to say what you think. _____ (frequency)

Question #38.
   Your friend asks you to buy seven hamburgers. You do not understand how many he wants. You ask him to start counting from zero and stop at the correct number. _____ (frequency)

Question #39.
   You are in a restaurant. The waitress does not understand what you want. You point to the item on the menu. _____ (frequency)

Question #40.
   You are in class. The teacher says something you do not understand. You pretend to understand and hope to get the information from the book later. _____ (frequency)

Question #41.
   You are at the dinner table with your family. Someone does not understand you. You say the same thing a different way. _____ (frequency)

Question #42.
  Someone who does not sign asks you for your phone number. You say each number and show the correct number of fingers as you speak. _____ (frequency)

Question #43.
  Two people are talking. You do not understand the conversation. You ask them to tell you the topic. _____ (frequency)

Question #44.
  You are talking with one person in a restaurant. His face is in the shadows. You know you could understand better if you changed seats with him. You ask to change seats. _____ (frequency)

Question #45.
  You are at the airport. You want to buy a ticket for a flight home. The clerk does not understand you. You write the information. _____ (frequency)

Question #46.
  You are visiting the doctor. He tells you what to do for your sickness. You do not understand his speech. You ask him to write. _____ (frequency)

Question #47.
  You are at a meeting. The speaker does not look at you when he talks. You feel angry but do nothing about it. _____ (frequency)

Question #48.
  You meet a deaf friend who is with another person. The other person talks to you but does not sign. You ask her to sign. _____ (frequency)

Question #49.
  You are at a meeting. You realize you are too far from the speaker to understand. There are empty seats in the front of the room. You change your seat. _____ (frequency)

Question #50.
  You are at a meeting at work. You are the only deaf person. You are afraid that you will not understand but you do not ask for help. You do the best you can. _____ (frequency)

Question #51.
  You are talking to the dentist. He speaks very fast. You cannot lipread him. You ask him to slow down. _____ (frequency)

Question #52.
  You are in class. The teacher talks while she writes on the board. You talk to her after class. You explain that you need to see her face in order to speechread. _____ (frequency)

Question #53.
  Your teacher likes to move around the room while she teaches. You have problems reading her signs. You ask her after class to lecture from one place so you can understand her signing. _____ (frequency)

Question #54.
  You are going to a series of meetings or lectures. The speaker does not sign. You ask the speaker to use the slides, pictures or the overhead projector whenever possible. _____ (frequency)

Question #55.

You are going to a series of meetings or lectures. The speaker does not sign. You ask him to find a person to take notes for you. _____ (frequency)

Question #56.

You are going to a series of meetings or lectures. The speaker does not sign. You ask for an interpreter. _____ (frequency)

Question #57.

You are going to a series of meetings or lectures. The speaker does not sign. You ask for an outline or a reading list. _____ (frequency)

Question #58.

You are going to a play. It will not be signed. You read the play or reviews of the play before you see it. _____ (frequency)

Question #59.

You are going to a job interview. You act out the situation in advance with a friend to prepare yourself for the experience. _____ (frequency)

Question #60.

You are talking with a clerk at the bank. A fire truck goes by. You ask him to stop talking until the noise stops. _____ (frequency)

Question #61.

You ask a person to repeat because you don't understand. He seems annoyed. You stop asking and pretend to understand. _____ (frequency)

Question #62.

You ask a stranger for directions to a place. You really want to understand his speech. You ask very specific questions like: "Is this place north or south of here?" "Do I turn left or right at the corner?" _____ (frequency)

Question #63.

You need to ask directions. You avoid asking a stranger because you think you will have trouble understanding him. _____ (frequency)

Question #64.

You must make a phone call to a hearing person. The person does not have a TDD. You ask a hearing friend to make the call and interpret for you. _____ (frequency)

Question #65.

You are at a store. You have trouble hearing the clerk because his voice is soft. You explain you are hearing impaired and ask him to talk louder. _____ (frequency)

Question #66.

You are at home. You ask your family to get your attention before they speak to you. _____ (frequency)

Question #67.

You are with five or six friends. No one is signing. You miss something important. You ask the person next to you what was said. _____ (frequency)

Question #68.
   You have trouble understanding a man who is chewing gum. You explain that you need to speechread. You politely ask him to remove the gum when he talks. _____ (frequency)

Question #69.
   You try to avoid people when you know you will have trouble hearing them. _____ (frequency)

Question #70.
   You hate to bother other people with your hearing problem. So, you pretend to understand. _____ (frequency)

Question #71.
   I avoid wearing my hearing aid because it makes me feel different. _____ (frequency)

SECTION III

Attitudes

Please read each situation. Decide if the sitution is true:
1. Almost always,
2. Sometimes, or
3. Almost never.

If you have not experienced this situation **DO NOT** answer the question. Go on to the next question.

Question #72.
   I feel embarrassed when I don't understand someone. _____ (frequency).

Question #73.
   I get upset when I can't follow a conversation. _____ (frequency)

Question #74.
   I become angry when people do not speak clearly enough for me to understand. _____ (frequency)

Question #75.
   I feel stupid when I misunderstand what a person is saying. _____ (frequency)

Question #76.
   It's hard for me to ask someone to repeat things. I feel embarrassed. _____ (frequency)

Question #77.
   Most people think I could understand better if I paid more attention. _____ (frequency)

Question #78.
   I get angry when people speak too softly or too fast. _____ (frequency)

Question #79.
   Sometimes I can't follow conversations at home. I still feel a part of family life. _____ (frequency)

Question #80.
   I feel frustrated when I try to communicate with hearing people. _____ (frequency)

Question #81.
  Most hearing people do not understand what it is like to be deaf. This makes me angry. _____ (frequency)

Question #82.
  I am ashamed of being hearing impaired. _____ (frequency)

Question #83.
  I get angry when someone speaks with his mouth covered or with his back to me. _____ (frequency)

Question #84.
  I prefer to be alone most of the time. _____ (frequency)

Question #85.
  I am uncomfortable with people who communicate differently than I do. _____ (frequency)

Question #86.
  My hearing loss makes me nervous. _____ (frequency)

Question #87.
  My hearing loss makes me feel depressed. _____ (frequency)

Question #88.
  My family understands my hearing loss. _____ (frequency)

Question #89.
  I get annoyed when people shout at me because I have a hearing loss._____ (frequency)

Question #90.
  People treat me like a stupid person when I don't understand their speech. _____ (frequency)

Question #91.
  People treat me like a stupid person when they don't understand me._____ (frequency)

Question #92.
  Members of my family don't get annoyed when I have trouble understanding them. _____ (frequency)

Question #93.
  People who know I have a hearing loss think I can hear when I want to. _____ (frequency)

Question #94.
  Members of my family don't leave me out of conversations. _____ (frequency)

Question #95.
  Hearing aids don't always help people understand speech, but they can help in other ways. _____ (frequency)

Question #96.
  I feel speechreading (lipreading) is helpful to me. _____ (frequency)

Question #97.
  I feel the only useful communication system for a deaf person is sign language. _____ (frequency)

Question #98.
   Even though people know I have a hearing loss, they don't help me by speaking clearly or repeating. _____ (frequency)

Question #99.
   My family is willing to make telephone calls for me. _____ (frequency)

Question #100.
   My family is willing to repeat as often as necessary when I don't understand them. _____ (frequency)

Question #101.
   Hearing people get frustrated when I don't understand what they say._____ (frequency)

Question #102.
   Hearing people get embarrassed when they don't understand my speech. _____ (frequency)

Question #103.
   Hearing people pretend to understand me when they really don't. _____ (frequency)

Question #104.
   I feel the only useful communications system for a deaf person is speech and lipreading. _____ (frequency)

Question #105.
   I feel embarrassed when hearing people don't understand my speech._____ (frequency)

Question #106.
   I do not mind repeating when people have trouble understanding my speech. _____ (frequency)

Question #107.
   I prefer to write when I communicate with hearing people because I am ashamed of my speech. _____ (frequency)

Question #108.
   I feel that most hearing people try to understand my speech. _____ (frequency)

Question #109.
   I feel that my family tries to understand my speech. _____ (frequency)

Question #110.
   I feel that strangers try to understand my speech. _____ (frequency)

■ INDEX ■